Cancer Gene Therapy

Contemporary Cancer Research

Jac A. Nickoloff, SERIES EDITOR

Cancer Gene Therapy

Edited by

David T. Curiel, MD, PhD

Joanne T. Douglas, PhD

*Division of Human Gene Therapy
and the Gene Therapy Center
University of Alabama at Birmingham
Birmingham, AL*

HUMANA PRESS ✳ TOTOWA, NEW JERSEY

© 2005 Humana Press Inc.
999 Riverview Drive, Suite 208
Totowa, New Jersey 07512

www.humanapress.com

This publication is printed on acid-free paper. ∞
ANSI Z39.48-1984 (American Standards Institute) Permanence of Paper for Printed Library Materials.

Cover design by Patricia F. Cleary
Cover illustration: Dendritic cells binding and activating T cells. (Artwork courtesy of Dr. Tanja de Gruijl.)

For additional copies, pricing for bulk purchases, and/or information about other Humana titles, contact Humana at the above address or at any of the following numbers: Tel: 973-256-1699; Fax: 973-256-8341; E-mail: humana@humanapr.com, or visit our Website: www.humanapress.com

Printed in the United States of America. 10 9 8 7 6 5 4 3 2 1

eISBN: 1-59259-785-8

Library of Congress Cataloging-in-Publication Data

Cancer gene therapy / edited by David T. Curiel, Joanne T. Douglas.
    p. ; cm. — (Contemporary cancer research)
  Includes bibliographical references and index.
  ISBN 1-58829-213-4 (alk. paper)
    1. Cancer—Gene therapy. [DNLM: 1. Gene Therapy. 2. Neoplasms—therapy. QZ 266 C21433 2004] I. Curiel, David. II. Douglas, Joanne T. III. Series.
  RC271.G45C355 2004
  616.99'40694—dc22
                                               2004010875

Preface

The field of cancer therapy is beginning to reap the benefits of our increasing understanding of the molecular basis of cancer. In contrast to conventional surgical interventions or cytotoxic chemotherapy and radiation therapy, a new generation of targeted cancer therapeutics is being specifically directed toward molecular pathways that underlie the malignant phenotype. In this regard, the management of patients with Philadelphia chromosome-positive chronic myeloid leukemia has been profoundly changed by Gleevec® (Novartis), a small molecule that specifically inhibits the Bcr-abl tyrosine kinase that is central to the pathogenesis of this disease. Particularly noteworthy is the rapid translation of this molecular targeted agent from the laboratory to clinical trials and thence to regulatory approval. Other novel targeted therapeutics that are currently approved by the FDA for treatment of patients with cancer include Rituxan® (Genentech), a humanized monoclonal antibody that binds to the CD20 antigen present on B-cell lymphomas and is currently approved for the treatment of patients with relapsed or refractory low-grade or follicular CD20-positive B-cell non-Hodgkin's lymphoma. The humanized anti-HER-2/neu monoclonal antibody Herceptin® (Genentech) is approved for use in patients with metastatic breast cancer that demonstrates overexpression of HER-2/neu. These therapies target specific tumor cell receptors or signaling events that are critical to tumor progression while reducing toxicity to normal cells.

Within this context of targeted molecular interventions with the potential to achieve a much higher level of specificity of action than afforded by conventional drug therapeutics, we can view cancer gene therapy as the transfer of genetic material to the cells of an individual with the goal of eradicating cancer cells. This can be accomplished directly by transferring genetic material into the cancer cells themselves to bring about their destruction, or indirectly, either by stimulating the immune system to recognize and eliminate the cancer cells or by targeting the nonmalignant stromal cells that support the growth and metastasis of cancer cells. Each of these approaches exploits our expanding knowledge of the genetic basis of cancer, thereby allowing rationally targeted interventions at the molecular level. These cancer gene therapy strategies are discussed in the first contributions to *Cancer Gene Therapy*.

Any gene therapy strategy is dependent on the safe and efficient transfer of the therapeutic gene selectively to the target cell. Indeed, one of the main lessons learned from the success of clinical gene therapy trials for monogenic inherited disorders, such as severe combined immunodeficiency and hemophilia, is that therapeutic advances are predicated on improvements in the design of gene delivery vehicles, or vectors. Hence, two chapters focus on the development of vectors for cancer gene therapy, both viral and nonviral, emphasizing how the properties of a given vector favor its application in a particular therapeutic approach.

The recognition of the limitations of replication-defective vectors, which are incapable of delivering therapeutic genes to more than a small proportion of cancer cells in a 3D tumor mass, has led to the development of a new class of anticancer therapeutic agents, oncolytic replication-competent viruses, which are also described. The safety of oncolytic viruses derives from the restriction of their replication to tumor cells, while sparing normal cells. A number of naturally occurring viruses possess intrinsic selectivity for replication in tumor cells, while advances in the molecular characterization of viruses and cancer cells have enabled other lytic viruses to be genetically engineered to selectively replicate in, and thus destroy, tumor cells.

It is apparent that therapeutic gene delivery designed to eradicate cancer cells in the clinical setting would benefit from noninvasive techniques to monitor the extent of gene transfer and disease regression during the course of treatment. Hence, a chapter describes imaging of cancer gene therapy. After a chapter discussing the lessons learned to date from clinical trials for cancer gene therapy, the final chapter reviews the regulatory guidelines with which future trials should comply.

Thus, the contributions to this book demonstrate that cancer gene therapy strategies are founded on an understanding of the molecular basis of disease that, together with improvements to the safety and efficacy of vectors, will provide a rational basis for their application in the clinic setting. It is anticipated that gene therapy will ultimately take its place in the clinic alongside other targeted molecular inventions for cancer.

David T. Curiel, MD, PhD
Joanne T. Douglas, PhD

Contents

Contributors

RAMON ALEMANY • *Gene Therapy Program, Institut Catalá d'Oncologia, Barcelona, Spain*

ROSEMARIE AURIGEMMA • *Biological Resources Branch, Developmental Therapeutics Program, National Cancer Institute, NCI-Frederick, Frederick, MD*

ANDREW BATEMAN • *Molecular Medicine Program and Department of Immunology, Mayo Clinic, Rochester, MN*

MALCOLM K. BRENNER • *Center for Cell and Gene Therapy, Baylor College of Medicine, Houston, TX*

J. MARTIN BROWN • *Division of Radiation and Cancer Biology, Department of Radiation Oncology, Stanford University School of Medicine, Stanford, CA*

STEVEN J. CHMURA • *Department of Radiation and Cellular Oncology, University of Chicago, Chicago, IL*

LELAND W. K. CHUNG • *Department of Urology, Molecular Urology and Therapeutics Program, Winship Cancer Institute, Emory University School of Medicine, Atlanta, GA*

STEPHEN CREEKMORE • *Biological Resources Branch, Developmental Therapeutics Program, National Cancer Institute, NCI-Frederick, Frederick, MD*

RONALD G. CRYSTAL • *Department of Genetic Medicine, Division of Pulmonary and Critical Care Medicine, Department of Medicine, Weill Medical College of Cornell University, New York, NY*

DAVID T. CURIEL • *Division of Human Gene Therapy, Departments of Medicine, Pathology, and Surgery, and Gene Therapy Center, University of Alabama at Birmingham, Birmingham, AL*

TYLER J. CURIEL • *Section of Hematology and Medical Oncology, Tulane Medical School, New Orleans, LA*

JOANNE T. DOUGLAS • *Division of Human Gene Therapy, Departments of Medicine, Pathology, and Surgery, and Gene Therapy Center, University of Alabama at Birmingham, Birmingham, AL*

AHMED EL-ZAWAHRY • *Department of Microbiology and Immunology, Medical University of South Carolina, Charleston, SC*

THOMAS A. GARDNER • *Departments of Urology, Microbiology, and Immunology, Walther Oncology Center, Indiana University Medical Center, Indianapolis, IN*

MICHAEL GAROFALO • *Department of Radiation and Cellular Oncology, University of Chicago, Chicago, IL*

JACK GAULDIE • *Department of Pathology and Molecular Medicine, McMaster University, Hamilton, Canada*

SUSAN F. GRAMMER • *Biotechwrite: Biomedical and Science Communications, Kalamazoo, MI*

TANJA D. DE GRUIJL • *Departments of Medical Oncology and Pathology, Vrije Universiteit Medical Center, Amsterdam, The Netherlands*

STEVE GYORFFY • *Department of Pathology and Molecular Medicine, McMaster University, Hamilton, Canada*

KEVIN HARRINGTON • *Molecular Medicine Program and Department of Immunology, Mayo Clinic, Rochester, MN*

AKSELI HEMMINKI • *Rational Drug Design, Department of Oncology, University of Helsinki, Helsinki, Finland*

KARI HEMMINKI • *German Cancer Research Center (DKFZ), Heidelberg, Germany; Department of Biosciences, Karolinska Institute, Stockholm, Sweden*

HARVEY R. HERSCHMAN • *Departments of Biological Chemistry and Pharmacology, University of California at Los Angeles, Los Angeles, CA*

DAVID H. HOLMAN • *Department of Microbiology and Immunology, Medical University of South Carolina, Charleston, SC*

JOHN A. HOWE • *Department of Molecular Biology and Biochemistry, Canji, Inc., San Diego, CA*

MIEN-CHIE HUNG • *Department of Molecular and Cellular Oncology, University of Texas M.D. Anderson Cancer Center, Houston, TX*

MARC L. HYER • *The Burnham Institute, La Jolla, CA*

JUAN ANTONIO JIMÉNEZ • *Departments of Urology, Microbiology and Immunology, Indiana University Medical Center, Indianapolis, IN*

CHINGHAI KAO • *Departments of Urology, Microbiology and Immunology, Walther Oncology Center, Indiana University Medical Center, Indianapolis, IN*

GINA M. KELLER • *Department of Microbiology and Immunology, Medical University of South Carolina, Charleston, SC*

DAVID J. KERR • *Department of Clinical Pharmacology, University of Oxford, Oxford, United Kingdom*

ROBERT J. KORST • *Division of Thoracic Surgery, Department of Cardiothoracic Surgery and Department of Genetic Medicine, Weill Medical College of Cornell University, New York, NY*

PHILIPPE LAMBIN • *Department of Experimental Radiation Oncology, University of Maastricht, Maastricht, The Netherlands*

PATRICK W. K. LEE • *Department of Microbiology and Infectious Diseases, University of Calgary, Calgary, Canada*

EMMANOUELA LINARDAKIS • *Molecular Medicine Program and Department of Immunology, Mayo Clinic, Rochester, MN*

SHIE-CHAU LIU • *Division of Radiation and Cancer Biology, Department of Radiation Oncology, Stanford University School of Medicine, Stanford, CA*

ALBERT F. LoBUGLIO • *Division of Hematology and Oncology, Department of Medicine and the Comprehensive Cancer Center, University of Alabama at Birmingham, Birmingham, AL*

PER EYSTEIN LØNNING • *Department of Oncology, University of Bergen, Norway*

R. SCOTT MCIVOR • *Department of Genetics, Cell Biology and Development, University of Minnesota, Minneapolis, MN*

ALAN MELCHER • *Molecular Medicine Program and Department of Immunology, Mayo Clinic, Rochester, MN*

ION NICULESCU-DUVAZ • *CRC Centre for Cancer Therapeutics at the Institute of Cancer Research, Sutton, United Kingdom*

KARA L. NORMAN • *Department of Microbiology and Infectious Diseases, University of Calgary, Calgary, Canada*

JAMES S. NORRIS • *Department of Microbiology and Immunology, Medical University of South Carolina, Charleston, SC*

DANIEL H. PALMER • *CR UK Institute for Cancer Studies, University of Birmingham, Birmingham, United Kingdom*

MEGAN K. PATRICK • *Department of Microbiology and Infectious Diseases, University of Calgary, Calgary, Canada*

VY PHAN • *Molecular Medicine Program and Department of Immunology, Mayo Clinic, Rochester, MN*

HERBERT M. PINEDO • *Department of Medical Oncology, Vrije Universiteit Medical Center, Amsterdam, The Netherlands*

SAMUEL D. RABKIN • *Molecular Neurosurgery Laboratory, Massachusetts General Hospital, Harvard Medical School, Charlestown, MA*

ROBERT RALSTON • *Department of Molecular Biology and Biochemistry, Canji, Inc., San Diego, CA*

MURALI RAMACHANDRA • *Department of Molecular Biology and Biochemistry, Canji, Inc., San Diego, CA*

KUNG-MING RAU • *Department of Molecular and Cellular Oncology, University of Texas M.D. Anderson Cancer Center, Houston, TX*

JOHN J. ROSSI • *Division of Molecular Biology, Beckman Research Institute of the City of Hope, Duarte, CA*

JACK A. ROTH • *W. M. Keck Center for Cancer Gene Therapy, Department of Thoracic and Cardiovascular Surgery, The University of Texas M.D. Anderson Cancer Center, Houston, TX*

SHERYL RUPPEL • *Biological Resources Branch, Developmental Therapeutics Program, National Cancer Institute, Bethesda, MD*

EDWARD A. SAUSVILLE • *Biopharmaceutical Development Program, SAID-Frederick/ NCI-Frederick, Frederick, MD*

RIK J. SCHEPER • *Departments of Medical Oncology and Pathology, Vrije Universiteit Medical Center, Amsterdam, The Netherlands*

LISA SCHERER • *Division of Molecular Biology, Beckman Research Institute of the City of Hope, Duarte, CA*

DENISE R. SHAW • *Division of Hematology and Oncology, Department of Medicine and the Comprehensive Cancer Center, University of Alabama at Birmingham, Birmingham, AL*

CAROLINE J. SPRINGER • *CRC Centre for Cancer Therapeutics at the Institute of Cancer Research, Sutton, United Kingdom*

A. KEITH STEWART • *Department of Experimental Therapeutics, Toronto General Research Institute/University Health Network; McLaughlin Centre for Molecular Medicine, University of Toronto, Toronto, Ontario, Canada*

THERESA V. STRONG • *Division of Hematology/Oncology, Department of Medicine, University of Alabama at Birmingham, Birmingham, AL*

COLIN L. SWEENEY • *Department of Genetics, Cell Biology and Development, University of Minnesota, Minneapolis, MN*

JAN THEYS • *Department of Experimental Radiation Oncology, University of Maastricht, The Netherlands*

TOMOKI TODO • *Department of Neurosurgery, University of Tokyo Hospital, Tokyo, Japan*

JOSEPH E. TOMASZEWSKI • *Toxicology & Pharmacology Branch, Developmental Therapeutics Program, National Cancer Institute, Bethesda, MD*

RICHARD VILE • *Molecular Medicine Program and Department of Immunology, Mayo Clinic, Rochester, MN*

ERNST WAGNER • *Department for Pharmacy, Ludwig-Maximillians-Universitaet, Muenchen, Germany*

GREG F. WALKER • *Department for Pharmacy, Ludwig-Maximillians-Universitaet, Muenchen, Germany*

HUI WANG • *Division of Clinical Pharmacology, Department of Pharmacology and Toxicology, University of Alabama at Birmingham, Birmingham, AL*

SHUANG WEI • *Section of Hematology and Medical Oncology, Tulane Medical School, New Orleans, LA*

RALPH R. WEICHSELBAUM • *Department of Radiation and Cellular Oncology, University of Chicago, Chicago, IL*

XIAO-YAN WEN • *Department of Experimental Therapeutics, Toronto General Research Institute/University Health Network; McLaughlin Centre for Molecular Medicine, University of Toronto, Toronto, Ontario, Canada*

DUEN-HWA YAN • *Department of Molecular and Cellular Oncology, University of Texas M.D. Anderson Cancer Center, Houston, TX*

RUIWEN ZHANG • *Division of Clinical Pharmacology, Department of Pharmacology and Toxicology, University of Alabama at Birmingham, Birmingham, AL*

WEIPING ZOU • *Section of Hematology and Medical Oncology, Tulane Medical School, New Orleans, LA*

1

Cancer Gene Therapy

Historical Perspective

Malcolm K. Brenner

1. INTRODUCTION

Although it is always tempting to skip the history of a field, this is particularly unwise for a discipline as young as cancer gene therapy. Indeed, it is the history of the last few years that is largely dictating the research directions that will likely be both profitable and permitted in the future. This brief introductory chapter outlines the early days of cancer gene therapy—the successes and the setbacks—and suggests how the remaining challenges may be faced.

2. BACKGROUND

When the possibility of human gene therapy was first mooted (and illicitly attempted) in the 1970s, it was assumed that inherited single-gene disorders would be the target of the approach *(1)*. The obvious elegance of repairing or replacing the root cause of a disease had and retains an enormous appeal to researchers, patients, and public alike. Unfortunately, it soon became obvious that the tools available were simply not up to the job.

Effective gene therapy of genetic disorders requires a vector that can efficiently transduce the desired cell type, in a targeted manner, preferably in vivo. Moreover, the gene product usually would need to be produced in substantial quantities for a long time, often in a regulated manner. Above all, the process and consequences of gene transfer should be safe.

Sadly, the gene transfer vectors available for clinical use, then as now, possess none of these desirable properties. They are diffusely targeted, inefficient at making transgene products, and difficult to regulate. As the gene therapy community has painfully learned, they are not even all that safe for they have the potential to produce immediate (adenovectors) or delayed (retroviral vectors) severe or lethal adverse events.

Many of these limitations were obvious to early workers in the field and led them to concentrate on disorders in which low-frequency transduction of stem cells would lead to a selective growth advantage and repopulation of the host and in which unregulated expression of even small quantities of the transgenic material would be of therapeutic benefit. The group of disorders that most clearly met these criteria was the inherited severe combined immunodeficiency syndromes. But, although these remain of great interest as a possible "proof of principle" for establishing the value of this new technology, they are exceedingly rare, and there was a strong feeling that the technology should be applied to more common conditions. Although these included more widespread inherited genetic disorders such as cystic fibrosis, the prospect of treating cancer with gene therapy grew increasingly justifiable in the 1980s.

From: *Contemporary Cancer Research*
Cancer Gene Therapy
Edited by: D. T. Curiel and J. T. Douglas © Humana Press Inc., Totowa, NJ

Several factors led to this change in perception:

1. The realization that cancer too was a genetic disorder, albeit one that was acquired and multigenic.
2. The existence of a profoundly unmet therapeutic need because conventional treatments were toxic, ineffective, or, most commonly, both.
3. The high incidence of the disorder, making it an appealing area for research and development support from industry.
4. The availability of an established community of researchers used to clinical trial development and monitoring.
5. A general agreement that the risk-to-benefit ratio was likely to be acceptable to patients, regulatory agencies, and the general public given the immediate life-threatening nature of most of these disorders and the paucity of safe alternatives.

As a consequence, the very first gene transfer protocol approved was in cancer patients *(2)*, and the dominance of this area in gene therapy has persisted to this day, with more than 80% of gene transfer subjects falling into this disease category *(3)*. However, it must also be pointed out that cancer gene therapy has a number of drawbacks, and as evident from the chapters in this book, these have led to an underappreciation of its achievements to date and an underestimation of its likely future importance.

Cancer, even of a single cell type in a single organ, is a molecularly heterogeneous disease. Although there is extensive categorization of the molecular basis of hematologic malignancies, this process is just beginning in solid tumors. Hence, no single therapeutic approach is likely to be effective in more than a minority of patients with a given broad histologic category of disease, so that a low success rate even for effective gene therapies is currently to be expected.

Even when effective, single therapies are rarely curative. Cancers evolve and escape from all therapeutic agents. Instead, combined modalities must be used in which resistance to one does not predicate resistance to the others. Although gene therapies have the great advantage of non-cross-resistance to most conventional treatments, combination clinical studies that convincingly show the benefits of adding gene therapy are slow and expensive to perform. End points are often either vague (e.g., increased tumor "response" rates) or delayed for months or years (e.g., prolongation of survival).

Most cancer patients have received multiple other toxic therapies. Their responsiveness to gene therapies designed, for example, to boost immunity may be deficient. Similarly, when toxic events occur, it may be difficult to discern whether they are attributable to the disease, to prior or concomitant therapy, or to the investigational gene drug.

It is these difficulties that lead to the failure or abandonment of many of the historically early studies in gene therapy. However, as is apparent from succeeding chapters, the ability to compensate for some of these problems now underlies many of the successes seen, together with improvements in the transgenes used and the ways in which they are delivered.

The earliest studies using gene transfer to treat cancer were all designed to compensate for the remarkable inefficiency of the available adenoviral, retroviral, and plasmid vectors. Gene-marking studies were the first out of the gate *(2,4–6)*. These were implemented not with any direct therapeutic intent, but rather to use the transferred marker gene as a means of tracking normal or malignant cells and help validate and improve interventions already in use. The principle of gene marking is the transfer and integration of a unique deoxyribonucleic acid (DNA) sequence (e.g., a nonhuman gene) into the DNA of a host cell (e.g., T cell, hematopoietic stem cell), allowing the gene or the gene product to be detected easily, thereby serving as a marker for these labeled cells *(5)*.

In 1988, Rosenberg proposed a protocol to genetically mark lymphocytes derived from tumor patients (tumor-infiltrating lymphocytes, TILs). These lymphocytes appeared to have antitumor activity and could be expanded ex vivo and returned to patients with tumors. However, it was unclear whether the infused cells were able to traffic to tumor sites and produce antitumor activity. Rosenberg's group planned to expand TIL cells ex vivo, transduce them with a Moloney retroviral vector encoding the neomycin phosphotransferase gene (*NEO* or, as it was then written, Neo^R) and return them to the patient. Any transduced cells infused and all their progeny could then be detected by subsequent analysis of blood, tissues, and tumor sites. This would in turn reveal whether these cells persisted in vivo, expanded, and trafficked to the tumor sites. If they did relocalize, it would also be possible to see whether their presence was associated with tumor regression.

Although simple in concept, this protocol, like all early gene therapy protocols, was exposed to intense, repetitious, and prolonged public and private scrutiny. At that time, all gene transfer protocols were examined locally by institutional review boards and biosafety committees before passing on to the Human Gene Therapy Subcommittee of the Recombinant DNA Advisory Committee (RAC) of the National Institutes of Health for public review.

Usually, after several reviews, each resulting in requested changes and additional data, protocols were forwarded to the RAC for public re-review. The RAC itself usually had requests and requirements before passing the protocol on to the director of the National Institutes of Health for approval. Next would come the submission to the Food and Drug Administration, which would generally also require public review by their own advisory panel before applying their standard internal review for investigational new drug applications, using staffers specializing in pharmacology/toxicology, product manufacturing, and clinical affairs. Although the review process has since simplified, it remains more complex than for other anticancer agents, even though many of these (such as alkylating agents) may have the potential to cause equivalent oncogenic, germline (transgenerational), and environmental harm.

Finally, patient accrual began on the first protocol, and the results were published in 1990 *(2)*. The study successfully showed the feasibility of human gene transfer in a clinical setting, and that marker studies could be safe. However, the low level of marking achieved and the limited expansion observed in vivo made it difficult to demonstrate clearly selective tumor homing or to correlate the presence of TILs with tumor response.

Later marking studies were more informative *(4,5,7–9)*. Autologous hematopoietic stem cell (HSC) transplantation had shown promise as an effective treatment for leukemias and lymphomas and some solid tumors *(10–13)*, but disease recurrence was the major cause of treatment failure. When the tumor originated from or involved the marrow, relapse could originate from malignant cells persisting in the patient, in the rescuing HSCs, or in both. Concern that the HSCs may contain residual malignant cells led to extensive evaluation of techniques for purging these cells *(14,15)*. However, it had been hard to show that this reduced the risk of relapse, and the purging techniques usually slowed engraftment because of damage to normal progenitor cells.

In three early 1990 studies, of acute myeloblastic leukemia, neuroblastoma, and chronic myeloid leukemia, autologous stem cells were marked, after they were harvested and prior to reinfusion, using murine retroviral vectors encoding the neomycin resistance gene. At relapse, the investigators looked to see whether the marker gene was present in the malignant cells *(7,16–18)*. In all three diseases, it proved possible to detect both the transferred marker and a tumor-specific marker in the same cells at the time of relapse, which provided unequivocal evidence that the residual malignant cells in the marrow were a source of malignant recurrence *(5)*. These studies also provided information on the transfer of marker genes to normal hematopoietic cells and showed that marrow autografts contribute to long-term hematopoietic reconstitution after transplant *(19)*. With more than 10 years follow-up, they have also so far proved safe.

Unfortunately, the poor transducibility of many other tumors by the available retroviral vectors prevented this technique from wide use in other tumor settings *(8,20)*. However, the approach was subsequently used in a series of protocols that demonstrated the safety, persistence, and effectiveness of viral and tumor-specific T lymphocytes *(9,21,22)*, which had been the intention of the first TIL protocol.

3. EARLY THERAPEUTIC STUDIES: THE NEED FOR AMPLIFICATION

Although informative, marker studies could never by themselves be considered gene therapy. But, the poor efficiency and lack of targeting of available vectors seemed to rule out using the transfer of directly therapeutic genes because too small a proportion of tumor cells would be affected for benefit to be seen. Instead, investigators tried to combine gene therapy with two modalities that could amplify the effects of gene transfer.

3.1. Prodrug Metabolizing Enzymes

In the first of these modalities, a gene was transferred that acted as an enzyme capable of splitting an inactive small molecule into a lethal cytotoxin. By intercellular (gap junction) and local extracellular spread, these newly formed toxic small molecules would be expected to diffuse locally and damage even tumor cells that had not been transduced, in a so-called bystander effect. Even before development of gene therapy, more than a dozen prodrug-metabolizing enzyme (PDME) systems had been described.

Of these, the herpes simplex virus thymidine kinase system was considered most appropriate for translation into a gene therapeutic. This gene phosphorylates small-molecule drugs such as acyclovir or ganciclovir to nucleoside analogs toxic to dividing cells. For the PDME approach to be tumor selective, either the vector or the prodrug product must be targeted to the malignant cell. The first clinical studies to test this novel strategy aimed for both types of selectivity by introducing a thymidine kinase gene into a tumor cell using a retroviral vector *(23,24)*. On exposure to ganciclovir, the transduced cells phosphorylate the drug. If the cell then divides, the product is incorporated into DNA with lethal consequences; nondividing cells are unaffected.

To maximize the therapeutic index of the approach, initial study of *Tk* gene transfer was made in patients with brain tumors; in this context, there is a particularly clear distinction between tumor cells (which divide and are destined to be killed by the ganciclovir) and normal neurons (which do not divide and should escape unharmed). Retroviral vectors offered additional tumor specificity in this system because they function only in dividing cells and therefore do not transduce normal neurons. In initial phase I and II studies introducing vector or vector producer cells, there appeared to be tumor regression and patient benefit. Unfortunately, this benefit was not seen in a larger scale, definitive, and extremely expensive phase III study, leading to abandonment of the approach by large pharma.

Other investigators have continued to use this system, delivering PDME genes with adenoviral vectors to sites such as the prostate, peritoneum, and lung. This loses the specificity for dividing cells at the level of infection (although retaining it at the level of drug activity), but the higher transducing efficiency of adenovectors is felt to be essential for efficacy. This approach remains in investigation for many tumors and is looking particularly promising when combined with the second amplification method, which uses the immune system.

3.2. Generation of Tumor Vaccines

Although current vectors lack the capacity to be targeted precisely and are poorly distributed, specificity and excellent biodistribution are almost the defining characteristics of the immune system. Tumor immunotherapy has had a long and somewhat tarnished history, but by the 1980s it was evident that many human tumor cells really did express tumor-associated or tumor-specific antigens, and that even when internal, these antigens could be processed to peptides and appear on the tumor cell surface. Most important perhaps, data from allogeneic stem cell transplantation and from newly developed monoclonal antibodies unequivocally demonstrated that an effectively manipulated immune system was indeed capable of eradicating even extensive malignancies.

Hence, there was great interest in using gene transfer to augment an otherwise ineffective antitumor immune response, which in turn would be sufficiently targeted and well distributed to destroy tumor sites regardless of their location in the patient. Murine studies showed that transduction of tumor cells with cytokine genes *(25)*, allogeneic major histocompatibility complex molecules *(26)*, or costimulatory molecules such as B7.1 or CD40 ligand *(27,28)* augmented immunogenicity. Injection of neoplastic cells in doses that would normally establish a tumor instead recruited immune system effector cells. In some models, established, nontransduced, parental malignant cells were also eradicated.

The first studies of this approach began in 1992 using autologous melanoma cells or allogeneic melanoma cell lines *(26,29)* expressing transgenic granulocyte-macrophage colony-stimulating factor or HLA-B7 (in HLA-B7-negative individuals). There were certainly clinical responses to these vaccines, but it has proved difficult to scale-up the projects and make them commercially viable. Nonetheless, the results were sufficiently encouraging that there have been well over 200 different tumor vaccine studies using a range of immunostimulatory molecules.

Results in diseases such as melanoma, renal cell carcinoma, and neuroblastoma showed that tumor cells transduced with the interleukin-2, granulocyte-macrophage colony-stimulating factor, or HLA-B7 gene can be given safely and produce immunomodulatory effects, including peripheral blood eosinophilia, a rise in natural killer and activated killer (AK) cell number and activity, and an increase in tumor-specific cytotoxic T-lymphocyte precursor frequency (29–34). There have been reports of clinical responses in distal tumor sites, although other metastases have continued to grow (perhaps because their phenotypic heterogeneity allowed them to evade the immune system). It is likely that the best application of this approach will be in the adjuvant setting to prevent relapse in patients with presumed minimal residual disease and/or in combination with cytoreductive, but not immunosuppressive, levels of chemotherapy. Unfortunately, the design, interpretation, and expense of such complex and lengthy studies represent major obstacles to drug development.

4. SELECTION OF TRANSDUCED CELLS

The application of gene therapy outside malignancy was predicated on the transduced cells having a survival advantage; hence, the earliest application to patients with inherited immunodeficiency states such as adenosine deaminase (ADA) deficiency (35). However, it was evident early on that one way of broadening these applications would be to build in a selectable marker along with the therapeutic gene of interest and then subsequently administer the selecting agent. Many cytotoxic drug resistance genes were discovered in the 1980s, making this approach a theoretical possibility.

Cancer patients were chosen to investigate the feasibility and toxicity of the selectable approach because one of the tenets of cancer therapy is that "more is better." There is certainly good evidence for some tumors that patients given more intense therapy for longer do better than those receiving less-intense or shorter treatments. Drug dosing is limited by toxicity to normal tissues, particularly marrow progenitor cells. Hence, if it were possible to transfer genes that rendered normal cells resistant to one or more cytotoxic drugs, it might enable them to resist the toxic consequences of the relevant agent. The multidrug resistance gene 1 (MDR-1) was the most widely considered gene for human therapy. Its product, *P*-glycoprotein, functions as an ATP binding cassette (ABC) transporter and is a potent drug efflux pump that confers resistance to many chemotherapeutic agents (36).

After extensive preclinical testing, a clinical protocol to test the approach began in 1994 (37). Patients with breast cancer were given marrow stem cells transduced with the MDR-1 gene via retroviral-mediated gene transfer and their response to chemotherapy with taxol as the selecting agent was measured. The investigators hoped to see a progressive rise in the numbers of MDR-1 transgenic cells after taxol therapy and ultimately the ability to sustain normal hemopoiesis even after extensive treatment. Unfortunately, the low efficiency of stem cell transduction and poor gene expression observed in the earliest clinical protocols resulted in no selection of gene-modified cells and hence no in vivo protection (37,38).

The approach has been pursued with different drug resistance genes in several different malignancies. Although transfer of such genes may find a place in treatment of malignant disease, it seems increasingly unlikely that it will ever be feasible to apply the technique in nonmalignant diseases as originally intended. The combination of retroviral gene transfer and cytotoxic drugs in patients without malignancy is one that now holds little appeal given the oncogenic events observed in the severe combined immunodeficiency (SCID) trials in France (39).

5. TUMOR CORRECTION

Although there is an attractive elegance to the strategy of introducing genetic material into a malignancy to correct the specific genetic defects contributing to the neoplastic phenotype, the lack of targeting and poor efficiency of gene transfer vectors was considered to render this approach clinically worthless: Transduction in vivo of 1–2% of tumor cells (an optimistic estimate) with a corrective gene would be of no patient benefit. There was therefore great resistance to an early protocol in which investigators proposed to replace a defective p53 gene in localized unresectable or recurrent carcinoma of the bronchus by injecting a retroviral vector encoding p53 *(40)*.

The protocol only went ahead after much debate, but to almost everyone's surprise, there were apparent tumor responses. Substitution of an adenoviral p53 vector apparently gave superior responses, and the approach appeared also to produce responses in localized head and neck cancer *(41)*. The effects occur regardless of whether the tumors are p53 mutant or wild type and certainly cannot be attributed to the low level of tumor transduction obtained with the vectors.

Although the mechanism of action remains uncertain, the results have been sufficiently encouraging to allow the implementation of a phase III clinical study. Regardless of the eventual outcome of these trials, the data make the important point that little is still understood of the biologic interactions between ourselves and our tumors, and that in the face of such ignorance, we should be careful about the predictions we make.

6. WHAT DID THE EARLY STUDIES TEACH US?

Above all else, of course, these early studies confirmed the obvious: Available vectors were simply inadequate for our needs. The past decade has seen an explosion of work identifying new vector systems, viral and nonviral. Of particular interest for cancer therapy has been the development of conditionally replication competent vectors capable of reproducing in malignant cells while sparing normal tissues. To date, these have been used clinically for their directly lytic properties, but the potential to incorporate therapeutic genes is obvious and may substantially boost the efficiency of almost all the approaches described in this chapter. Many other groups are working on vector targeting and on transgene regulation. They have made substantial advances that are described elsewhere in this volume and that will soon be showing up in clinical trials.

The issue of vector and transgene immunogenicity is also a concern. Although an adjuvantlike effect may enhance some cancer gene therapies, readministration is severely curtailed in the presence of a neutralizing immune response. The ability to deal with this problem may ultimately be the most important factor in determining the value of cancer gene therapy.

Perhaps the most important conceptual message from these early studies is that, although a single gene therapy approach alone can undoubtedly induce a tumor response, it is unlikely to eradicate disease successfully. Instead, inter- and intrapatient tumor heterogeneity means that several different therapeutic methods will need to be combined. As discussed in this book, efforts to combine gene therapies with conventional modalities are proceeding, as are efforts to combine different types of gene therapies themselves. For example, if Tk gene transfer (followed by ganciclovir) is combined with cytokine gene transfer, the patient may benefit from both a direct cytotoxic and an immune-mediated antitumor effect.

Undoubtedly, gene therapy has had a difficult first 12 years. Understandable excitement about the approach lead to unrealistic expectations about the time it would take to apply the technology successfully, and intense scrutiny of adverse events (predominantly those in nonmalignant conditions) has been discouraging to many in academia and in industry. A brief study of the history of every other novel cancer therapy, including cytotoxic drugs, radiation, or monoclonal antibodies, reveals a 20-year gap between discovery and truly successful implementation. The complexity of gene therapies and of the current regulatory environment means that much the same can be expected of this technology. Although many industrial partners have dropped from the race, it seems likely that eventual success will encourage a resurrection of interest.

One final lesson of this early history, however, is that ultimately the successful model for cancer gene therapy may not always be the pharmaceutical one. Instead, investigators may need to assemble components from a number of suppliers and provide an institution-based manufacturing process—the model of organ transplantation and indeed of surgery and radiotherapy in general.

7. CONCLUSION

Although the history of cancer gene therapy has emphasized individual investigators and industrial sponsors, the future is more likely to accentuate the importance of interdisciplinary teams and the institutions in which they work.

REFERENCES

1. Friedmann, T. (1999) The origins, evolution and directions of human gene therapy. In *The Development of Human Gene Therapy* (Friedmann, T., ed.), Cold Spring Harbor Laboratory Press, Cold Spring Harbor, NY, pp. 1–20.
2. Rosenberg, S. A., Aebersold, P., Cornetta, K., et al. (1990) Gene transfer into humans—immunotherapy of patients with advanced melanoma, using tumor-infiltrating lymphocytes modified by retroviral gene transduction. *N. Engl. J. Med.* **323,** 570–578.
3. Rosenberg, S. A., Blaese, R. M., Brenner, M. K., et al. (2000) Human gene marker/therapy clinical protocols. *Hum. Gene Ther.* **11,** 919–979.
4. Brenner, M. K., Rill, D. R., Moen, R. C., et al. (1993) Gene-marking to trace origin of relapse after autologous bone marrow transplantation. *Lancet* **341,** 85–86.
5. Brenner, M. K., Rill, D. R., Holladay, M. S., et al. (1993) Gene marking to determine whether autologous marrow infusion restores long-term haemopoiesis in cancer patients. *Lancet* **342,** 1134–1137.
6. Deisseroth, A. B., Zu, Z., Claxton, D., et al. (1994) Genetic marking shows that Ph+ cells present in autologous transplants of chronic myelogenous leukemia (CML) contribute to relapse after autologous bone marrow in CML. *Blood* **83,** 3068–3076.
7. Deisseroth, A. B., Kantarjian, H., Talpaz, M., et al. (1991) Autologous bone marrow transplantation for CML in which retroviral markers are used to discriminate between relapse which arises from systemic disease remaining after preparative therapy vs relapse due to residual leukemia cells in autologous marrow: A pilot trial. *Hum. Gene Ther.* **2,** 359–376.
8. Dunbar, C. E., Cottler-Fox, M., O'Shaunessy, J. A., et al. (1995) Retrovirally marked CD34-enriched peripheral blood and marrow cells contribute to long term engraftment after autologous transplantation. *Blood* **85,** 3048–3057.
9. Heslop, H. E., Ng, C. Y. C., Li, C., et al. (1996) Long-term restoration of immunity against Epstein-Barr virus infection by adoptive transfer of gene-modified virus-specific T lymphocytes. *Nat. Med.* **2,** 551–555.
10. Gorin, N. C. (1998) Autologous stem cell transplantation in acute myelocytic leukemia. *Blood* **92,** 1073–1090.
11. To, L. B., Haylock, D., Simmons, P. J., and Juttner, C. A. (1997) The biology and clinical uses of blood stem cells. *Blood* **89,** 2233–2258.
12. Nieto, Y. and Shpall, E. J. (1999) Autologous stem-cell transplantation for solid tumors in adults. *Hematol. Oncol. Clin. North Am.* **13,** 939–968, vi.
13. Johnston, L. J. and Horning, S. J. (1999) Autologous hematopoietic cell transplantation in non-Hodgkin's lymphoma. *Hematol. Oncol. Clin. North Am.* **13,** 889–918.
14. Bensinger, W. I. (1998) Should we purge? *Bone Marrow Transplant.* **21,** 113–115.
15. Zwicky, C. S., Maddocks, A. B., Andersen, N., and Gribben, J. G. (1996) Eradication of polymerase chain reaction detectable immunoglobulin gene rearrangements in non-Hodgkin's lymphoma is associated with decreased relapse after autologous bone marrow transplantation. *Blood* **88,** 3314–3322.
16. Brenner, M., Mirro, J. Jr., Hurwitz, C., et al. (1991) Autologous bone marrow transplant for children with AML in first complete remission: use of marker genes to investigate the biology of marrow reconstitution and the mechanism of relapse. *Hum. Gene Ther.* **2,** 137.
17. Santana, V. M., Brenner, M. K., Ihle, J., et al. (1991) A phase I trial of high-dose carboplatin and etoposide with autologous marrow support for treatment of stage D neuroblastoma in first remission: use of marker genes to investigate the biology of marrow reconstitution and the mechanism of relapse. *Hum. Gene Ther.* **3,** 257–272.
18. Cornetta, K., Tricot, G., Broun, E. R., et al. (1992) Retroviral-mediated gene transfer of bone marrow cells during autologous bone marrow transplantation for acute leukemia. *Hum. Gene Ther.* **3,** 305–318.
19. Brenner, M. K., Rill, D. R., Heslop, H. E., et al. (1994) Gene marking after bone marrow transplantation. *Eur. J. Cancer* **30A,** 1171–1176.
20. Cornetta, K., Srour, E. F., Moore, A., et al. (1996) Retroviral gene transfer in autologous bone marrow transplantation for adult acute leukemia. *Hum. Gene Ther.* **7,** 1323–1329.
21. Rooney, C. M., Smith, C. A., Ng, C., et al. (1995) Use of gene-modified virus-specific T lymphocytes to control Epstein-Barr virus-related lymphoproliferation. *Lancet* **345,** 9–13.

22. Rooney, C. M., Smith, C. A., Ng, C. Y. C., et al. (1998) Infusion of cytotoxic T cells for the prevention and treatment of Epstein-Barr virus-induced lymphoma in allogeneic transplant recipients. *Blood* **92,** 1549–1555.
23. Culver, K. W., Ram, Z., Wallbridge, S., Ishii, H., Oldfield, E. H., and Blaese, R. M. (1992) In vivo gene transfer with retroviral vector-producer cells for treatment of experimental brain tumors. *Science* **256,** 1550–1552.
24. Ram, Z., Culver, K. W., Oshiro, E. M., et al. (1997) Therapy of malignant brain tumors by intratumoral implantation of retroviral vector-producing cells. *Nature Med.* **3,** 1354–1361.
25. Dranoff, G. and Mulligan, R. C. (1995) Gene transfer as cancer therapy. *Adv,. Immunol.* **58,** 417–454.
26. Nabel, G. J., Nabel, E. G., Yang, Z. Y., et al. (1993) Direct gene transfer with DNA-liposome complexes in melanoma: expression, biologic activity, and lack of toxicity in humans. *Proc. Natl. Acad. Sci. USA* **90,** 11,307–11,311.
27. Townsend, S. E. and Allison, J. P. (1993) Tumor rejection after direct costimulation of CD8$^+$ T cells by B7-transfected melanoma cells. *Science* **259,** 368–370.
28. Dilloo, D., Brown, M., Roskrow, M., et al. (1997) CD40 ligand induces an anti-leukemia immune response in vivo. *Blood* **90,** 1927–1933.
29. Soiffer, R., Lynch, T., Mihm, M., et al. (1998) Vaccination with irradiated autologous melanoma cells engineered to secrete human granulocyte-macrophage colony-stimulating factor generates potent antitumor immunity in patients with metastatic melanoma. *Proc. Natl. Acad. Sci. USA* **95,** 13,141–13,146.
30. Schreiber, S., Kampgen, E., Wagner, E., et al. (1999) Immunotherapy of metastatic malignant melanoma by a vaccine consisting of autologous interleukin 2-transfected cancer cells: outcome of a phase I study. *Hum. Gene Ther.* **10,** 983–993.
31. Bowman, L., Grossmann, M., Rill, D., et al. (1998) IL-2 adenovector-transduced autologous tumor cells induce anti-tumor immune responses in patients with neuroblastoma. *Blood* **92,** 1941–1949.
32. Bowman, L. C., Grossmann, M., Rill, D., et al. (1998) IL-2 gene-modified allogeneic tumor cells for treatment of relapsed neuroblastoma. *Hum. Gene Ther.* **9,** 1303–1311.
33. Simons, J. W., Jaffe, E. M., Weber, C. E., et al. (1997) Bioactivity of autologous irradiated renal cell carcinoma vaccines generated by ex-vivo granulocyte-macrophage colony-stimulating factor gene transfer. *Cancer Res.* **57,** 1537–1546.
34. Simons, J. W., Mikhak, B., Chang, J. F., et al. (1999) Induction of immunity to prostate cancer antigens: results of a clinical trial of vaccination with irradiated autologous prostate tumor cells engineered to secrete granulocyte-macrophage colony-stimulating factor using ex vivo gene transfer. *Cancer Res.* **59,** 5160–5168.
35. Blaese, R. M., Culver, K. W., Miller, A. D., et al. (1995) T lymphocyte-directed gene therapy for ADA—SCID: initial trial results after 4 years. *Science* **270,** 475–480.
36. Pastan, I. and Gottesman, M. M. (1991) Multidrug resistance. *Annu. Rev. Med.* **42,** 277.
37. Hanania, E. G., Giles, R. E., Kavanagh, J., et al. (1996) Results of MDR-1 vector modification trial indicate that granulocyte/macrophage colony-forming unit cells do not contribute to posttransplant hematopoietic recovery following intensive systemic therapy. *Proc. Natl. Acad. Sci. USA* **93,** 15,346–15,351.
38. Hesdorffer, C., Ayello, J., Ward, M., et al. (1998) Phase I trial of retroviral-mediated transfer of the human MDR1 gene as marrow chemoprotection in patients undergoing high-dose chemotherapy and autologous stem-cell transplantation. *J. Clin. Oncol.* **16,** 165–172.
39. Hacein-Bey-Abina, S., von Kalle, C., Schmidt, M., et al. (2003) A serious adverse event after successful gene therapy for X-linked severe combined immunodeficiency. *N. Engl. J. Med.* **348,** 255–256.
40. Roth, J. A., Nguyen, D., Lawrence, D. D., et al. (1996) Retrovirus-mediated wild-type p53 gene transfer to tumors of patients with lung cancer. *Nat. Med.* **2,** 985–991.
41. Swisher, S. G., Roth, J. A., Nemunaitis, J., et al. (1999) Adenovirus-mediated p53 gene transfer in advanced non-small-cell lung cancer. *J. Natl. Cancer Inst.* **91,** 763–771.

2

The Genetic Basis of Cancer

Akseli Hemminki and Kari Hemminki

1. INTRODUCTION

Cancer is a genetic disease in which malignant cells have undergone mutations and epigenetic changes but maintain the transformed phenotype even when cultured or when injected into immunologically tolerant experimental animals *(1,2)*. However, most of the genetic events in tumors are somatic (i.e., not hereditary), brought about environmentally or randomly, and the identified inherited (often referred to as "genetic") causes account for a small proportion of all cancers.

Specifically, the genes with mutations that are relevant to the carcinogenic process, fall into two classes: tumor suppressor genes and oncogenes. The distinction between heritable and environmental causes may be easily made if a hereditary cancer syndrome or an environmental exposure, such as tobacco smoking or human papilloma virus, poses a high risk. For most common cancers, this is not the case, and they are therefore considered complex diseases caused by many underlying and interacting genetic and environmental factors. Heritable effects would lead to a clustering of cancer in families *(3,4)*. However, familial clustering can also be caused by shared environment or lifestyle, and an increased familial risk does not tell whether the reason is heritable or environmental *(5)*.

In this chapter, we discuss causes of cancer and the underlying molecular mechanisms from the point of view of potential gene therapy approaches. Improved understanding of the causes of cancer will be helpful for scientific, clinical, and cancer preventive measures. A certain notion of cancer causation, often implicit, is embedded in many science and health policy decisions.

2. THE GENETIC BACKGROUND OF CARCINOGENESIS

In a nutshell, cancer can be considered a disease caused by mutations and epigenetic changes (e.g., methylation defects) in tumor suppressor genes and oncogenes *(6)*. Mutations may be the more common of the two types of changes and can be missense (altered amino acid), frameshift (altered reading frame), or nonsense (truncation of protein product). Sometimes, mutations do not affect the amino acid sequence, but rather influence the promoter or splice sites. Deoxyribonucleic acid (DNA) sequence variations that do not have a direct unequivocal link to the phenotype of interest but may play a role are called *polymorphisms*.

There are various mechanisms that can cause mutations. These include deletions of small or large DNA segments, inversions, translocations, looping leading to truncated sequence, and so on. The initial causes for these mechanisms range from ultraviolet radiation to chemical and viral carcinogens, but for most cases of cancer, causation remains poorly defined. Probably, diet and other environmental causes play a major role, but cause–effect relationships are difficult to demonstrate conclusively because of the long time between initiation of a tumor and clinical presentation. Hereditary mutations have also been identified as a cause of cancer and are discussed here.

From: *Contemporary Cancer Research*
Cancer Gene Therapy
Edited by: D. T. Curiel and J. T. Douglas © Humana Press Inc., Totowa, NJ

By definition, genetic changes important for carcinogenesis (i.e., can be detected as clonal changes in malignant tumors) inactivate tumor suppressor genes or activate oncogenes. Both groups include dozens of well-defined members, and hundreds probably remain poorly characterized. A classic example of an oncogene is *RAS*, which was initially identified as a gene activated in the process of virally induced tumorigenesis. Later, mutations of *RAS* have been commonly found in a wide variety of cancers. Most protein products of oncogenes are involved in signal transduction and growth regulation. An activating mutation of one allele is usually sufficient.

The normal functions of proteins coded by tumor suppressor genes are often related to important regulatory or housekeeping functions crucial to the integrity of cellular functions, including cell division and programmed cell death. Therefore, the loss of these functions is beneficial to malignant progression. In most cases, both alleles of a tumor suppressor gene must be lost for loss of function of the protein product. Often, one allele is lost because of a "local" mutation; the other allele is lost because of a large deletion (loss of heterozygosity). Classic tumor suppressor genes include *p53* and *APC* (adenomatous polyposis *coli*). The former has a wide variety of functions associated with cell cycle control and programmed cell death (apoptosis). Mutations of *p53* have been identified in more than half of all cancers.

APC was initially identified as the gene harboring germline mutations in patients with familial adenomatous polyposis, a hereditary disorder that leads to formation of hundreds of intestinal polyps that, when untreated, eventually undergo malignant transformation and cause death at a young age. *APC* has multiple functions involved with cellular signaling and adhesion. The *APC* example is interesting for two reasons. First, it is a useful example of a rare genetic disorder revealing the molecular background of common disease. Although familial adenomatous polyposis is rare, mutations of *APC* (or members of its signaling pathway) were consecutively identified in virtually all colorectal cancers. In fact, the same is true for most of the cancer syndromes discussed in this chapter. Although the syndromes are rare, the causative genes are commonly involved in sporadic carcinogenesis as well.

Second, studies (many of which were performed by Bert Vogelstein and colleagues at Johns Hopkins in Baltimore, MD) of *APC* and the genetic basis of colorectal cancer have revealed another aspect that may be common for many types of malignant tumors. Inactivation of *APC* may be the initial or an early step in many colorectal cancers, but it is not the only change found in advanced tumors. Instead, carcinogenesis may often be a multistep process in which additional mutations confer features useful for increased growth and decreased susceptibility to growth regulation (Fig. 1).

It is unlikely that all occurring mutations are beneficial to the malignant clone. Instead, the majority may give rise to subclones that have reduced viability or perhaps increased detection by the immune system. Nevertheless, the rare beneficial changes gain a growth advantage and can thus be detected in the end product of the multistep process of carcinogenesis, which in most cases is an aggressively growing tumor capable of invasion and metastasis.

The gene that sustains the initial mutation that allows the carcinogenic process to proceed has been called the gatekeeper gene (Gene 1 in Fig. 1). The theory is that each cell type may have a crucial growth regulatory circuit; its inactivation may be necessary for carcinogenesis. For example, *APC* has been suggested as the gatekeeper for the colorectal epithelium. Another suggested class of tumor suppressor genes is the caretaker genes; their inactivation may facilitate the multistep process of carcinogenesis by allowing rapid accumulation of further mutations *(2)*. These genes are often involved with DNA repair and maintaining the integrity of the genome.

For gene therapists, an important question is how many steps of the multistep process need to be blocked for effective intervention? Presently, the complete answer is not known. Nevertheless, most available evidence suggests that correction of a single defect, such as replacement of a defective tumor suppressor gene or inactivation of an overactive oncogene, can be sufficient for controlling the malignant process. For example, when *p53* is expressed in *p53* mutant cancer cells (with many other mutations as well), the cells undergo apoptosis and may in fact trigger neighboring cancer cells to do the same.

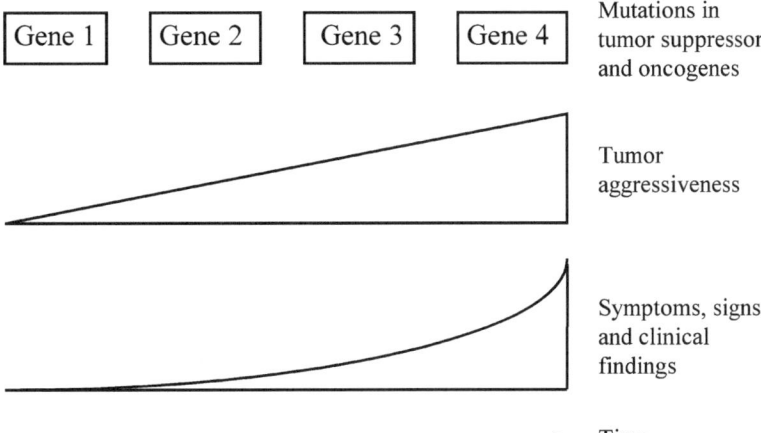

Fig. 1. The multistep nature of cancer. Mutations accumulating in tumor suppressor genes and oncogenes result in increasingly aggressive behavior, that is, the capacity for invasion and metastasis. Together with increasing size, these features usually eventually result in clinical symptoms and findings. Most organs and body compartments have significant reserve capacity; therefore, symptoms often arise late in the evolution of the tumor.

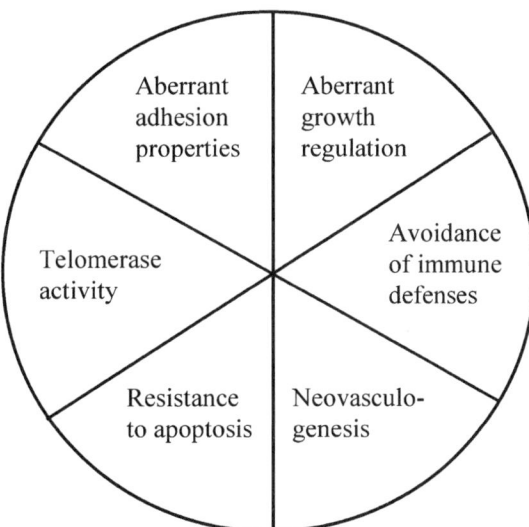

Fig. 2. Common features of advanced cancers.

Thus, perhaps the malignant phenotype can be compared to a house of cards, for which removal of any card causes the whole structure to collapse. This is not completely surprising considering the various defenses the human body has against malignant cells. Fittingly, malignant cells can be detected circulating in healthy individuals who never develop cancer. Further, cancer typically arises in advanced age, when the body's defense mechanisms have slowed, but the cancer has had decades to develop a delicately balanced combination of features that allow sustained growth while remaining undetected by the immune system.

An increasing number of genes are identified as tumor suppressor and oncogenes, and the respective protein products seem to have a wide variety of functions *(1,6)*. Nevertheless, many cancer-associated genetic changes seem to fall into six categories (Fig. 2), which include (1) aberrant adhesion

Table 1
Heritable Effects of Cancer and Some Involved Genes

Cancer site	Proportion of variance attributed to heritable effects		
	From twins	From families	Known genes
Stomach	0.28	0.01[a]	E-cadherin
Colorectum	0.35[a]	0.13[a]	Mismatch repair, *APC, LKB1*
Pancreas	0.36	—	*CDKN2A*
Lung	0.26	0.08[a]	Metabolic low-penetrance genes
Breast	0.27[a]	0.25[a]	*BRCA1/2, ATM* (ataxia telangiectasia mutated)
Cervix uteri	0	0.22[a]	Immune response genes?
Corpus uteri	0	—	Mismatch repair, *PTEN*
Ovary	0.22	—	*BRCA1/2*, mismatch repair
Prostate	0.42[a]	—	Candidate loci
Bladder	0.31	0.07[a]	Metabolic low-penetrance genes
Leukemia	0.21	0.09[a]	*ATM*, helicase

Source: Based on a Nordic twin *(7)* and a Swedish family study *(8)*.
[a]95% confidence interval does not include 0.0; that is, the estimate is statistically significant.

properties (e.g., loss of contact inhibition), (2) exaggerated or unphysiological response to growth-promoting signals and reduced responsiveness to growth-regulating signals, (3) failure to undergo programmed cell death on genetic damage (dysfunction of cell cycle checkpoints), (4) immortalization (gain of telomerase activity), (5) avoidance of immune defenses, and (6) factors promoting neo-vasculogenesis (rapidly growing tumors need an ample supply of oxygen and nutrients). Importantly, all of these features are distinct from characteristics found in most nonmalignant cells and thus may allow intervention.

3. APPORTIONING CANCER CAUSATION

Although most cases of cancer are somatic, that is, they do not have an identifiable familial component, studies of hereditary syndromes have produced or initiated much of today's understanding of cancer as a genetic disease. It is not unreasonable to assume that this will be true in the future as well; therefore, we briefly discuss hereditary cancer here.

Two studies have provided unique insight into the familial component of various common cancers. The first study used the classic twin design, that is, comparison of correlation of cancer in monozygotic and dizygotic twins from three Nordic countries *(7)*. In this model, it is assumed that both types of twins equally share the environmental effects; monozygotic twins are genetically identical, whereas dizygotic twins are like any siblings, sharing by average 50% of their genes. The second study was based on the nationwide Swedish Family-Cancer Database of 3 million families *(8)*. It compared correlation of cancers between all family members using the same statistical model used in the twin study. It had a much higher statistical power than the twin study because the whole Swedish population and its 1 million tumors were scrutinized. On the other hand, most sex-specific cancers could not be assessed in the model.

The results from both models are presented in Table 1. For stomach cancer, heritability was estimated to account for 28% from the twin study and 1% from the family study. The remainder, 72% and 99%, respectively, could be the total environmental effect, of which the majority were because of nonshared or random environment. The twin study gave statistically significant heritability estimates (for which the 95 % confidence interval did not include zero) only for cancers of the colorectum (35%), breast (27%), and prostate (42%). The family study gave an identical estimate for the breast, but a lower estimate for the colorectum. The heritability of cervical cancer was 22%, but that of lung and bladder cancer and leukemia was less than 10%.

Caution should be used in overinterpreting these estimates from statistical modeling. However, certain common cancers showed a much higher range of heritability than that observed by comparing familial risks between first-degree relatives *(9)*. If the estimates for colorectal, breast, and prostate cancers, showing 27–42% heritability, are confirmed, there are major gaps in the understanding of the genetic basis of these neoplasms.

Some of the genes that transmit familial risks are indicated in Table 1 *(2)*. The frequencies of mutations in the well-known high-risk susceptibility genes *BRCA1* and *BRCA2* in breast cancer and DNA mismatch repair genes in hereditary nonpolyposis colorectal cancer (HNPCC) are so low that they explain at most 10% of the heritability noted, and 90% remain unaccounted *(10,11)*. For prostate cancer, candidate genes have been mapped, but not identified *(12–16)*. These findings suggest that other genes are yet to be identified, but because their polymorphisms are likely to be relatively common and confer only a modest risk increase, their identification will be difficult.

4. CANCER MODELS

Well-characterized cancer syndromes, such as familial retinoblastoma, *BRCA*-linked breast cancer, and HNPCC, follow a dominant Mendelian pattern of inheritance, with high penetrance (proportion of genotype carriers with phenotype); therefore, close to 50% of the offspring of an affected parent present with the disease. Nevertheless, these syndromes are rare, and the frequency of the mutant gene is on the order of 1/1000 (carrier frequency = 1/500) or less. The most common cancer syndromes *BRCA1* and *BRCA2* and HNPCC are thought to account for 1–3% all breast and colorectal cancers, respectively *(10,17,18)*. Bloom syndrome, ataxia telangiectasia, and xeroderma pigmentosum are examples of Mendelian recessive cancer syndromes. About 25% of the offspring of two heterozygote parents display symptoms, including neoplasms. It is relatively easy to estimate the proportion of all cancer because of such well-characterized monogenic syndromes conferring a high risk, and 1% appears to be a good estimate *(19)*.

Most common cancers are caused by alterations in many genes. According to the multistage theory of cancer, the clonal tumor emerges as a result of a number of mutations in a single cell *(20–27)*. The first mutations occur in normal cells, creating a slow-growing preneoplastic colony. Additional changes in a cell of the preneoplastic colony are believed to be necessary to create a neoplastic cell capable of growing as a malignant tumor. The number of required mutations may vary and probably depends on the genes and cell types affected. This is probably true for cases arising as a result of hereditary mutations as well. The initial gatekeeper mutation may confer a growth advantage and thus increase the target size (number of cells with the initiating defect) for subsequent promotional mutations. Mathematical adoption of known mutation rates, number of stem cells, and normal human life-span can accommodate a carcinogenic process with three or more mutations, such as two in the initiation stage and one or more in the promotional stage *(24,25)*.

When two or more genes are involved, it is difficult to observe Mendelian inheritance in pedigrees *(27)* because the likelihood decreases that an offspring will inherit the parental set of disease genes. Therefore, it is difficult to distinguish multifactorial inheritance from low-penetrance single-gene or environmental effects, which is a major challenge to current segregation analyses *(28–30)*. In the twin model, polygenic inheritance would be expressed as a much higher risk among monozygotic than dizygotic twins *(3,31)*. Another model in which polygenic inheritance could be distinguished is in multiple primary cancers in the same individual *(32,33)*.

5. CANCER GENES

Only a small proportion of cancer is because of single-gene, dominant traits *(6,34)*. However, the affected families have been helpful in the efforts of gene identification, and the majority of the tumor-related high-penetrance genes have been described from such families *(2)*. Results can be obtained even for rare cancer syndromes, such as Peutz-Jeghers or skin and uterine leiomyomas if the families are homogeneous and the risk is high *(35,36)*. An interesting aspect of the leiomyoma study was that the gene turned out to be fumarate hydratase coding for an enzyme in the tricarboxylic acid cycle. Another enzyme in this metabolic pathway, succinate dehydrogenase, was implicated in hereditary paragangiomas and pheochromocytomas *(37)*. These data have widened the scope of tumor-related genes to metabolic, housekeeping genes from the earlier cell cycle regulator, DNA repair, and signal transduction paradigms.

5.1. High-Risk, Rare Genes

Many forms of cancer in which a single gene poses a high risk have been identified. Of the 4700 dominant and 2800 recessive human genetic traits known in the early 1990s *(31)*, some 440 were single-gene traits in which cancer was a complication; many of them were extremely rare, with a few identified families worldwide *(38)*. Most known cancer syndromes are dominant at the population level (although recessive at the molecular level; *19*), the gene carriers are type Aa, where a = mutant gene. In tumors, the normal allele is lost (loss of heterozygosity), and the tumor is therefore hemizygous a or homozygous aa if another mutation occurs instead of allele loss. In dominant cancer syndromes, the penetrance is typically high, often approaching 100%, which facilitates identification of the dominant pattern because cases are found in all generations.

Some rare cancer syndromes, such as xeroderma pigmentosum, ataxia telangiectasia, and Bloom syndrome, are recessive (aa) at both population and molecular levels. The detection of recessive conditions is difficult because the cases appear apparently randomly in pedigrees, but often reveal consanguinity at a closer inspection. Population geneticists have raised questions about the relatively small number of known human recessive syndromes. In species of experimental animals, recessive traits predominate, as opposed to humans, for whom dominant traits are more common *(31)*. It is not excluded that this is an observation bias because of difficulties in identifying a recessive pattern. A further complication is that, in many cancer syndromes, the mutations are *de novo* germline mutations lacking familial pattern. This is the case for most disorders for which cancer occurs early; thus, the propagation of the defect to further generations is reduced. Examples include Wilms tumor, retinoblastoma, and neurofibromatoses 1 and 2 *(39)*.

The relative risks (RRs) of cancer may be very high (<1000) in the rare cancer syndromes. In fact, if the penetrance is close to 100%, RR depends on the population frequency of the disease only. Most known syndromes affect young individuals, for which the population incidence is low, resulting in excessive RRs. The unusual risk of rare cancers in young individuals has facilitated identification of syndromes, including Li-Fraumeni, multiple endocrine neoplasia 2 (MEN2), and HNPCC *(40,41)*. The RR of childhood cancers in Li-Fraumeni syndrome (hereditary *p53* mutation) has been estimated at >100 *(42)* and that of colorectal cancer in HNPCC at 70 *(17)*. The estimates from the Swedish Family-Cancer Database give RRs of 30 for endometrial cancer in HNPCC and 5000 for medullary thyroid cancer in MEN2 *(43,44)*.

The proportion of gene carriers depends on the population, and the most accurate estimates are available for Europeans and European Americans. Among the known dominant cancer syndromes, the frequency of gene carriers is highest for HNPCC, about 1/500, and BRCA1 and BRCA2, each about 1/1000. For most others, such as Li-Fraumeni, MEN1 and 2, neurofibromatosis 1 and hereditary renal cell cancer (caused by mutation in VHL), retinoblastoma, Wilms, and Gorlin cancers, the frequency of carriers ranges from 1/3000 to 1/50,000 *(39)*. In recessive conditions, such as xeroderma pigmentosum and ataxia telangiectasia, the frequency of diseased (a^2) is low (1/1 million and 1/40,000, respectively), but the carrier frequency (2Aa) of ataxia telangiectasia has been estimated at 1–5% in the US population *(45)*. If heterozygotes are at risk for cancer, the impact may be significant. Ataxia telangiectasia heterozygotes may have an elevated risk of various cancers, such as breast cancer, and because of the large number of carriers, calculations argue that the attributable proportion of ataxia telangiectasia in breast cancer is higher than that of *BRCA1* and *BRCA2* *(46,47)*.

A further aspect of familial cancer syndromes is that they often affect cancers at multiple sites, even though detected through cancers at a particular "index" site. Li-Fraumeni syndrome is an example, with more than a 100-fold RR at the index sites (childhood sarcomas), but a modest RR for more common diseases such as breast cancer. Further examples are HNPCC, *BRCA1*, and *BRCA2*. In the recessive cancer syndromes, including ataxia telangiectasia and Bloom, the affected individuals can present with almost any kind of malignancy *(45,48)*.

Another aspect relating to the identification of a clinical entity is the presentation of other diseases in many of the known syndromes. Patients with recessive cancer syndromes are severely handicapped, as indicated by some of their descriptive names. Severe noncancer diseases beset even dominant conditions such as NF1 and NF2, MEN 1 and 2, and hereditary renal cell cancer.

5.2. Low-Risk, Common Genes

Familial effects in cancer are not only because of high-risk gene defects as discussed previously, but most likely there is contribution by more common low-risk defects, which may be frequent enough to be called polymorphisms (sometimes defined as the variant present in more than 1% of the population). Many polymorphisms have been described in the areas of drug and carcinogen metabolism, with some recent data also on hormone receptors and DNA repair genes *(49–51)*. Although it is likely that a large number of low-risk genes modulate the carcinogenic process in humans, there has been much controversy in the current literature on the role of metabolism genes in cancer *(52)*.

Immune surveillance plays an important role in cancer, as has been observed in immunosuppressed patients who are at a marked risk of lymphomas and many types of squamous cell carcinomas *(53,54)*. Milder forms of immunodeficiencies probably explain some familial patterns of non-Hodgkin's lymphoma, Hodgkin's disease, cervical cancer, and squamous cell skin cancer *(53,55,56)*. Suppressed immune function is also likely to modulate host response to virus, such as human papilloma virus and Epstein-Barr virus *(57–60)*.

6. CONCLUSION

There are no data available on the etiology of cancer that would refute the predominant role of environment as a causative factor. However, since the epochal review by Doll and Peto in 1981 *(61)*, disappointingly little progress has been seen in the search for new causes of environmental carcinogenesis. One likely reason is that environmental carcinogenesis is because of the interaction of external and host factors, which cannot be unraveled by epidemiological or molecular biological means alone. There is hope that merging of these approaches into molecular epidemiology or, even better, into molecular genetic epidemiology will tool the exogenous/endogenous interphase of human carcinogenesis. Nevertheless, there is little doubt that, regardless of the causative agents, on the molecular level the malignant process manifests as mutations and epigenetic changes in tumor suppressor and oncogenes. Further, the accumulation of mutations in these genes gradually increases the aggressiveness of the clone and therefore constitutes the multistep process of carcinogenesis.

All the main types of cancer appear to have a familial component with a frequency that varies, but often ranges from 1 to 5%. Familial risks observed among twins and among patients with multiple primary cancers provide support for the multistage carcinogenesis in human cancers at a population level *(27,30)*. There are at least three practical implications from such findings. One is that, in the search for new susceptibility factors in cancer, low-penetrance genes may be better identified in association studies with a case–control design than in linkage studies *(62–64)*. The second implication is that, in clinical counseling, polygenic and recessive conditions imply uncertainty *(30)*. The disease strikes apparently randomly even though there is an inherited background.

The third problem that may have implications for gene therapy approaches involves a question: If many genes contribute to each case of cancer, is blocking or repair of one defect sufficient for reverting the malignant phenotype? Current evidence suggests that removing one "card" (mutation) from the "house of cards" (advanced malignant tumor) can be enough. Nevertheless, considering the awesome capacity of cancers to acquire resistance, a cytostatic effect may not be desirable, and rapid killing of cells may be required instead. In addition to resistance on the cellular level, tumors can acquire resistance on the tissue level. This implies the existence of subclones that are not sensitive to the treatment. Therefore, removing multiple cards simultaneously or consecutively could have advantages.

Identification of cancer as a disease caused by mutations and epigenetic changes in genes immediately suggested gene therapy as a logical means for intervention. Thus, if the causative defects can be corrected or blocked, the disease phenotype can be reversed. Alternatively, the genetic changes present in cancer cells offer a variety of characteristics that separate them from noncancer cells. These features include dysregulated promoters and enhancers, aberrant expression of receptors and epitopes, and loss of antiviral defense mechanisms. As discussed in this book, these features can be utilized in the planning of gene therapy strategies aimed at direct killing of cancer cells.

REFERENCES

1. Hanahan, D. and Weinberg, R. (2000) The hallmarks of cancer. *Cell* **100,** 57–70.
2. Vogelstein, B. and Kinzler, K. (2002) *The Genetic Basis of Human Cancer*, 2nd ed., McGraw-Hill, New York.
3. Risch, N. (2001) The genetic epidemiology of cancer: interpreting family and twin studies and their implications for molecular genetic approaches. *Cancer Epidemiol. Biomarkers Prev.* **10,** 733–741.
4. Hemminki, K. (2002) Re: Genetic epidemiology of cancer: interpreting family and twin studies and their implications for molecular genetic approaches. *Cancer Epidemiol. Biomarkers Prev.* **11,** 423.
5. Hemminki, K., Dong, C., and Vaittinen, P. (2001) Cancer risks to spouses and offspring in the Family-Cancer Database. *Genet. Epidemiol.* **20,** 247–257.
6. Futreal, P. A., Coin, L., Marshall, M., et al. (2004) A census of human cancer genes. *Nat. Rev. Cancer* **4,** 177–183.
7. Lichtenstein, P., Holm, N., Verkasalo, P., et al. (2000) Environmental and heritable factors in the causation of cancer. *N. Engl. J. Med.* **343,** 78–85.
8. Czene, K., Lichtenstein, P., and Hemminki, K. (2002) Environmental and heritable causes of cancer among 9.6 million individuals in the Swedish Family-Cancer Database. *Int. J. Cancer* **99,** 260–266.
9. Hemminki, K. and Czene, K. (2002) Attributable risks of familial cancer from the Family-Cancer Database. *Cancer Epidemiol. Biomarkers Prev.* **11,** 1638–1644.
10. Peto, J., Collins, N., Barfoot, R., et al. (1999) Prevalence of BRCA1 and BRCA2 gene mutations in patients with early-onset breast cancer. *J. Natl. Cancer Inst.* **91,** 943–949.
11. Salovaara, R., Loukola, A., Kristo, P., et al. (2000) Population-based molecular detection of hereditary nonpolyposis colorectal cancer. *J. Clin. Oncol.* **18,** 2193–2200.
12. Gronberg, H., Smith, J., Emanuelsson, M., et al. (1999) In Swedish families with hereditary prostate cancer, linkage to the HPC1 locus on chromosome 1q24–25 is restricted to families with early-onset prostate cancer. *Am. J. Hum. Genet.* **65,** 134–140.
13. Gibbs, M., Stanford, J., McIndoe, R., et al. (1999) Evidence for a rare prostate cancer-susceptibility locus at chromosome 1p36. *Am. J. Hum. Genet.* **64,** 776–787.
14. Berry, R., Schaid, D. J., Smith, J. R., et al. (2000) Linkage analyses at the chromosome 1 loci 1q24–25 (HPC1), 1q42.2–43 (PCAP), and 1p36 (CAPB) in families with hereditary prostate cancer. *Am. J. Hum. Genet.* **66,** 539–546.
15. Wang, L., McDonnell, S. K., Elkins, D. A., et al. (2001) Role of HPC2/ELAC2 in hereditary prostate cancer. *Cancer Res.* **61,** 6494–6499.
16. Xu, J., Zheng, S. L., Carpten, J. D., et al. (2001) Evaluation of linkage and association of HPC2/ELAC2 in patients with familial or sporadic prostate cancer. *Am. J. Hum. Genet.* **68,** 901–911.
17. Aarnio, M., Sankila, R., Pukkala, E., et al. (1999) Cancer risk in mutation carriers of DNA-mismatch-repair genes. *Int. J. Cancer* **81,** 214–218.
18. Syrjäkoski, K., Vahteristo, P., Eerola, H., et al. (2000) Population-based study of *BRCA1* and *BRCA2* mutations in 1035 unselected Finnish breast cancer patients. *J. Natl. Cancer Inst.* **92,** 1529–1531.
19. Fearon, E. R. (1997) Human cancer syndromes: clues to the origin and nature of cancer. *Science* **278,** 1043–1050.
20. Armitage, P. and Doll, R. (1954) The age distribution of cancer and a multi-stage theory of carcinogenesis. *Br. J. Cancer* **8,** 1–12.
21. Armitage, P. and Doll, R. (1957) A two-stage theory of carcinogenesis in relation to the age distribution of human cancer. *Br. J. Cancer* **9,** 161–169.
22. Moolgavkar, S. and Knudson, A. Jr. (1981) Mutation and cancer: a model for human carcinogenesis. *J. Natl. Cancer Inst.* **66,** 1037–1052.

23. Moolgavkar, S. and Luebeck, E. (1992) Multistage carcinogenesis: population-based model for colon cancer. *J. Natl. Cancer Inst.* **84,** 610–618.
24. Herrero-Jimenez, P., Thilly, G., Southam, P., et al. (1998) Mutation, cell kinetics, and subpopulations at risk for colon cancer in the United States. *Mut. Res.* **400,** 553–578.
25. Herrero-Jimenez, P., Tomita-Mitchell, A., Furth, E., Morgenthaler, S., and Thilly, W. (2000) Population risk and physiological rate parameters for colon cancer. The union of an explicit model for carcinogenesis with the public health records of the United States. *Mut. Res.* **447,** 73–116.
26. Loeb, L. (2001) A mutator phenotype in cancer. *Cancer Res.* **61,** 3230–3239.
27. Hemminki, K. and Mutanen, P. (2001) Genetic epidemiology of multistage carcinogenesis. *Mut. Res.* **473,** 11–21.
28. Sham, P. (1998) *Statistics in Human Genetics.* Wiley, New York.
29. Aitken, J., Baailey-Wilson, J., Green, A., MacLennen, R., and Martin, N. (1998) Segregation analysis of cutaneous melanoma in Queensland. *Genet. Epidemiol.* **15,** 391–401.
30. Pharoah, P. D., Antoniou, A., Bobrow, M., Zimmern, R. L., Easton, D. F., and Ponder, B. A. (2002) Polygenic susceptibility to breast cancer and implications for prevention. *Nat. Genet.* **31,** 33–36.
31. Vogel, F. and Motulsky, A. (1996) *Human Genetics: Problems and Approaches.* Springer, Heidelberg, Germany.
32. Hemminki, K. (2001) Genetic epidemiology: science and ethics on familial cancers. *Acta Oncol.* **40,** 439–444.
33. Dong, C. and Hemminki, K. (2001) Multiple primary cancers at colon, breast and skin (melanoma) as models for polygenic cancers. *Int. J. Cancer* **92,** 883–887.
34. Lynch, H., Fusaro, R., and Lynch, J. (1995) Hereditary cancer in adults. *Cancer Detect. Prev.* **19,** 219–233.
35. Hemminki, A., Markie, D., Tomlinson, I., et al. (1998) A serine/threonine kinase gene defective in Peutz-Jeghers syndrome. *Nature* **391,** 184–187.
36. Tomlinson, I. P., Alam, N. A., Rowan, A. J., et al. (2002) Germline mutations in *FH* predispose to dominantly inherited uterine fibroids, skin leiomyomata and papillary renal cell cancer. *Nat. Genet.* **30,** 406–410.
37. Astuti, D., Latif, F., Dallol, A., et al. (2001) Gene mutations in the succinate dehydrogenase subunit *SDHB* cause susceptibility to familial pheochromocytoma and to familial paraganglioma. *Am. J. Hum. Genet.* **69,** 49–54.
38. Mulvihill, J., Davis, S., and Fromkin, K. (1996) The catalog of human genes predisposing to neoplasia. In *Familial Cancer Management* (Weber, W., Narid, S., and Mulvihill, J., eds.), CRC Press, Boca Raton, FL, pp. 203–237.
39. Vogelstein, B. and Kinzler, K. W. (eds.). (1998) *The Genetic Basis of Human Cancer.* McGraw-Hill, New York, 1998.
40. Lynch, H. and Smyrk, T. (1996) Hereditary nonpolyposis colorectal cancer (Lynch syndrome). *Cancer* **78,** 1149–1167.
41. Li, F. (1995) Phenotypes, genotypes, and interventions for hereditary cancers. *Cancer Epidemiol. Biomarkers Prev.* **4,** 579–582.
42. Malkin, D. (1998) The Li-Fraumeni syndrome. In *The Genetic Basis of Human Cancer* (Vogelstein, B. and Kinzler, K., eds.), McGraw-Hill, New York, pp. 393–407.
43. Hemminki, K., Vaittinen, P., and Dong, C. (1999) Endometrial cancer in the Family-Cancer Database. *Cancer Epidemiol. Biomarkers Prev.* **8,** 1005–1010.
44. Hemminki, K. and Dong, C. (2000) Familial relationships in thyroid cancer by histopathological type. *Int. J. Cancer* **85,** 201–205.
45. Gatti, R. (1998) Ataxia-telangiectasia. In *The Genetic Basis of Human Cancer* (Vogelstein, B. and Kinzler, K., eds.), McGraw-Hill, New York, pp. 275–300.
46. Broeks, A., Urbanus, J., Floore, A., et al. (2000) ATM-heterozygous germline mutations contribute to breast cancer-susceptibility. *Am. J. Hum. Genet.* **66,** 494–500.
47. Olsen, J., Hahnemann, J., Börresen-Dale, A.-L., et al. (2001) Cancer in patients with ataxia-telangiectasia and in their relatives in the Nordic countries. *J. Natl. Cancer Inst.* **93,** 121–127.
48. German, J. and Ellis, N. (1998) Bloom syndrome. In *The Genetic Basis of Human Cancer* (Vogelstein, B. and Kinzzler, K., eds.), McGraw-Hill, New York, pp. 301–315.
49. Dunning, A., Healy, C., Pharoah, P., Teare, D., Ponder, B., and Easton, D. (1999) A systematic review of genetic polymorphisms and breast cancer risk. *Cancer Epidemiol. Biomarkers Prev.* **8,** 843–854.
50. Berwick, M. and Vineis, P. (2000) Markers of DNA repair and susceptibility to cancer in humans: an epidemiological review. *J. Natl. Cancer Inst.* **92,** 874–897.
51. Garte, S., Gaspari, L., Alexandrie, A. K., et al. (2001) Metabolic gene polymorphism frequencies in control populations. *Cancer Epidemiol. Biomarkers Prev.* **10,** 1239–1248.
52. Ioannidis, J. P., Ntzani, E. E., Trikalinos, T. A., and Contopoulos-Ioannidis, D. G. (2001) Replication validity of genetic association studies. *Nat. Genet.* **29,** 306–309.
53. Birkeland, S., Storm, H., Lamm, L., et al. (1995) Cancer risk after renal transplantation in the Nordic countries, 1964–1986. *Int. J. Cancer* **60,** 183–189.
54. IARC. (1996) *IARC Monographs on the Evaluation of Carcinogenic Risks to Humans.* IARC, Lyon, France.
55. Hemminki, K., Dong, C., and Vaittinen, P. (1999) Familial risks in cervix cancer: is there a hereditary component? *Int. J. Cancer* **82,** 775–781.

56. Hemminki, K. and Vaittinen, P. (1998) Familial risks in in situ cancers from the Family-Cancer Database. *Cancer Epidemiol. Biomarkers Prev.* **7,** 865–868.
57. IARC. (1995) *Human Papillomaviruses.* IARC, Lyon, France.
58. IARC. (1997) IARC Monographs on the Evaluation of Carcinogenic Risks to Humans. Epstein-Barr Virus and Kaposi's Sarcoma. Herpesvirus/Human Herpesvirus 8. IARC, Lyon, France.
59. Dong, C. and Hemminki, K. (2001) Second primary neoplasms in 633,964 cancer patients in Sweden, 1958–1996. *Int. J. Cancer* **93,** 155–161.
60. Hemminki, K. and Boffetta, P. (2004) Multiple primary cancers as clues of environmental and heritable causes of cancer and of mechanisms of carcinogenesis. *IARC Sci.* **157,** 289–297.
61. Doll, R. and Peto, R. (1981) The causes of cancer. *J. Natl. Cancer Inst.* **66,** 1191–1309.
62. Risch, N. and Merikangas, K. (1996) The future of genetic studies of complex diseases. *Science* **273,** 1516–1517.
63. Easton, D. (1999) How many more breast cancer predisposition genes are there? *Breast Cancer Res.* **1,** 14–17.
64. Reich, D. E. and Lander, E. S. (2001) On the allelic spectrum of human disease. *Trends Genet.* **17,** 502–510.

3

Tumor Suppressor Gene Replacement for Cancer

Jack A. Roth and Susan F. Grammer

1. INTRODUCTION

Long before the genetic basis of cancer was accepted and over half a century before the term tumor suppressor gene (TSG) was coined, German biologist Theodor Boveri *(1)* suggested "the presence of definite chromosomes which inhibit division." Writing in 1914 (translation published in 1929), Boveri ventured that "cells of tumors with unlimited growth would arise if those 'inhibiting chromosomes' were eliminated." Over half a century later, molecular analysis of human tumors revealed that, in every case of cancer, at least one of the multiple genetic alterations found is in an "inhibiting chromosome," now known as a TSG. During the 1980s, molecular biology and cancer genetics (*see* Chapters 1 and 2) transformed Boveri's theoretical inhibiting chromosomes into powerful tools for the study of the molecular pathogenesis of cancer and then, during the 1990s, propelled them from the laboratory bench to the bedside. Between 1994 and the end of 2002, more than 25 clinical trials for TSG replacement therapy were initiated, and results indicated a promising future for TSG in the management of cancer.

Because the base of knowledge of human TSG is expanding so rapidly, this chapter includes only a superficial summary of TSG biology and provides direction to several excellent reviews for additional details. Likewise, data from preclinical studies and clinical trials accumulate daily, so discussion of the development of gene therapy strategies for TSG replacement for the most part is limited to a synopsis of the application of gene therapy to one of the most commonly altered TSGs, *p53*.

2. TUMOR SUPPRESSOR GENES: FROM THE LABORATORY BENCH TO THE BEDSIDE

Once the rapidly advancing fields of molecular biology and genetics provided tools to tease apart the inner workings of normal and malignant cells, an intricate web of biochemical pathways began to emerge. The laborious process of untangling that web involved piecing together bits of information gleaned from various lines of inquiry, a process that at times seemed unlikely to yield definitive answers to questions about the biochemistry of cancer. Watson summarized a 1977 textbook chapter on control of cell proliferation with a mix of optimism and skepticism *(2)*:

> The fact that some reproducible differences are at last beginning to be seen between normal and cancer cells tells us that the study of cancer at the molecular level is no longer a premature Don Quixotic science. ...On the other hand, we must not deceive ourselves that, because we can measure the amount of cAMP and, if we are more clever, that of cGMP, we are in any sense close to being on top of the cancer problem ... much cancer research will continue to resemble a search for a coin lost along a path only occasionally illuminated by street lights. Of necessity we look under the lighted regions for, no matter how long you look into the dark, the search will never be successful. Thus, as long as most components of the normal cell membrane remain essentially black boxes, the biochemistry of cancer may remain a mystery for some still future generation to understand.

From: *Contemporary Cancer Research*
Cancer Gene Therapy
Edited by: D. T. Curiel and J. T. Douglas © Humana Press Inc., Totowa, NJ

Just a few years later, refined techniques for manipulating biological molecules shed additional light on those black boxes, gradually revealing detailed biochemical information about the web of pathways governing cellular processes and revealing that many genes involved in regulation of normal cellular processes of growth (cell division, differentiation, and cell death) were altered in tumor cells.

The ability to compare normal and malignant cells at the gene level quickly led to the implication of dominant oncogenes in the etiology of cancer, but information on members of the TSG family was more elusive *(3)*. Although biological evidence for the existence of genes that suppressed tumorigenesis had emerged from several lines of inquiry in the 1970s and 1980s *(4–7)*, the study of TSG biology and biochemistry at the molecular level required more advanced strategies than did the study of oncogene biology, and elucidation of the role of TSGs in normal cell processes and in cancer lagged behind. During the 1990s, though, loss of function of several TSGs was found to be common in many different cancers, answering questions about the molecular pathogenesis of cancer and leading to the current genetic paradigm: Cancer results from multiple genetic lesions accumulating over the lifetime of an individual. Loss of function of TSGs predisposes to cancer, either "familial cancer," in which one altered allele is inherited as a germline mutation and the other is acquired later, or "sporadic cancer," which occurs as a result of somatic mutation of both alleles of a critical gene during the lifetime of the individual.

Despite confirmation of the genetic basis of tumorigenesis, gene replacement therapy was not initially considered a likely strategy for cancer treatment. Because multiple genetic lesions result in unique genetic profiles in nearly every tumor, the possibility of finding one gene that would have an impact on a large subset of tumors seemed unlikely. Even after lesions in some TSGs, such as *p53*, were shown to be common to many different types of tumors, the possibility that correcting only one of the multiple lesions in a tumor would cause tumor regression also seemed improbable. Studies of TSG replacement in cell lines and in laboratory animals in the late 1980s and early 1990s, however, proved these suspicions false, and three clinical trials of *p53* gene replacement in colon and lung cancer were initiated in 1994. By late 2002, 25 protocols for TSG replacement had been approved, including seven phase II trials and two multisite phase II–III trials.

Results of early clinical trials quickly delivered "proof of principle" by demonstrating delivery of TSG to tumor cells, gene expression in targeted cells, minimal toxic effects, and finally evidence of regression or stabilization of treated tumors. Subsequent trials demonstrated that TSG replacement also rendered some tumor cells more sensitive to the effects of conventional deoxyribonucleic acid (DNA)-damaging therapies, extending the potential application of TSG replacement to protocols combining TSG replacement therapy with chemotherapy and radiation.

As these promising results were emerging in the clinic, work at the laboratory bench did not slow, and results of laboratory studies aimed at uncovering new TSGs suggested that damage to TSGs occurs relatively early in the sequence of genetic lesions that lead to cancer *(8–11)*. Damage to candidate TSGs was detected in normal lung epithelium and in preneoplastic lesions, suggesting that TSGs, in addition to offering therapeutic benefit to cancer patients, may also hold possibilities for prevention and early detection of cancer.

3. BIOLOGY AND BIOCHEMISTRY OF TSGs

In normal cells, the function of genes of the TSG family is to maintain appropriate cell numbers through inhibition of proliferation, induction of apoptosis, or detection and repair of damaged DNA. TSGs regulate signaling pathways involved in nearly every normal cell process, including cell cycle, cell death, angiogenesis, cell adhesion, and cytoskeletal and cell membrane processes. The list of genes in the TSG family is growing rapidly, so this chapter does not include an exhaustive review. Instead, the several excellent reviews *(12,13)* and a two-volume comprehensive overview of the biology of known tumor suppressor pathways *(14,15)* provide additional information.

3.1. Gatekeepers and Caretakers

As the list of TSGs grew, it became apparent that some TSGs function mainly as gatekeepers for the cell; others exhibit more caretaker-like properties *(16)* (*see* Table 1). Some TSGs, like *p53 (17)*, exhibit both gatekeeper and caretaker functions. In general, gatekeeper TSGs directly regulate cellular functions involved in cell growth, differentiation, and cell death; caretaker genes control cellular processes involved in repair of damaged genes and maintain genomic integrity.

Mutations in gatekeepers directly predispose to cancer by allowing uncontrolled proliferation and disrupting apoptosis induction; inactivation of caretaker genes leads to genetic instability, resulting in mutation of other genes, including gatekeeper TSGs. Examples of gatekeepers are *p53, p73, PTEN, Fhit* (fragile histidine triad), *Rb* (retinoblastoma), vonHippel Lindau, *APC* (adenomatous polyposis), and *NF1* (neurofibromatosis type 1). Caretaker genes include *ATM* (ataxia telangiectasia mutated), *BRCA1, BRCA2, ATR* (*ATM* and *Rad3* related), and mismatch repair genes. A brief summary of the functions of some of the TSGs most commonly altered in cancer and the diseases associated with them is included in Table 1.

TSGs that can induce apoptosis or suppress tumor cell growth, most often gatekeeper genes, have been the most attractive targets for developing gene replacement strategies thus far. Several have already been shown to induce apoptosis or cause cell cycle arrest when introduced into tumor cells, including *APC (18)*, *Rb (19,20)*, *p16 (21)*, *p21 (22)*, *E2F1 (23)*, *PTEN (24)*, *Fhit (25–27)*, *p73 (28)*, and, most notably so far, *p53 (29)*.

3.2. TSGs, Growth Arrest Pathways, and Programmed Cell Death

The myriad roles TSGs play in normal cell function cannot be detailed in this chapter; however, a brief summary focused on the role of *p53* in cellular pathways will lead to better understanding of the rationale behind *p53* gene replacement therapy and provide insight into the rationale behind replacement of other TSGs.

Expression of some gene products, including growth factors, oncogenes, cyclins, and cyclin-dependent kinases (CDKs) drive a cell toward proliferation. Expression of TSGs and other inhibitors of CDKs induces cell cycle arrest when appropriate, maintaining the cell number at an appropriate level for the particular tissue. Mammalian cell proliferation, for the most part, is regulated by two interconnected pathways, the Rb pathway and the p53 pathway, which are both in turn regulated at the protein level by oncogenes and other TSGs. In general, the Rb protein (the product of the retinoblastoma TSG) regulates maintenance of, and release from, the G1 phase, and the p53 protein monitors cellular stress and DNA damage, either effecting growth arrest and repair or inducing apoptosis *(30)*. Damage to one or more genes in either of these pathways can drive the cell to utilize an alternative pathway for regulating proliferation or, if no alternative pathway remains genetically uncompromised, begin to proliferate out of control.

When a cell is stressed by oncogene activation, hypoxia, or DNA damage, it is the task of the "guardian of the genome," *p53*, to determine whether the cell will receive a signal to halt at the G1 stage of the cell cycle, whether it will be signaled to attempt repair, or whether it will self-destruct via apoptosis. Apoptosis plays a key role in numerous normal cellular mechanisms, from embryogenesis to self-policing of DNA damage caused by random mutations, ionizing radiation, and DNA-damaging chemicals and has been implicated as a major mechanism of cell death because of DNA-damaging cancer therapies, such as chemotherapy and radiation. A precisely maintained balance between two types of signals received by a cell at any given time—proapoptotic vs prosurvival (antiapoptotic)—determines whether apoptosis will be induced.

Although these signals determine the actions of p53 protein, expression of many of the genes that generate these critical signals is in turn regulated by the activation status of *p53*, forming an elaborate feedback loop. P53 carries out housekeeping duties by targeting the prosurvival (or antiapoptotic)

Table 1
TSGs Commonly Disrupted in Cancer: Normal Function and Diseases Associated With Loss of Function

Gene	Function	Diseases associated with loss of unction
Rb (retinoblastoma)	Inhibition of transcription of genes required for DNA replication and cell division; role in apoptosis induction	Retinoblastoma, osteosarcoma, prostate cancer, breast cancer
P53	Transcription factor targeting p21, bax, PIG8, mdm2, GADD45, DR5, others; repress expression of bcl02 and PCNA; control G1 and G2 checkpoints; apoptosis induction via transcriptional activation of proapoptotic genes	*Germline inherited:* Li-Fraumeni syndrome (breast cancer, lung cancer, soft tissue tumors, brain tumors, osteosarcoma, leukemia) *Somatic mutations:* Various cancers
P16/INK4a	Gatekeeper gene; maintain normal Rb function by inhibiting CDK4 and CDK6 and promoting G1/S transition; stabilizes and activates p53 by binding mdm2	*Germline inherited:* Familial melanomas *Somatic mutation:* Pancreatic cancer, brain cancer
PTEN (also known as MMAC1 and TEP1)	Gatekeeper gene; maintains low level of PIP-3 by acting as lipid phosphatase	*Germline inherited:* Multiple benign tumors; increased susceptibility to breast, thyroid, and brain cancer *Somatic mutation:* Glioblastoma, endometrial cancer, prostate cancer, melanoma
BRCA1	Caretaker gene; expression increased in S phase of cell cycle; interacts with many proteins involved in DNA damage repair	Breast cancer and ovarian cancer
BRCA2	Caretaker gene; DNA damage repair	Breast cancer and male breast cancer
APC	Multiple cellular functions; signal transduction, intercellular adhesion, cytoskeletal stabilization, possibly cell cycle and apoptosis regulation	Hereditary and sporadic colon cancer
Neurofibromatosis type 1	Suppress cell growth by controlling wnt signaling pathway; ras signaling pathway	*Germline inherited mutation:* Benign peripheral nerve sheath tumors; predisposition to astrocytoma, glioblastoma, optic gliomas, pheochromocytomas, myeloid leukemia
FHIT	Not understood	Various primary tumors, including lung, stomach, breast, colon, cervix, head and neck; 80% of small cell lung tumors; 40% of nonsmall cell lung tumors

Source: From ref. *13.*

genes, including the proto-oncogenes *bcl-2, bcl-X2, bcl-w*, and *CED9*, and the proapoptotic genes, such as *bax, bad*, and *bid (31)*. Available transcripts of each of these genes interact with one another to form heterodimers, and the relative ratio of proapoptotic to prosurvival proteins in these heterodimers determines activity of the resulting molecule, thereby determining whether the cell lives or is directed to undergo apoptosis.

The p53 pathway is regulated at the protein level by other TSGs and by several oncogenes *(30)*. For example, mdm2 (product of the proto-oncogene *mdm2*) normally binds to the N-terminal transactivating domain of p53, prohibiting p53 activation and leading to its rapid degradation. In the event of genotoxic stress, resulting DNA damage causes phosphorylation of serines on p53, weakening binding to mdm2 and destabilizing the p53/mdm2 interaction. The resulting increase in p53 DNA-binding activity leads to an array of downstream signals that switch other genes on or off. In the normal cell, mdm2 is inhibited by proto-oncogenes that induce expression of *p19ARF*, a TSG encoded by the same gene locus as *p16INK4a*, but read in an alternate reading frame *(32)*.

Because activated p53 has a very short half-life in the cell (20 minutes), binding of mdm2 ensures tight control of a very low level of active p53 in the normal cell, thereby maintaining the required balance between proliferation and cell cycle arrest or apoptosis. Both *Rb* and *p53* are commonly altered in cancer, as are several other TSG and proto-oncogenes involved in these pathways. For example, deletion of the TSG *p19ARF* results in increased levels of mdm2 and subsequent inactivation of p53, resulting in inappropriate progression through the cell cycle.

4. TSG REPLACEMENT IN CANCER

Success of gene replacement strategies for cancer rests first on successful delivery of a therapeutic gene to the intended target tissue and then on expression of the gene at adequate levels with acceptably low toxicity. Only when these requirements are met can the desired therapeutic benefit, tumor regression, be measured. Several of the TSGs mentioned here have shown potential application in preclinical laboratory and animal studies, and several are in clinical trials. Because most clinical trials to date involve replacement of the TSG most commonly altered in cancer, *p53*, discussion of preclinical laboratory studies and subsequent clinical trials focuses on this gene. This summary of progress on *p53* gene replacement also provides insight into understanding the potential applications of other TSGs to cancer gene therapy.

4.1. TSG Replacement Therapy: The Case of p53

4.1.1. Rationale

Loss of function of *p53* is observed in over 50% of all malignant tumors, making it the most common genetic lesion in cancer. It follows, then, that insertion of a copy of a "wild-type" gene might be sufficient to restore the normal balance of cell proliferation and cell death to a tumor cell. In addition, the critical role of *p53* in the induction of programmed cell death or apoptosis indicates that replacement of this gene might restore or enhance sensitivity to therapeutic agents, such as chemotherapy and radiation therapy, that depend on DNA damage and subsequent p53-dependent apoptosis as a mechanism of tumor cell destruction.

4.1.2. Preclinical Studies of p53 Gene Replacement

Early laboratory studies in an orthotopic human lung cancer model demonstrated that the TSG *p53*, delivered via a retroviral expression vector, restored suppression of tumor growth *(33)*. Similarly, restoration of functional p53 suppressed the growth of some, but not all, human lung cancer cell lines *(34)*. Although successful gene transfer of tumor cell growth suppression was demonstrated with the retroviral expression vector, the transduction efficiency of the vector was limiting, as is generally true of retroviral vectors. Unlike retroviruses, adenoviruses can be produced at high titers and are capable of infecting both dividing and nondividing cells, so subsequent trials were carried out with adenoviral vectors. Because adenoviruses do not integrate into the genome, expression is transient, a situation not considered a disadvantage in cancer therapy as it would be in gene therapy for some diseases because destruction of cancer cells is the desired end point of therapy.

Initially, it was feared that the effectiveness of gene therapy for cancer might be limited by the inability of a vector to transduce every cell within a tumor, but Fujiwara, Cusack, and their respective colleagues *(35,36)* demonstrated in three-dimensional cancer cell matrices and subcutaneous xenografts that therapeutic genes were likely to spread beyond the immediate intratumoral injection site to nontransduced tumor cells via a "bystander effect." Bystander killing appears to involve mechanisms more elaborate than the mere spread of vector away from the injection site. Several proposed mechanisms include angiogenesis *(37,38)*, immune upregulation *(39–41)*, and secretion of soluble proapoptotic proteins *(42)*.

Transfer of *p53* into lung cancer cells by an adenoviral vector was demonstrated by Zhang and coworkers *(43)*, and in subsequent studies this gene/vector combination *(Adp53)* induced apoptosis in cancer cells with nonfunctional *p53* without significantly affecting proliferation of normal cells *(44)*. *Adp53* also inhibited tumor growth in a mouse model of human orthotopic lung cancer *(45)* and induced apoptosis and suppression of proliferation in pancreatic cancer cell lines *(46)*, colorectal cancer cell lines *(47)*, and human breast tumors *(48)*. In vivo studies of *p53* gene transfer in mouse xenograft tumor models also showed significant suppression of human tumor growth *(47,49)*. Other TSGs have also suppressed tumor growth in cell culture and in animal models.

4.1.3. Clinical Trials of p53 Gene Replacement

Early preclinical studies of retroviral p53 described in Section 4.1.2. led to approval of the first clinical trial protocol for *p53* gene-replacement. A retroviral vector expressing wild-type *p53* under control of the β-actin promoter *(50)* was introduced into tumors of nine patients with unresectable non-small cell lung cancer (NSCLC) that had already proved resistant to other interventions. No vector-related toxicity was observed, and three of the nine patients had evidence of antitumor activity, demonstrating the feasibility and safety of gene therapy *(51,52)*. For the reasons described in Section 4.1.2., further clinical trials of *p53* gene transfer utilized an adenoviral expression vector.

Twenty-eight patients with NSCLC whose cancers had not responded to conventional treatments enrolled in a phase I clinical trial; successful gene transfer was demonstrated in 80% of evaluable patients *(53)*. Vector-specific *p53* DNA was detected in 46%, and apoptosis was demonstrated in all but 1 of the patients expressing the gene. Most important, despite up to six injections per patient, no significant toxic effects related to transfer of the vector appeared. In addition, more than a 50% reduction in tumor size was observed in two patients. One patient remained free of tumor more than a year after the conclusion of therapy, and another experienced nearly complete regression of an upper lobe endobronchial tumor that had resisted chemotherapy, radiotherapy, and laser treatment.

A phase I study of 33 patients with head and neck squamous cell carcinoma also concluded that transfer of the *p53* construct caused little toxicity; again, significant clinical response was observed in 9 of 18 clinically evaluable patients *(54)*. A subsequent phase II clinical trial of *p53* in over 200 patients with recurrent or refractory head and neck squamous cell carcinoma resulted in demonstration of complete or partial responses in approx 10% of patients, with some evidence of antitumor activity observed in 60% of patients *(55,56)*.

These studies and others established *P53* gene transfer as a clinically feasible strategy resulting in successful gene transfer and expression, low toxicity, and strong indications for tumor regression. Registered clinical trials of TSG replacement, including trials involving *p53, Rb, mda7, BRCA1,* and *p16* are summarized in Table 2 *(57)*. All clinical trials involving recombinant DNA carried out at institutions receiving federal funds must be approved by the National Institutes of Health (NIH) Recombinant DNA Advisory Committee (RAC), and investigators not receiving federal funds are encouraged to register protocols as well as report adverse effects of treatment for inclusion in the NIH database.

Table 2
Clinical Trials of TSG Replacement[a]

RAC protocol	TSG/other therapeutic	Vector	Disease	Route of administration	Phase/year approved
9812-275	p53	Adenovirus serotype 5	Advanced cancers	Intravenous	I/1998
9601-195	Rb	Adenovirus serotype 5	Bladder	Intravesicular	I/1996
9710-219	P53	Adenovirus serotype 5	Bladder	Intravesicular	I/1997
9808-263	P53	Adenovirus serotype 5	Brain/glioma	Intratumoral	I/1998
9709-216	P53/chemotherapy	Adenovirus serotype 5	Breast	Intralesional	I/1997
9904-305	P53/to purge cancer cells from stem cell preparation	Stem cells	Breast	Intravenous with stem cells	I/1999
0101-455	P53/chemotherapy	Adenovirus serotype 5	Breast	Intratumoral	I/2001
0104-171	Mda7	Adenovirus serotype 5	Breast	Intratumoral	I/2001
9412-097	P53	Adenovirus serotype 5	Colon with liver metastasis	Intrahepatic/hepatic artery	I/1994
9905-318	P53/chemotherapy	Adenovirus serotype 5	Colon with liver metastasis	Intrahepatic/hepatic artery	II/1999
9403-031	P53/Ras oncogene	Adenovirus serotype 5	Lung	Intratumoral	I/1994
9406-079	P53/chemotherapy	Adenovirus serotype 5	Lung	Intratumoral	I/1994
9710-220	P53/chemotherapy	Adenovirus serotype 5	Lung (nonsmall cell)	Intratumoral	II/1997
9804-250	P53/radiotherapy	Adenovirus serotype 5	Lung (nonsmall cell)	Intratumoral	I-II/1998
9902-287	P53	Adenovirus serotype 5	Lung (bronchoalveolar)	Respiratory tract	I/1999
9902-288	P53/radiotherapy	Adenovirus serotype 5	Lung (nonsmall cell)	Intratumoral	I/1999
0101-448	P53/radiation and chemotherapy	Adenovirus serotype 5	Lung (nonsmall cell)	Intratumoral	II-III/2001
0201-513[b]	P53	Liposome gene complex	Lung (NSCLC)	Intravenous	I/2002[a]
9603-149	BRCA-1	Retrovirus	Ovarian	Intraperitoneal	I/1996
9806-255	P53	Adenovirus serotype 5	Ovarian	Intraperitoneal	I/1998
9807-262	P53	Adenovirus serotype 5	Ovarian (chemotherapy-resistant)	Intraperitoneal	I/1998
9901-280	P53/chemotherapy	Adenovirus serotype 5	Ovarian	Intraperitoneal	II-III/1999
9909-339	BRCA-1	Retrovirus	Ovarian	Intraperitoneal	I-II/1999
9706-192	P53	Adenovirus serotype 5	Prostate	Intratumoral	I/1997
9710-217	P53	Adenovirus serotype 5	Prostate	Intratumoral	I-II/1997
9909-338	P16	Adenovirus serotype 5	Prostate	Intratumoral	I/1999
	P53/radioactive seed implant	Adenovirus serotype 5	Prostate	Percutaneous/transperineal implant	II/2000
9412-096	P53	Adenovirus serotype 5	Head and neck (squamous cell)	Intratumoral	I/1994
9709-214	P53	Adenovirus serotype 5	Head and neck (squamous cell)	Intratumoral	II/1997
9712-226	P53	Adenovirus serotype 5	Head and neck (squamous cell)	Intratumoral	II/1997
9912-366	P53	Adenovirus serotype 5	Head and neck (squamous cell)	Intratumoral	III/1999
0009-412	P53/chemotherapy	Adenovirus serotype 5	Head and neck (squamous cell)	Intratumoral	III/2000
0101-445[b]	P53	Adenovirus serotype 5	Head and neck (squamous cell)	Intratumoral	I/II/2001
0101-454	P53/chemoradiotherapy	Adenovirus serotype 5	Head and neck (squamous cell)	Intratumoral	II/2001

[a]Source: Summary of protocols approved by the RAC as of December 2002 (57).
[b]Reviewed with recommendations; not open for enrollment.

4.2. p53 *Gene Replacement in Combination*
With Conventional DNA-Damaging Agents

4.2.1. Rationale for Combination Therapy

Many cancer patients fail conventional therapy because their tumors are resistant to DNA-damaging agents such as chemotherapy and radiation therapy. Once apoptosis was implicated as the normal mechanism of cell destruction in response to these DNA-damaging agents, it followed that a defect in the normal apoptotic pathway might confer resistance to some tumor cells. Often missing or nonfunctional in radiation- and chemotherapy-resistant tumors, *p53* is known to play a key role in detecting damage to DNA and directing repair or destruction through apoptosis. The link between *p53* and apoptosis made therapeutic strategies combining *p53* gene replacement and conventional DNA-damaging therapies a natural extension of earlier studies. The low toxicity (less than 5% incidence of serious adverse events) of *p53* in initial trials suggested that *p53* gene therapy could be combined with other anticancer treatments without significant increases in treatment-related toxicity *(58)*.

4.2.2. Preclinical Studies

Several in vitro studies *(59–61)* demonstrated that overexpression of *p53* in wild-type *p53* transfected cell lines could drive cells into apoptosis. Subsequent in vitro and animal studies examining apoptosis in tumor cells treated with radiation or chemotherapeutic agents also supported a link between apoptosis induction and functional p53 expression *(62–67)*.

Preclinical studies of *p53* gene therapy combined with cisplatin in cultured NSCLC cells and in human xenografts in nude mice demonstrated that sequential administration of cisplatin and *p53* gene therapy resulted in enhanced expression of the *p53* gene product *(65,68)*. Over 50% of the cells pretreated with cisplatin were apoptotic 12 hours after gene transfer, with over 90% of the cells undergoing apoptosis at 24 hours; cells not pretreated with cisplatin prior to gene transfer demonstrated only 19 and 68% apoptotic cells at 12 and 24 hours, respectively. Studies of systemic cisplatin treatment prior to *p53* gene transfer in nude mice resulted in at least a 55% further reduction in final tumor size in cisplatin-pretreated mice when compared to mice receiving only *p53* gene transfer.

Similarly, preclinical studies of *p53* gene transfer combined with radiotherapy indicated that delivery of *p53* to *p53*-deficient tumor cells, both in vitro and in vivo, increased their sensitivity to radiation *(47)*. When in vitro cultured human colorectal carcinoma cells were gamma irradiated, 55% of the tumor cells survived; transfection of the cells with *p53* prior to irradiation, however, lowered the survival rate to 23% and increased apoptosis. Significant tumor suppression was also observed in an animal tumor model when animals received *p53* followed by radiation; regrowth of tumors was delayed 2 days when tumors were treated with radiation alone and 15 days when treated with *p53* gene transfer alone, but tumors of animals receiving the *p53* gene followed by radiation treatment required 37 days to reach pretreatment size.

Numerous other studies have generated additional supporting evidence for a critical link between radiation sensitivity and the ability of a cell to induce apoptosis *(69–73)*; however, the radiosensitivity of some tumor types (e.g., epithelioid tumors) does not appear to be correlated with *p53* status *(74–76)*.

4.2.3. Clinical Trials of TSG Replacement Combined With Chemotherapy

A phase I trial of *p53* in sequence with cisplatin *(77)* enrolled 24 patients with NSCLC carcinoma previously unresponsive to conventional treatments. Of the patients, 75% entered into the trial had previously demonstrated tumor progression on cisplatin- or carboplatin-containing regimens. Up to six monthly courses of intravenous cisplatin, each followed 3 days later with intratumoral injection of *p53*, resulted in 17 patients remaining stable for at least 2 months, 2 patients achieving partial responses, and 4 patients continuing to exhibit progressive disease (1 patient was unevaluable because of progressive disease). Analysis of apoptotic activity in tumor biopsies resulted in 79% showing an increase in number of apoptotic cells, 14% indicating no change, and 7% demonstrating a decrease in apoptosis.

A phase II study evaluated two comparable lesions in each enrolled patient with metastatic NSCLC *(78)*. All patients received chemotherapy, either three cycles of carboplatin plus paclitaxel or three cycles of cisplatin plus vinorelbine. *P53* was injected directly into one lesion; the other lesion was used as a control and was not injected. The goal of the study was to demonstrate enhanced radiologic response in the injected lesion compared to the noninjected lesion. *P53* treatment resulted in minimal vector-related toxicity and no increase in chemotherapy-related adverse events. Statistical analysis of the combined data indicated that *p53* did not provide additional benefit to patients receiving an effective first-line chemotherapy. Examination of results with the less-successful cisplatin and vinorelbine regimen only, however, indicated that mean local tumor regression as measured by size was significantly greater in the *p53*-injected lesion as compared to the control lesion.

A phase I/II clinical study by Buller and coworkers of patients with recurrent ovarian cancer demonstrated safety and tolerability of single-dose and multiple-dose intraperitoneal *p53* in combination with platinum-based chemotherapy *(79)*. A long-term follow-up study of these patients indicated that individuals who received multiple-dose *p53* with chemotherapy had a median survival of 12–13 months, compared to only 5 months for those treated with a single dose of *p53 (80)*. More than 20 months after multiple-dose treatment for recurrent disease, there were 10 long-term survivors, but only 2 patients receiving a single dose of *p53* were long-term survivors.

4.2.4. Clinical Trials of TSG Replacement Combined With Radiation Therapy

Successful preclinical studies suggesting that *p53* gene replacement might confer radiation sensitivity to some tumors *(47,69,71–73)* led to the initiation of a phase II clinical trial of adenoviral-mediated *p53* gene transfer in conjunction with radiation therapy *(81)*. Preliminary data from 19 patients with localized NSCLC revealed a complete response in 1 patient (5%), partial response in 11 patients (58%), stable disease in 3 patients (16%), and progressive disease in 2 patients (11%). Two patients (11%) were nonevaluable because of tumor progression or early death. Three months following completion of therapy, biopsies revealed no viable tumor in 12 patients (63%) and viable tumor in 3 patients (16%). Tumors of 4 patients (21%) were not biopsied because of tumor progression, early death, or weakness. The 1-year progression-free survival rate was 45.5%. Among 13 evaluable patients, 5 (38%) had a complete response, and 3 (23%) had a partial response or disease stabilization. Most of the treatment failures were caused by metastatic disease, but not by local progression.

5. FUTURE DIRECTIONS

Although these early trials of TSG replacement clearly demonstrated proof of principle, TSG therapy is not widely applicable in its current form. TSGs can currently be delivered only to tumors accessible via needle or endoscope, making improvement in gene delivery systems a critical area for future development. In addition, strategies to take advantage of bystander effects are under development, and combination of TSG therapy with transfer of genes aimed at blocking angiogenesis or enhancing the immune system are also on the horizon. Continued exploration of TSG replacement as an adjuvant to conventional chemotherapy, radiation therapy, and surgery continues to look positive.

5.1. Bystander Effect

"Bystander killing" of nontransduced tumor cells is considered an important factor in the success of gene replacement therapy thus far, and strategies to enhance this effect are under investigation. Suggested mechanisms of bystander killing include inhibition of angiogenesis *(37,38,82)*, upregulation of various immune system components *(39–41)*, and secretion of soluble proapoptotic proteins *(42)*.

5.2. Vector Development

Promising approaches to gene therapy used to date in clinical studies have utilized retroviral, adenoviral, and herpes vectors for intratumoral gene delivery, but the larger problem in cancer is treatment of disseminated disease of the lung, breast, and colon, requiring systemic administration of genes. Viral vectors present real and theoretical problems because of induction of immune responses and related toxicity. Preliminary studies suggested that extruded liposomes can efficiently deliver genes systemically to distant sites with acceptable vector-associated toxicity *(83)*; in further studies of these liposomes, two TSGs (*p53* and *Fhit*) were delivered to tumor cells in vitro and in animal models of murine and human disseminated lung tumors *(84)*. Transgene expression was observed in 25% of the cells in each tumor, and significant suppression was seen in both primary and metastatic lung disease. Repeated treatments resulted in a 2.5-fold increase in gene expression and an increase in therapeutic efficacy compared to single treatments. The study demonstrated that liposome-mediated delivery of at least two TSGs can suppress tumor growth in vivo when administered either systemically or locally, that there were no toxic effects associated with this treatment, and that the delivery system was not restricted by gene or tumor type. In addition, the results demonstrated the potential for multiple treatments without development of resistance.

5.3. Tissue Targeting

Other approaches to extending the application of gene therapy beyond the reach of needles and endoscopes have involved attempts to target recombinant adenoviral vectors to specific types of cells by manipulating cell surface-binding properties of the viral particle. Bifunctional fusion proteins consisting of an antibody fragment specific to the fiber protein of the virus and a ligand, epidermal growth factor *(85)*, were constructed; addition of fusion proteins to the adenovirus enhanced the transduction efficiency of an epidermoid carcinoma cell line 16-fold compared with infection with native adenovirus vector.

Another approach to targeting genes directly to endothelial cells involved a cell surface molecule, the integrin $\alpha v\beta 3$, which potentiates internalization of adenoviruses. A cationic nanoparticle coupled to an integrin-targeting ligand was able to deliver genes selectively to angiogenic blood vessels in tumor-bearing mice *(86)*.

5.4. TSG Replacement Combined With Other Gene Therapy Strategies

Complementary TSGs, delivered together, might cooperate to induce apoptosis more efficiently. Introduction of the TSGs *p16INK4* and *p53* in combination resulted in a synergistic effect on the induction of apoptosis in hepatocellular carcinoma cells (mutated *p53*) and colon carcinoma cells (very low expression of *p53*) in vitro. Delivery of TSG in combination with various oncogenes is also under evaluation.

5.5. Identification of New TSGs

Methods for screening large portions of the genome for candidate TSGs have revealed numerous genes potentially useful as prognostic or early diagnostic indicators, in monitoring of prevention efforts and in development of novel therapeutic strategies *(87–89)*. Multiple contiguous genes that may exhibit tumor suppressor activity in vitro and in vivo were identified, and it has been proposed that the genes in a particular 120-kb region of the human chromosome 3p21.3 may cooperate as a "tumor suppressor region" by functional activation of tumor suppressor pathways *(89)*.

6. BEYOND CLINICAL TRIALS: GENE REPLACEMENT THERAPY AS A STANDARD OF CARE?

TSG replacement therapy is rapidly becoming a reality with the potential to impact the general population in the foreseeable future. It seems, therefore, a critical time to address societal issues that can have an impact on successful application of gene therapy. Manipulation of DNA in the last decade has raised new and complex scientific, medical, ethical, and social issues that must be addressed as carefully and completely as the basic science and technical questions if gene therapy is to take its place as the standard of care for cancer. Gene therapy technologies, no matter how flawless, will be of little use to a public which does not understand, and is therefore not willing to accept, its benefits.

The path to acceptance of this new and sometimes intimidating technology by society may have as many obstacles to overcome as did the scientific development of the strategy. The aura of discomfort surrounding all types of gene manipulation, even those not involving transfer of genes to humans, is likely to linger until medical science can assure the public that gene therapy will be safe and responsibly applied. Release of accurate information (both positive and negative) from clinical trials and honest discussion of the limitations—as well as the promises—of gene therapy are critical. In the United States, an official step to further this communication was taken in 1974 when the NIH RAC was formed in answer to public concerns about the safety of gene manipulation. All recombinant DNA clinical protocols carried out in federally funded institutions must be submitted to the RAC for approval. Reports of adverse side effects must also be submitted and are accessible to researchers, physicians, and the public *(90)*.

Use of this information, as well as acceptance of evidence from clinical trials, requires a basic understanding of the concepts of molecular biology, something that many potential patients do not have. Soon, this understanding will be critical for patients and their families to make informed decisions at the time of cancer diagnosis. Education can empower individuals to appreciate the potential impact of cancer gene therapy on quality of life for all health care consumers and is critical to facilitate the exchange of ideas among the public, the medical community, and governing bodies as they work together to decide how best to develop gene therapy technology in an ethical and responsible manner.

7. SUMMARY

Although initial predictions about potential application of TSG therapy to cancer were less than optimistic, virus-assisted gene transfer has been shown to be even more efficient in cancer cells than in normal tissue cells, and viral vectors appear to spread readily through a tumor and to cause cell death via apoptosis. Postinjection gene expression can be documented and occurs even in the presence of an antiadenovirus immune response. Clinical trials of *p53* gene replacement have demonstrated that direct intratumor injection can cause tumor regression or prolonged stabilization of local disease, and the low toxicity associated with gene transfer indicates that TSG replacement can be readily combined with existing and future treatments. Initial concerns that the wide diversity of genetic lesions in cancer cells would prevent the application of gene therapy to cancer appear unfounded; on the contrary, correction of a single genetic lesion has, repeatedly, yielded significant tumor regression, and successful early clinical trials of *p53* gene replacement provided information that will be useful in the design of future gene therapy strategies.

In spite of the obvious promise evident in the results of the clinical trials of TSG gene transfer, it is critical to recognize that there are still gaps in knowledge and technology that must be filled before the most finely tuned gene therapy strategies can emerge. Unresectable tumors are a prominent problem in oncology, with proven therapies such as radiotherapy and chemotherapy controlling less than 50% of lung cancers. Although technical limitations currently prevent the widespread application of gene therapy to cancer, development of more efficient vectors, novel genes, and combined modality approaches are on the horizon and promise to widen the applicability of gene therapy to disseminated cancer. Many studies suggest great potential for combining TSG therapy with pharmaceutical, immunological, and radiotherapeutic approaches to kill cells more effectively and in greater numbers. TSG replacement therapy targets the etiology of the disease, so may even lead to potentially viable strategies for cancer prevention.

ACKNOWLEDGMENTS

This work was partially supported by grants from the National Cancer Institute and the NIH (PO1 CA7877-01A1) and SPORE (2P50-CA70970-04); by gifts to the Division of Surgery from Tenneco and Exxon for the Core Laboratory Facility; by the University of Texas M. D. Anderson Cancer Center Support Core Grant (CA 16672); by a grant from the Tobacco Settlement Funds as appropriated by the Texas State Legislature (Project 8), the W. M. Keck Foundation, and a sponsored research agreement with Introgen Therapeutics Inc. (SR93-004-1).

REFERENCES

1. Boveri, T. (1929) *The Origin of Malignant Tumors.* Williams and Wilkins, Baltimore, MD.
2. Watson, J. D. (1977) The awful incompleteness of eucaryotic cell biochemistry. In *Molecular Biology of the Gene* (Watson, J. D., ed.), W. A. Benjamin, Reading, PA, p. 584–585.
3. Bishop, J. M. (1991) Molecular themes in oncogenesis. *Cell* **64,** 235–248.
4. Sager, R. (1989) Tumor suppressor genes: the puzzle and the promise. *Science* **246,** 1406–1412.
5. Knudson, A. G. Jr. (1971) Mutation and cancer: statistical study of retinoblastoma. *Proc. Natl. Acad. Sci. USA* **68,** 820–823.
6. Marshall, C. J. (1991) How does p21-ras transform cells? *Trends Genet.* **7,** 91–95.
7. Weinberg, R. A. (1991) Tumor suppressor genes. *Science* **254,** 1138–1146.
8. Ji, L., Nishizaki, M., Gao, B., et al. (2002) Expression of several genes in the human chromosome 3p21.3 homozygous deletion region exhibit tumor suppressor activities in vitro and in vivo. *Cancer Res.* **62,** 2715–2720.
9. Park, I. W., Wistuba, I. I., Maitra, et al. (1999) Multiple clonal abnormalities in the bronchial epithelium of patients with lung cancer. *J. Natl. Cancer Inst.* **91,** 1863–1868.
10. Wistuba, I. I., Behrens, C., Virmani, A. K., et al. (2000) High resolution chromosome 3p allelotyping of human lung cancer and preneoplastic/preinvasive bronchial epithelium reveals multiple, discontinuous sites of 3p allele loss and three regions of frequent breakpoints. *Cancer Res.* **60,** 1949–1960.
11. Wistuba, I. I., Berry, J., Behrens, C., et al. (2000) Molecular changes in the bronchial epithelium of patients with small cell lung cancer. *Clin. Cancer Res.* **6,** 2604–2610.
12. Levine, A. J. (1997) p53, the cellular gatekeeper for growth and division. *Cell* **88,** 323–331.
13. Hakem, R. and Mak, T. W. (2001) Animal models of tumor-suppressor genes. *Annu. Rev. Genet.* **2001,** 209–241.
14. El-Deiry, W. (2003) *Tumor Suppressor Genes, Volume 1, Pathways and Isolation Strategies.* Humana Press, Totowa, NJ.
15. El-Deiry, W. (2003) *Tumor Suppressor Genes, Volume 2, Regulation, Function and Medicinal Applications.* Humana Press, Totowa, NJ.
16. Kinzler, K. W. and Vogelstein, B. (1997) Gatekeepers and caretakers. *Nature* **386,** 761–763.
17. Vogelstein, B., Lane, D., and Levine, A. J. (2000) Surfing the p53 network. *Nature* **408,** 307–310.
18. Morin, P. J., Vogelstein, B., and Kinzler, K. W. (1996) Apoptosis and APC in colorectal tumorigenesis. *Proc. Natl. Acad. Sci. USA* **93,** 7950–7954.
19. Nikitin, A. Y., Juarez-Perez, M. I., Li, S., Huang, L., and Lee, W. H. (1999) RB-mediated suppression of spontaneous multiple neuroendocrine neoplasia and lung metastases in Rb+/− mice. *Proc. Natl. Acad. Sci. USA* **96,** 3916–3921.
20. Demers, G. W., Harris, M. P., Wen, S. F., Engler, H., Nielsen, L. L., and Maneval, D. C. (1998) A recombinant adenoviral vector expressing full-length human retinoblastoma susceptibility gene inhibits human tumor cell growth. *Cancer Gene Ther.* **5,** 207–214.
21. Sandig, V., Brand, K., Herwig, S., Lukas, J., Bartek, J., and Strauss, M. (1997) Adenovirally transferred p16(INK4/CDKN2) and p53 genes cooperate to induce apoptotic tumor cell death. *Nat. Med.* **3,** 313–319.
22. Tsao Y. P., Huang, S., Chang, J., Hsieh, J. T., Pong, R. C., and Chen, S. (1999) Adenovirus-mediated p21 (WAF1/SDII/CIP1) gene transfer induces apoptosis of human cervical cancer cell line. *J. Virol.* **73,** 4983–4990.
23. Dong, Y., Yang, H., Elliott, M., and McMasters, K. M. (2002) Adenovirus-mediated E2F-1 gene transfer sensitizes melanoma cells to apoptosis induced by topoisomerase II inhibitors. *Cancer Res.* **62,** 1776–1783.
24. Tanaka, M., Koul, D., Davies, M., Liebert, M., Steck, P. A., and Grossman, H. B. (2000) MMAC1/PTEN inhibits cell growth and induces chemosensitivity to doxorubicin in human bladder cancer cells. *Oncogene* **19,** 5406–5412.
25. Dumon, K., Ishii, H., Vecchione, A., et al. (2001) Fragile histidine triad expression delays tumor development and induces apoptosis in human pancreatic cancer. *Cancer Res.* **6,** 4827–4836.
26. Ji, L., Fang, B., Yen, N., Fong, K., Minna, J. D., and Roth, J. A. (1999) Induction of apoptosis and inhibition of tumorigenicity and tumor growth by adenovirus vector-mediated fragile histidine triad (FHIT) gene overexpression. *Cancer Res.* **59,** 3333–3339.
27. Dumon, K. R., Ishii, H., Fong, L., et al. (2001) FHIT gene therapy prevents tumor development in Fhit-deficient mice. *Proc. Natl. Acad. Sci. USA* **98,** 3346–3351.

28. Sasaki, Y., Morimoto, I., Ishida, S., Yamashita, T., Imai, K., and Tokino, T. (2001) Adenovirus-mediated transfer of the p53 family genes, p73 and p51/p63 induces cell cycle arrest and apoptosis in colorectal cancer cell lines: potential application to gene therapy of colorectal cancer. *Gene Ther.* **8,** 1401–1408.

29. Spitz, F. R., Nguyen, D., Skibber, J. M., Meyn, R. E., Cristiano, R. J., and Roth, J. A. (1996) Adenoviral-mediated wild-type p53 gene expression sensitizes colorectal cancer cells to ionizing radiation. *Clin. Cancer Res.* **2,** 1665–1671.

30. Burns, T. and El-Deiry, W. (1999) The p53 pathway and apoptosis. *J. Cell. Physiol.* **181,** 231–239.

31. Adams, J. M. and Cory, S. (1998) The Bcl-2 protein family: arbiters of cell survival. *Science* **281,** 1322–1326.

32. Kamijo, T., Zindy, F., Roussel, M. F., et al. (1997) Tumor suppression at the mouse INK4a locus mediated by the alternative reading frame product p19ARF. *Cell* **91,** 649–659.

33. Fujiwara, T., Cai, D. W., Georges, R. N., Mukhopadhyay, T., Grimm, E. A., and Roth, J. A. (1994) Therapeutic effect of a retroviral wild-type p53 expression vector in an orthotopic lung cancer model. *J. Natl. Cancer Inst.* **86,** 1458–1462.

34. Cai, D. W., Mukhopadhyay, T., and Roth, J. A. (1993) *A Novel Ribozyme for Modification of Mutated p53 Pre-mRNA in Non-small Cell Lung Cancer Cell Lines.* Third Antisense Workshop presented Nov. 13, 1993.

35. Fujiwara, T., Grimm, E. A., Mukhopadhyay, T., Cai, D. W., Owen-Schaub, L. B., and Roth, J. A. (1993) A retroviral wild-type p53 expression vector penetrates human lung cancer spheroids and inhibits growth by inducing apoptosis. *Cancer Res.* **53,** 4129–4133.

36. Cusack, J. C., Spitz, F. R., Nguyen, D., Zhang, W. W., Cristiano, R. J., and Roth, J. A. (1996) High levels of gene transduction in human lung tumors following intralesional injection of recombinant adenovirus. *Cancer Gene Ther.* **3,** 245–249.

37. Miyashita, T. and Reed, J. C. (1995) Tumor suppressor p53 is a direct transcriptional activator of human bax gene. *Cell* **80,** 293–299.

38. Dameron, K. M., Volpert, O. V., Tainsky, M. A., and Bouck, N. (1994) Control of angiogenesis in fibroblasts by p53 regulation of thrombospondin-1. *Science* **265,** 1582–1584.

39. Molinier-Frenkel, V., Le Boulaire, C., Le Gal, F. A., et al. (2000) Longitudinal follow-up of cellular and humoral immunity induced by recombinant adenovirus-mediated gene therapy in cancer patients. *Human Gene Ther.* **11,** 1911–1920.

40. Yen, N., Ioannides, C. G., Xu, K., et al. (2000) Cellular and humoral immune responses to adenovirus and p53 protein antigens in patients following intratumor injection of an adenovirus vector expressing wild-type p53 (Ad-p53) *Cancer Gene Ther.* **7,** 530–536.

41. Carroll, J. L., Nielsen, L. L., Pruett, S. B., and Mathis, J. M. (2001) The role of natural killer cells in adenovirus-mediated p53 gene therapy. *Mol. Cancer Ther.* **1,** 49–60.

42. Owen-Schaub, L. B., Zhang, W., Cusack, J. C., et al. (1995) Wild-type human p53 and a temperature-sensitive mutant induce Fas/APO-1 expression. *Mol. Cell. Biol.* **15,** 3032–3040.

43. Zhang, W. W., Fang, X., Mazur, W., French, B. A., Georges, R. N., and Roth, J. A. (1994) High-efficiency gene transfer and high-level expression of wild-type p53 in human lung cancer cells mediated by recombinant adenovirus. *Cancer Gene Ther.* **1,** 5–13.

44. Wang, J., Bucana, C. D., Roth, J. A., and Zhang, W. W. (1995) Apoptosis induced in human osteosarcoma cells is one of the mechanisms for the cytocidal effect of Ad5CMV-p53. *Cancer Gene Ther.* **2,** 9–17.

45. Georges, R. N., Mukhopadhyay, T., Zhang, Y., Yen, N., and Roth, J. A. (1993) Prevention of orthotopic human lung cancer growth by intratracheal instillation of a retroviral antisense K-ras construct. *Cancer Res.* **53,** 1743–1746.

46. Bouvet, M., Fang, B., Ekmekcioglu, S., et al. (1998) Suppression of the immune response to an adenovirus vector and enhancement of intratumoral transgene expression by low-dose etoposide. *Gene Ther.* **5,** 189–195.

47. Spitz, F. R., Nguyen, D., Skibber, J., Meyn, R., Cristiano, R. J., and Roth, J. A. (1996) Adenoviral mediated p53 gene therapy enhances radiation sensitivity of colorectal cancer cell lines. *Proc. Am. Assoc. Cancer Res.* **37,** 347.

48. Xu, M., Kumar, D., Srinivas, S., et al. (1997) Parenteral gene therapy with p53 inhibits human breast tumors in vivo through a bystander mechanism without evidence of toxicity. *Hum. Gene Ther.* **8,** 177–185.

49. Nielsen, L. L., Dell, J., Maxwell, E., Armstrong, L., Maneval, D., and Catino, J. J. (1997) Efficacy of p53 adenovirus-mediated gene therapy against human breast cancer xenografts. *Cancer Gene Ther.* **4,** 129–138.

50. Roth, J. A., Nguyen, D., Lawrence, D. D., et al. (1996) Retrovirus-mediated wild-type p53 gene transfer to tumors of patients with lung cancer. *Nat. Med.* **2,** 985–991.

51. Roth, J. A. (1996) Clinical protocol: modification of mutant K-ras gene expression in non-small cell lung cancer (NSCLC). *Hum. Gene Ther.* **7,** 875–889.

52. Roth, J. A. (1996) Clinical protocol: modification of tumor suppressor gene expression and induction of apoptosis in non-small cell lung cancer (NSCLC) with an adenovirus vector expressing wildtype p53 and cisplatin. *Hum. Gene Ther.* **7,** 1013–1030.

53. Swisher, S. G., Roth, J. A., Nemunaitis, J., et al. (1999) Adenovirus-mediated p53 gene transfer in advanced non-small cell lung cancer. *J. Natl. Cancer Inst.* **91,** 763–771.

54. Clayman, G. L., El-Naggar, A. K., Lippman, S. M., et al. (1998) Adenovirus-mediated p53 gene transfer in patients with advanced recurrent head and neck squamous cell carcinoma. *New Frontiers Res. Treat. Aerodigestive Tract Cancers* **41,** 109–110.

55. Goodwin, W. J., Esser, D., Clayman, G. L., Nemunaitis, J., Yver, A., and Dreiling, L. K. (1999) Randomized phase II study of intratumoral injection of two dosing schedules using a replication-deficient adenovirus carrying the p53 gene (AD5CMV-P53) in patients with recurrent/refractory head and neck cancer. *Proc. Am. Soc. Clin. Oncol.* **19,** 445a.

56. Bier-Laning, C. M., VanEcho, D., Yver, A., and Dreiling, L. K. (1999) A phase II multi-center study of AD5CMV-P53 administered intratumorally to patients with recurrent head and neck cancer. *Proc. Am. Soc. Clin. Oncol.* **18,** 444a.

57. National Institute of Health, Recombinant DNA Advisory Committee. (2002) *Gene Therapy Protocols by Disease.* NIH, Washington, D.C.

58. Yver, A., Dreiling, L. K., Mohanty, S., et al. (1999) Tolerance and safety of RPR/INGN 201, an adeno-viral vector containing a p53 gene, administered intratumorally in 309 patients with advanced cancer enrolled in phase I and II studies world-wide. *Proc. Am Soc. Clin. Oncol.* **19,** 460a.

59. Yonish-Rouach, E., Resnitzky, D., Lotem, J., Sachs, L., Kimchi, A., and Oren, M. (1991) Wild-type p53 induces apoptosis of myeloid leukemic cells that is inhibited by interleukin-6. *Nature* **352,** 345–347.

60. Ramqvist, T., Magnusson, K. P., Wang, Y., Szekeley, L., and Klein, G. (1993) Wild-type p53 induces apoptosis in a Burkitt lymphoma (BL) line that carries mutant p53. *Oncogene* **8,** 1495–1500.

61. Shaw, P., Bovey, R., Tardy, S., Sahli, R., Sordat, B., and Costa, J. (1992) Induction of apoptosis by wild-type p53 in a human colon tumor-derived cell line. *Proc. Natl. Acad. Sci. USA* **89,** 4495–4499.

62. Dewey, W. C., Ling, C. C., and Meyn, R. E. (1995) Radiation induced apoptosis: relevance to radiotherapy. *Int. J. Radiat. Oncol. Biol. Phys.* **33,** 781–796.

63. Roth, J. A. (1995) Review: clinical protocol for modification of tumor suppressor gene expression and induction of apoptosis in non-small cell lung cancer (NSCLC) with an adenovirus vector expressing wildtype p53 and cisplatin. *Hum. Gene Ther.* **6,** 252–255.

64. Meyn, R. E., Stephens, L. C., Hunter, N. R., and Milas, L. (1997) Apoptosis in murine tumors treated with chemotherapy agents. *Anticancer Drugs* **6,** 443–450.

65. Fujiwara, T., Grimm, E. A., Mukhopadhyay, T., Zhang, W. W., Owen-Schaub, L. B., and Roth, J. A. (1994) Induction of chemosensitivity in human cancer cells in vivo by adenovirus-mediated transfer of the wild-type p53 gene. *Surg. Forum* **45,** 524–526.

66. Nguyen, D. M., Spitz, F. R., Yen, N., Cristiano, R. J., and Roth, J. A. (1996) Gene therapy for lung cancer: enhancement of tumor suppression by a combination of sequential systemic cisplatin and adenovirus-mediated p53 gene transfer. *J. Thorac. Cardiovasc. Surg.* **112,** 1372–1377.

67. Hamada, M., Fujiwara, T., Hizuta, A., et al. (1996) The p53 gene is a potent determinant of chemosensitivity and radiosensitivity in gastric and colorectal cancers. *J. Cancer Res. Clin. Oncol.* **122,** 360–365.

68. Nguyen, D., Spitz, F., Kataoka, M., Wiehle, S., Roth, J. A., and Cristiano, R. (1996) Enhancement of gene transduction in human carcinoma cells by DNA-damaging agents. *Proc. Am. Assoc. Cancer Res.* **37,** 347.

69. Jasty, R., Lu, J., Irwin, T., Suchard, S., Clarke, M. F., and Castle, V. P. (1998) Role of p53 in the regulation of irradiation-induced apoptosis in neuroblastoma cells. *Mol. Genet. Metab.* **65,** 155–164.

70. Akimoto, T., Hunter, N. R., Buchmiller, L., Mason, K., Ang, K. K., and Milas, L. (1999) Inverse relationship between epidermal growth factor receptor expression and radiocurability of murine carcinomas. *Clin. Cancer Res.* **5,** 2884–2890.

71. Feinmesser, M., Halpern, M., Fenig, E., et al. (1994) Expression of the apoptosis-related oncogenes bcl-2, bax, and p53 in Merkel cell carcinoma: can they predict treatment response and clinical outcome? *Hum. Pathol.* **30,** 1367–1372.

72. Broaddus, W. C., Liu, Y., Steele, L. L., et al. (1999) Enhanced radiosensitivity of malignant glioma cells after adenoviral p53 transduction. *J. Neurosurg.* **91,** 997–1004.

73. Sakakura, C., Sweeney, E. A., Shirahama, T., et al. (1996) Overexpression of bax sensitizes human breast cancer MCF-7 cells to radiation-induced apoptosis. *Int. J. Cancer* **67,** 101–105.

74. Brachman, D. G., Becket, M., Graves, D., Haraf, D., Vokes, E., and Weichselbaum, R. R. (1993) p53 mutation does not correlate with radiosensitivity in 24 head and neck cancer cells lines. *Cancer Res.* **53,** 3667–3669.

75. Slichenmyer, W. J., Nelson, W. G., Slebos, R. J., and Kastan, M. B. (1993) Loss of a p53-associated G1 checkpoint does not decrease cell survival following DNA damage. *Cancer Res.* **53,** 4164–4168.

76. Danielsen, T., Smith-Sorensen, B., Gronlund, H. A., Hvidsten, M., Borresen-Dale, A. L., and Rofstad, E. K. (1994) No association between radiosensitivity and TP53 status, G(1) arrest or protein levels of p53, myc, ras or raf in human melanoma lines. *Int. J. Radiat. Biol.* **75,** 1149–1160.

77. Nemunaitis, J., Swisher, S. G., Timmons, T., et al. (2000) Adenovirus-mediated p53 gene transfer in sequence with cisplatin to tumors of patients with non-small cell lung cancer. *J. Clin. Oncol.* **18,** 609–622.

78. Schuler, M., Herrmann, R., De Greve, J. L., et al. (2001) Adenovirus-mediated wild-type p53 gene transfer in patients receiving chemotherapy for advanced non-small-cell lung cancer: results of a multicenter phase II study. *J. Clin. Oncol.* **19,** 1750–1758.

79. Buller, R., Runnebaum, I., Karlan, B., et al. (2002) A phase I/II trial of rAd/p53 (SCH 58500) gene replacement in recurrent ovarian cancer. *Cancer Gene Ther.* **9,** 553–566.

80. Buller, R. E., Shahin, M. S., Horowitz, J. A., et al. (2002) Long term follow-up of patients with recurrent ovarian cancer after Ad p53 gene replacement with SCH 58500. *Cancer Gene Ther.* **9,** 567–572.

81. Swisher, S., Roth, J. A., Komaki, R., et al. (2000) A phase II trial of adenoviral mediated p53 gene transfer (RPR/INGN 201) in conjunction with radiation therapy in patients with localized non-small cell lung cancer (NSCLC). *Am. Soc. Clin. Oncol.* **19,** 461a.

82. Nishizaki, M., Fujiwara, T., Tanida, T., et al. (1999) Recombinant adenovirus expressing wild-type p53 is antiangiogenic: a proposed mechanism for bystander effects. *Clin. Cancer Res.* **5,** 1015–1023.

83. Templeton, N. S., Lasic, D. D., Frederik, P. M., Strey, H. H., Roberts, D. D., and Pavlakis, G. N. (1997) Improved DNA: liposome complexes for increased systemic delivery and gene expression. *Nat. Biotechnol.* **15,** 647–652.

84. Ramesh, R., Saeki, T., Templeton, N. S., et al. (2001) Successful treatment of primary and disseminated human lung cancers by systemic delivery of tumor suppressor genes using an improved liposome vector. *Mol. Ther.* **3,** 337–350.

85. Shimizu, T., Chen, J., Gamou, S., and Takayanagi, A. (1996) Immunogene approach toward cancer therapy using epidermal growth factor receptor-mediated gene delivery. *Cancer Gene Ther.* **3,** 113–120.

86. Hood, J. D., Bednarski, M., Frausto, R., et al. (2002) Tumor regression by targeted gene delivery to the neovasculature. *Science* **296,** 2404–2407.

87. Kondo, M., Ji, L., Kamibayashi, C., et al. (2001) Overexpression of candidate tumor suppressor gene FUS1 isolated from the 3p21.3 homozygous deletion region leads to G1 arrest and growth inhibition of lung cancer cells. *Oncogene* **20,** 6258–6262.

88. Ji, L., Nishizaki, M., Gao, B., et al. (2002) Expression of several genes in the human chromosome 3p21.3 homozygous deletion region by an adenovirus vector results in tumor suppressor activities in vitro and in vivo. *Cancer Res.* **62,** 2715–2720.

89. Lerman, M. I. and Minna, J. D. (2000) The 630-kb lung cancer homozygous deletion region on human chromosome 3p21.3: identification and evaluation of the resident candidate tumor suppressor genes. The International Lung Cancer Chromosome 3p21.3 Tumor Suppressor Gene Consortium. *Cancer Res.* **60,** 6116–6133.

90. National Institutes of Health and Office of Biomedical Affairs. (2002) Recombinant DNA and gene transfer Web site. NIH/NCI. 11-25-0002.

4

Antisense Technology

Ruiwen Zhang and Hui Wang

1. INTRODUCTION

Antisense therapy is designed to deliver to the target cells antisense molecules that can hybridize and specifically inhibit the expression of pathogenic genes (Fig. 1). In the past, the term *antisense* included several distinct but related approaches, including classical antisense or anticode, ribozyme or catalytic ribonucleic acid (RNA), triplex or antigene, and aptamer technologies (Table 1). A unified terminology has not yet been developed to describe technologies in this field. For the purpose of this chapter, we use *antisense therapy* to refer to the classical antisense approach. Other chapters in this book provide further information and discussions on ribozyme and aptamer approaches (*see* Chapter 5).

Antisense nucleic acids are single-stranded oligonucleotides complementary to the sequence of a target RNA or deoxyribonucleic acid (DNA). Zamecnik and Stephenson first introduced antisense therapy over 25 years ago *(1,2)*. In addition, naturally occurring antisense RNA was found to be a means of regulation of gene expression in living cells *(3)*. However, these striking discoveries were not translated to exciting research as the development of antisense therapeutics experienced a very slow growing period in the 1970s and 1980s.

After a major breakthrough in automated oligonucleotide synthesis yielded oligonucleotides in sufficient amounts and high quality for in vitro and in vivo studies, including human studies, antisense technology has rapidly developed and been widely applied for investigating gene function and regulation, modulation of gene expression, and validation of new drug targets *(4–9)*. There is now a large body of published studies suggesting the potential use of antisense oligonucleotides in the treatment of various human diseases, such as hypertension and other cardiovascular diseases, cancer, genetic disorders, and viral infections *(4–9)*.

The first antisense drug, Vitravene, has been approved for the treatment of patients with cytomegalovirus-induced retinitis *(10)*. Several antisense oligonucleotides have entered phase I–III clinical trials as anticancer agents administered alone or in combination with conventional chemotherapy *(4,5,9,11–15*; Table 2).

Another closely related area is RNA interference (RNAi) technology *(16,17)*. RNAi was first discovered as a cellular-protecting mechanism against invasion by foreign genes in *Caenorhabditis elegans* and subsequently observed in various eukaryotes, such as insects, plants, fungi, and vertebrates. RNAi is a powerful intracellular mechanism for sequence-specific, posttranscriptional gene silencing initiated by double-stranded RNAs homologous to suppression of the gene. Double-stranded RNAs are processed by Dicer, a cellular ribonuclease III, to generate duplexes of about 21 nt with 3'-overhangs called small interfering RNA (siRNA) that mediate sequence-specific messenger RNA (mRNA) degradation. The siRNA molecules in mammalian cells are also capable of specifically silencing gene expression. Thus, RNAi technology has been used as a new and powerful alternative to other gene-silencing technologies, such as antisense and ribozymes.

From: *Contemporary Cancer Research*
Cancer Gene Therapy
Edited by: D. T. Curiel and J. T. Douglas © Humana Press Inc., Totowa, NJ

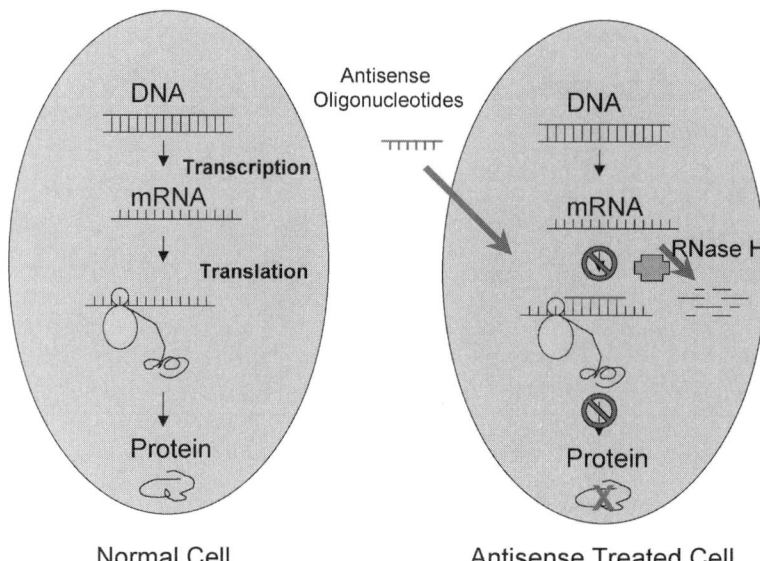

Fig. 1. Simplified presentation of gene expression process and mechanisms of action of antisense oligo-nucleotides. Antisense oligonucleotide is complementary to the target RNA sequence. It specifically hybridizes with target RNA, resulting in translational arrest and increased RNA degradation by activating RNase H and/or decreased RNA anabolism by inhibiting RNA splicing.

Table 1
Major Characteristics of Antisense and RNAi Technologies

Technology	Active molecule	Molecular target	Cellular site of action[a]	Suggested mechanisms of action	Status of drug discovery and development
Antisense	DNA or RNA	RNA[b]	Cytoplasm	Translation arrest, RNase H activation, inhibition of splicing, disruption of RNA structure	Clinical use[c], clinical trials
Ribozyme	RNA	RNA	Cytoplasm	Translation arrest, destruction of RNA structure	Clinical trials
Triplex-forming-oligo-nucleotides	DNA	DNA	Nucleus	Blockage of transcription	Preclinical
Aptamer	DNA or RNA	Protein	Nucleus, cytoplasm, or extracellular	Interference with protein function	Clinical phase I trial
RNAi	RNA	RNA	Cytoplasm	Promoting RNA degradation	In vitro study, limited in vivo study

[a]Site of action refers to the initial site of interaction of active molecule with its target molecule and may not be the same as biological activity occurs.

[b]Any kind of RNA can be targeted: pre-RNA, mRNA, or viral RNA.

[c]The first antisense drug, Vitravene, has been approved for the treatment of patients with cytomegalovirus-induced retinitis. Several other antisense oligonucleotides have entered clinical phase I–III trials (*see* Table 2).

Table 2
Examples of Antisense Oligonucleotides as Anticancer Agents in Clinical Trials

Target gene	Oligonucleotide sequence[a]	Target diseases
First-generation antisense (phosphorothioate) oligonucleotides		
bcl-2	5'-TCTCCCAGCGTGCGCCAT-3'	Lymphoma, prostate cancer, melanoma
bcr-abl	5'-CGCTGAAGGGCTTCTTCCTTATTGAT-3'	Chronic myeloid leukemia.
bcr-abl	5'-CGCTGAAGGGCTTTTGAACTGTGCTT-3'	Chronic myeloid leukemia
c-myb	5'-TATGCTGTGCCGGGGTCTTCGGGC-3'	Chronic myeloid leukemia
c-myc	5'-GCTAACGTTGAGGGGCAT-3'	Restenosis
c-raf-1	5'-TCCCGCCTGTGACATGCATT-3'	Colon cancer, renal carcinoma, ovarian cancer, pancreatic cancer
Ha-ras	5'-GGGACTCCTCGCTACTGCCT-3'	Sarcoma, pancreatic cancer, colon cancer, melanoma
IGF-IR	5'-GGACCCTCCTCCGGAGCC-3'	Malignant astrocytomas
PKC-α	5'-GTTCTCGCTGGTGAGTTTCA-3'	Lymphoma, nonsmall cell lung cancer, ovarian cancer
p53	5'-CCCTGCTCCCCCCTGGCTCC-3'	Acute myeloid leukemia, myelodysplastic syndrome
Second-generation (mixed-backbone) antisense oligonnucleotides		
PKA-RIa	5'-**GCGU**GCCTCCTCAC**UGGC**-3'	Solid tumors

PKC, Protein kinase C; PKA-RIα regulatory subunit Iα of cAMP-dependent protein kinase A.

[a]All the sequences contain phosphorothioate internucleotide linkages; roman and bold letters indicate deoxy- and 2'-*O*-methyl-ribonucleosides, respectively.

However, this technology is also associated with limitations; using siRNA molecules to modulate expression of a specific gene depends on target accessibility and effective delivery of siRNAs into target cells. Most reports on siRNA technology are results from in vitro studies, and its in vivo efficacy and long-term utility are uncertain. Other chapters in this book provide further information and discussions on various RNAi or siRNA approaches (*see* Chapter 5).

2. ANTISENSE TECHNOLOGY

2.1. Antisense Chemistry

Both antisense RNA and DNA have been used in studying gene function by silencing target gene expression (Table 1).

2.1.1. Antisense RNA

Natural antisense RNA has been demonstrated to be involved in gene regulation in normal organisms *(3)*. Synthesized antisense RNAs have also been used for in vitro studies. As RNAs are extremely sensitive to nuclease degradation, the potential pharmacological uses of antisense RNA are limited.

In the past, two major approaches were employed to apply antisense RNA into living cells: nuclear expression of antisense RNA by engineered antisense genes and microinjection of synthesized antisense RNA into cells. Chemically modified antisense RNAs have been studied as stable antisense RNA molecules in downregulation of cancer-related genes.

For example, a 30-mer antisense 2'-*O*-methyl RNA targeting thymidylate synthase (TS) mRNA has been shown to be an effective antisense agent in vitro *(18)*. TS is a key enzyme in nucleoside metabolism, and its expression is controlled by its own protein end product TS in a negative autoregulatory manner *(18)*. Disruption of this regulation results in increased synthesis of TS and may lead to the development of cellular drug resistance to TS-directed anticancer agents such as 5-fluorouracil. This antisense 2'-*O*-methyl RNA was designed to target directly the 5' upstream *cis*-acting regulatory element (nucleotides 80–109) of TS mRNA, and it inhibited TS expression in human colon cancer RKO cells in a dose-dependent manner. TS expression was unaffected by treatment with sense or mismatched controls.

The investigators also demonstrated that an 18-mer antisense 2'-*O*-methyl RNA targeting the same core sequence also inhibited TS expression. However, further reduction in the oligonucleotide size resulted in loss of antisense activity. Following antisense RNA treatment, TS protein levels were reduced in a time-dependent manner, with maximal reduction occurring after 24-hour exposure to the oligonucleotide. However, Northern blot analysis demonstrated that TS mRNA was not affected by the antisense RNA treatment, and the half-life of TS protein was unchanged after antisense treatment, suggesting that the mechanism of action for antisense RNA is mediated through a process of translational arrest not associated with mRNA stability. These findings indicate that short-length, chemically modified antisense RNAs may have potential in gene silencing. However, in vivo application of these antisense RNAs is largely unknown.

2.1.2. Antisense DNA

Antisense oligodeoxynucleotides are short sequences of single-stranded DNA and can be produced in large quantity using automated synthetic organic chemistry with various modified linkages or terminal groups. Thus, antisense DNAs now are used much more frequently than antisense RNA and ribozymes. Examples of clinically tested antisense DNAs are listed in Table 2.

2.1.3. Unmodified Phosphodiester Oligodeoxynucleotides

The early antisense investigations began with phosphodiester oligodeoxynucleotides (PO-oligos) *(1)*. With high affinity to their targets, PO-oligos bind stably to the target mRNA, and the melting temperature T_m of the PO-oligos:RNA duplex is high. PO-oligos also activate RNase H, resulting in mRNA degradation (Fig. 1). The major disadvantages of PO-oligos are sensitivity to nucleases and poor cell uptake. Therefore, the application of PO-oligos is very limited.

2.1.4. Oligonucleotide Analogs With Backbone Modifications

Many studies have demonstrated that backbone modifications improve the cell uptake and increase resistance to nucleases of antisense oligonucleotides. Among them, phosphothioate oligonucleotides (PS-oligos) and methylphosphonate oligonucleotides (MP-oligos) have been investigated extensively. MP-oligos, for which $-CH_3$ replaces $-O$, were first synthesized in the late 1970s by Miller and colleagues *(19)* and have been confirmed to be much more resistant to extra- and intracellular nucleases. The melting temperature of the MP-oligos:RNA duplex is also higher than that of PO-oligos. As one kind of uncharged oligonucleotides, MP-oligos pass through cytoplasm membrane much better than PO-oligos.

The major disadvantages of MP-oligos are relatively poor hybridization efficiency and inability to activate RNase H *(20)*. Isosteric substitution of sulfur for oxygen on the phosphorus residue of DNA generates PS-oligos. Like unmodified oligonucleotides, PS-oligos retain the negative charge and thus are more aqueous soluble than MP-oligos. PS-oligos also are resistant to nucleases and readily activate RNase H. The disadvantages of PS-oligos are less cellular uptake and nonspecific toxicities in vivo. Thus far, most clinically tested antisense oligonucleotides are PS-oligos (Table 2).

2.1.5. Oligonucleotides With Terminal Modification

Studies have shown that antisense oligonucleotides can be degraded from 3' and 5' ends or both *(21)*. To enhance cellular uptake and nuclease resistance of oligonucleotides, different terminal modification at the 5' or 3' terminus of oligonucleotides has been attempted. For example, polylysine, avidin (such as acridine), and cholesterol have been used to improve cellular uptake and antisense effects of oligonucleotides *(22)*. However, the value of these modifications remains uncertain, especially in in vivo settings.

2.1.6. Mixed-Backbone Oligonucleotides

To improve the properties of antisense oligonucleotides further, we have designed mixed-backbone oligonucleotides (MBOs) *(23–31)*. One kind contains phosphorothioate segments at the 3' and 5' ends and has a modified oligodeoxynucleotide or oligoribonucleotide segment located in the central portion of the oligonucleotide. Some MBOs have been shown to have improved properties compared with PS-oligos with respect to affinity to RNA, RNase H activation, and antitumor activity. In addition, more acceptable pharmacological, in vivo degradation, and pharmacokinetic profiles were obtained with these MBOs *(23–30)*. One of these MBOs has entered clinical trials *(30*; Table 2) Another example of MBOs contains 2'-5'-ribo- and 3'-5'-deoxyribonucleotide segments *(31)*.

Thermal melting studies of the phosphodiester MBOs indicated that 2'-5'-ribonucleoside incorporation into 3'-5'-oligodeoxyribonucleotides reduces binding to the target strands compared to an all 3'-5'-oligodeoxyribonucleotide of the same sequence and length. Increasing the number of 2'-5' linkages (from six to nine) further reduces binding to the DNA target strand than to the RNA target strand. PS-analogs of MBOs destabilize the duplex with the DNA target strand more than the duplex with the RNA target strand. These MBOs exhibited moderately higher stability against nucleases.

Although 2'-5' modification does not evoke RNase H activity, it does not affect the RNase H activation property of the 3'-5'-deoxyribonucleotide segment adjacent to the modification. There is less effect on cell proliferation, clotting prolongation, and hemolytic complement lysis than with control PS-oligos *(31)*. These results suggest that a limited number of 2'-5' linkages could be used in conjunction with PS-oligos to modulate further the properties of antisense oligonucleotides as therapeutic agents.

2.2. Antisense Mechanisms

The exact mechanism of action for antisense oligonucleotides is not fully understood, but may be complex *(2,5–9,12–15,24,32–36)*. There is increasing evidence to support that the biological activity of a given antisense oligonucleotide may be influenced by various factors at molecular, cellular, organ/tissue, and whole body levels. For instance, those factors may include the concentration of oligonucleotide at the target site (RNA), the concentration of the target RNA, the metabolism of the RNA, and the mechanisms of the interaction between the oligonucleotide and its target RNA.

Many mechanisms of antisense action have been proposed, with two major mechanisms, hybrid-arrest and RNase H activation, generally accepted (Fig. 1). Early studies suggested that antisense oligonucleotides bind to and interact with the code region, cause blockade of ribosomal read-through mRNA, and stop translation (Fig. 1). Later, it was demonstrated that antisense oligonucleotides also can be targeted to the initiation code region and to inhibit downstream gene expression more efficiently. Moreover, antisense oligonucleotides may produce antisense effects through binding to the 5' cap region, 3' poly A, and/or the splicing site of the pre-RNA, the last interfering with RNA splicing, maturation, and transport *(33)*.

Another major mechanism of action is RNase H activation by several types of antisense oligonucleotides, such as PS-oligo, that may bind with their target RNA to form an RNA:DNA duplex, while activating enzyme RNase H, which results in target RNA degradation. Other types of oligonucleotides, such as MP-oligo, however, do not possess this property *(37)*.

Human RNase H has been cloned and characterized *(38)*, which may facilitate the investigation of antisense mechanisms *(38–40)*. Human RNase H1 shares many enzymatic properties with *Escherichia coli* RNase H1. The human enzyme cleaves RNA in a DNA:RNA duplex, resulting in products with 5'-phosphate and 3'-hydroxy termini, can cleave overhanging single-stranded RNA adjacent to a DNA:RNA duplex, and is unable to cleave substrates in which either the RNA or DNA strand has 2' modifications at the cleavage site. The human enzyme has a greater initial rate of cleavage of a heteroduplex-containing RNA-phosphorothioate DNA than an RNA:DNA duplex. The minimum RNA: DNA duplex length that supports cleavage is 6 bp, and the minimum RNA:DNA "gap size" that supports cleavage is 5 bp *(38)*. These finding may facilitate the design of RNase H-dependent antisense oligonucleotides.

In general, RNAi can be considered an antisense mechanism of action that utilizes a double-stranded RNase to promote hydrolysis of the target RNA. Vickers et al. compared the efficacy of optimized antisense oligonucleotides designed to work by an RNAi mechanism to oligonucleotides designed to work by an RNase H-dependent mechanism in human cells *(40)*. They found that these oligonucleotides are comparable in terms of potency, maximal effectiveness, duration of action, and sequence specificity. Furthermore, activity of both siRNA oligonucleotides and RNase H-dependent oligonucleotides is affected by the secondary structure of the target mRNA. Examination of 80 siRNA oligonucleotide duplexes designed to bind to RNA from four distinct human genes revealed that, in general, activity correlated with the activity to RNase H-dependent oligonucleotides targeted to the same site *(40)*. One major difference between the two approaches is that RNase H-dependent oligonucleotides are active when directed against targets in the pre-mRNA, whereas siRNAs have no activity. These findings suggest that both siRNA-based and RNase H-dependent antisense technologies are valid approaches to evaluating gene functions, at least in cell-based assays. However, whether these findings can be translated to in vivo efficacy remains to be determined.

2.3. Principles of Antisense Design

Although the design of antisense oligonucleotides is theoretically simple and straightforward (to identify a complementary oligonucleotide on the basis of the nucleotide sequence of the mRNA), the selection of an effective and specific antisense oligonucleotide is largely based on investigators' experience and trial-based experiments. In addition, because certain oligonucleotide sequences, such as CpG and GGGG, have been shown to have sequence-dependent, non-antisense effects, these sequences should be avoided to identify sequence-specific antisense drugs *(24)*. Several general approaches to selecting optimal antisense sequences are discussed next.

2.3.1. Random "Sequence-Walking" Approach

The random sequence-walking method is based on Watson-Crick base pairing rules and a known sequence of the target gene, and it uses a linear, sequence-walking approach to design and select antisense oligonucleotides. Usually, a relatively large number of "random" oligonucleotides (10–100, depending on the length of the gene of interest) with a certain length (15–25 mer, for example), targeted to various regions of the target mRNA, are synthesized individually, and their antisense activity is determined using a defined cell-free or cell-based in vitro screening assay. This conventional method has been used in many antisense experiments and has yielded good results, although it is expensive and time and labor consuming (only fewer than 5% of the oligonucleotides are generally found to be effective) *(41,42)*.

2.3.2. Computer-Aided Target Selection

Using the above methods (*see* Section 2.3.1.), it is frequently seen that a single or a few base shifts have no significant change in oligonucleotide:RNA binding, but may have large differences in antisense activity. The binding efficiency of complementary oligonucleotide to target RNA is suggested to be mainly determined by the secondary and tertiary structures of the target RNA *(43)*. Therefore, the antisense efficacy of antisense oligonucleotides may be largely associated with the possibility of targeting accessible sites of the targeted RNA. Accessible sites in mRNAs may be predicted using computer programs through various approaches to predict the secondary structure of RNA *(44)*. For example, using an RNA-folding program such as MFOLD (Genetics Computer Group, Madison, WI), antisense oligonucleotides may be designed to target against the regions of mRNA predicted to be free from intramolecular base pairing and therefore accessible to the designed oligonucleotides *(43)*.

2.3.3. Oligonucleotide Scanning Arrays

Advances in DNA array technologies have led to the development of oligonucleotide scanning arrays as a novel approach for identifying active antisense oligonucleotides *(45)*. This method allows combinatorial synthesis of a large number of oligonucleotides and parallel measurement of the binding strength of all oligonucleotides to the target mRNA. There may also be a correlation between the binding strength and the antisense activity, providing a basis for optimization of antisense oligonucleotides *(45)*. However, this method has not been widely tested in antisense research.

2.3.4. RNase H Digestion-Based Screening

As discussed in Section 2.2., RNase H activation is one of the major antisense mechanisms, especially for PS-oligos. RNase H screening assays can be used in combination with a random or semirandom oligonucleotide library to optimize lead oligonucleotides *(46,47)*. The target mRNA is transcribed in vitro, end labeled, and mixed with the oligonucleotide library; the RNase H cleavage sites are then identified by gel electrophoresis. However, this method may not precisely define the accessible sites of the target mRNA because RNase H cleavage can occur at more than one location; therefore, it will be difficult to predict the antisense activity solely based on RNase mapping.

3. PRINCIPLES OF ANTISENSE EVALUATION

Like any new drugs, antisense oligonucleotide therapeutics need to undergo an extensive, systematic evaluation in various preclinical and clinical settings (Figs. 2 and 3). The biological activity of a given antisense drug, including desired and undesired effects, may be influenced by various factors at the molecular, cellular, organ/tissue, and whole body levels (Tables 3 and 4). Antisense oligonucleotides may exert their biological effects on target genes through several distinct mechanisms, including both antisense and non-antisense mechanisms in target and nontarget cells or tissues *(4–9,11–15,23,24)*.

In addition, the delivery of antisense drugs to target cells is a key issue in success. In in vitro studies, lipids are frequently used to facilitate the cellular uptake of oligonucleotides. Of note, the ratio of lipids to oligonucleotides will affect the results of uptake and likely the biological activity. The cytotoxicity of certain lipids alone may affect the interpretation of in vitro results. In contrast, the in vivo uptake of oligonucleotides seems much better than that in settings in vitro *(25–30)*, making the use of a special carrier unnecessary. Reviews of drug delivery of antisense oligonucleotides provide further information *(48,49)*.

3.1. Pharmacological Evaluation

There is a large body of reports describing pharmacokinetic properties of various antisense oligonucleotides *(4,5,7,8,15,25–30)*. Antisense oligonucleotides with various lengths and base compositions have been investigated in various species, including rats, mice, rabbits, monkeys, and humans and following various routes of administration (e.g., intravenous, intraperitoneal, subcutaneous, intradermal, oral, and inhalation). In most cases, quantification of parent oligonucleotides (and degraded products, in some cases) was reported using plasma samples.

In some studies, tissue distribution of oligonucleotides was carried out *(25–30)*. In general, PS-oligos have a short plasma distribution half-life $t_{1/2}\alpha$ of less than 1 hour and a prolonged elimination half-life $t_{1/2}\beta$ in the range of 40–60 hours *(25–30)*. The plasma pharmacokinetics of oligonucleotides is not associated with the length or primary sequence, but with the backbone modification and specific segments at the 3' and/or 5' ends. Antisense oligonucleotides have a wide tissue distribution, with the highest concentrations found in the liver and kidneys. Urinary excretion is believed to be the major elimination pathway *(25–30)*.

The retention of oligonucleotides in target tissues and normal tissues is directly associated with in vivo stability. To increase therapeutic effects, it is desirable to increase the retention time of intact oligonucleotides in the body by increasing in vivo stability and decreasing elimination. Studies in our

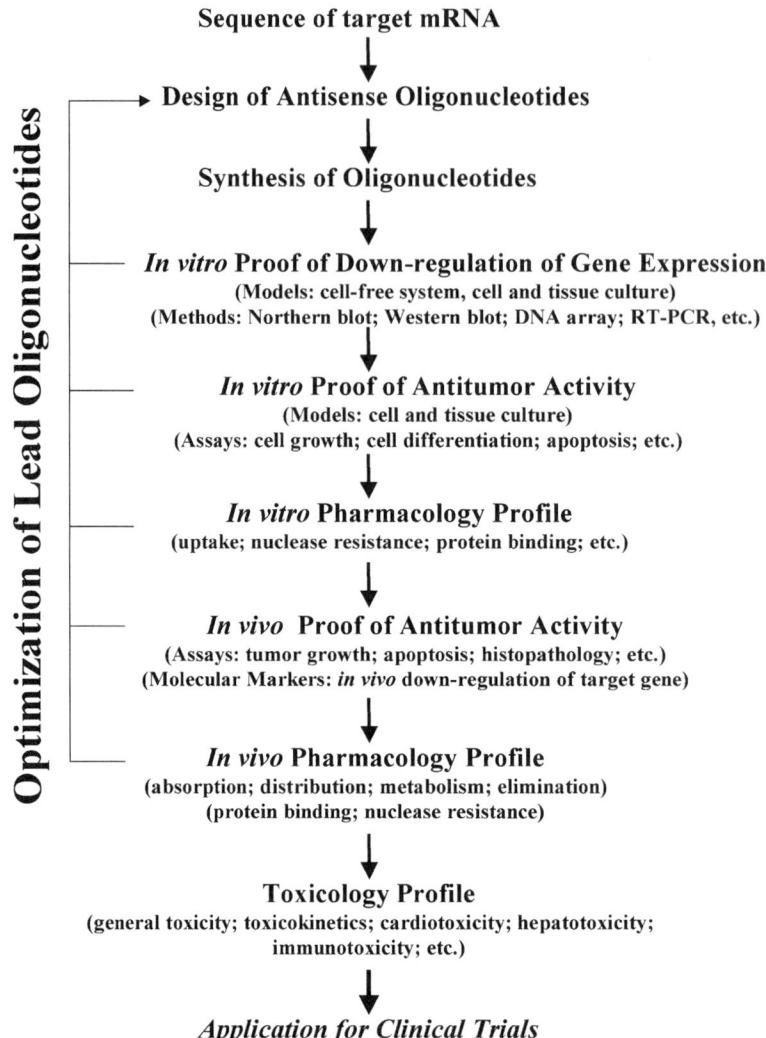

Fig. 2. Preclinical evaluation of antisense oligonucleotides as anticancer drugs.

laboratory have shown that MBOs have prolonged tissue retention compared with PS-oligos *(25–30)*. However, because of nonspecific tissue distribution and accumulation, high levels and prolonged retention of oligonucleotides in host tissue may increase the risk of toxicity, and such a risk may increase further because of individual disease status and organ functions, such as liver and renal functions.

3.2. Evaluation of Antisense Efficacy

Perhaps the most important aspects of pharmacological evaluation of antisense oligonucleotides are target effectiveness and specificity of these antisense agents (Fig. 2; Table 3). Designed oligonucleotides are usually tested at both in vitro and in vivo levels (Fig. 2). In vitro, cell-free or cell-based assays have been routinely employed to establish the basis for further investigation. Cellular uptake of test oligonucleotides may depend on cell type, drug concentrations, cell culture conditions, and delivery system. It is generally accepted that the majority of oligonucleotides can cross the cell membrane and distribute to cytosol in sufficient quantities to exert the desired effect.

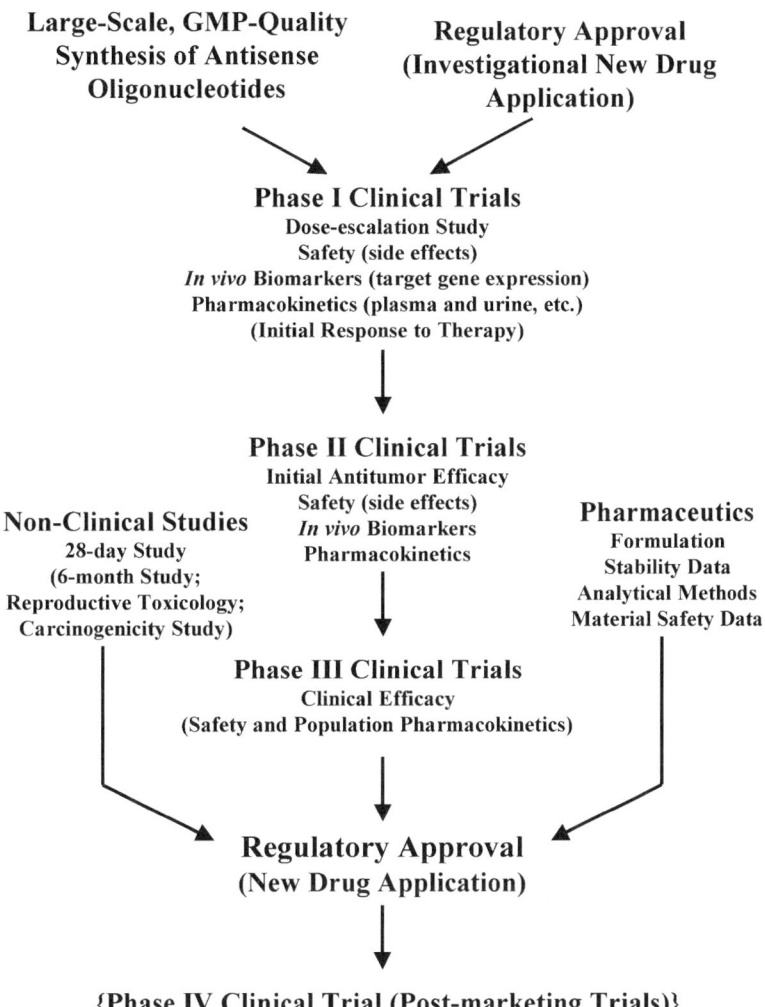

Fig. 3. Clinical evaluation of antisense oligonucleotides as anticancer drugs. GMP, good manufacturing practice.

To increase cellular uptake in vitro, several means of delivery, such as liposomes or phospholipids, have now been routinely used to avoid the use of extremely high concentration found in early days of antisense research. To demonstrate the specificity of test oligonucleotides, the expression levels of target genes are usually analyzed using Western blot, reverse transcriptase polymerase chain reaction (RT-PCR), and/or Northern blot analyses. If inhibition of protein expression and impact on mRNA metabolism of target genes are demonstrated in a time-, dose-, sequence-dependent manner, an antisense-specific effect is indicated. Proper controls (untreated, mismatched oligo, lipids) are usually included. To demonstrate further the specificity of test antisense oligonucleotides, control proteins or housekeeping genes such as actin are usually analyzed simultaneously.

Assays to determine cell variability, proliferation, and apoptosis are used to illustrate antitumor activity of test oligonucleotides compared with controls. However, these assays may produce false-positive and false-negative results. For example, some lipids used to increase oligonucleotide uptake have cytotoxicity *per se*. Therefore, proper (e.g., negative, positive, and mismatch) controls are needed. Dose-, time-, and sequence-dependent responses are better evidence for antisense effects and desirable to establish a basis for further in vivo evaluation of the test oligonucleotides.

Table 3
Factors That May Influence Preclinical Experimental Results and Interpretation

Category	Factors or conditions
Molecular targets	Specificity of mRNA sequence chosen
	Concentration of mRNA
	Rate and synthesis of mRNA
	Degradation of mRNA
	Other related/unrelated genes
Oligonucleotides	Purity and impurity
	Sequence and structure
	Chemistry and modifications
	Microbial test
	Special carrier/conjugates
In vitro study	Stability of oligonucleotides
	Test system
	Cellular uptake and distribution
	Cell type and culture conditions
	Concentrations of oligonucleotides
	Control oligonucleotides
	Delivery approach (microinjection, lipids, and so on)
	Assay to determine the mRNA and protein levels of targets
In vivo study	In vivo stability of oligonucleotides
	Binding to protein and/or other macromolecules
	Pharmacokinetics: absorption, distribution, metabolism, and elimination
	Toxicokinetics
	Pharmacodynamics: interaction of oligonucleotides and mRNA target
	Dose-dependent effects
	Dose-independent effects
	Pharmaceutical issues: Formulations and delivery
	Test system and disease model
	Animal use and care
	Dose, schedule, and duration of treatment
	Combination therapy
	Assay to determine the mRNA and protein levels of targets
	End points of therapeutic effects (tumor growth, toxicity, and so on)
Mechanisms of action	Antisense sequence-specific effects
	Non-antisense, sequence-dependent effects
	Nonspecific effects
	RNase H activity

Evidence for in vivo antitumor activity of antisense oligonucleotides is critical in the development pipeline, but it is relatively harder to produce convincing, reproducible results compared to in vitro testing. Various murine models, such as xenograft models in nude and SCID mice and transgenic mouse models, are most used prior to clinical trials. For example, human cancer cell lines are xenoplanted into nude mice or SCID mice. The end points for efficacy can be tumor mass, metastasis, survival, molecular markers, and histopathological evaluation.

Three types of test models can be used, depending on the treatment schedule and time. First, the effect on tumor onset and formation of oligonucleotides can be determined using an ex vivo protocol in which cells are treated with test antisense oligonucleotide prior to xenoplantation or an in vivo treatment protocol in which oligonucleotide treatment begins immediately after cell xenoplantation. The rate of tumor formation and growth inhibition can be used as major end points in these models.

Table 4
Factors That May Influence Clinical Trial Results and Interpretation

Category	Factors or conditions
Subjects/patients	Expression levels of the target gene
	Disease and stage
	Host conditions/status
	Demographics
	Prior or concurrent treatment
Oligonucleotides	Purity
	Impurities
	Formulation
	In vivo stability of oligonucleotides
Pharmacology	Binding to protein or other macromolecules
	Pharmacokinetics: absorption, distribution, metabolism, and elimination
	Toxicokinetics
	Pharmacodynamics: interaction of oligonucleotides and mRNA target
Treatment and effects	Dose-dependent effects
	Dose-independent effects
	Dose, schedule, and duration of treatment
	Combination therapy
	Assay to determine the mRNA and protein levels of targets
	End points of therapeutic effects (response, survival, and so on)
	Adverse effects

Second, the inhibitory effects on tumor growth of test oligonucleotides can be assayed using an in vivo treatment protocol in which oligonucleotide treatment begins in an early stage of tumor growth, usually when the tumor mass reaches 50–100 mg. In these models, tumor growth inhibition and molecular/pathology markers can be major end points.

Third, the antitumor activity of oligonucleotides can also be tested in the late stage of tumors using a protocol in which oligonucleotide treatment begins when the tumor mass reaches 500–1000 mg, depending on tumor type. In these models, tumor growth inhibition and survival can be major end points.

It is very important to establish dose–response relations in in vivo models. Proper (e.g., untreated, vehicle, oligonucleotide) controls should be included. In vivo evidence for blocking of specific gene expression is also desirable. It should be pointed out that in vivo antitumor activity of a given antisense oligonucleotide is not necessarily the result of antisense mechanism and can be associated with nonspecific activity and/or sequence-specific non-antisense activity.

3.3. Combination Therapy

Although most antisense oligonucleotides are tested in vivo as monotherapy, combination treatment of antisense oligonucleotides and conventional chemotherapeutic agents, anticancer antibodies, and radiation therapy has also been widely investigated. There are a number of preclinical studies demonstrating that downregulation of specific gene products with antisense oligonucleotides sensitizes cancer cells to chemotherapeutic agents, resulting in an additive or synergistic anticancer activity. These antisense targets include mouse double minutes 2 (MDM2) *(50–55)* epidermal growth factor receptor *(56)*, cyclic adenosine monophosphate (cAMP)-dependent protein kinase *(30,57–60)* c-myc *(61)*, protein kinase Cα *(62)*, and *Bcl-2 (63)*. These antisense oligonucleotides increase the therapeutic effects of such chemotherapeutic agents as paclitaxel, 5-fluorouracil, cisplatin, carboplatin, taxotere, camptothecin, irinotecan, leucovorin, gemcitabin, mefosfamide, doxorubicin, adriamycin, and dacarbazine.

However, the mechanisms responsible for such additive or synergistic effects between antisense oligonucleotides and chemotherapeutic agents are not fully understood. Both pharmacokinetic and pharmacodynamic factors may be involved (Table 3). The synergy between the two classes of agents may result from interaction on several mechanisms, such as cell cycle arrest, induction of apoptosis, induction of immune responses, and production of cytokines. Although most studies showed such additive or synergistic effects are sequence specific, other studies demonstrated that antisense oligonucleotides could also potentiate the antitumor activity of irinotecan in a sequence-independent manner *(50,51,64)*, presumably through an interaction at the pharmacokinetic and/or metabolic level to increase the conversion of the active metabolite *(51)*.

3.4. Clinical Trials

Compared with preclinical studies, far fewer clinical studies of oligonucleotides have been reported *(4,9,11*; Table 2). Most clinically tested antisense antitumor oligonucleotides are PS-oligos that have been shown to have an acceptable safety profile and initial anti-tumor efficacy in humans. Antisense oligonucleotides have been tested as monotherapy and in combination with chemotherapeutic agents *(65)*.

In most published phase I trials, antisense oligonucleotides had favorable safety profiles. Side effects included thrombocytopenia, prolongation of activated partial thromboplastin time, and slight elevation in liver enzymes. No significant liver and renal toxicity has been reported. Pharmacokinetic studies have been carried out in patients, indicating a short plasma distribution half-life and prolonged elimination half-life. Urinary excretion represents the major pathway of excretion, with mainly degraded products observed. Antisense oligonucleotides have now been shown to inhibit expression of targeted genes and initial antitumor response specifically. Limited phase II and III trials have been reported. Further studies are needed. In fact, the future of antisense therapy depends on successful proof of efficacy in clinical trials.

3.5. Safety Evaluation

Thorough toxicity studies are key components of antisense drug development. There are limited reports on toxicity evaluation of antisense oligonucleotides, although a number of phosphorothioates have been studied extensively for their safety profiles in several species, including mice, rats, monkeys, and humans. The dose-dependent side effects in experimental rats and mice included thrombocytopenia, splenomegaly, and elevation of transaminases *(66,67)*. Histopathology changes included mononuclear cell infiltration in tissues such as liver, kidney, and spleen and reticuloendothelial cell and lymphoid cell hyperplasia. The severity of side effects was dependent on the dose, frequency, and duration of the administration of oligonucleotides. In general, the toxicity profiles of PS-oligos are similar with various lengths and base compositions, with exceptions in the presence of certain sequence motifs, such as CpG-dinucleotides *(66,68)* and poly-G motifs *(69)*, which contribute to the severity of toxicity.

Preclinical toxicity studies are used to guide a starting dose and dose escalation scheme of clinical trials and are expected to be conducted in accordance with current good laboratory practices. To support clinical phase I trials, animal toxicity studies using two animal species are usually conducted in one rodent species and one nonrodent species. For antisense oligonucleotides, nonhuman primates have often been used. In addition, special toxicity studies have been suggested to determine cardiotoxicity, hepatotoxicity, and immunotoxicity. A review provides details *(70)*.

4. CONCLUSION

Although significant progress has been made in the last decade, antisense oligonucleotides have not been developed as a valid therapeutic approach. One of the most important aspects of the development of therapeutic oligonucleotides is validation of the drug target and improving the targeting effectiveness and specificity of these antisense drugs. With an increasing number of antisense anticancer oligonucleotides evaluated in the clinic, there are promising therapeutic agents used alone or in combination with other therapeutic agents. Future studies are needed not only to provide the proof of principle for antisense technology in vitro and in vivo, but also to meet the full requirement for antisense therapy as an established therapeutic approach. More basic research is needed to uncover the mechanisms of action for various biological activities (antisense, sequence dependent non-antisense, and non-sequence specific) of oligonucleotides responsible. With new generations of antisense drugs created and tested, therapeutic effectiveness and safety profiles of these new agents are expected to be significantly improved.

ACKNOWLEDGMENT

This project was supported by a grant (R01 CA 80698) from the National Institutes of Health, National Cancer Institute to R. Zhang.

REFERENCES

1. Zamecnik, P. C. and Stephenson, M. L. (1978) Inhibition of Rous sarcoma virus replication and cell transformation by a specific oligodeoxynucleotide. *Proc. Natl. Acad. Sci. USA* **75,** 280–284.
2. Zamecnik, P. C. (1996) History of antisense oligonucleotides. In *Antisense Therapeutics* (Agrawal, S., ed.). Humana, Totowa, NJ, pp. 1–12.
3. Simons, R. W. (1988) Naturally occurring antisense RNA control, a brief review. *Gene* **72,** 35–44.
4. Wickstrom, E. (1998) *Clinical Trials of Genetic Therapy With Antisense DNA and DNA Vectors.* Marcel Dekker, New York.
5. Stein, C. A. and Krieg, A. M. (1998) *Applied Antisense Oligonucleotide Technology.* Wiley-Liss, New York.
6. Agrawal, S. and Zhao, Q. (1998) Antisense therapeutics. *Curr. Opin. Chem. Biol.* **2,** 519–528.
7. Phillips, M. I. (2000) Antisense technology: Part B: Applications. In *Methods in Enzymology.* Academic, San Diego, CA, Vol. 314.
8. Crooke, S. T. (2001) *Antisense Drug Technology, Principles, Strategies, and Applications.* Marcel Dekker, New York.
9. Wang, H., Prasad, G., Buolamwini, J. K., and Zhang, R. (2001) Antisense anticancer oligonucleotide therapeutics. *Curr. Cancer Drug Targets* **1,** 177–196.
10. Crooke, S. T. (1998) Vitravene—another piece in the mosaic. *Antisense Nucleic Acid Drug Dev.* **8,** vii–viii.
11. Agrawal, S. (1996) Antisense oligonucleotides: towards clinical trial. *Trends Biotechnol.* **14,** 376–387.
12. Kushner, D. M. and Silverman, R. H. (2000) Antisense cancer therapy: the state of the science. *Curr. Oncol. Rep.* **2,** 23–30.
13. Monia, B. P., Holmlund, J., and Dorr, F. A. (2000) Antisense approaches for the treatment of cancer. *Cancer Invest.* **18,** 635–650.
14. Gewirtz, A. M. (2000) Oligonucleotide therapeutics: a step forward. *J. Clin. Oncol.* **18,** 1809–1811.
15. Crooke, S. T. (2000) Potential roles of antisense technology in cancer chemotherapy. *Oncogene* **19,** 6651–6659.
16. Shuey, D. J., McCallus, D. E., and Giordano, T. (2002) RNAi: gene-silencing in therapeutic intervention. *Drug Discov. Today* **7,** 1040–1046.
17. Scherr, M., Morgan, M. A., and Eder, M. (2003) Gene silencing mediated by small interfering RNAs in mammalian cells. *Curr. Med. Chem.* **10,** 245–256.
18. Schmitz, J. C., Yu, D., Agrawal, S., and Chu, E. (2001) Effect of 2'-*O*-methyl antisense ORNs on expression of thymidylate synthase in human colon cancer RKO cells. *Nucleic Acids Res.* **29,** 415–422.
19. Miller, P. S., McParland, K. B., Jayaraman, K., and Ts'o, P. O. P. (1981) Biochemical and biological effects of nonionic nucleic acid methylphosphonates. *Biochemisty* **20,** 1874–1880.
20. Carter, G. and Lemoine, N. R. (1993) Antisense technology for cancer therapy: does it make sense? *Br. J. Cancer* **67,** 869–876.
21. Temsamani, J., Roskey, A., Chaix, C., and Agrawal, S. (1997) In vivo metabolic profile of a phosphorothioate oligodeoxyribonucleotide. *Antisense Nucleic Acid Drug Dev.* **7,** 159–165.
22. Nechers, L. M. (1993) Cellular internalization of oligodeoxynucleotides. In *Antisense Research and Applications* (Crooke, S. T. and Lebleu, B., eds.), CRC Press, Boca Raton, FL, pp. 451–460.
23. Agrawal, S. (1999) Importance of nucleotide sequence and chemical modifications of antisense oligonucleotides. *Biochim. Biophys. Acta* **1489,** 53–68.
24. Agrawal, S. and Kandimalla, E. R. (2000) Antisense therapeutics: is it simple as complementary base recognition? *Mol. Med. Today* **6,** 72–81.

25. Agrawal, S. and Zhang, R. (1997) Pharmacokinetics of phosphorothioate oligonucleotide and its novel analogs. In *Antisense Oligodeoxynucleotides and Antisense RNA as Novel Pharmacological and Therapeutic Agents* (Weiss, B., ed.), CRC Press, Boca Raton, FL, pp. 58–78.

26. Agrawal, S. and Zhang, R. (1997) Pharmacokinetics of oligonucleotides. *Ciba Sym.* **209**, 60–78.

27. Agrawal, S. and Zhang, R. (1998) Pharmacokinetics and bioavailability of oligonucleotides following oral and colorectal administrations in experimental animals. In *Antisense Research and Applications* (Crooke, S., ed.), Springer-Verlag, Heidelberg, Germany, pp. 525–543.

28. Agrawal, S., Jiang, Z., Zhao, Q., et al. (1997) Mixed-backbone oligonucleotides as second generation antisense oligo-nucleotides: in vitro and in vivo studies. *Proc. Natl. Acad. Sci. USA* **94**, 2620–2625.

29. Agrawal, S., Zhang, X., Zhao, H., et al. (1995) Absorption, tissue distribution and in vivo stability in rats of a hybrid antisense oligonucleotide following oral administration. *Biochem. Pharm.* **50**, 571–576.

30. Wang, H., Cai, Q., Zeng, X., Yu, D., Agrawal, S., and Zhang,R. (1999) Anti-tumor activity and pharmacokinetics of a mixed-backbone antisense oligonucleotide targeted to RIα subunit of protein kinase A after oral administration. *Proc. Natl. Acad. Sci. USA* **96**, 13,989–13,994.

31. Kandimalla, E. R., Manning, A., Zhao, Q., et al. (1997) Mixed backbone antisense oligonucleotides: design, biochem-ical and biological properties of oligonucleotides containing 2'-5'-ribo- and 3'-5'-deoxyribonucleotide segments. *Nucleic Acids Res.* **25**, 370–378.

32. Lebedeva, I. and Stein, C. (2001) Antisense oligonucleotides: promise and reality. *Ann. Rev. Pharm. Toxicol.* **41**, 403–419.

33. Crooke, S. T. (1999) Molecular mechanisms of action of antisense drugs. *Biochim. Biophys. Acta* **1489**, 31–44.

34. Crooke, S. T. (2000) Comments on evaluation of antisense drugs in the clinic. *Antisense Nucleic Acid Drug Dev.* **10**, 225–227.

35. Crooke, S. T. (2000) Progress in antisense technology: the end of beginning. *Methods Enzymol.* **313**, 3–45.

36. Diasio, R. B. and Zhang, R. (1997) Pharmacology of therapeutic oligonucleotides. *Antisense Nucleic Acid Drug Dev.* **7**, 239–243.

37. Boiziau, C., Thuong, N. T., and Toulmé, J. J. (1992) Mechanisms of the inhibition of reverse transcription by antisense oligonucleotides. *Proc. Natl. Acad. Sci. USA* **89**, 768–772.

38. Wu, H., Lima, W. F., and Crooke, S. T. (1999) Properties of cloned and expressed human RNase H1. *J. Biol. Chem.* **274**, 28,270–28,278.

39. Wu, H., Lima, W. F., and Crooke, S. T. (2001) Investigating the structure of human RNase H1 by site-directed muta-genesis. *J. Biol. Chem.* **276**, 23,547–23,553.

40. Vickers, T. A., Koo, S., Bennett, C. F., Crooke, S. T., Dean, N. M., and Baker, B. F. (2003) Efficient reduction of target RNAs by small interfering RNA and RNase H-dependent antisense agents. A comparative analysis. *J. Biol. Chem.* **278**, 7108–7118.

41. Peyman, A., Helsberg, M., Kretzschmar, G., Mag, M., Grabley, S. and Uhlmann, E. (1995) Inhibition of viral growth by antisense oligonucleotides directed against the IE110 and the UL30 mRNA of herpes simplex virus type-1. *Biol. Chem. Hoope-Seyler* **376**, 195–198.

42. Monia, B. P., Johnson, J. F., Geiger, T., Muller, M., and Fabbro, D. (1996) Antitumor activity of a phosphorothioate anti-sense oligodeoxynucleotide targeted against C-raf kinase. *Nat. Med.* **2**, 668–675.

43. Milner, N., Mir, K. U., and Southern, E. M. (1997) Selecting effective antisense reagents on combinatorial oligonucle-otide arrays. *Nat. Biotechnol.* **15**, 537–541.

44. Zuker, M. (1989) On finding all suboptimal folding of an RNA molecule. *Science* **244**, 48–52.

45. Elder, J. K., Johnson, M., Milner, N., Mir, K. U., Sohail, M., and Southern, E. M. (1999) Antisense oligonucleotide scanning arrays. In *DNA Microarrays: A Practical Approach* (Schena, M., ed.), IRL, Oxford, UK, pp. 77–99.

46. Ho, S. P., Bao, Y., Lesher, T., et al. (1998) Mapping of RNA accessible sites for antisense experiments with oligonu-cleotide libraries. *Nat. Biotechnol.* **16**, 59–63.

47. Lima, W. F., Brown-Driver, V., Fox, M., Hanecak, R., and Bruice, T. (1997) Combinatorial screening and rational optimization for hybridisation to folded hepatitis C virus RNA of oligonucleotides with biological antisense activity. *J. Biol. Chem.* **272**, 626–638.

48. Agrawal, S. and Akhtar, S. (1995) Advances in antisense efficacy and delivery. *T. I. B. Tech.* **13**, 197–199.

49. Dokka, S. and Rojanasakul, Y. (2000) Novel non-endocytic delivery of antisense oligonucleotides. *Adv. Drug Delivery Rev.* **44**, 35–39.

50. Wang, H., Nan, L., Yu, D., Agrawal, S., and Zhang, R. (2001) Antisense anti-MDM2 oligonucleotides as a novel therapeutic approach to human breast cancer: in vitro and in vivo activities and mechanisms. *Clin. Cancer Res.* **7**, 3613–3624.

51. Wang, H., Wang, S., Nan, L., Yu, D., Agrawal, S., and Zhang, R. (2002) Antisense anti-MDM2 mixed-backbone oligonucleotides enhance therapeutic efficacy of topoisomerase I inhibitor irinotecan in nude mice bearing human cancer xenografts: in vivo activity and mechanisms. *Int. J. Oncol.* **20**, 745–752.

52. Prasad, G., Wang, H., Agrawal, S., and Zhang, R. (2002) Antisense oligonucleotides targeted to MDM2 oncogene as a novel approach to the treatment of glioblastoma multiforme. *Anticancer Res.* **22**, 107–116.

53. Wang, H., Nan, L., Yu, D., Lindsey, J. R., Agrawal, S., and Zhang, R. (2002) Anti-tumor efficacy of a novel antisense anti-mdm2 mixed-backbone oligonucleotide in human colon cancer models: p53-dependent and p53-independent mechanisms. *Mol. Med.* **8,** 185–199.

54. Wang, H., Yu, D., Agrawal, S., and Zhang, R. (2003) Experimental therapy of human prostate cancer by inhibiting MDM2 expression with novel mixed-backbone antisense oligonucleotides: in vitro and in vivo activities and mechanisms. *Prostate* **54,** 194–205.

55. Tortora, G., Caputo, R., Damiano, V., et al. (2000) Novel MDM2 anti-sense oligonucleotide has anti-tumor activity and potentiates cytotoxic drugs acting by different mechanisms in human colon cancer. *Int. J. Cancer* **88,** 804–809.

56. Ciardiello, F., Caputo, R., Troiani, T., et al. (2001) Antisense oligonucleotides targeting the epidermal growth factor receptor inhibit proliferation, induce apoptosis, and cooperate with cytotoxic drugs in human cancer cell lines. *Int. J. Cancer* **93,** 172–178.

57. Wang, H., Yu, D., Agrawal, S., and Zhang, R. (2002) Antisense mixed-backbone oligonucleotide targeted to cAMP-dependent protein kinase (GEM231) improves therapeutic efficacy of topoisomerase I irinotecan in nude mice bearing human cancer xenografts: in vivo activities, pharmacokientics and toxicity. *Int. J. Oncol.* **21,** 73–80.

58. Tortora, G., Caputo, R., Damiano, V., et al. (1998) Cooperative antitumor effect of mixed backbone oligonucleotides targeting protein kinase A in combination with cytotoxic drugs or biologic agents. *Antisense Nucleic Acid Drug Dev.* **8,** 141–145.

59. Tortora, G., Caputo, R., Damiano, V., et al. (1997) Synergistic inhibition of human cancer cell growth by cytotoxic drugs and mixed backbone antisense oligonucleotide targeting protein kinase A. *Proc. Natl. Acad. Sci. USA* **94,** 12,586–12,591.

60. Tortora, G., Caputo, R., Pomatico, G., et al. (1999) Cooperative inhibitory effect of novel mixed backbone oligonucleotide targeting protein kinase A in combination with docetaxel and anti-epidermal growth factor-receptor antibody on human breast cancer cell growth. *Clin. Cancer Res.* **5,** 875–881.

61. Akie, K., Dosaka-Akita, H., Murakami, A., and Kawakami, Y.A. (2000) Combination treatment of C-myc antisense DNA with all-trans-retinoic acid inhibits cell proliferation by downregulating C-myc expression in small cell lung cancer. *Antisense Nucleic Acid Drug Dev.* **10,** 243–249.

62. Geiger, T., Muller, M., Dean, N. M., and Fabbro, D. (1998) Antitumor activity of a PKC-alpha antisense oligonucleotide in combination with standard chemotherapeutic agents against various human tumors transplanted into nude mice. *Anticancer Drug Des.* **13,** 35–45.

63. Lopes de Menezes, D. E., Hudon, N., McIntosh, N., and Mayer, L. D. (2000) Molecular and pharmacokinetic properties associated with the therapeutics of bcl-2 antisense oligonucleotide G3139 combined with free and liposomal doxorubicin. *Clin. Cancer Res.* **6,** 2891–2902.

64. Agrawal, S., Kandimalla, E. R., Yu, D., et al. (2001) Potentiation of antitumor activity of irinotecan by chemically modified oligonucleotides. *Int. J. Oncol.* **18,** 1061–1069.

65. Jansen, B., Wacheck, V., Heere-Ress, E., et al. (2000) Chemosensitisation of malignant melanoma by BCL2 antisense therapy. *Lancet* **356,** 1728–1733.

66. Agrawal, S., Zhao, Q., Jiang, Z., et al. (1997) Toxicologic effects of an oligodeoxynucleotide phosphorothioate and its analogs following intravenous administration in rats. *Antisense Nucleic Acid Drug Dev.* **7,** 575–584.

67. Henry, S. P., Zuckerman, J. E., Rojko, J., et al. (1997) Toxicological properties of several novel oligonucleotide analogs in mice. *Anticancer Drug Des.* **12,** 1–14.

68. Agrawal, S. and Zhao, Q. (1998) Mixed backbone oligonucleotides: Improvement in oligonucleotide-induced toxicity in vivo. *Antisense Nucleic Acid Drug Dev.* **8,** 135–139.

69. Agrawal, S., Iadarola, P. L., Temsamani, J., Zhao, Q., and Shaw, D. R. (1996) Effect of G-rich sequences on the synthesis, purification, binding, cell uptake, and hemolytic activity of oligonucleotides. *Bioorg. Med. Chem. Lett.* **6,** 2219–2224.

70. Ahn, C. H. and DeGeorge, J. J. (1998) Preclinical development of antisense oligonucleotide therapeutics for cancer: regulatory aspects. In *Clinical Trials of Genetic Therapy With Antisense DNA and DNA Vectors* (Wickstrom, E., ed.), Marcel Dekker, New York, pp. 39–52.

5

Cancer Therapeutic Applications of Ribozymes and RNAi

Lisa Scherer and John J. Rossi

1. INTRODUCTION

1.1. Ribozymes

Ribozymes are ribonucleic acid (RNA) molecules capable of acting as enzymes even in the complete absence of proteins. They have the catalytic activity of breaking and/or forming covalent bonds with extraordinary specificity, accelerating the rate of these reactions. The ability of RNA to serve as a catalyst was first shown for the self-splicing group I intron of *Tetrahymena* and the RNA moiety of RNAse P *(1–3)*. Subsequent to the discovery of these two RNA enzymes, RNA-mediated catalysis has been associated with the self-splicing group II introns of yeast, fungal, and plant mitochondria (as well as chloroplasts) *(4)*; single-stranded plant viroid and virusoid RNAs *(5–7)*; hepatitis delta virus *(8)*; and a satellite RNA from *Neurospora* mitochondria *(9)*. It is rather clear that the RNA component of the larger ribosomal subunit is functioning as a peptidyltransferase as well *(10–13)*. The potential functioning of spliceosomal smaller nuclear (sn)RNAs as a ribozyme in complex with the pre-messenger RNA (pre-mRNA) to catalyze pre-mRNA splicing has also been proposed *(14)*. It is highly likely that additional RNA catalytic motifs and new roles for RNA-mediated catalysis will also be found as more is learned about the genomes of a variety of organisms.

Ribozymes occur naturally, but can also be artificially engineered and synthesized to target specific sequences in *cis-* or *trans-*. New biochemical activities are under development using in vitro selection protocols as well *(15)*. Ribozymes can easily be manipulated to act on novel substrates. These custom-designed RNAs have great potential as therapeutic agents and are becoming a powerful tool for molecular biologists. Catalytic hammerhead and hairpin ribozymes represent the most popular choices for therapeutic applications and are depicted in Fig. 1.

1.2. RNA Interference

RNA interference (RNAi) is a gene-silencing mechanism originally elucidated in plants (in which it was known as posttranscriptional gene silencing), *Caenorhabditis elegans*, and *Drosophila (16–20)*. In the current model, the RNAi pathway is activated by a double-stranded RNA (dsRNA) "trigger," which is then processed into short, 21- to 22-nt dsRNAs, referred to as small interfering RNAs (siRNAs) by the cellular enzyme Dicer (Fig. 2A). The siRNAs become incorporated into the RNA-induced silencing complex (RISC), in which the siRNA serves as a guide to identify the homologous mRNA for destruction *(19)*. In mammalian cells, dsRNA longer than 30 nts triggers the interferon pathway, activating PKR and 2'-5'-oligoadenylate synthetase rather than RNAi. However, shorter siRNAs exogenously introduced into mammalian cells or transcribed endogenously bypass the Dicer

From: *Contemporary Cancer Research*
Cancer Gene Therapy
Edited by: D. T. Curiel and J. T. Douglas © Humana Press Inc., Totowa, NJ

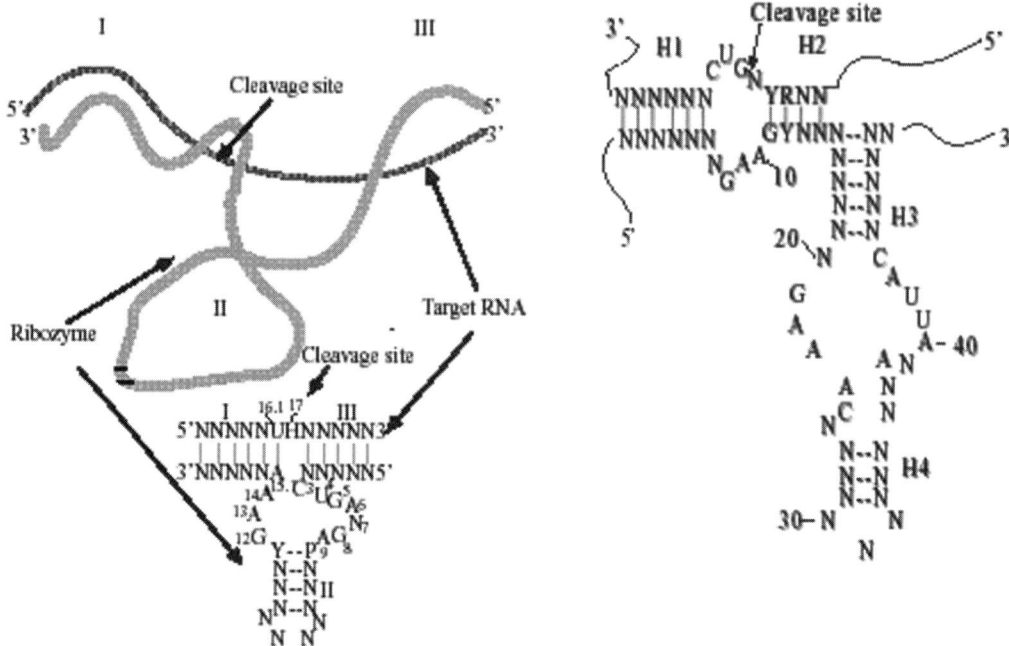

Fig. 1. The commonly used hammerhead and hairpin catalytic ribozymes. Secondary structures for the hammerheadand hairpin ribozymes are depicted. N, any nucleotide; R, purine; and Y, pyrimidine. A diagram of the tertiary structure of the hammerhead ribozyme is depicted beside the secondary structure model. The corresponding stems I, II, and III in both structures are shown. In the hammerhead ribozyme, H is A, C, or U at the cleavage site. In the hairpin ribozymes, H1, H2, and so on refer to the helical regions of the RNA structure.

step and directly activate homologous mRNA degradation without initiating the interferon response (Fig. 2B) *(21,22)*.

2. RIBOZYME APPLICATIONS

Ribozymes have been applied as antiviral agents, for the treatment of cancer and genetic disorders, and as tools for pathway elucidation and target validation. Initial uses of ribozymes focused on antiviral considerations, primarily for the treatment of human immunodeficiency virus (HIV) *(23–26)*. Viruses that go through a genomic RNA intermediate in their replication cycle, such as HIV, hepatitis B virus, and hepatitis C virus, are attractive targets because a single species of ribozyme can target both viral genomic RNA and mRNAs. Ribozymes have also been widely used to target cellular genes, including those aberrantly expressed in cancers.

One early ribozyme target was the *bcr-abl* fusion transcript created from the Philadelphia chromosome associated with chronic myelogenous leukemia *(27–30)*. This chromosome is characterized by a translocation that results in the expression of a transforming *bcr-abl* fusion protein. In this case, ribozymes have been designed to target the fusion mRNA specifically and not the normal *bcr* or *abl* mRNAs, preventing the function of *bcr-abl* oncogenes. The mutation at codon 12 in c-H-*ras* from GGU to GUU creates a site for hammerhead ribozyme-mediated cleavage. An endogenously expressed ribozyme targeted to this site was effective in preventing focus formation in about 50% of NIH3T3 cells transfected with this activated *ras* gene. In contrast, cells expressing this same ribozyme but transfected with an activated *ras* in which the codon change was at position 61 instead of 12 were not protected from foci formation by the ribozyme *(31,32)*. Ribozymes targeting overexpressed *HER-2/neu* in breast carcinoma cells effectively reduced the tumorigenicity of these cells in mice *(33)*.

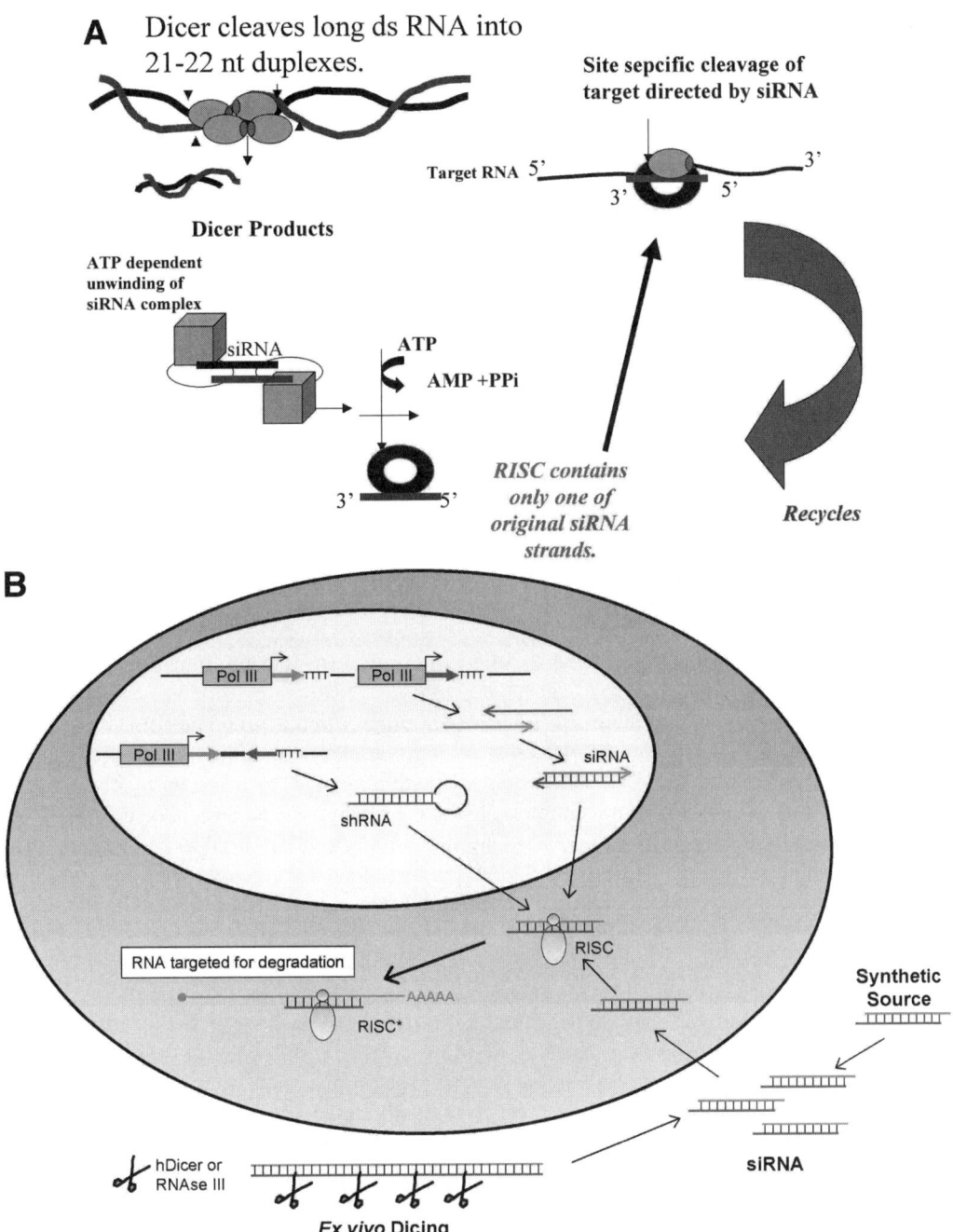

Fig. 2. Mechanism of siRNA-directed degradation target mRNA in mammalian cells. (**A**) dsRNAs greater than 30 bp are cleaved by the RNAse III family member Dicer into 21- to 22-nt siRNAs that have 2 base 3' over-hangs. The siRNAs are unwound by a helicase complex that has yet to be characterized, and the antisense strand is paired with the target by a complex called the RNA-induced silencing complex (RISC). RISC directs site-specific cleavage of target RNA and recycles. (**B**) A single synthetic siRNA or a mixture of enzymatically derived siRNAs derived from the target RNA can be supplied exogenously. Alternatively, siRNA can be generated endogenously using either a dual-cassette system, in which sense and antisense strands are separately transcribed and subsequently anneal, or a single-cassette system, in which the siRNA is transcribed as a hairpin loop. It is not known how the loop of shRNAs are processed.

In addition to targeting oncogenes directly, ribozymes have also been applied more indirectly as anticancer therapies. For example, ribozymes targeting the multiple drug resistance gene 1 (MDR-1) *(34–36)* or fos mRNAs *(37,38)* in cancer cell lines effectively made the cells more sensitive to chemotherapeutic agents. Alternatively, a ribozyme targeting *bcl-2* triggered apoptosis in oral cancer cells *(39)*.

Factors required for metastasis are also attractive targets for ribozymes. Ribozymes targeted against *CAPL/mts (40)*, matrix metalloproteinase-9 *(41)*, pleiotrophin *(42)*, and VLA-6 integrin *(43,44)* all reduced the metastatic potential of the respective tumor cells. Angiogenesis is also an important target for cancer therapy and has been blocked in mice by ribozymes targeting fibroblast growth factor-binding protein *(45)* and pleiotrophin *(42)*.

Ribozyme-based therapies have also been tested in animals to inhibit other proliferative disorders, such as coronary artery restenosis *(46–48)*. Antitelomerase RNA ribozymes are also being tested for possible applications in cancer gene therapy *(49)*. The use of ribozymes as possible therapeutic agents in a variety of cancers has been reviewed *(50)*.

2.1. Delivery

Whatever type of ribozyme is chosen, it must be introduced into its target cells. Two general mechanisms exist for introducing catalytic RNA molecules into cells: exogenous delivery of the preformed ribozyme and endogenous expression from a transcriptional unit. Preformed ribozymes can be delivered into cells using liposomes, electroporation, or microinjection.

Many exciting developments in the chemical synthesis of RNA and modified forms of RNA have taken place over the past several years. Molecules with long-term stability in serum or intracellular environments have been synthesized *(51–53)*. Several of these backbone-modified ribozymes still maintain the site specificity and catalytic turnover features of unmodified RNAs, and some have enhanced catalytic properties, making them candidates for ex vivo delivery. Chemically modified ribozymes have been shown capable of delivery without encapsulation and can be taken up by cells *(53)*.

Stable intracellular expression of transcriptionally active ribozymes can be achieved by viral vector-mediated delivery. Currently, retroviral vectors are the most commonly used in cell culture, primary cells ,and transgenic animals *(54)*. Retroviral vectors have the advantage of stable integration into a dividing host cell genome, and the absence of any viral gene expression reduces the chance of an immune response in animals. In addition, retroviruses can be easily pseudotyped with a variety of envelope proteins to broaden or restrict host cell tropism, thus adding an additional level of cellular targeting for ribozyme gene delivery. Adenoviral vectors can be produced at high titers and provide very efficient transduction, but they do not integrate into the host genome; consequently, expression of the transgenes is only transient in actively dividing cells *(55)*. Other viral delivery systems are actively being pursued, such as the adeno-associated virus, alpha viruses, and lentiviruses *(15,56–60)*. Adeno-associated virus is attractive as a small, nonpathogenic virus that can stably integrate into the host genome. An alpha virus system, using recombinant Semliki Forest virus, provides high transduction efficiencies of mammalian cells along with cytoplasmic ribozyme expression *(61)*.

Another vehicle for the ex vivo delivery of ribozyme genes is cationic lipids *(62)*. Because there are a variety of formulations for these lipids, it is usually best to test a panel of lipids for those that provide the highest efficiency of gene transfer with the least toxicity.

3. TRANSGENIC ANIMALS EXPRESSING RIBOZYMES

Therapeutics and target validation studies will certainly be tested in animals. Ribozymes have been used in transgenic mice to create disease models, such as for diabetes, by selectively downregulating the hexokinase mRNA in pancreatic islets *(63)*. In this case, the ribozyme expression was under the control of the insulin promoter and was therefore only expressed in the pancreatic β-cells. Retroviral delivery of ribozymes targeted against neuregulin 1 in a chick blastoderm resulted in the same embryonic lethal phenotype as a gene knockout *(64)*. Localized retroviral delivery of the same ribozyme later in development allowed dissection of the neuregulin biochemical pathway *(65)*. The use of a heat-inducible ribozyme against *Fushi tarzu* in *Drosophila* allowed the developmentally timed disruption of this gene function in *Drosophila* embryos *(66)*.

4. RIBOZYME-MEDIATED RNA REPAIR

A novel therapeutic application of ribozymes exploits the *trans*-splicing activity of the *Tetrahymena* ribozyme. This ribozyme has been used to repair defective mRNAs by *trans*-splicing onto these RNAs a functional sequence *(67,68)*. These ribozymes are designed to bind and cleave the target RNAs 5' of the undesired mutation. Because the ribozyme in this case is an intron, it is engineered to carry with it the correct RNA sequence as the 3' exon. Following cleavage of the mutant target RNA, the ribozyme catalyzes ligation of wild-type sequence onto the cleaved transcript. This was first successfully demonstrated with the correction of a mutant *lacZ* transcript *(69)* in bacteria and subsequently with the correction of a sickle cell message in erythroid cells *(70)*.

5. RIBOZYME EVOLUTION

The discovery of the ribozyme sparked new debate on the "RNA world" hypothesis, by which all biological processes are carried out by RNA-based enzymes. Since then, RNA evolution has been forced in vitro to come up with RNA enzymes capable of carrying out a wide variety of biochemical reactions, as far-reaching as carbon–carbon bond and peptide bond formation. In vitro RNA evolution has been used to create RNA-cleaving ribozymes with smaller catalytic domains, deoxyribonucleic acid (DNA)-cleaving ribozymes, and new catalytic motifs *(71)*. Even RNA-cleaving DNAzymes have been generated through in vitro evolution *(72)*. These "evolved" enzymes exemplify the power of in vitro evolution and will no doubt find many applications.

It is reasonable to conclude that achieving effective ribozyme–substrate interactions and ribozyme function in an intracellular environment is not a straightforward task, and that new strategies for expression and localization of ribozymes in the intracellular milieu will be required to permit the general utility of ribozymes as therapeutic agents.

6. OTHER CONSIDERATIONS

Although base pairing specificity confers target selectivity, minimizing the potential for general toxicity, the question of toxicity must be rigorously tested because mispairing by a ribozyme to a nontargeted substrate could elicit undesired antisense inhibitory effects. Because every ribozyme sequence has different potential base pairing interactions, an accumulation of data from many different ribozyme experiments will be required to assess this potential problem rigorously. Some of the potential sources of toxicity are nonspecific interactions of ribozymes with cellular proteins, the generation of high intracellular concentrations of the cleavage products, and the inhibitory effects on cellular metabolism of various chemically generated backbone modifications used to stabilize presynthesized ribozymes.

One of the potential advantages of ribozymes vs antisense RNAs is their catalytic activity, which could theoretically lead to inactivation of multiple targeted substrates. It has yet to be demonstrated that this type of catalytic activity can occur intracellularly. Protein facilitation of hammerhead ribozyme-mediated cleavage *(73–75)* suggested that intracellular ribozyme-mediated substrate turnover may be possible. Experiments designed to exploit the protein facilitation of ribozyme turnover intracellularly are currently under way in several laboratories. The inclusion of RNA-binding proteins in in vitro evolution strategies to enrich for ribozyme-protein combinations with enhanced catalytical activities should also be exploited. Finally, the design and chemical synthesis of ribozymes capable of high catalytic turnover as a consequence of specific base and backbone modifications is a distinct possibility.

7. FUTURE PROSPECTS

The notion that ribozymes could be used as therapeutic agents has only been around for a few years, yet there is a great deal of interest in deploying clinically useful ribozymes in the very near future. At this time, it is premature to conclude that ribozymes will have a place in the repertoire of therapeutic agents available to modern medicine. A great deal more must be learned about the movement of RNA inside the cells as well as the cellular factors that can impede or enhance ribozyme utilization. These are not simple problems, but they are not confined to those studying the application of ribozymes. As techniques in cell biology become more refined, answers to some of these problems will be forthcoming.

The transformation of ribozyme sequences from naturally occurring, *cis*-cleaving (and -ligating) molecules to target-specific, *trans*-cleaving (and -ligating) reagents has stimulated a great deal of interest in their potential applications. Ribozymes targeting viral genes are now in clinical evaluation, ribozymes targeting cellular genes are moving into transgenic animals, and the use of ribozymes is expanding into RNA evolution, mRNA repair, and gene discovery.

For ribozymes to become realistic therapeutic agents, several obstacles first need to be overcome. These obstacles are the efficient delivery to a high percentage of the cell population, efficient expression of the ribozyme from a vector or intracellular ribozyme concentration, colocalization of the ribozyme with the target, specificity of the ribozyme for the desired mRNA, and an enhancement of ribozyme-mediated substrate turnover. As knowledge of RNA structure, secondary and tertiary, increases, RNAs will be targeted more rationally, which may help with the problems of specificity. At the same time, the understanding of the physical localization of RNA in cells and its tracking as it moves from the nucleus to the cytoplasm will also help ensure colocalization of the ribozyme and target. Modifications of the ribozymes, (e.g., the 2' ribose) with various agents, such as methyl, allyl, fluoro, and amino groups, increase the stability to nucleases quite dramatically. Similarly, chimeric DNA-RNA ribozymes increase the stability. The efficiency of delivery to cells with viral vectors or liposomes is also continually improving. These molecules must retain their catalytic potential, reach an accessible site on the substrate, and effectively impact the steady-state levels of target molecules to be useful either as surrogate genetic tools or as therapeutic agents. Great progress has been made in all of these areas and should allow extensive use of the highly specific reagents for downregulating expression of target RNAs.

7.1. RNA Interference

We focus on some of the most recent advances using RNAi-based technologies in mammalian systems, with a focus on applications in cancer research. Finally, we briefly compare the use of siRNA- and ribozyme-based approaches in downregulating specific mRNA targets.

The siRNAs are the functional entities produced by the enzymatic cleavage of longer dsRNAs by the enzyme Dicer. The most commonly used lengths are 21- and 22-nt duplexes that have two base 3' overhangs. Both siRNAs and short hairpin RNAs (shRNAs) can be chemically synthesized and introduced exogenously or expressed endogenously from a promoter (Fig. 2B) In vitro transcription kits for producing siRNAs are commercially available, as are supplies of chemically synthesized siRNAs. The following are useful Web sites for these suppliers and approaches:

http://www.ambion.com/techlib/misc/siRNA_design.html
http://www.qiagen.com/jp/siRNA/sirna_design.asp
http://www.dharmacon.com/
http://www.biobase.dk/embossdocs/sirna.html

For expression, two basic siRNA cassette designs have been used successfully. The first mimics the natural Dicer product and consists of two 21-nt RNAs, typically with a 2-nt overhang at each 3' end. The classic overhang consists of two uridines, but the overhang may also be derived from the intended target sequence. Longer siRNA stems, up to 29 nts long, can be used without triggering the interferon response in mammalian cells. The second design, referred to as an shRNA, consists of a single transcript containing both the target sense and antisense sequences connected by a hairpin loop. Loops as small as 4 nts have been part of effective siRNAs, but larger loops, up to 9 nts, are more reliable.

The pol III promoters have been particularly effective in transcribing siRNAs and shRNAs (ultimately processed to siRNAs), which elicit target-specific mRNA degradation *(76,77)*. The U6 + 1 promoter has a number of characteristics that make it particularly suitable for expressing siRNAs. U6 + 1 is an external promoter driving high expression in many cell types. Transcription begins at a specific initiating guanosine and terminates at a run of four or more sequential uridines in the transcript, leaving a 3' polyU overhang recognized by the RISC machinery. Finally, it is a relatively small promoter, easily introduced into numerous vector backbones. Additional pol III promoters have also been explored *(78)*, and pol II promoters are under development *(79)*.

Standard plasmid vectors can be used for transient endogenous expression of siRNAs. Stable expression has been achieved with both episomal *(80)* and retroviral *(81)* vectors. There have been several reports using lentiviral vectors *(82–85)* for long-term expression of siRNAs; packaged lentiviral vectors have the advantage that they can transduce both dividing and nondividing cells.

7.2. RNAi and Cancer Applications

SiRNA is currently under exploration as a tool to downregulate the product of the Philadelphia chromosome, which is the result of a reciprocal translocation between the unrelated BCR gene on chromosome 22 and ABL on chromosome 9, creating an oncogenic fusion gene. The resulting BCR/ABL gene and transcript is present in nearly all patients with chronic myeloid leukemia (CML), as well as in 30% of adults with acute lymphoblastic leukemia, who respond poorly to conventional therapies. Two versions can be defined by differing breakpoints in BCR: M-BCR and m-BCR, producing M-BCR/ABL and m-BCR/ABL oncoproteins of 210 kDa and 190 kDa, respectively*(86,87)*. The hybrid protein has elevated kinase activity compared to the normal cellular ABL homologue, which is thought to be part of the cascade of effects leading to oncogenic growth and inhibition of apoptosis.

Wilda and coworkers *(88)* used the human K652 chronic myelogenous leukemia cell line expressing M-BCR/ABL mRNA to test the ability of a synthetic siRNA to specifically downregulate the corresponding message and protein and increase susceptibility of the cells to apoptosis. Transiently transfected siRNA directed against the region spanning the M-BCR/ABL fusion joint specifically lowered p210 levels without affecting the endogenous ABL or vimentin proteins; a control siRNA with mismatches in both strands corresponding to seventh and eighth bases of the antisense strand had no effect. More important, the siRNA-induced reduction of the oncogenic transcript resulted in a desired physiological effect: The cells became more susceptible to apoptosis. Increased apoptosis was not observed with sense or antisense oligonucleotides alone, the mutant M-BCR/ABL siRNA, or an siRNA directed against the analogous target in the m-BCR/ABL fusion (not present in these cells). M-BCR/ABL siRNA induced similar levels of apoptosis as the chemotherapeutic agent STI 571 by 72 hours, although with slower kinetics. They did not observe an additive effect using both STI 571 and siRNA; however, only one concentration of STI 571 was tested, which may have induced near maximal levels of apoptosis. Reciprocal dose–response profiles for the M-BCR/ABL siRNA and STI 571 might have revealed cooperativity. Nonetheless, these results provide evidence that siRNA can specifically reduce levels of an oncogenic transcript and partially reverse an oncogenic growth characteristic in a cell line model system.

Scherr et al. *(89)* confirmed specific reduction of M-BCR/ABL mRNA in K562 cells by electroporation of the same siRNA and showed that endogenous c-bcr and c-abl levels were unchanged (with respect to cellular GAPDH). In addition, transfection of siRNA into murine TonB210.1 cells containing an inducible M-BCR/ABL reduced both mRNA and protein levels after induction; cell viability also declined in parallel, to approximately the same extent as STI 571 in previous experiments *(88)*. The authors also tested whether M-BCR/ABL siRNA could reduce cytokine-induced proliferation as well as bcr/abl-driven proliferation in TonB cells. Addition of interleukin 3 (IL-3) reversed both siRNA- and STI 571-induced growth inhibition, although the reduction of BCR/ABL mRNA levels was the same for siRNA-treated cells with or without IL-3; therefore, M-BCR/ABL siRNA reduces bcr/abl-dependent, but not cytokine-dependent, growth inhibition.

This result was particularly interesting in light of subsequent experiments in primary cells. Electroporation of M-BCR/ABL siRNA into PBMCs or purified $CD34^+$ cells derived from six patients with chronic myeloid leukemia with siRNA reduced levels of the oncogenic transcript by 50–79%. However, there was no growth inhibition or reduction in colony formation when primary cells were transfected with siRNA followed by growth in cytokine-supplemented liquid or semisolid media for cell proliferation assays or colony formation assays, respectively; in contrast, control treatment with STI571 was effective. The absence of M-BCR/ABL siRNA-dependent growth reduction in primary cells may reflect dilution of the siRNA over the experimental time period or, alternatively, interference by the cytokine cocktail used to culture the cells, reminiscent of the results in TonB cells. However, in TonB cells, IL-3 overcame both the siRNA and STI 571 effects; STI 571 was still inhibitory in the colony formation assays. This situation may be clarified by repeating the experiments with stably expressed M-BCR-ABL siRNA from a lentiviral backbone, for instance. Taken together, these experiments illustrate that siRNA can be a powerful method for reducing a specific oncogenic transcript; however, results in tissue culture cells may not automatically translate to primary cells or a physiological setting.

Similarly, siRNA is under testing to target the ALM1/MTG8 fusion oncogene resulting from translocation between chromosomes 21 and 8, which occurs in 10–15% of all patients with *de novo* AML *(89)*. The ALM1/MTG8 fusion converts the normal function of AML1 as a transcriptional activator regulating hematopoiesis to a constitutive and transdominant repressor, which may predispose cells to oncogenic transformation.

To understand better the role of AML/MTG8 in leukemogenesis, siRNA was used to study the effects of suppressing the oncogenic protein in human leukemic cell lines Kasumi-1 and SKNO-1. The authors designed several siRNAS that specifically target the AML/MTG8 fusion mRNA, analogous to the experiments with BCR/ABL. At 16 hours after transformation of Kasumi-1 cells, RNAse protection assays showed that 200-nM AML/MTG8 siRNAs specifically reduced the oncogene mRNA relative to endogenous AML1 compared to irrelevant and mutant AML1/MTG8 siRNAs. Similar results were observed in both SKNO-1 and Kasumi-1 cells as assayed by real-time reverse transcriptase polymerase chain reaction normalized to cellular GAPDH. Suppression of the oncogenic transcript persisted for 5 days and was paralleled by a major decrease of the corresponding protein for at least 4 days posttransfection; cellular AML was unaffected.

Next, the AML/MTG8 siRNAs were used to examine secondary effects induced by downregulation of the protein. Previous experiments have implicated the oncogenic protein in interfering with normal cytokine-induced upregulation of CD11 and macrophage colony-stimulating factor (M-CSF) receptor and, by inference, myelomonocytic differentiation in Kasumi-1 and SKNO-1 cells. Specifically, AML1/MTG8 binds to the transforming growth factor-β (TGF-β)-activated transcription factor SMAD3, potentially causing a block in TGF-β/vitamin D_3-mediated myeloid differentiation *(90)*. Likewise, the fusion protein binds to C/EBP-α, which is essential for granulocytic development *(91)*. The authors used AML1/MTG8 siRNA to connect downregulation of the protein directly with the reappearance of differentiation characteristics. AML1/MTG8 siRNA alone caused a small increase in the number of CD11b-positive Kasumi-1 cells. However, when AML1/MTG8siRNA was combined with TGF-β_1 and vitamin D_3 treatment, Kasumui-1 cells displayed decreased clonogenic growth; an increase in the number of cells carrying the myeloid differentiation marker CD11b-positive cells from a maximum of 20% (TGF-$\beta_{1-\beta}$/vitamin D-$\beta_{3-\beta}$ alone) to 40–60%; a substantial increase in surface M-CSF receptor expression; and a 60-fold increase in cellular C/EBP-α levels (over 15-fold with AML1/MTG8 siRNA alone). These results are consistent with a role of AML1/MTG8 in suppressing cytokine-driven induction of myeloid differentiation and maintaining the leukemic blast cell state and demonstrate the application of siRNA in gene functional analyses.

As a final example, RNAi has been used to target the product of the translocation t(11;22)(q24;q12), which produces the oncogenic EWS/Fli-1 fusion protein detected in 85% of Ewing's sarcoma and primitive neuroectodermal tumor cells. Two overlapping siRNAs asymmetrically targeting the fusion joint were expressed from the U6 + 1 promoter in the Ewing's sarcoma cell line TC135 *(92)*. Both EWS/Fli-1 siRNAS specifically reduced the fusion mRNA relative to cellular β-actin. However, the site II siRNA containing 17 bases of homology to Fli-1 also partially reduced endogenous Fli-1 mRNA. However, the converse did not occur; the site I siRNA containing 17 bases of homology with cellular EWS specifically downregulated only the oncogenic transcript. These results highlight the importance of monitoring potential cross-suppression of endogenous transcripts when using RNAi. TC135 cells cotransfected with the specific site I EWS/Fli-1 siRNA and an eGFP expression vector (to allow for FACS sorting of transfected cells) exhibited reduced rates of growth in culture for 3 weeks. In addition, c-Myc expression, which is activated by the EWS/Fli-1 protein, was also reduced by siRNA treatment.

In summary, siRNAs have been very effective in reducing levels of oncogenic fusion proteins such as M-BCR/ABL, AML/MTG8, and EWS/Fli-1. These results demonstrate the possibility of using siRNA as a therapeutic agent in these cancers, perhaps in conjunction with standard drug therapies. The success of this approach will depend in part on whether siRNAs can mediate both the reduction of target oncogenic transcripts and the desired downstream physiological changes in primary cancer cells.

7.3. SiRNA vs Ribozymes

SiRNA has emerged as a powerful tool to knock down mRNA transcripts specifically to a few percent of their original levels. This raises the question of when to choose siRNA or another nucleic acid-based technology. As a partial response, we end with a brief commentary on the use of ribozymes vs siRNAs, with a comparison of the potential advantages of each approach.

Currently, much more is known about tolerance to modifications that extend half-life and efficacy in transient applications of ribozymes than of siRNAs. Initial experiments indicated that fully 2'-*O*-methylated siRNAs are inactive *(21)*. More recent experiments have shown that limited 2'-*O*-methyl or phosphorothioate modifications at the ends of siRNAs only minimally reduce activity; comparable allyl modifications result in greater loss of activity *(93)*. Fluorine-derivatized siRNAs have also been used successfully *(94)*. Further research will be required to determine the degree and type of chemical modifications that can be tolerated by siRNAs.

Published evidence indicated that siRNA functions primarily, and possibly exclusively, in the cytoplasm *(95)*; consequently, siRNAs cannot target introns. Therefore, the only siRNA target site in a specific mRNA isoform is a unique exon–exon junction, which may be problematic if the site is refractory to siRNA degradation. Ribozymes can theoretically be designed against sequences anywhere in an isoform-specific intron, increasing the probability of finding a susceptible site, although the kinetics of splicing may limit effectiveness in any given instance. By the same token, ribozymes can be used when it is highly advantageous to degrade mRNA before it reaches the cytoplasm. For instance, early stages of cellular HIV replication tend to be more easily controlled by nucleic acid inhibitors as the mRNAs coding for the regulatory proteins are less abundant than the later structural genes. Also, inhibiting export of early viral RNAs coding for the early Tat and Rev regulatory proteins may prevent the initiation of active viral replication. For example, an anti-HIV ribozyme that was directed to the nucleolar compartment successfully inhibited HIV replication *(96)*.

Finding an effective target site within an mRNA can be problematic for both siRNA and ribozyme design. However, if the choice of target sites is limited, use of a ribozyme may not be possible if the site does not contain an appropriate triplet cleavage site, which is not a limitation of siRNA design. That aside, if a specific target site is refractive to siRNA, there are currently no options for improving cleavage of that site. A number of colocalization options exist to improve ribozyme accessibility by direction to specific cell compartments and sequence-directed colocalization with the target *(95–97)*. Moreover, a ribozyme appended to nonadjacent target antisense sequences can both colocalize the target and ribozyme and facilitate structural changes that make a target site more accessible (L. Scherer, 2003, unpublished data). The size requirement of siRNAs precludes the use of appended sequences, although there are exceptions *(99)*, and more may emerge as the biochemical processing pathways of siRNAs and the related microRNAs are better understood. Characterization of hybrid RNAs sharing both microRNA and siRNA characteristics has already begun *(100)*.

The use of siRNA will only continue to expand, especially as the biochemical mechanisms are better understood; however, RNAi is unlikely to supplant the use of ribozymes, aptamers, and related approaches completely. Besides the issues already raised, the RNAi apparatus appears to be saturable; consequently, the number of simultaneous mRNAs that can be targeted by RNAi may be limited. SiRNAs provide an additional tool that may be even more powerful combined with other nucleic acid-based therapies.

ACKNOWLEDGMENT

J. J. R. was supported by the National Institutes of Health (AI 29329 and AI 42552).

REFERENCES

1. Bevilacqua, P. C. and Turner, D. H. (1991) Comparison of binding of mixed ribose-deoxyribose analogues of CUCU to a ribozyme and to GGAGAA by equilibrium dialysis: evidence for ribozyme specific interactions with 2' OH groups. *Biochemistry* **30**, 10,632–10,640.
2. Guerrier-Takada, C. and Altman, S. (1992) Reconstitution of enzymatic activity from fragments of M1 RNA. *Proc. Natl. Acad. Sci. USA* **89**, 1266–1270.
3. Kruger, K., Grabowski, P. J., Zaug, A. J., Sands, J., Gottschling, D. E., and Cech, T. R. (1982) Self-splicing RNA: autoexcision and autocyclization of the ribosomal RNA intervening sequence of *Tetrahymena. Cell* **31**, 147–157.
4. Costa, M. and Michel, F. (1995) Frequent use of the same tertiary motif by self-folding RNAs. *EMBO J.* **14**, 1276–1285.
5. Hutchins, C. J., Rathjen, P. D., Forster, A. C., and Symons, R. H. (1986) Self-cleavage of plus and minus RNA transcripts of avocado sunblotch viroid. *Nucleic Acids Res.* **14**, 3627–3640.
6. Buzayan, J. M., McNinch, J. S., Schneider, I. R., and Bruening, G. (1987) A nucleotide sequence rearrangement distinguishes two isolates of satellite tobacco ringspot virus RNA. *Virology* **160**, 95–99.
7. Buzayan, J. M., Hampel, A., and Bruening, G. (1986) Nucleotide sequence and newly formed phosphodiester bond of spontaneously ligated satellite tobacco ringspot virus RNA. *Nucleic Acids Res.* **14**, 9729–9743.
8. Kumar, P. K., Suh, Y. A., Miyashiro, H., et al. (1992) Random mutations to evaluate the role of bases at two important single-stranded regions of genomic HDV ribozyme. *Nucleic Acids Res.* **20**, 3919–3924.
9. Saville, B. J. and Collins, R. A. (1990) A site-specific self-cleavage reaction performed by a novel RNA in *Neurospora* mitochondria. *Cell* **61**, 685–696.
10. Cech, T. R. (2000) Structural biology. The ribosome is a ribozyme. *Science* **289**, 878–879.
11. Moore, P. B. and Steitz, T. A. (2002) The involvement of RNA in ribosome function. *Nature* **418**, 229–235.
12. Moore, P. B. and Steitz, T. A. (2003) After the ribosome structures: how does peptidyl transferase work? *RNA* **9**, 155–159.
13. Nissen, P., Hansen, J., Ban, N., Moore, P. B., and Steitz, T. A. (2000) The structural basis of ribosome activity in peptide bond synthesis. *Science* **289**, 920–930.
14. Setlik, R. F., Shibata, M., Sarma, R. H., et al. (1995) Modeling of a possible conformational change associated with the catalytic mechanism in the hammerhead ribozyme. *J. Biomol. Struct. Dyn.* **13**, 515–522.
15. Lipkowitz, M. S., Hanss, B., Tulchin, N., et al. (1999) Transduction of renal cells in vitro and in vivo by adeno-associated virus gene therapy vectors. *J. Am. Soc. Nephrol.* **10**, 1908–1915.
16. Ullu, E., Djikeng, A., Shi, H., and Tschudi, C. (2002) RNA interference: advances and questions. *Philos. Trans. R. Soc. Lond. B Biol. Sci.* **357**, 65–70.
17. Boutla, A., Delidakis, C., Livadaras, I., Tsagris, M., and Tabler, M. (2001) Short 5'-phosphorylated double-stranded RNAs induce RNA interference in *Drosophila. Curr. Biol.* **11**, 1776–1780.

18. Vaucheret, H., Beclin, C., and Fagard, M. (2001) Post-transcriptional gene silencing in plants. *J. Cell Sci.* **114,** 3083–3091.
19. Hannon, G. J. (2002) RNA interference. *Nature* **418,** 244–251.
20. Banerjee, D. and Slack, F. (2002) Control of developmental timing by small temporal RNAs: a paradigm for RNA-mediated regulation of gene expression. *Bioessays* **24,** 119–129.
21. Elbashir, S. M., Harborth, J., Lendeckel, W., Yalcin, A., Weber, K., and Tuschl, T. (2001) Duplexes of 21-nucleotide RNAs mediate RNA interference in cultured mammalian cells. *Nature* **411,** 494–498.
22. Elbashir, S. M., Lendeckel, W., and Tuschl, T. (2001) RNA interference is mediated by 21- and 22-nucleotide RNAs. *Genes Dev.* **15,** 188–200.
23. Rossi, J. J. (1992) Ribozymes. *Curr. Opin. Biotechnol.* **3,** 3–7.
24. Rossi, J. J. (1995) Therapeutic antisense and ribozymes. *Br. Med. Bull.* **51,** 217–225.
25. Rossi, J. J. (1997) Therapeutic applications of catalytic antisense RNAs (ribozymes). *CIBA Found. Symp.* **209,** 195–204.
26. Rossi, J. J. (1999) Ribozymes, genomics and therapeutics. *Chem. Biol.* **6,** R33–R37.
27. Snyder, D. S., Wu, Y., McMahon, R., Yu, L., Rossi, J. J., and Forman, S. J. (1997) Ribozyme-mediated inhibition of a Philadelphia chromosome-positive acute lymphoblastic leukemia cell line expressing the p190 bcr-abl oncogene. *Biol. Blood Marrow Transplant.* **3,** 179–186.
28. Snyder, D. S., Wu, Y., Wang, J. L., et al. (1993) Ribozyme-mediated inhibition of bcr-abl gene expression in a Philadelphia chromosome-positive cell line. *Blood* **82,** 600–605.
29. Kuwabara, T., Warashina, M., Tanabe, T., Tani, K., Asano, S., and Taira, K. (1998) A novel allosterically trans-activated ribozyme, the maxizyme, with exceptional specificity in vitro and in vivo. *Mol. Cell* **2,** 617–627.
30. Lange, W. (1995) Cleavage of BCR/ABL mRNA by synthetic ribozymes—effects on the proliferation rate of K562 cells. *Klin. Paediatr.* **207,** 222–224.
31. Hertel, K. J., Pardi, A., Uhlenbeck, O. C., et al. (1992) Numbering system for the hammerhead. *Nucleic Acids Res.* **20,** 3252.
32. Kijima, H., Tsuchida, T., Kondo, H., et al. (1998) Hammerhead ribozymes against gamma-glutamylcysteine synthetase mRNA down-regulate intracellular glutathione concentration of mouse islet cells. *Biochem. Biophys. Res. Commun.* **247,** 697–703.
33. Czubayko, F., Liaudet-Coopman, E.D., Aigner, A., Tuveson, A. T., Berchem, G. J., and Wellstein, A. (1997) A secreted FGF-binding protein can serve as the angiogenic switch in human cancer. *Nat. Med.* **3,** 1137–1140.
34. Kobayashi, H., Dorai, T., Holland, J. F., and Ohnuma, T. (1994) Reversal of drug sensitivity in multidrug-resistant tumor cells by an MDR1 (PGY1) ribozyme. *Cancer Res.* **54,** 1271–1275.
35. Scanlon, K. J., Ishida, H., and Kashani-Sabet, M. (1994) Ribozyme-mediated reversal of the multidrug-resistant phenotype. *Proc. Natl. Acad. Sci. USA* **91,** 11,123–11,127.
36. Wang, F. S., Kobayashi, H., Liang, K. W., Holland, J. F., and Ohnuma, T. (1999) Retrovirus-mediated transfer of anti-MDR1 ribozymes fully restores chemosensitivity of P-glycoprotein-expressing human lymphoma cells. *Hum. Gene Ther.* **10,** 1185–1195.
37. Funato, T., Shitara, T., Tone, T., Jiao, L., Kashani-Sabet, M., and Scanlon, K. J. (1994) Suppression of H-ras-mediated transformation in NIH3T3 cells by a ras ribozyme. *Biochem. Pharmacol.* **48,** 1471–1475.
38. Funato, T. (1997) [Circumventing multidrug resistance in human cancer by anti-ribozyme]. *Nippon Rinsho* **55,** 1116–1121.
39. Gibson, S. A., Pellenz, C., Hutchison, R. E., Davey, F. R., and Shillitoe, E. J. (2000) Induction of apoptosis in oral cancer cells by an anti-bcl-2 ribozyme delivered by an adenovirus vector. *Clin. Cancer Res.* **6,** 213–222.
40. Maelandsmo, G. M., Hovig, E., Skrede, M., et al. (1996) Reversal of the in vivo metastatic phenotype of human tumor cells by an anti-CAPL (mts1) ribozyme. *Cancer Res.* **56,** 5490–5498.
41. Sehgal, G., Hua, J., Bernhard, E. J., Sehgal, I., Thompson, T. C., and Muschel, R. J. (1998) Requirement for matrix metalloproteinase-9 (gelatinase B) expression in metastasis by murine prostate carcinoma. *Am. J. Pathol.* **152,** 591–596.
42. Czubayko, F., Riegel, A. T., and Wellstein, A. (1994) Ribozyme-targeting elucidates a direct role of pleiotrophin in tumor growth. *J. Biol. Chem.* **269,** 21,358–21,363.
43. Yamamoto, H., Irie, A., Fukushima, Y., et al. (1996) Abrogation of lung metastasis of human fibrosarcoma cells by ribozyme-mediated suppression of integrin alpha6 subunit expression. *Int. J. Cancer* **65,** 519–524.
44. Feng, B., Rollo, E. E., and Denhardt, D. T. (1995) Osteopontin (OPN) may facilitate metastasis by protecting cells from macrophage NO-mediated cytotoxicity: evidence from cell lines down-regulated for OPN expression by a targeted ribozyme. *Clin. Exp. Metastasis* **13,** 453–462.
45. Czubayko, F., Downing, S. G., Hsieh, S. S., et al. (1997) Adenovirus-mediated transduction of ribozymes abrogates HER-2/neu and pleiotrophin expression and inhibits tumor cell proliferation. *Gene Ther.* **4,** 943–949.
46. Frimerman, A., Welch, P. J., Jin, X., et al. (1999) Chimeric DNA-RNA hammerhead ribozyme to proliferating cell nuclear antigen reduces stent-induced stenosis in a porcine coronary model. *Circulation* **99,** 697–703.
47. Gu, J. L., Pei, H., Thomas, L., et al. (2001) Ribozyme-mediated inhibition of rat leukocyte-type 12-lipoxygenase prevents intimal hyperplasia in balloon-injured rat carotid arteries. *Circulation* **103,** 1446–1452.
48. Jarvis, T. C., Alby, L. J., Beaudry, A. A., et al. (1996) Inhibition of vascular smooth muscle cell proliferation by ribozymes that cleave c-myb mRNA. *RNA* **2,** 419–428.

49. Yokoyama, Y., Wan, X., Shinohara, A., Takahashi, Y., and Tamaya, T. (2001) Hammerhead ribozymes to modulate telomerase activity of endometrial carcinoma cells. *Hum. Cell* **14,** 223–231.
50. Kashani-Sabet, M. (2002) Ribozyme therapeutics. *J. Investig. Dermatol. Symp. Proc.* **7,** 76–78.
51. Heidenreich, O., Benseler, F., Fahrenholz, A., and Eckstein, F. (1994) High activity and stability of hammerhead ribozymes containing 2'-modified pyrimidine nucleosides and phosphorothioates. *J. Biol. Chem.* **269,** 2131–2138.
52. Burgin, A. B. Jr., Gonzalez, C., Matulic-Adamic, J., et al. (1996) Chemically modified hammerhead ribozymes with improved catalytic rates. *Biochemistry* **35,** 14,090–14,097.
53. Flory, C. M., Pavco, P. A., Jarvis, T. C., et al. (1996) Nuclease-resistant ribozymes decrease stromelysin mRNA levels in rabbit synovium following exogenous delivery to the knee joint. *Proc. Natl. Acad. Sci. USA* **93,** 754–758.
54. Morgan, R. A. and Anderson, W. F. (1993) Human gene therapy. *Annu. Rev. Biochem.* **62,** 191–217.
55. Perlman, H., Sata, M., Krasinski, K., Dorai, T., Buttyan, R., and Walsh, K. (2000) Adenovirus-encoded hammerhead ribozyme to Bcl-2 inhibits neointimal hyperplasia and induces vascular smooth muscle cell apoptosis. *Cardiovasc. Res.* **45,** 570–578.
56. Giordano, V., Jin, D. Y., Rekosh, D., and Jeang, K. T. (2000) Intravirion targeting of a functional anti-human immunodeficiency virus ribozyme directed to pol. *Virology* **267,** 174–184.
57. Horster, A., Teichmann, B., Hormes, R., Grimm, D., Kleinschmidt, J., and Sczakiel, G. (1999) Recombinant AAV-2 harboring gfp-antisense/ribozyme fusion sequences monitor transduction, gene expression, and show anti-HIV-1 efficacy. *Gene Ther.* **6,** 1231–1238.
58. Kunke, D., Grimm, D., Denger, S., et al. (2000) Preclinical study on gene therapy of cervical carcinoma using adeno-associated virus vectors. *Cancer Gene Ther.* **7,** 766–777.
59. L'Huillier, P. J., Soulier, S., Stinnakre, M. G., et al. (1996) Efficient and specific ribozyme-mediated reduction of bovine alpha-lactalbumin expression in double transgenic mice. *Proc. Natl. Acad. Sci. USA* **93,** 6698–6703.
60. Welch, P. J., Yei, S., and Barber, J. R. (1998) Ribozyme gene therapy for hepatitis C virus infection. *Clin. Diagn. Virol.* **10,** 163–171.
61. Smith, S. M., Maldarelli, F., and Jeang, K. T. (1997) Efficient expression by an alphavirus replicon of a functional ribozyme targeted to human immunodeficiency virus type 1. *J. Virol.* **71,** 9713–9721.
62. Castanotto, D., Bertrand, E., and Rossi, J. (1997) Exogenous cellular delivery of ribozymes and ribozyme encoding DNAs. *Methods Mol. Biol.* **74,** 429–439.
63. Efrat, S., Leiser, M., Wu, Y. J., et al. (1994) Ribozyme-mediated attenuation of pancreatic beta-cell glucokinase expression in transgenic mice results in impaired glucose-induced insulin secretion. *Proc. Natl. Acad. Sci. USA* **91,** 2051–2055.
64. Tang, J. and Breaker, R. R. (1998) Mechanism for allosteric inhibition of an ATP-sensitive ribozyme. *Nucleic Acids Res.* **26,** 4214–4221.
65. Zhao, J. J. and Lemke, G. (1998) Selective disruption of neuregulin-1 function in vertebrate embryos using ribozyme-tRNA transgenes. *Development* **125,** 1899–1907.
66. Zhao, J. J. and Pick, L. (1993) Generating loss-of-function phenotypes of the fushi tarazu gene with a targeted ribozyme in *Drosophila. Nature* **365,** 448–451.
67. Sullenger, B. A. (1996) Ribozyme-mediated repair of RNAs encoding mutant tumor suppressors. *Cytokines Mol. Ther.* **2,** 201–205.
68. Watanabe, T. and Sullenger, B. A. (2000) RNA repair: a novel approach to gene therapy. *Adv. Drug Deliv. Rev.* **44,** 109–118.
69. Sullenger, B. A. and Cech, T. R. (1994) Ribozyme-mediated repair of defective mRNA by targeted, trans-splicing. *Nature* **371,** 619–622.
70. Chaulk, S. G. and MacMillan, A. M. (1998) Caged RNA: photo-control of a ribozyme reaction. *Nucleic Acids Res.* **26,** 3173–3178.
71. Hager, A. J. and Szostak, J. W. (1997) Isolation of novel ribozymes that ligate AMP-activated RNA substrates. *Chem. Biol.* **4,** 607–617.
72. Santoro, S. W. and Joyce, G. F. (1998) Mechanism and utility of an RNA-cleaving DNA enzyme. *Biochemistry* **37,** 13330.
73. Coetzee, T., Herschlag, D., and Belfort, M. (1994) Escherichia coli proteins, including ribosomal protein S12, facilitate in vitro splicing of phage T4 introns by acting as RNA chaperones. *Genes Dev.* **8,** 1575–1588.
74. Bertrand, E., Pictet, R., and Grange, T. (1994) Can hammerhead ribozymes be efficient tools to inactivate gene function? *Nucleic Acids Res.* **22,** 293–300; published erratum appears in *Nucleic Acids Res.* **22,** 1326.
75. Sioud, M. (1996) Ribozyme modulation of lipopolysaccharide-induced tumor necrosis factor-alpha production by peritoneal cells in vitro and in vivo. *Eur. J. Immunol.* **26,** 1026–1031.
76. Lee, N. S., Dohjima, T., Bauer, G., et al. (2002) Expression of small interfering RNAs targeted against HIV-1 rev transcripts in human cells. *Nat. Biotechnol.* **20,** 500–505.
77. Paul, C. P., Good, P. D., Winer, I., and Engelke, D. R. (2002) Effective expression of small interfering RNA in human cells. *Nat. Biotechnol.* **20,** 505–508.
78. Paul, C. P., Good, P. D., Li, S. X., Kleinhauer, A., Rossi, J. J., and Engelke, D. R. (2003) Localized expression of small RNA inhibitors in human cells. *Mol. Ther.* **7,** 237–247.

79. Xia, X., Mao, Q., Paulson, H. L., and Davidson, B. L. (2002) siRNA-mediated gene silencing in vitro and in vivo. *Nat. Biotechnol.* **20**, 1006–1010.
80. Wilson, J. A., Jayasena, S., Khvorova, A., et al. (2003) RNA interference blocks gene expression and RNA synthesis from hepatitis C replicons propagated in human liver cells. *Proc. Natl. Acad. Sci. USA* **100**, 2783–2788.
81. Barton, G. M. and Medzhitov, R. (2002) Retroviral delivery of small interfering RNA into primary cells. *Proc. Natl. Acad. Sci. USA* **99**, 14,943–14,945.
82. Abbas-Terki, T., Blanco-Bose, W., Deglon, N., Pralong, W., and Aebischer, P. (2002) Lentiviral-mediated RNA interference. *Hum. Gene Ther.* **13**, 2197–2201.
83. Qin, X. F., An, D. S., Chen, I. S., and Baltimore, D. (2003) Inhibiting HIV-1 infection in human T cells by lentiviral-mediated delivery of small interfering RNA against CCR5. *Proc. Natl. Acad. Sci. USA* **100**, 183–188.
84. Rubinson, D. A., Dillon, C. P., Kwiatkowski, A. V., et al. (2003) A lentivirus-based system to functionally silence genes in primary mammalian cells, stem cells and transgenic mice by RNA interference. *Nat. Genet.* **33**, 401–406.
85. Tiscornia, G., Singer, O., Ikawa, M., and Verma, I. M. (2003) A general method for gene knockdown in mice by using lentiviral vectors expressing small interfering RNA. *Proc. Natl. Acad. Sci. USA* **100**, 1844–1848.
86. Hooberman, A. L., Rubin, C. M., Barton, K. P., and Westbrook, C. A. (1989) Detection of the Philadelphia chromosome in acute lymphoblastic leukemia by pulsed-field gel electrophoresis. *Blood* **74**, 1101–1107.
87. Rubin, C. M., Larson, R. A., Bitter, M. A., et al. (1987) Association of a chromosomal 3;21 translocation with the blast phase of chronic myelogenous leukemia. *Blood* **70**, 1338–1342.
88. Wilda, M., Fuchs, U., Wossmann, W., and Borkhardt, A. (2002) Killing of leukemic cells with a BCR/ABL fusion gene by RNA interference (RNAi). *Oncogene* **21**, 5716–5724.
89. Scherr, M., Battmer, K., Winkler, T., Heidenreich, O., Ganser, A., and Eder, M. (2003) Specific inhibition of bcr-abl gene expression by small interfering RNA. *Blood* **101**, 1566–1569.
90. Jakubowiak, A., Pouponnot, C., Berguido, F., et al. (2000) Inhibition of the transforming growth factor beta 1 signaling pathway by the AML1/ETO leukemia-associated fusion protein. *J. Biol. Chem.* **275**, 40,282–40,287.
91. Pabst, T., Mueller, B. U., Zhang, P., et al. (2001) Dominant-negative mutations of CEBPA, encoding CCAAT/enhancer binding protein-alpha (C/EBPalpha), in acute myeloid leukemia. *Nat. Genet.* **27**, 263.
92. Dohjima, T., Lee, N. S., Li, H., Ohno, T., and Rossi, J. J. (2003) Small interfering RNAs expressed from a Pol III promoter suppress the EWS/Fli-1 transcript in an Ewing sarcoma cell line. *Mol. Therapy* **7**, 811–816.
93. Amarzguioui, M., Holen, T., Babaie, E., and Prydz, H. (2003) Tolerance for mutations and chemical modifications in a siRNA. *Nucleic Acids Res.* **31**, 589–595.
94. Capodici, J., Kariko, K., and Weissman, D. (2002) Inhibition of HIV-1 infection by small interfering RNA-mediated RNA interference. *J. Immunol.* **169**, 5196–5201.
95. Zeng, Y. and Cullen, B. R. (2002) RNA interference in human cells is restricted to the cytoplasm. *RNA* **8**, 855–860.
96. Michienzi, A., Cagnon, L., Bahner, I., and Rossi, J. J. (2000) Ribozyme-mediated inhibition of HIV 1 suggests nucleolar trafficking of HIV-1 RNA. *Proc. Natl. Acad. Sci. USA* **97**, 8955–8960.
97. Lee, N. S., Sun, B., Williamson, R., Gunkel, N., Salvaterra, P. M., and Rossi, J. J. (2001) Functional colocalization of ribozymes and target mRNAs in Drosophila oocytes. *FASEB J.* **15**, 2390–2400.
98. Castanotto, D., Scherr, M., and Rossi, J. J. (2000) Intracellular expression and function of antisense catalytic RNAs. *Methods Enzymol.* **313**, 401–420.
99. Kawasaki, H., Suyama, E., Iyo, M., and Taira, K. (2003) siRNAs generated by recombinant human Dicer induce specific and significant but target site-independent gene silencing in human cells. *Nucleic Acids Res.* **31**, 981–987.
100. Zeng, Y., Wagner, E. J., and Cullen, B. R. (2002) Both natural and designed micro RNAs can inhibit the expression of cognate mRNAs when expressed in human cells. *Mol. Cell* **9**, 1327–1333.

6

Fusogeneic Membrane Glycoproteins for Cancer Gene Therapy

A Better Class of Killer

Andrew Bateman, Vy Phan, Alan Melcher,
Emmanouela Linardakis, Kevin Harrington, and Richard Vile

1. INTRODUCTION

There are currently no vector systems available that are efficient enough or targeted enough to transduce all of the tumor cells in a patient with even a single copy of a therapeutic gene *(1–4)*. Ideally, therefore, the genes used for gene transfer therapy of cancer should be able to achieve two major goals. The first is to kill tumor cells locally with high efficiency. The second is to stimulate potent antitumor immunity such that distant metastases, to which genes cannot be delivered, can also be eradicated.

Several different classes of genes have been used for the direct killing of tumor cells at a local site, including immune stimulatory genes *(5,6)* and the suicide genes, such as the herpes simplex virus thymidine kinase (HSV-TK) and cytosine deaminase genes *(7)*. The genes used so far have very different forms and functions, but most focus on destruction of the target cells *(8–18)*. That destruction may be brought about through direct cytotoxicity of the protein encoded by the gene, by the initiation of cellular signaling pathways that induce apoptosis, or by expression of a protein that stimulates immune cells to recognize and kill the tumor cells. However, although there are literally hundreds of different genes that can kill the cells in which they are expressed, perhaps the most pertinent issue at the moment is how to kill those cells in which the gene is not expressed. This is a critical clinical question and currently dominates the field of gene therapy of cancer because of the problems encountered in finding delivery vehicles sufficiently efficient and targeted to deliver genes to every tumor cell. Even at the level of delivery to localized, inoperable tumors, this issue is highly problematic; when the treatment of systemically distributed metastases is considered, however, the problems associated with gene delivery (or the lack of it) become daunting.

There are, however, steps that can be taken to improve the efficacy of gene therapy even in the absence of the elusive "magic bullet" vector. There are two principal areas in which the activity of the gene can help to compensate for the paucity of its delivery into tumors. The first is that it should have a potent local bystander killing effect; that is, expression of the gene in a single cell can lead to killing of close neighbors without the need for it to be expressed directly by those cells. The second is that it should induce strong systemic bystander effects. Here, tumor cells in completely separate deposits from those that are accessible and targetable by gene delivery vectors can be killed as a result of localized expression of the gene. Such systemic bystander effects usually operate through stimulation of immune effector cells that, once activated against tumor antigens, can circulate systemically

From: *Contemporary Cancer Research*
Cancer Gene Therapy
Edited by: D. T. Curiel and J. T. Douglas © Humana Press Inc., Totowa, NJ

and selectively find, recognize, and destroy residual tumor cells. The specificity of appropriately activated T cells makes them the key players in generating systemic bystander responses, and most molecular immunotherapies are aimed at stimulating T-cell responses against tumor-associated antigens. Alternatively, systemic bystander killing effects can also be raised using genes that interfere with crucial processes central to tumor development, such as angiogenesis. Hence, genes encoding systemic factors, such as angiostatin or endostatin, which inhibit endothelial cell proliferation, can also be effective against distant tumor deposits by effectively starving them of their developing blood supplies.

The early clinical trials of genes designed to kill tumor cells—including cytokines and HSV-TK—showed that the potency of the bystander effects seen in rodent animal models is clearly much reduced in the clinical setting of patients with advanced tumors and, frequently, suppressed immune systems. Therefore, we explored the possibilities to kill tumor cells using genes that have much greater levels of potency in cell killing at the levels of (1) direct tumor cell killing, (2) local bystander cell killing, and (3) systemic bystander cell killing.

2. FUSOGENIC MEMBRANE GLYCOPROTEINS

2.1. A Novel Cytotoxic Gene

It has long been known that some viruses infect cells by expressing envelope proteins that can bind to receptors on target cells and then mediate fusion of the virus with the target cell membrane, thereby releasing the viral core particle into the cell's cytoplasm. In addition, expression of the envelope gene in newly infected cells allows the generation of new viral particles and their subsequent release for further rounds of infection. However, a byproduct of cellular envelope expression is that neighboring, uninfected cells expressing the viral receptor can also bind to the envelope, leading to fusion between the infected and uninfected cells. This fusion can occur between a single envelope-expressing cell and many surrounding cells as long as they express the receptor. The result is the formation of large, multinucleated syncytia, which will eventually become nonviable and die. This characteristic—the recruitment of multiple bystander cells into structures ultimately destined to die—is exactly what we hope to achieve with gene transfer into tumor cells at the local bystander killing level.

Over the last 5 years, we have shown that transfer of genes encoding viral fusogenic membrane glycoproteins (FMGs) into tumor cells can provide a new approach to cytoreductive gene therapy for cancer that has shown potent antitumor efficacy both in vitro and in vivo *(19–22)*. We initially used three examples of these envelope genes and showed that their ability to kill cells locally is indeed greatly enhanced over other commonly used genes, such as HSV-TK. In culture experiments, expression of the gibbon ape leukemia virus (GALV) retroviral FMG, the vesicular stomatitis virus G (VSV-G) protein, or the measles virus F and H proteins by a single cell was able to recruit over 200 bystander cells into syncytia and thereby kill them (Figs. 1 and 2). In contrast, every cell expressing HSV-TK was able to kill only about 10 other cells through the metabolic conversion, and cell–cell transfer, of ganciclovir into its toxic derivative *(20,21)* (Fig. 3).

Therefore, our data showed that FMG transfection is a much more effective treatment for killing human tumor lines in vitro than commonly used suicide genes (Fig. 3). Killing is cell density dependent, is independent of cell division, and does not require administration of a prodrug, thereby alleviating the problems of drug delivery and bioavailability. In addition, we have shown that delivery of a hyperfusogenic mutant of either the GALV or the measles virus F and H protein combination in the context of plasmid or viral vectors leads to therapeutic reductions in the growth of human tumor xenografts in nude mice *(20,21)* despite the relatively low efficiency of gene transfer (Fig. 4A,B). Therefore, FMG delivery directly to tumors growing *in vivo* offers the potential for direct tumor killing and improved local control of tumor growth.

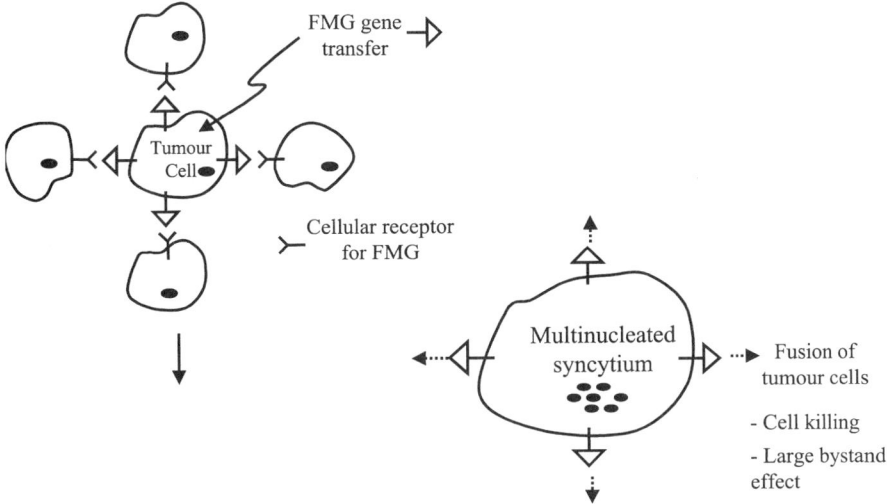

Fig. 1. FMG for gene therapy of cancer: local bystander killing.

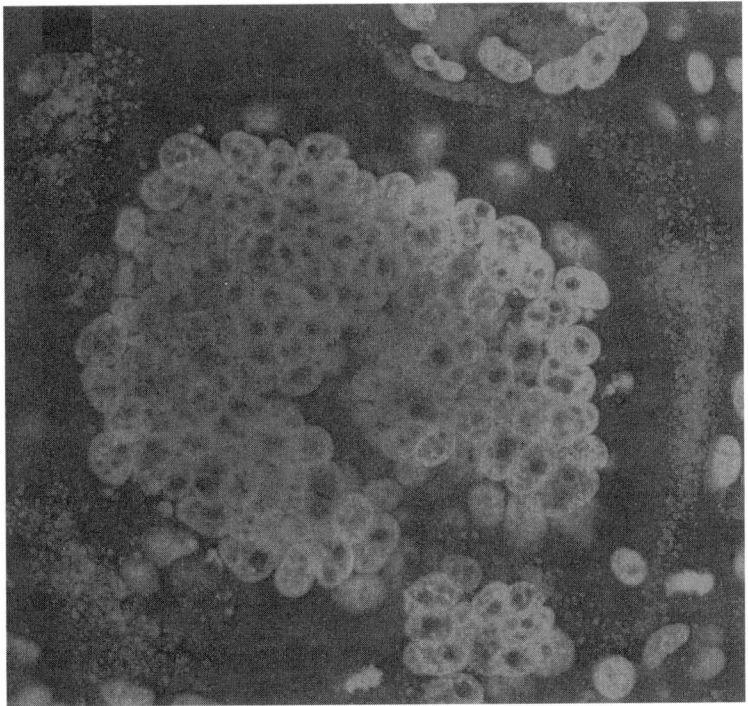

Fig. 2. A multinucleated syncytium consisting of nuclei from about 200 cells that have been fused together by expression of an FMG.

2.2. *Pathological-like Tumor Cell Killing From a Single Gene*

Although the extent of direct and local bystander cell death *per se* has a significant bearing on the outcome of any cytoreductive gene therapy approach, no vector system can at present reliably deliver therapeutic transgenes systemically to metastatic cancer deposits disseminated throughout the body *(3)*. Therefore, strategies that prime a systemic immune response against untransduced tumor cells and metastatic deposits offer the most immediate prospect of clinically beneficial gene therapy *(23)*.

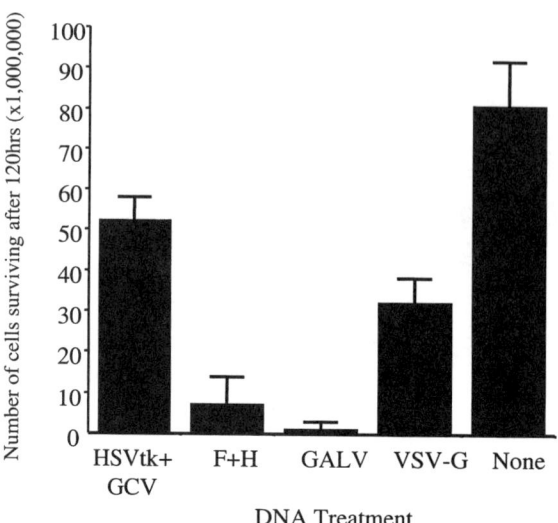

Fig. 3. In vitro killing: FMG vs suicide genes (GCV, ganciclovir).

In this respect, work in our laboratory as well as elsewhere has demonstrated that the biochemical mechanisms by which cancer cells are killed are very important to the subsequent immunogenicity of that death *(24–27)*. In general terms, cell death by the highly ordered process of apoptosis, with subsequent phagocytosis of neatly packaged cellular fragments by macrophages, escapes detection by the immune system and is actually immunosuppressive *(28,29)*. In contrast, cancer cell death through nonapoptotic (necrotic/oncotic) mechanisms—separate from nonphysiological processes such as freeze-thaw processes or osmotic shock—is proinflammatory and has the potential to prime the generation of a systemic antitumor immune response *(24–27,29)* (Fig. 5).

For these reasons, we set out to characterize the mechanisms by which FMG-mediated syncytial formation leads to cell killing. Many different biochemical pathways leading to apoptosis have been described, and it is becoming increasingly unclear exactly what constitutes apoptotic as opposed to nonapoptotic death *(30–32)*. However, by multiple different criteria, syncytia-associated cell death proceeds through pathways that lack the morphological, cytogenetic, or biochemical markers of classical apoptosis *(30,31,33,34)*. We could not detect significant changes in the level of expression of pro- or antiapoptotic genes at any point through syncytial formation (0–24 hours after transfection), development (24–72 hours), and disintegration (72–120 hours) *(35)*. FMG-mediated cytotoxicity was not inhibited by the pan-caspase inhibitor Z-Val-Ala-Asp-fluoromethyl ketone (ZVAD-fmk), and there was minimal activation of pro-caspase 3 or cleavage of poly(ADP-ribose) polymerase (PARP), typical indicators of caspase-dependent apoptotic cell death.

DNA (deoxyribonucleic acid) analysis of syncytia indicated a G2-M block occurring with time following initiation of syncytial formation and a lack of accumulation of cells in a sub-G1 peak, again indicating a lack of apoptotic death. TUNEL and DNA laddering assays were uniformly negative with the exception at very late stages of the killing process when the majority of tumor cells were dead. We also observed that syncytial development is structurally a highly ordered process *(35)*. However, at late stages, disintegration of the syncytia occurs, marked usually by nuclear fusion, severe depletion of cellular adenosine triphosphate (which is known to inhibit many apoptotic pathways), and the appearance of multiple acidified vacuoles that resemble lysosomes. Subsequent death of the syncytia is rapid, probably through a process that is most akin to autophagy *(32,36,37)*. The precise triggers that turn a viable, ordered syncytium into a self-digesting, dying aggregate may include the increasing volume of the syncytium, cell cycle-associated signals, or the severe meta-

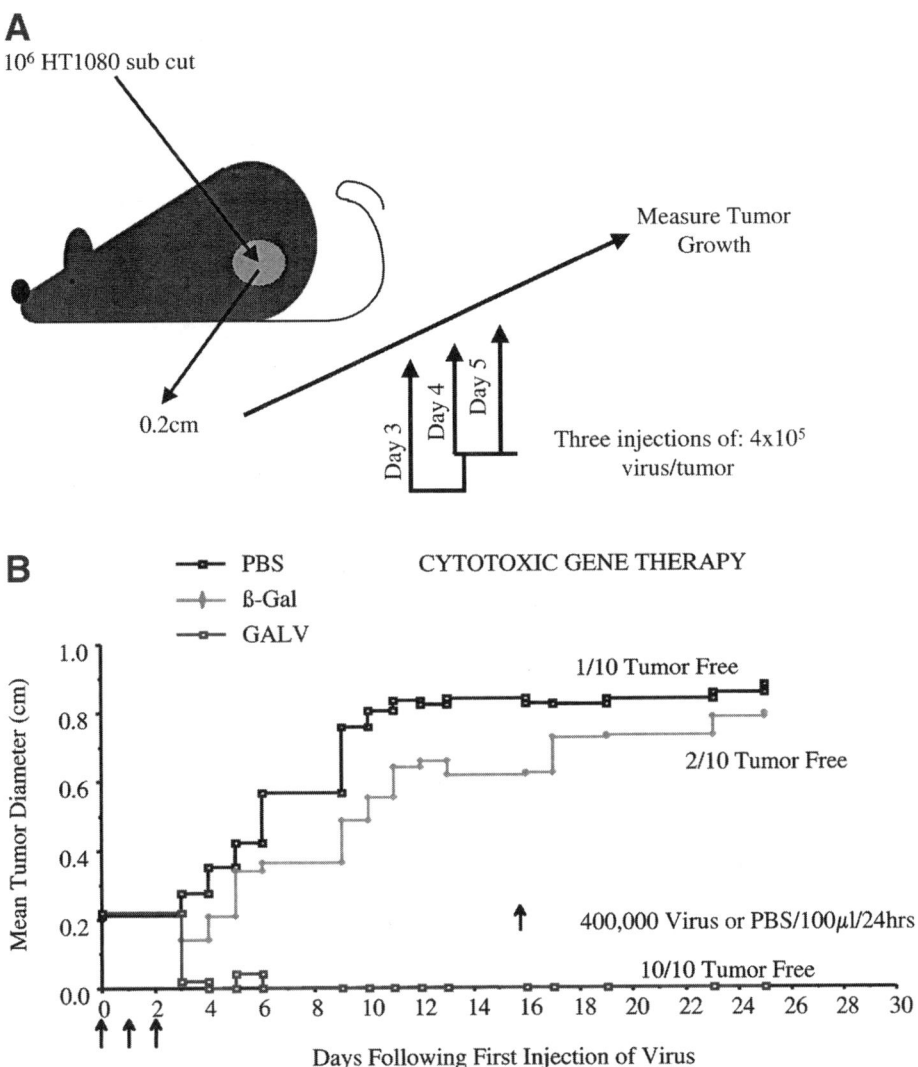

Fig. 4. (A) In vivo gene therapy with Lenti-GALV virus. **(B)** Cytotoxic gene therapy.

bolic depletion that occurs as a result of trying to maintain such a huge cellular structure. Importantly, these mechanisms are independent of the five different cell types that we tested and were similar for two different FMGs *(35)* (Table 1).

We and others have shown that direct killing of tumor cells in vivo with the HSV-TK suicide gene system can, in some cases, stimulate antitumor immunity *(14,24,38)*. In particular, the mechanisms by which tumor cells are killed is critical to the attraction of professional antigen-presenting cells (APCs)—such as dendritic cells (DCs) and macrophages–to the site of killing *(25,29,39)*. In general, large amounts of apoptotic death that overwhelms the local phagocytic capacity to clear it *(25,28, 40,41)* or nonapoptotic cell death associated with activation of stress response programs *(24,26,27, 29,42)* lead to activation of antitumor immune responses (Fig. 5). Therefore, we hypothesized that the nonapoptotic killing of tumor cells that we observed with FMG may have significant immunostimulatory properties.

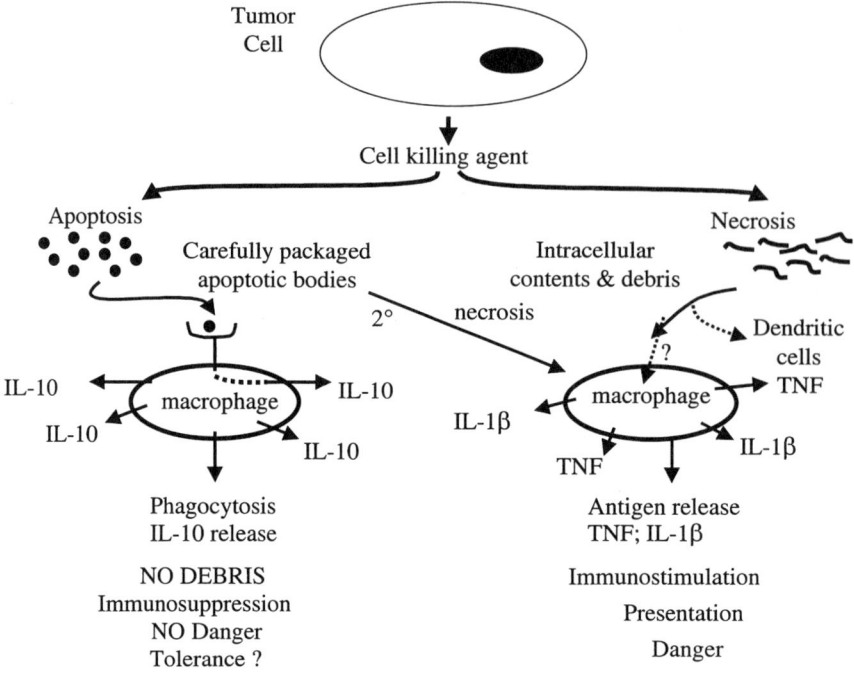

Fig. 5. The different immunological consequences of apoptotic or necrotic cell death.

Table 1
Characteristics of FMG-Mediated Cell Death

Nonapoptotic by classical markers: TUNEL, EM, ZVAD, PARP cleavage, procaspase 3 activation,
 morphology, cytochrome-*c* release, RPA for proapoptotic genes
Associated with increasing cell volume
Autophagic markers
Metabolic depletion: ATP depletion, fructose inhibition
Induction of hsp70
Vacuolation and blebbing: reminiscent of exosomes?

We observed that fusing tumor cells release increased numbers of tumor-derived, exosomelike vesicles *(43,44)* compared to normal cells growing in culture or tumor cells killed through irradiation, osmotic shock, or freezing-thawing *(35)* (Fig. 6). Moreover, exosomes from FMG-mediated fusion are also of a significantly enhanced quality in terms of their ability to transfer tumor-derived material into immature DCs. Finally, we observed that this loading of DCs is immunologically relevant because it allows the cross-presentation by DCs of gp100, a known tumor antigen. This cross presentation was significantly more reproducible and effective than using tumor-derived exosomes from other sources of cell killing, including irradiation and HSV-TK/ganciclovir-mediated killing. For these reasons, we believe that the exosomes produced from FMG-mediated fusing tumor cells *(syncytiosomes)* are qualitatively different from exosomes derived from other sources in ways that enhance their recognition, uptake, and loading abilities regarding DCs *(35)*.

These observations are particularly provocative given the increasing interest in the concept that cells can communicate with each other via the release of secreted vesicles. Such vesicles, in different

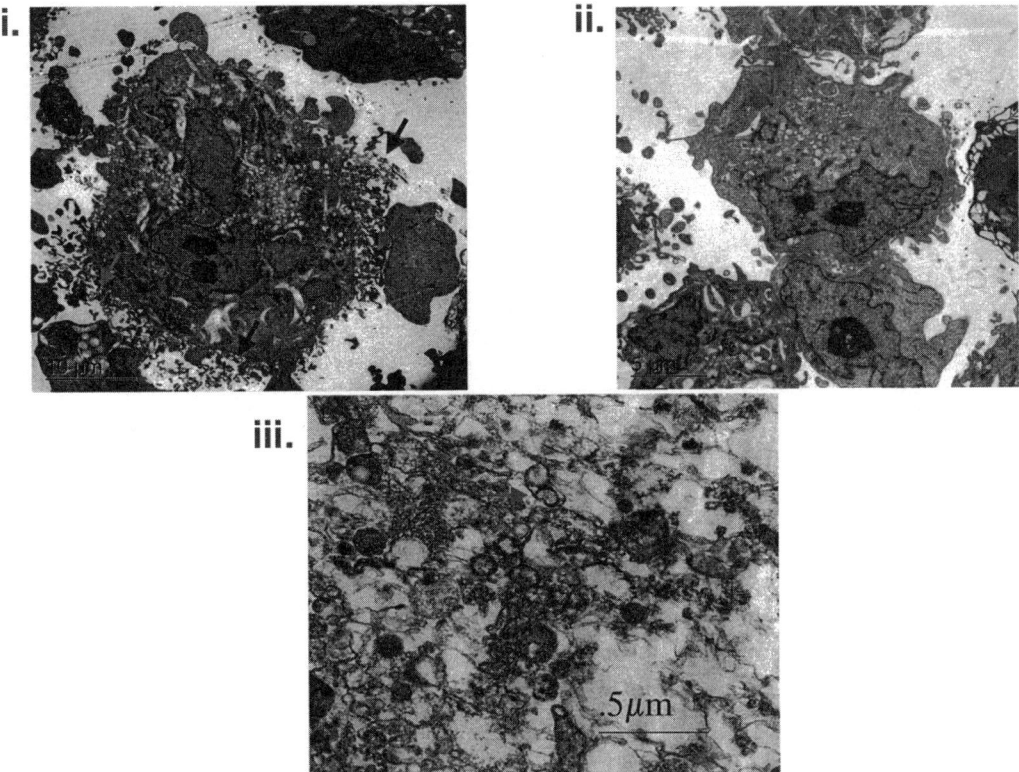

Fig. 6. Electron microscopy of fusing tumor cells (**i**) shows release of numerous membrane vesicles that are seen in greatly reduced number of normal cells (**ii**). In (**iii**), purification of these particles shows a population of exosome-like vesicles.

forms, have been proposed to act as intercellular messengers for, among other things *(45)*, membrane exchange of major histocompatibility complex class I molecules to downregulate T-cell responses, antigen transfer into APCs to stimulate antitumor immune responses *(43,46)*, immune evasion and increased tumorigenesis *(47)*, and sampling of peripheral tissue self-antigens by DCs as a means to maintain tolerance to self-antigens *(48,49)*. It may even be possible that viral shedding is some form of parasitisation of normal cellular membrane vesicle secretion pathways *(50)*. Therefore, the identification and characterization of a novel family of such cellular-secreted vesicles, such as we described with syncytiosome production *(35)*, may represent an important new addition to the concept of membrane vesicles as intercellular messengers.

Taken together, our studies have indicated that syncytial cell killing not only promotes antigen release, but also allows entry of the antigen into the class I antigen-processing pathways for (cross) presentation by DCs. These data are significant in several ways. First, they demonstrate that syncytial killing occurs through a nonapoptotic pathway associated with an enhanced ability to deliver antigens into DCs for cross-presentation to T cells. This may represent a natural immunological adaptation to viral infection that allows the immune system to see viral-induced cell fusion as an immunogenic event *(42)*. Second, these results highlight the possibility that transfer of cellular antigens to DCs following infections with fusogenic viruses also may play a role in the etiology of some autoimmune diseases by helping to break tolerance to self-antigens *(51)*. Third, specific mechanisms must also exist in the few situations when physiological cell fusion occurs, both to prevent cell killing and to prevent the immunostimulatory nature of syncytiosome release from inducing potent autoimmune disease. Foremost among such examples is the formation of the syncytiotrophoblasts involved in placental formation, for which endogenous retroviral FMGs have been mechanistically implicated *(52,53)*. Finally, and of direct relevance to our studies discussed here, the functional efficiency of transfer of cellular tumor antigens into DCs using syncytiosomes may allow insights into mechanisms of antigen loading and presentation that will allow simpler, cell-free methods for the generation of cancer cell vaccines.

2.3. Liberating Tumor Antigens for Better Vaccine Production

Given the observations discussed in the previous sections, we reasoned that fusing tumor cells to each other, with the associated immune stimulatory mechanisms of cell killing, may provide an effective method to liberate relevant tumor antigens from cancer vaccine cells along with several additional immune-potentiating benefits. Consistent with this hypothesis, we observed that a single gene modification of a tumor cell vaccine line (VSV-G-induced tumor cell fusion) is effective in generating both rejection of established tumor as well as long-term T-cell-mediated protection responses (Fig. 7) *(54)*. Syncytia of tumor cells are likely to be good targets for natural killer and other nonspecific immune effector killing mechanisms through expression of the viral immunogen VSV-G *(55–57)*.

In addition, direct syncytial-mediated cell killing will release immune-stimulatory molecules at the vaccine site that will recruit and activate host APCs *(27)*, and stress proteins expressed within the syncytia *(20)* should contribute directly to immune stimulation *(24,26,29,58)*. Thus, released tumor-associated antigens will then become available for cross-presentation by host APCs *(59–62)*.

Our hypothesis is that the activation of cellular stress programs in response to VSV-G-mediated fusion *(20,22)* may mimic a pathological-type situation, which is sensed by the cell as an immunologically relevant situation *(25,42)*. Consistent with this view, we observed that macrophages recruited to the subcutaneous site of fusing cell vaccination are significantly activated *in situ* by the presence of fusing cells, permitting initiation of a more effective antitumor immune response *(29)*.

Clinically, these data offer new opportunities for the design of tumor cell vaccines. By modifying either patient-recovered tumor explants or established allogeneic cell lines with a gene for an FMG, fusing tumor cell vaccines can be produced in vitro for patient use (Fig. 8).

3. MORE OPPORTUNITIES IN AN ALREADY BROAD PORTFOLIO

We are currently exploring additional situations for which the expression of an FMG in different cell types may allow the development of improved protocols and treatments over and above currently existing options.

3.1. Tumor Cell-DC Hybrids

The fusion of tumor cells with APCs has been proposed as an efficient method to render antigenic tumor cells highly immunogenic *(63)*. This would be achieved by virtue of the ability of the hybrids to express a full repertoire of tumor antigens (from the tumor fusion partner) along with the costimulatory and antigen-presenting machinery (class I and II major histocompatibility complex molecules) of the APC partner. The immunotherapeutic advantage of such an approach is that, in principle, it covers the entire range of tumor-associated antigens without having to clone them individually and allows the hybrids to present both class I- and class II-associated epitopes of these antigens directly to T cells to induce tumor-specific cytotoxic T-cell responses *(64,65)*.

Hybrid cell vaccines have shown considerable promise in a variety of preclinical model systems *(66,67)*. The APC partners of the fusions have been either B cells *(66)* or DCs *(67)*. In addition, the DC component of the fusion vaccine can be either autologous or allogeneic *(64,68)*. Either way, such approaches have demonstrated eradication of established tumors dependent on the generation of T-cell memory *(66,68–74)*. Moreover, this technology has now entered clinical trials in patients with malignant melanoma *(75)* and glioma *(76)*.

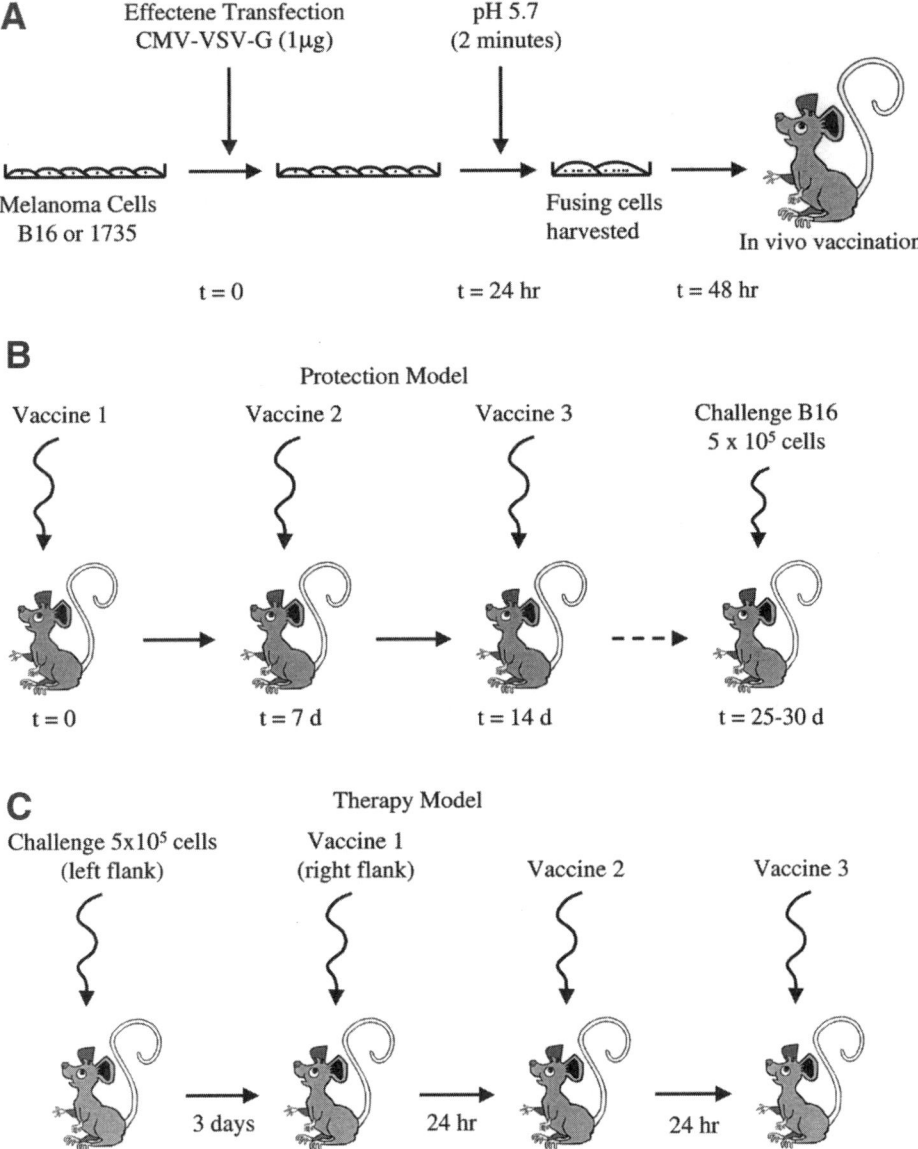

Fig. 7. Fusing cell vaccine protocol (B16 model). (**A**) The protocol for in vitro production of fusing cell vaccines that are often used in either a prophylactic vaccination model against challenge with live tumor (**B**) or in a therapeutic vaccination model following the establishment of subcutaneous tumor (**C**).

The methodology to achieve hybrid cell formation has so far relied on the use of chemical reagents such as polyethylene glycol *(77)* or physical techniques such as electrofusion *(78,79)*. However, in both of these methodologies, the nature of the cell fusion event is difficult to characterize and, in some cases, to standardize. In addition, the levels of cell fusion are somewhat difficult to assess. Most studies have used FACS analysis to determine the percentage of fusion that occurs within the cultures using coalescence of fluorescent dyes or costaining with tumor cell- and APC-derived markers *(80,81)*. However, these techniques are still somewhat difficult to interpret in terms of the quantity and the quality of the fusion produced. These difficulties arise from false positivity because of leakage of dyes between

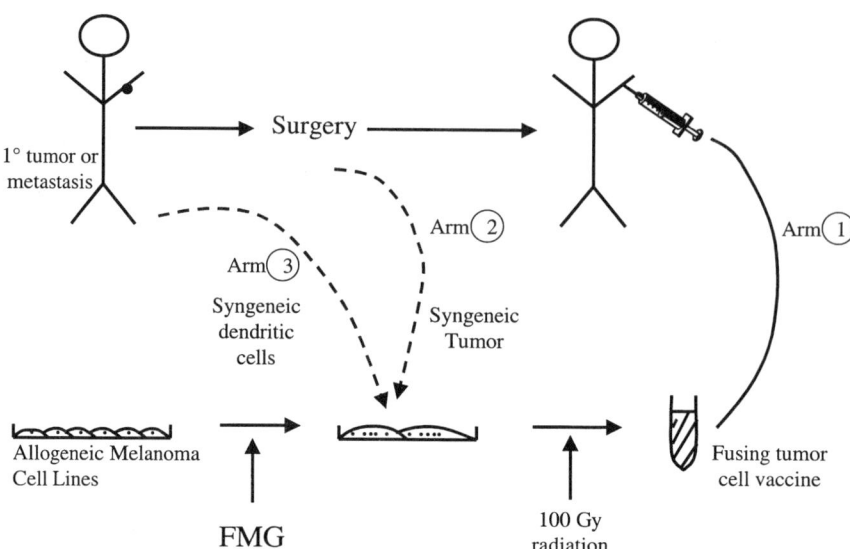

Fig. 8. Clinical protocol for use of fusing tumor cell vaccines.

cells, the phagocytosis by (unfused) DCs of debris from dying tumor cells, and the problems of making accurate distinctions between aggregated and fused cells by FACS.

Given our work with tumor cell–tumor cell fusion, we hypothesized that we might be able to exploit FMG gene transfer to mediate the fusion between tumor cells and DCs for the generation of hybrid cell vaccines. We demonstrated that FMG gene transfer to tumor cells followed by admixing with DCs generates a population of small (2–4 nuclei), short-lived tumor cell/DC hybrids that retain their ability to traffic to lymph nodes, are extremely potent in their ability to present a model antigen to T cells in vitro, and are highly immunogenic in vivo. We detected hybrid formation dependent on the provision of tumor cell-specific transcription factors into the cytoplasm/nucleus of the DC to activate expression of a tumor-tissue-specific promoter stably integrated into the genome of the DC. Only on cell fusion is the promoter activated. This assay therefore differentiates genuine fusion—in which cell contents become mixed—from other effects, such as cell aggregation.

3.2. Making Replicating Vectors Better

Most of the clinical trials of in vivo gene delivery have been disappointing in terms of the levels of transduction of human tumors compared to the preclinical studies in fast-growing rodent systems *(82,83)*. Significant advances, therefore, are required to make gene therapy a realistic prospect for cancer treatment, including development of vector systems to increase the efficiency, coupled with targeting, of gene transfer to human tumors *in situ*. Acceptance of this has led to increasing advocacy of the use of replicating viruses for delivery to both local and disseminated tumors *(3,4,84–93)*. However, problems associated with achieving effective tumor targeting remain even with replicating constructs *(4,92)*.

There are now both established and growing portfolios of replicating viral systems with proposed tumor-selective, oncolytic properties *(86,91,94–96)*. In particular, the development of conditionally replication-competent adenoviral vectors *(86,91,92,97)* offers the chance to combine several different levels of both targeting and therapeutic approaches. Surface *(98)*, transcriptional *(99)*, and cancer cell-specific genetic targeting *(100,101)* have all been described with vectors derived from this virus *(86,91)*. In addition, the virus is lytic, and a wide variety of therapeutic genes of all of the classes described above can be incorporated *(86,97)*. Nonetheless, it is still very clear that methods are still

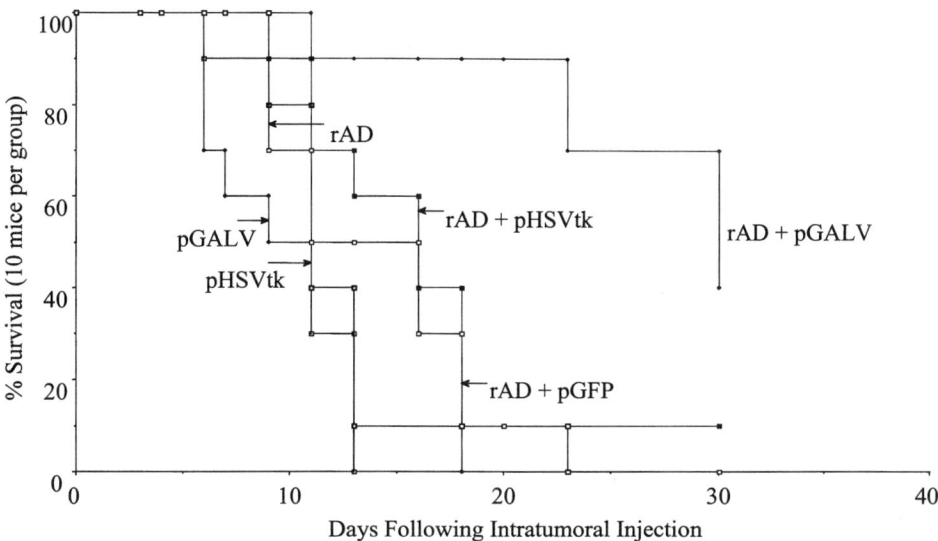

Fig. 9. Intratumoral expression of GALV enhances the efficacy of replicating adenovirus therapy in well-established LnCap tumors.

required to improve the efficiency and selectivity of replicating adenoviruses because of the problems of immune inactivation of vector and poor levels of viral spread through the tumor *(3,91,92)*.

Regarding the last point, therapeutic improvements, therefore, will derive from virus designs that enhance virus release and spread through a tumor. Our studies *(102)* showed that the FMG-mediated syncytial formation significantly enhances the efficacy of replicating adenoviral therapy through modest increases in total viral titers (total virus produced from infected cells); greater viral release from cultures of infected syncytial cultures compared to normal nonfusing monolayers; and, consistent with a report regarding use of the human immunodeficiency virus gp120 FMG *(103)*, enhanced spread of adenoviral particles through the tumor cell cultures.

Interestingly, we have observed that syncytial death is associated with metabolic depletion caused by very high metabolic activity of syncytia *(22)*. Moreover, expression of several different transgenes is significantly increased from syncytial cultures *(53,104)*. Therefore, the increased metabolic activity induced by syncytial formation appears to convert syncytia into transient protein production factories associated with increased levels of translation of preexisting messenger ribonucleic acids that, in this case, lead to increased levels of E1A and viral production. These effects may reflect a mechanism by which syncytial-inducing viruses ensure maximal levels of viral protein and particle production before the death of the parasitized cell.

As well as the overall increase in viral titer, syncytial formation is also associated with increased release of adenoviral particles on a per-cell basis. Most probably this is caused at least in part by lysis of infected cells releasing intracellular particles that would otherwise remain cell associated for longer. Therefore, the increased level of viral production coupled with accelerated release of viral particles and the resultant dispersal through tumor cell cultures would suggest that combination therapy with FMG expression and replicating adenovirus infection may overcome some of the problems associated with the use of replicating adenovirotherapy that have been seen to date.

Indeed, the efficacy of intratumoral injection of replicating adenovirus is greatly enhanced by the coinjection of an FMG-encoding plasmid *(102)* (Fig. 9). This combinatorial approach was sufficient to eradicate very small established tumors at viral doses in which injection of the virus or plasmid alone was not effective. Intratumoral injections into large, established, slow-growing tumors was also significantly more effective than either low-dose plasmid GALV or replication-competent adeno-virus (rAD) therapy alone (Fig. 9). These data suggest that replicating adenoviruses expressing the GALV FMG will be significantly more potent than viruses lacking the transgene. However, in addition, there is potential value in keeping the FMG component of the therapy separate from the replicating virus. Cotransduction of virus and plasmid as described here allows the use of significantly lower doses of both components (FMG plasmid and virus). In addition, should systemic release of virus or plasmid occur, the chances of them being carried together significant distances to normal tissues is low, thereby reducing the overall chances of toxicity associated with either type of treatment.

Finally, in addition to these studies with adenoviruses, the GALV FMG has also been expressed in the context of an oncolytic HSV, resulting in significantly enhanced antitumoral effects of the virus. Tumor specificity of the virus was maintained by expressing the FMG from a late viral promoter only activated following initiation of viral DNA replication *(105)*. Such results indicate that the value of FMG expression within viral vectors is unlikely to be restricted to a single virus type.

4. CONCLUSION: A MULTIFUNCTIONAL ANTICANCER DRUG FOR ONCOLOGISTS, IMMUNOLOGISTS, AND VIROLOGISTS

Expression of FMG genes in tumor cells leads to tumor cell killing that proceeds through syncytial formation, metabolic exhaustion, and autophagic degeneration. This is very efficient at killing tumor cells directly and has a large bystander effect. Equally important, the killing process is potentially highly immunostimulatory because it is accompanied by release of tumor-derived syncytiosomes capable of loading DCs with defined tumor antigens and leading to their processing and cross presentation by the DCs.

In particular, we believe that FMG-mediated syncytial formation mimics a pathological-type infection to which tumor cells react with activation of stress-related programs *(29)* that alert the immune system to the cell death in a potent immunostimulatory fashion *(25,26,42,106)*. These properties, along with several other potential uses of the FMG, make it clear that gene transfer of FMG-encoding genes represents an exciting new area to improve direct tumor cell killing, antitumor immune activation, cancer cell vaccine design, and development of more potent vector systems. As a result, FMG-mediated gene delivery, both alone and in combination with other genes, offers great potential as a treatment for both locally recurrent and systemically disseminated cancer.

REFERENCES

1. Verma, I. and Somia, N. (1977) Gene therapy—promises, problems and prospects. *Nature* **389,** 239–242.
2. Vile, R. G., Sunassee, K., and Diaz, R. M. (1998) Strategies for achieving multiple layers of selectivity in gene therapy. *Mol. Med. Today* **4,** 84–92.
3. Vile, R. G., Russell, S. J., and Lemoine, N. R. (2000) Cancer gene therapy: hard lessons and new courses. *Gene Ther.* **7,** 2–8.
4. Harrington, H., Alvarez-Vallina, L., Crittenden, M., et al. (2002) Cells as vehicles for cancer gene therapy: the missing link between targeted vectors and systemic delivery? *Hum. Gene Ther.* **13,** 1263–1280.
5. Colombo, M. P. and Forni, G. (1996) Immunotherapy: cytokine gene transfer strategies. *Cancer Metastasis Rev.* **15,** 317–328.
6. Vile, R. G. and Chong, H. (1996) Immunotherapy: combinatorial molecular immunotherapy—a synthesis and suggestions. *Cancer Metastasis Rev.* **15,** 351–364.
7. Moolten, F. L. (1994) Drug sensitivity ("suicide") genes for selective cancer chemotherapy. *Cancer Gene Ther.* **1,** 279–287.
8. Vile, R. G. and Hart, I. R. (1994) Targeting of cytokine gene expression to malignant melanoma cells using tissue-specific promoter sequences. *Ann. Oncol.* **5,** S59–S65.
9. Castleden, S. A., Chong, H., Garcia-Ribas, I., et al. (1997) A family of bicistronic vectors to enhance both local and systemic anti tumour effects of HSVtk or cytokine expression in a murine melanoma model. *Hum. Gene Ther.* **8,** 2087–2102.

10. Chong, H., Hutchinson, G., Hart, I. R., and Vile, R. G. (1998) Expression of B7 co-stimulatory molecules by B16 melanoma results in a natural killer cell-dependent local anti tumour response, but induces T cell-dependent systemic immunity only against B7-expressing tumours. *Br. J. Cancer* **78**, 1043–1050.

11. Diaz, R. M., Todryk, S., Chong, H., et al. (1998) Rapid adenoviral transduction of freshly resected tumour explants with therapeutically useful genes provides a rationale for genetic immunotherapy for colorectal cancer. *Gene Ther.* **5**, 869–879.

12. Vile, R. G. and Hart, I. R. (1993) In vitro and in vivo targeting of gene expression to melanoma cells. *Cancer Res.* **53**, 962–967.

13. Vile, R. G. and Hart, I. R. (1993) Use of tissue-specific expression of the herpes simplex virus thymidine kinase gene to inhibit growth of established murine melanomas following direct intratumoral injection of DNA. *Cancer Res.* **53**, 3860–3864.

14. Vile, R. G., Nelson, J. A., Castleden, S., Chong, H., and Hart, I. R. (1994) Systemic gene therapy of murine melanoma using tissue specific expression of the HSVtk gene involves an immune component. *Cancer Res.* **54**, 6228–6234.

15. Vile, R. G., Miller, N., Chernajovsky, Y., and Hart, I. R. (1994) A comparison of the properties of different retroviral vectors containing the murine tyrosinase promoter to achieve transcriptionally targeted expression of the HSVtk or IL-2 genes. *Gene Ther.* **1**, 307–316.

16. Chong, H., Todryk, S., Hutchinson, G., Hart, I. R., and Vile, R. G. (1998) Tumour cell expression of B7 costimulatory molecules and interleukin-12 or granulocyte-macrophage colony stimulating factor induces a local antitumour response and may generate systemic protective immunity. *Gene Ther.* **5**, 223–232.

17. Chester, J., Ruchatz, A., Gough, M., et al. (2002) Tumor antigen-specific induction of transcriptionally targeted retroviral vectors from chimeric immune receptor-modified T cells. *Nat. Biotechnol.* **20**, 256–263.

18. Harrington, K. J., Melcher, A. A., Bateman, A. R., Ahmed, A., and Vile, R. G. (2002) Cancer gene therapy: Part 2. Candidate transgenes and their clinical development. *Clin. Oncol. (R. Coll. Radiol.)* **14**, 148–169.

19. Fielding, A. K., Chapel-Fernandes, S., Chadwick, M. P., et al. (2000) A hyperfusogenic gibbon ape leukaemia envelope glycoprotein: targeting of a cytotoxic gene by ligand display. *Hum. Gene Ther.* **11**, 817–826.

20. Bateman, A., Bullough, F., Murphy, S., et al. (2000) Fusogenic membrane glycoproteins as a novel class of genes for the local and immune-mediated control of tumor growth. *Cancer Res.* **60**, 1492–1497.

21. Diaz, R. M., Bateman, A., Emiliusen, L., et al. (2000) A lentiviral vector expressing a fusogenic glycoprotein for cancer gene therapy. *Gene Ther.* **7**, 1656–1663.

22. Higuchi, H., Bronk, S., Bateman, A., Harrington, K. J., Vile, R. G., and Gores, G. J. (2000) Viral fusogenic membrane glycoprotein expression causes syncytia formation with bioenergetic cell death: implications for gene therapy. *Cancer Res.* **60**, 6396–6402.

23. Pardoll, D. M. (1995) Paracrine cytokine adjuvants in cancer immunotherapy. *Annu. Rev. Immunol.* **13**, 399–415.

24. Melcher, A. A., Todryk, S., Hardwick, N., Ford, M., Jacobson, M., and Vile, R. G. (1998) Tumor immunogenicity is determined by the mechanism of cell death via induction of heat shock protein expression. *Nat. Med.* **4**, 581–587.

25. Melcher, A. A., Gough, M. J., Todryk, S., and Vile, R. G. (1999) Apoptosis or necrosis for tumour immunotherapy—what's in a name? *J. Mol. Med.* **77**, 824–833.

26. Basu, S., Binder, R. J., Suto, R., Anderson, K. M., and Srivastava, P. K. (2000) Necrotic but not apoptotic cell death releases heat shock proteins, which deliver a partial maturation signal to dendritic cells and activate the NF-kappaB pathway. *Int. Immunol.* **12**, 1539–1546.

27. Gallucci, S., Lolkema, M., and Matzinger, P. (1999) Natural adjuvants: endogenous activators of dendritic cells. *Nat. Med.* **5**, 1249–1255.

28. Savill, J. and Fadok, V. (2000) Corpse clearance defines the meaning of cell death. *Nature* **407**, 784–788.

29. Gough, M. J., Melcher, A. A., Ahmed, A., et al. (2001) Macrophages orchestrate the immune response to tumor cell death. *Cancer Res.* **61**, 7240–7247.

30. Leist, M. and Jaattela, M. (2001) Four deaths and a funeral: from caspases to alternative mechanisms. *Nat. Rev. Mol. Cell Biol.* **2**, 589–598.

31. Kitanaka, C. and Kuchino, Y. (1999) Caspase-independent programmed cell death with necrotic morphology. *Cell Death Differ.* **6**, 508–515.

32. Clarke, P. G. (1990) Developmental cell death: morphological diversity and multiple mechanisms. *Anat. Embryol. (Berl.)* **181**, 195–213.

33. Hengartner, M. O. (2000) The biochemistry of apoptosis. *Nature* **407**, 770–776.

34. Denecker, G., Vercammen, D., Declercq, W., and Vandenabeele, P. (2001) Apoptotic and necrotic cell death induced by death domain receptors. *Cell Mol. Life Sci.* **58**, 356–370.

35. Bateman, A., Harrington, K., Kottke, T., et al. (2002) Viral fusogenic membrane glycoproteins kill solid tumor cells by non-apoptotic mechanisms which promote cross presentation of tumor antigens by dendritic cells. *Cancer Res.* **62**, 5466–6578.

36. Dunn, W. A. J. (1994) Autophagy and related mechanisms of lysosome-mediated protein degradation. *Trends Cell Biol.* **4**, 139–143.

37. Liang, X. H., Jackson, S., Seaman, M., et al. (1999) Induction of autophagy and inhibition of tumorigenesis by beclin 1. *Nature* **402,** 672–676.
38. Freeman, S. M., Ramesh, R., and Marrogi, A. J. (1997) Immune system in suicide gene therapy. *Lancet* **349,** 2–3.
39. Reiter, I., Krammer, B., and Schwamberger, G. (1999) Cutting edge: differential effect of apoptotic versus necrotic tumor cells on macrophage antitumor activities. *J. Immunol.* **163,** 1730–1732.
40. Albert, M. L., Sauter, B., and Bhardwaj, N. (1998) Dendritic cells acquire antigen from apoptotic cells and induce class I-restricted CTLs. *Nature* **392,** 86–89.
41. Bellone, M., Iezzi, G., Rovere, P., et al. (1997) Processing of engulfed apoptotic bodies yields T cell epitopes. *J. Immunol.* **159,** 5391–5399.
42. Matzinger, P. (1994) Tolerance, danger and the extended family. *Annu. Rev. Immunol.* **12,** 991–1045.
43. Wolfers, J., Lozier, A., Raposo, G., et al. (2001) Tumor-derived exosomes are a source of shared tumor rejection antigens for CTL cross-priming. *Nat. Med.* **7,** 297–303.
44. Clayton, A., Court, J., Navabi, H., et al. (2001) Analysis of antigen presenting cell derived exosomes, based on immunomagnetic isolation and flow cytometry. *J. Immunol. Methods* **247,** 163–174.
45. Thery, C., Zitvogel, L., and Amigorena, S. (2002) Exosomes: composition, biogenesis and function. *Nat. Rev. Immunol.* **2,** 569–579.
46. Andre, F., Schartz, N. E., Movassagh, M., et al. (2002) Malignant effusions and immunogenic tumour-derived exosomes. *Lancet* **360,** 295–305.
47. Dolo, V., Ginestra, A., Cassara, D., et al. (1998) Selective localisation of matrix metalloproteinase 9, beta 1 integrins, and human lymphocyte antigen class I molecules on membrane vesicles shed by 8701-BC breast carcinoma cells. *Cancer Res.* **58,** 4468–4474.
48. Karlsson, M. (2001) Tolerosomes are produced by intestinal epithelial cells. *Eur. J. Immunol.* **31,** 2892–2900.
49. Steinman, R. M., Turley, S., Mellman, I., and Inaba, K. (2000) The induction of tolerance by dendritic cells that have captured apoptotic cells [comment]. *J. Exp. Med.* **191,** 411–416.
50. Brown, G., Aitken, J., Rixon, H. W., and Sugrue, R. J. (2002) Caveolin-1 is incorporated into mature respiratory syncytial virus particles during virus assembly on the surface of virus infected cells. *J. Gen. Virol.* **83,** 611–621.
51. Marrack, P., Kappler, J., and Kotzin, B. L. (2001) Autoimmune disease: why and where it occurs. *Nat. Med.* **7,** 899–905.
52. Blond, J. L., Lavillette, D., Cheynet, V., et al. (2000) An envelope glycoprotein of the human endogenous retrovirus HERV-W is expressed in the human placenta and fuses cells expressing the type D mammalian retrovirus receptor. *J. Virol.* **74,** 3321–3329.
53. Mi, S., Lee, X., Li, X., et al. (2000) Syncytin is a captive retroviral envelope protein involved in human placental morphogenesis. *Nature* **403,** 785–789.
54. Linardakis, E., Bateman, A., Phan, V., et al. (2002) Enhancing the efficacy of a weak allogeneic melanoma vaccine by viral fusogenic membrane glycoprotein-mediated tumor cell-tumor cell fusion. *Cancer Res.* **62,** 5495–5504.
55. Mandelboim, O., Lieberman, N., Lev, M., et al. (2001) Recognition of haemagglutinins on virus-infected cells by NKp46 activates lysis by human NK cells. *Nature* **409,** 1055–1060.
56. Eslahi, N. K., Muller, S., Nguyen, L., et al. (2001) Fusogenic activity of vesicular stomatitis virus glycoprotein plasmid in tumors as an enhancer of IL-12 gene therapy. *Cancer Gene Ther.* **8,** 55–62.
57. Schirrmacher, V., Haas, C., Bonifer, R., Ahlert, T., Gerhards, R., and Ertel, C. (1999) Human tumor cell modification by virus infection: an efficient and safe way to produce cancer vaccine with pleiotropic immune stimulatory properties when using Newcastle disease virus. *Gene Ther.* **6,** 63–73.
58. Prehn, R. T. (1993) Two competing influences that may explain concomitant tumor resistance. *Cancer Res.* **53,** 3266–3269.
59. Cavallo, F., Giovarrelli, M., Gulino, A., et al. (1992) Role of neutrophils and CD4+ T lymphocytes in the primary and memory response to nonimmunogenic murine mammary adenocarcinoma made immunogenic by IL-2 gene transfer. *J. Immunol.* **149,** 3627–3635.
60. Cayeux, S., Richter, G., Becker, C., Pezzutto, A., Dorken, B., and Blankenstein, T. (1999) Direct and indirect T cell priming by dendritic cell vaccines. *Eur. J. Immunol.* **29,** 255–234.
61. Huang, A. Y. C., Bruce, A. T., Pardoll, D. M., and Levitsky, H. I. (1996) In vivo cross-priming of MHC class I-restricted antigens requires a TAP transporter. *Immunity* **4,** 349–355.
62. Forni, G., Lollini, P. L., Musiani, P., and Colombo, M. P. (2000) Immunoprevention of cancer: is the time ripe? *Cancer Res.* **60,** 2571–2575.
63. Walden, P. (2000) Hybrid cell vaccination for cancer immunotherapy. *Adv. Exp. Med. Biol.* **465,** 347–354.
64. Stuhler, G. and Walden, P. (1994) Recruitment of helper T cells for induction of tumour rejection by cytolytic T lymphocytes. *Cancer Immunol. Immunother.* **39,** 342–345.
65. Stuhler, G., Trefzer, U., and Walden, P. (1998) Hybrid cell vaccination in cancer immunotherapy. Recruitment and activation of T cell help for induction of antitumour cytotoxic T cells. *Adv. Exp. Med. Biol.* **451,** 277–282.
66. Guo, Y., Wu, M., Chen, H., et al. (1994) Effective tumor vaccine generated by fusion of hepatoma cells with activated B cells. *Science* **263,** 518–520.

67. Gong, J., Avigan, D., Chen, D., et al. (2000) Activation of antitumor cytotoxic T lymphocytes by fusions of human dendritic cells and breast carcinoma cells. *Proc. Natl. Acad. Sci. USA* **97**, 2715–2718.

68. Tanaka, Y., Koido, S., Chen, D., Gendler, S. J., Kufe, D., and Gong, J. (2001) Vaccination with allogeneic dendritic cells fused to carcinoma cells induces antitumor immunity in MUC1 transgenic mice. *Clin. Immunol.* **101**, 192–200.

69. Gong, J., Chen, D., Kashiwaba, M., and Kufe, D. (1997) Induction of antitumor activity by immunization with fusions of dendritic and carcinoma cells. *Nat. Med.* **3**, 558–561.

70. Homma, S., Toda, G., Gong, J., Kufe, D., and Ohno, T. (2001) Preventive antitumor activity against hepatocellular carcinoma (HCC) induced by immunization with fusions of dendritic cells and HCC cells in mice. *J. Gastroenterol.* **36**, 764–771.

71. Gong, J., Apostolopoulos, V., Chen, D., et al. (2000) Selection and characterization of MUC1-specific CD8+ T cells from MUC1 transgenic mice immunized with dendritic-carcinoma fusion cells. *Immunology* **101**, 316–324.

72. Gong, J., Chen, D., Kashiwaba, M., et al. (1998) Reversal of tolerance to human MUC1 antigen in MUC1 transgenic mice immunized with fusions of dendritic and carcinoma cells. *Proc. Natl. Acad. Sci. USA* **95**, 6279–6283.

73. Souberbielle, B. E., Westby, M., Ganz, S., et al. (1998) Comparison of four strategies for tumour vaccination in the B16-F10 melanoma model. *Gene Ther.* **5**, 1447–1454.

74. Dunnion, D. J., Cywinski, A. L., Tucker, V. C., et al. (1999) Human antigen-presenting cell/tumour cell hybrids stimulate strong allogeneic responses and present tumour-associated antigens to cytotoxic T cells in vitro. *Immunology* **98**, 541–550.

75. Trefzer, U., Weingart, G., Chen, Y., et al. (2000) Hybrid cell vaccination for cancer immune therapy: first clinical trial with metastatic melanoma. *Int. J. Cancer* **85**, 618–626.

76. Kikuchi, T., Akasaki, Y., Irie, M., Homma, S., Abe, T., and Ohno, T. (2001) Results of a phase I clinical trial of vaccination of glioma patients with fusions of dendritic and glioma cells. *Cancer Immunol. Immunother.* **50**, 337–344.

77. Koido, S., Tanaka, Y., Chen, D., Kufe, D., and Gong, J. (2002) The kinetics of in vivo priming of CD4 and CD8 T cells by dendritic/tumor fusion cells in MUC1-transgenic mice. *J. Immunol.* **168**, 2111–2117.

78. Scott-Taylor, T. H., Pettengell, R., Clarke, I., et al. (2000) Human tumour and dendritic cell hybrids generated by electrofusion: potential for cancer vaccines. *Biochim. Biophys. Acta* **1500**, 265–279.

79. Trefzer, U., Herberth, G., Sterry, W., and Walden, P. (2000) The hybrid cell vaccination approach to cancer immunotherapy. *Ernst Schering Res. Found. Workshop* 154–166.

80. Kugler, A., Stuhler, G., Walden, P., et al. (2000) Regression of human metastatic renal cell carcinoma after vaccination with tumor cell-dendritic cell hybrids. *Nat. Med.* **6**, 332–336.

81. Trefzer, U., Weingart, G., Sterry, W., and Walden, P. (2000) Hybrid cell vaccination in patients with metastatic melanoma. *Methods Mol. Med.* **35**, 469–475.

82. Plautz, G. E., Yang, Z.-Y., Wu, B.-Y., Gao, X., Huang, L., and Nabel, G. J. (1993) Immunotherapy of malignancy by in vivo gene transfer into tumors. *Proc. Natl. Acad. Sci. USA* **90**, 4645–4649.

83. Ram, Z., Culver, K. W., Oshiro, E. M., et al. (1997) Therapy of malignant brain tumors by intratumoral implantation of retroviral vector-producing cells. *Nat. Med.* **3**, 1354–1361.

84. Russell, S. J. (1994) Replicating vectors for cancer therapy: a question of strategy. *Semin. Cancer Biol.* **5**, 437–443.

85. Russell, S. J. (1994) Replicating vectors for gene therapy of cancer: risks, limitations and prospects. *Eur. J. Cancer* **30A**, 1165–1171.

86. Alemany, R., Balague, C., and Curiel, D. T. (2000) Replicative adenoviruses for cancer therapy. *Nat. Biotechnol.* **18**, 723–727.

87. Curiel, D. T. (2000) The development of conditionally replicative adenoviruses for cancer therapy. *Clin. Cancer Res.* **6**, 3395–3399.

88. Nemunaitis, J., Khuri, F., Ganly, I., et al. (2001) Phase II trial of intratumoral administration of ONYX-015, a replication-selective adenovirus, in patients with refractory head and neck cancer. *J. Clin. Oncol.* **19**, 289–298.

89. Heise, C., Hermiston, T., Johnson, L., et al. (2000) An adenovirus E1A mutant that demonstrates potent and selective systemic anti-tumoral efficacy. *Nat. Med.* **6**, 1134–1139.

90. Kirn, D. H. (2000) A tale of two trials: selectively replicating herpesviruses for brain tumors. *Gene Ther.* **7**, 815–816.

91. Kirn, D., Martuza, R. L., and Zwiebel, J. (2001) Replication-selective virotherapy for cancer: biological principles, risk management and future directions. *Nat. Med.* **7**, 781–787.

92. Vile, R. G. (2001) Vironcology-not yet, but soon? *Nat. Biotechnol.* **19**, 1020–1022.

93. Vile, R. G., Ando, D., and Kirn, D. H. (2002) The oncolytic virotherapy treatment platform for cancer: unique biological and biosafety points to consider. *Cancer Gene Ther.* **9**, 1062–1067.

94. Logg, C. R., Tai, C. K., Logg, A., Anderson, W. F., and Kasahara, N. (2001) A uniquely stable replication-competent retrovirus vector achieves efficient gene delivery in vitro and in solid tumors. *Hum. Gene Ther.* **12**, 921–932.

95. Grote, D., Russell, S. J., Cornu, T. I., et al. (2001) Live attenuated measles virus induces regression of human lymphoma xenografts in immunodeficient mice. *Blood* **97**, 3746–3754.

96. Peng, K.-W., Ahmann, G. J., Pham, L., Greipp, P. R., Cattaneo, R., and Russell, S. J. (2001) Systemic therapy of myeloma xenografts by an attenutaed measles virus. *Blood* **98**, 2002–2007.

97. Freytag, S. O., Khil, M., Stricker, H., et al. (2002) Phase I study of replication-competent adenovirus-mediated double suicide gene therapy for the treatment of locally recurrent prostate cancer. *Cancer Res.* **62,** 4968–4976.
98. Krasnykh, V., Belousova, N., Korokhov, N., Mikheeva, G., and Curiel, D. T. (2001) Genetic targeting of an adenovirus vector via replacement of the fiber protein with the phage T4 fibritin. *J. Virol.* **75,** 4176–4183.
99. Rodriguez, R., Schuur, E. R., Lim, H. Y., Henderson, G. A., Simons, J. W., and Henderson, D. R. (1997) Prostate attenuated replication competent adenovirus (ARCA) CN706: a selective cytotoxic for prostate-specific antigen-positive prostate cancer cells. *Cancer Res.* **57,** 2559–2563.
100. Bischoff, J., Kirn, D. H., Williams, A., et al. (1996) An adenovirus mutant that replicates selectively in p53-deficient human tumor cells. *Science* **274,** 373–376.
101. Ramachandra, M., Rahman, A., Zou, A., et al. (2001) Reengineering adenovirus regulatory pathways to enhance oncolytic specificity and efficacy. *Nat. Biotechnol.* **19,** 1035–1041.
102. Ahmed, A., Suzuki, K., Kottke, T., et al. (2003) Intratumoral expression of a fusogenic membrane glycoprotein enhances the efficacy of replicating adenovirus therapy. *Gene Ther.* **10,** 1663–1671.
103. Li, H., Haviv, Y. S., Derdeyn, C. A., et al. (2001) Human immunodeficiency virus type 1-mediated syncytium formation is compatible with adenovirus replication and facilitates efficient dispersion of viral gene products and De Novo-synthesized virus particles. *Hum. Gene Ther.* **12,** 2155–2165.
104. Bateman, A. (2002) FMG: a cancer gene therapy. Ph.D. thesis, Open University, London, UK.
105. Fu, X., Tao, L., Jin, A., Vile, R., Brenner, M. K., and Zhang, X. (2003) Expression of a fusogenic membrane glycoprotein by an oncolytic herpes simplex virus provides potent synergistic anti-tumor effect. *Mol. Ther.* **7,** 784–786.
106. Sauter, B., Albert, M. L., Francisco, L., Larsson, M., Somersan, S., and Bhardwaj, N. (2000) Consequences of cell death: exposure to necrotic tumor cells, but not primary tissue cells or apoptotic cells, induces the maturation of immunostimulatory dendritic cells. *J. Exp. Med.* **191,** 423–434.

7

Suicide Gene Therapy

Caroline J. Springer and Ion Niculescu-Duvaz

1. INTRODUCTION

Chemotherapy is used alongside surgery and radiotherapy in the treatment of malignant diseases. Unfortunately, their efficacy is often hampered by an insufficient therapeutic index, lack of specificity, and the emergence of drug-resistant cell subpopulations. Emerging technologies such as genomics and proteomics, discovering proteins specific for various types of cancer cells that may be used as targets, are ways to address these hurdles (1). Alternatives aimed at enhancing the selectivity of cancer chemotherapy for solid tumors rely on targeting cancer cells with chemoimmunoconjugates, antibody-directed enzyme prodrug therapy (ADEPT) (2,3), or gene-directed enzyme prodrug therapy (GDEPT) (4–6).

Gene therapy may be broadly defined as a technology aimed at modifying the genetic component of cells to obtain therapeutic benefits. In cancer gene therapy, both malignant and nonmalignant cells can be targeted for a therapeutic gain. The possibility of rendering cancer cells more sensitive to chemotherapeutics or toxins by introducing "suicide genes" was suggested in the late 1980s. This approach has two alternatives: toxin gene therapy, by transfecting genes that express toxic molecules, or enzyme-activating prodrug therapy, by transfecting genes able to express enzymes that can activate specific prodrugs selectively. The latter approach is known as suicide gene therapy, GDEPT (7,8), virus-directed enzyme prodrug therapy (VDEPT) (9), or genetic prodrug activating therapy (GPAT) (10).

In this chapter, we focus on GDEPT, which is a two-step treatment for solid tumors. In the first step, the gene for a foreign enzyme is administered and targeted in a variety of ways to the tumor for expression. In the second step, a prodrug is administered that is activated to the cytotoxic drug selectively by the foreign enzyme expressed in the tumor. GDEPT potentially represents a major advantage over conventional prodrug therapy in terms of selectivity and the ability to deliver higher drug concentrations to the tumor target.

Ideally, the enzyme gene should be expressed exclusively or with a relatively high ratio in the tumor cells compared to normal tissues and blood and should achieve a concentration sufficient to activate prodrug for clinical benefit. The catalytic activity of the expressed protein must be sufficient for activation of the prodrug under physiological conditions.

Because expression of the foreign enzymes will not occur in all cells of a targeted tumor in vivo, a bystander effect (BE) is required by which the prodrug is cleaved to an active drug that kills not only the tumor cells in which it is formed, but also neighboring tumor cells that do not express the foreign enzyme. Mechanisms of BE have not been fully elucidated, but include the generation and export of cytotoxic metabolites able to kill nontransfected neighboring cells as well as immune responses in in vivo models. These general principles are illustrated in Fig. 1.

From: *Contemporary Cancer Research*
Cancer Gene Therapy
Edited by: D. T. Curiel and J. T. Douglas © Humana Press Inc., Totowa, NJ

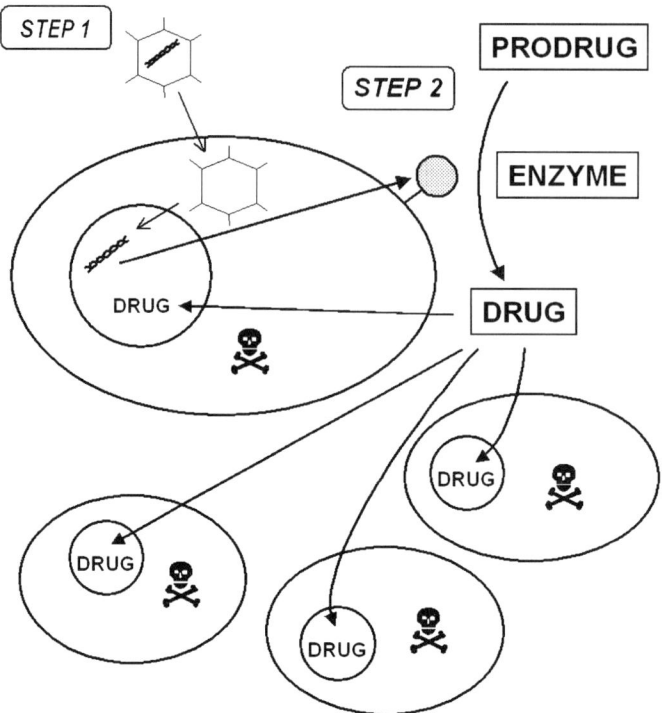

Fig. 1. Gene-directed enzyme prodrug therapy (DGEPT).

2. SUICIDE GENE THERAPY

The goal for successful anticancer agents has been to design drugs with intrinsic specificity for specific types of cancer cells. Many compounds have failed, but successful examples occur, such as Gleevec, which is extremely effective in acute myeloid leukemia *(11)*. However, an important concept is the design of technologies that target cancer cells without important side effects.

One methodology is the use of chemoimmunoconjugates to utilize the specificity of tumor antigens by targeting an antibody-linked anticancer agent to the tumor *(12)*. This area suffers from the difficulties of insufficient density and irregular distribution of the antigens on the malignant cells and the need for the internalization of the antibody conjugates. There are also potential problems linked to the release of the drugs from the conjugates and the absence of BEs *(2)*.

A different technology was the development of ADEPT, in which the antibody–enzyme conjugates were used to activate subsequently administered prodrugs *(13–15)*. This approach offers at least two consistent advantages over chemoimmunoconjugates. One is the amplification effect because one molecule of enzyme-antibody conjugate, acting as a catalyst, is able to activate a large number of prodrug molecules. A BE effect was observed in ADEPT experiments both in vitro and in vivo. The fact that there is no need for antibody conjugate or prodrug internalization for activation is a second important advantage *(2)*.

Suicide gene therapy has some of the same advantages as ADEPT. The difference is that the vector that delivers the therapeutic enzyme gene provides the targeting to cancer cells, and the length of time the therapeutic enzyme resides at the tumor is likely to be longer than with ADEPT. A comparison of these two systems is summarized in Table 1.

The genes can be engineered for expression of their product intracellularly, extracellularly, or by secretion in the recipient cells *(7,16–18)*. There are advantages for each approach. When the enzyme

Table 1
Comparison Between ADEPT and GDEPT Systems

Parameters	ADEPT	GDEPT	
		Internal expression	External expression
Selectivity	Determined by antigen expression and density on the cells surface, affinity and avidity of antibody	Determined by the delivery system and the translational specificity	
Targeting	Based on antigen–antibody interactions	Can be achieved with retargeted viruses, bacteria, or nonviral vectors	
Amplification effect		Very important property of ADEPT and GDEPT systems	
Bystander effect	Prodrugs activated extracellularly; comparable with enzyme surface-tethered expression in GDEPT	Export outside the cells of the active drugs is required to achieve the BE	Presumed better compared to GDEPT intracellular expression as no export of drug from the cell is required
Prodrug design	Prodrugs with suitable pharmacokinetic properties have been designed to achieve sufficient tumor concentration; internalization of the released drugs is necessary for cell kill	Internalization of the prodrugs is required for activation	As for ADEPT because internalization is not required
Immunogenicity	Immunogenicity is described as a negative factor in clinical trials because it precludes antibody-conjugate repeated treatments; may be overcome using human fusion proteins of antibody with enzyme	Immunogenicity described as positive factor in experimental protocols because it may result in an immune response against the tumor	
Potential leakage of the drug outside the tumor	Potential risk depending on the nature of the active drugs and their half-lives	Minimal risks because of an extra barrier to be crossed by the active drug	Potential risk depending on the nature of the active drugs and their half-lives
Efficacy of the system in clinical trials	Four phase I clinical trials to date; responses have been reported in first	Encouraging results have been obtained in glioma, head and neck, ovarian cancers; Thirty-four clinical trials are ongoing	Not performed to date
Miscellaneous	Clearance of antibody-enzyme conjugate from normal body tissues can be achieved using a second clearing antibody prior to administration of the prodrug; efficacy can be enhanced with an antiangiogenic agent	Therapeutic effect can be enhanced by combining two suicide genes, adding immunostimulatory genes, or mutating the active site of the enzyme to obtain greater specificity for the substrate prodrug	

is intracellularly expressed, the prodrug must enter the cells for activation; subsequently, the active drug must diffuse through the interstitium across the cell membrane to elicit a BE. Cells in which the enzyme is expressed in a secretory form or tethered to their outer surface are able to activate the prodrug extracellularly. A more substantial BE could therefore be generated in the last systems because the prodrug does not have to enter cells for activation. A leak-back of the active drug to the general circulation is a possible disadvantage of this approach.

A number of factors are important for efficacy in GDEPT. The gene must be "carried" in a vehicle or vector, which is also responsible for the specificity of targeting and for the efficient transfection of the therapeutic genes into the cancer cells. The vectors for gene therapy can be divided in two major classes: viral and nonviral. The first category includes all types of viruses (such as adenoviruses, retroviruses, adeno-associated viruses, lentiviruses, baculoviruses) *(19–24)* as well as bacteria *(25,26)*, which can be engineered to carry one or several therapeutic genes. These vectors can also be engineered to be replicative competent (e.g., the oncolytic viruses ONYX 015 or ONYX 411) *(27–30)* or replicative defective. The targeting of cancer cells is based on structural changes of the envelope for retargeting, which allows specific interactions with elements overexpressed on, or characteristic for, the surface of the cancer cell receptors *(31)*. Other alternatives for achieving specificity toward cancer cells are specific transcriptional regulation (using tissue-specific or inducible promoters) *(31,32)*, alternative splicing *(33)*, translational control *(34,35)* or specific delivery strategies. The main advantage of viral vectors is good transfection efficiencies; their main weaknesses are the safety issues, toxicity, and immunogenicity.

Bacteria (*Salmonella typhimurium, Clostridia,* and *Bifidobacterium longum*) *(25,26,36–39)* are another rapidly expanding category of vectors that accumulate in tumors and can be engineered to carry therapeutic genes. The reasons for this accumulation are not fully understood, although a putative mechanism is in the area of hypoxia. Concentrations of bacteria up to 2×10^8 bacteria/gram tumor were obtained with *Clostridia sporogenes (40)*. This property can be exploited to activate prodrugs selectively in an approach similar to GDEPT. However, because infection of the therapeutic genes in a cancer cell does not occur, this therapy is described as bacteria-directed enzyme prodrug therapy.

Much effort has been made in the development of nonviral vectors, including naked deoxyribonucleic acid (DNA), liposomes, polymers, peptides, and proteins *(41–43)*. Their main advantages concern safety, lower chance of eliciting immunogenic effect, and low toxicity. Their main drawback is that there is often insufficient transfer efficacy in vivo.

Other important factors for the efficiency of the GDEPT system are the transport of prodrugs to the tumor and its uptake into malignant cells, the kinetics of prodrug activation, the extent of the BE, the potency of the released drugs and their mechanism of action, and the propensity of the released drug to target dividing and nondividing cells and to induce resistance. Beneficial immune effects may be induced either by stimulation of the host immune system or by the use of additional cytokine gene therapy. Finally, clinically feasible treatment schedules are another important consideration.

2.1. Suicide Gene Therapy Systems

A number of reviews covered many aspects of GDEPT technologies *(4–6,44–50)*. This chapter focuses on the qualitative and quantitative aspects related to GDEPT and the methods for taking advantage of them for improving this technology. There are many enzyme/prodrug systems for GDEPT (*see* Table 2).

The enzymes used must meet specific requirements by which they must catalyze scission or other types of reactions, such as phosphorylations, ribosyl transfer, redox reactions, or β-elimination, and should be different from any circulating endogenous enzymes. They should be expressed in sufficient concentrations and have high catalytic activity, preferably without the need for cofactors.

The enzymes proposed for GDEPT can be characterized into two categories. The first comprises "foreign" enzymes of nonmammalian origin with or without human homologs, such as viral tyrosine

Table 2
Enzyme/Prodrug Systems

Names and codes	Enzyme			Prodrug systems		Potential of activation (fold)	Degree of activation (fold)	Clinical trials
	Origin	Expression	Mutation	Prodrugs	Released (pro)drugs			
Carboxyl esterase (CE)	Human, rabbit	Intracellular	No	Irinotecan, 7-ethyl-10-[4-(1-piperidino)-1-piperidino]-carbonyloxy-(20S)-camptothecin	SN-38, 7-ethyl-10-hydroxy-(20S)-camptothecin	150–3000	7–17	1
Carboxypeptidase A (CPA)	Human	Intracellular and extracellular secreted	Yes, for secreted or surface-tethered expression and modified substrates	MTX-α-peptides	MTX	>1000	>400	—
Carboxypeptidase G2 (CPG2), EC 3.4.22.12	*Pseudomonas str.*	Intracellular and extracellular surface tethered	Yes, for extracellular expression	CMDA, ZD2767P, self-immolative	CMBA, phenol-bisiodo nitrogen mustard; alkylating agents, anthracycline antibiotics	21–400	11–115	1
Cytochrome P450; human CYP2B1, CYP2B6, CYP2C8, CYP2C9, CYP2C18, and CYP3A; rat CYP2B1; rabbit 4B1 (with or without P450 reductase)	Human, rat, rabbit	Intracellular	No	Oxazaphosphorines, ipomeanol, 2-amino-anthracene (2-AA); acetaminophen	Alkylating agents toxic metabolites, *N*-acetyl benzoquinoneimine (NABQI)	?	5–100	2
Cytosine deaminase (CD), EC 3.5.4.1 (with or without UPRT)	*E. coli*, yeast	Intracellular and extracellular	Yes, for secreted expression	5-fluorocytosine (5-FC)	5-fluorouracil (5-FU)	1000–8000	70–1000	1

(continued)

85

Table 2 (Continued)

| Names and codes | Enzyme | | | Prodrug systems | | Potential of activation (fold) | Degree of activation (fold) | Clinical trials |
	Origin	Expression	Mutation	Prodrugs	Released (pro)drugs			
D-amino-acid oxidase	*Rodhotorula gracilis* (yeast)	Intracellular	No	D-Alanine	Hydrogen peroxide	—	—	—
Deoxycytidine kinase (dCK), EC.2.7.1.21	Human	Intracellular	No	Cytosine arabinoside	Cytosine arabinoside monophosphate	—	—	—
Deoxyribonucleotide kinase (*Dm*NK)	*Drosophila melanogaster*	Intracellular	No	Analogs of pyrimidine and purine 2′-deoxy-nucleosides	Analogs of pyrimidine and purine 2′-deoxy-nucleotide monophosphates	?	?	No
DT-d, EC 1.6.99.2	Human, rat	Intracellular	No	Bioreductive agents: EO9, etc;; mitomycin C	Reduced forms?	—	—	No
β-Gal, EC 3.2.1.23	*E. coli*	Intracellular	No	Self-immolative prodrugs from anthracyclin antibiotics	Anthracyclin antibiotics	—	—	No
β-Glu	Human	Intracellular and extracellular	Yes, for secreted expression	Self-immolative, HM-1826, Dox-GA3, 9-amino-camptothecin glucuronide	Doxorubicin, 9-amino-camptothecin	235	4–5	No
β-Lactamase	Bacterial	Extracellular, secreted, or surface tethered	Yes	Self-immolative (cephem prodrugs) antibiotics	Alkylating agents, *Vinca* alkaloids, anthracycline	—	—	—

86

Enzyme	Source	Location	Improve kinetics	Substrate	Product			Clinical trials
Methionine-α,γ-lyase (MET)	Pseudomonas putida	Intracellular	No	Selenomethionine	Methylselenol	?	400	No
Multiple drug activating enzyme (MDAE)	Tomato	Intracellular	No	Acetylated 6-TG and other purines	6-TG, cytotoxic purines	—	—	No
Nitroreductase (NR)	E. coli	Intracellular	No	CB1954 and analogs; self-immolative	Alkylating agents, pyrazolidines, enediynes	>50,000	14–10,000	1
Penicillin G amidase (PGA)	Bacterial	Extracellular	Yes	—	—	—	—	No
Purine nucleotide phosphorylase (PNP), EC2.4.2.1	E. coli	Intracellular	No	Purine nucleosides, flutarabine	6-Methylpurine, 2-fluoroadenine	25–1000	40	No
Uracil phospho-ribosyl transferase	E. coli	Intracellular	No	5-FU	5-Fluorouracil triphosphate	—	—	—
Thymidine kinase (TK), EC 2.7.1.21	Herpes simplex or varicella zoster virus	Intracellular	Yes, to improve phosphorylation kinetics	Modified pyrimidine nucleosides: GCV, ACV, valacyclovir, lobucavir, pencciclovir; FIAU, purine nucleosides; tricyclic analogs of ACV and GCV	Monophosphate nucleotide analogs	—	20–1000	>25; one phase III
Thymidine phosphorylase (TP), EC2.4.2.4	Human	Intracellular	No	Pyrimidine analogs, 5-DFUR	5-Fluorodeoxyuridine monophosphate, 5-FdRMP	7000	165	No
Xanthine-guanine phosphoribosyl transferase	E. coli	Intracellular	No	6-Thiopurines	6-Thiopurine nucleoside	—	—	No

ACV, acyclovir; CB1954, 5-aziridinyl-2,4-dinitrobenzamide; β-Gal, β-galactosidase; β-Glu, β-glucuronidase; CMBA, N,N-(2-chloroethyl)(2-mesyloxyethyl)aminobenzoic acid; CMDA, N,N-(2-chloroethyl)(2-mesyloxyethyl)aminobenzoyl-L-glutamic acid; 5'-FUdR, 5'-deoxy-5-fluorouridine; DT-d, DT-diaphorase; EO9, 3-hydroxy-5-aziridinyl-L-methyl-(1H-indole-4,7-dione)-propenol; FIAU, 1-(2'-deoxy-2'-fluoro-β-D-arabinofuranosyl)-5-iodouracil; GCV, ganciclovir; HM-1826, N-(4-β-glucuronyl-3-nitro-benzyloxy-carbonyl)-doxorubicin; MET, methionine-α, γ-lyase; 6-TG, 6-thioguanine; ZD2767P, 4-[bis(2-iodoethyl)aminophenyl]-oxycarbonyl-L-glutamic acid.

kinase (TK), bacterial cytosine deaminase (CD), carboxypeptidase G2 (CPG2), purine nucleotide phosphorylase (PNP), D-amino-acid oxidase, α- and β-galactosidase (α- and β-Gal), β-lactamase, methionine-α,γ-lyase (MET), nitroreductase (NR), rabbit cytochrome P450, and xanthine-guanine phosphoribosyltransferase. The second category consists of enzymes of human origin: carboxypeptidase A (CPA), deoxycytidine kinase (dCK), DT-diaphorase (DT-d), thymidine phosphorylase (TP), β-glucuronidase (β-Glu), carboxylesterase (CA), cytochrome P450 reductase (HRE-P450), and several cytochrome P450 (CYP) isophorms (CYP1A2, CYP3A, CYP2B, CYP2B1, CYP2C, and CYP2D6) *(5,6,47)*. Some of these enzymes are absent or are expressed only at low concentrations in tumor cells (e.g., dCK, CA, TP, and CYP).

The human homologs of the first category have different substrate structural requirements in comparison to the "foreign" enzymes. Their main disadvantage is their potential to elicit an immune response in humans, although this may provide benefits to therapy *(vide infra)*. The main advantage of enzymes belonging to the second category resides in the reduction of their potential for inducing an immune response. However, the presence of these enzymes in normal tissues is likely to preclude specific activation of the prodrugs only in tumors.

The number of enzyme/prodrug systems has expanded rapidly. Approximately 22–30 enzyme/prodrug systems have been reported *(3,6)*. The systems have been expanded by the discovery of more effective enzymes and by synthesizing better prodrugs. Improving the prodrugs has been an active area of research. New prodrugs have been designed for activation by herpes simplex virus TK (HSV-TK), NR, CPA, CPG2, CYP450, and DT-d enzymes *(see also* Section 2.4. and Table 2). New enzyme/prodrug systems have been described. The horseradish peroxidase/indole-3-acetic acid (IAA) system was designed for use in hypoxic cells *(51)*. The system is effective in T24 bladder cell carcinoma lines *(52)*. Prodrugs based on the IAA structure have also been synthesized, and the fluorinated analog (5F-IAA) was claimed to be more active than IAA *(51)*.

A system based on transfecting the human flavoprotein HRE-P450 gene under the control of the hypoxia-regulated promoter and the nitro-imidazole prodrug RB-6145 (1-[3-(2-bromoethylamino)-2-hydroxypropyl]-2-nitroimidazole) was described *(53)*. A 30-fold increase in oxic/hypoxic cytotoxicity, as compared to controls, was obtained after activation of the prodrug to the corresponding RSU-1069 drug in HT-1080 human fibrosarcoma cells expressing HRE-P450. In vivo data, using GFP/R9 xenografts in mice expressing the same enzyme showed that regressions (50% free of tumor survivors at 100 days) were achieved when RB-6145 was combined with a reduced radiotherapy dose of 10 Gy *(53)*.

A different GDEPT system exploited the toxic properties of methyl-selenol, which is released from selenomethionine (SeMET) following its activation by MET. In the cells transduced with the MET gene, the cytotoxicity of SeMET was increased 1000-fold. A strong BE was also observed. Treatment of rat hepatoma R1S1 ascites with adenoviral MET gene followed by SeMET administration significantly prolonged the survival of animals, with 3/5 animals alive at 72 days; the controls survived only 24 days *(54)*.

It has been reported that the system hypoxanthine-guanine phosphoribosyltransferase/allopurinol may be of some utility in non-small cell lung carcinoma. The enzyme converts allopurinol to cytotoxic metabolites, and it was demonstrated that five nonsmall cell lung carcinoma cell lines were twofold to eightfold more sensitive to the prodrug when infected with *Trypanosoma brucei* containing the hypoxanthine-guanine phosphoribosyltransferase gene *(55)*.

Other GDEPT systems reported include β-Glu/9-aminocamptothecin glucuronide, which releases 9-aminocampthotecin *(56)*; DT-d/mitomycin C *(57)*; and PNP/flutarabine, which releases 2-fluoroadenine *(58)*.

In addition to improving the enzyme/prodrug systems, the performance of GDEPT can be enhanced using stronger promoters or a combination of enhancer-promoters. A 30-fold increase in efficacy of yeast CD/5-fluorocytosine (5-FC) under the control of a combination of a carcinoembryonic antigen promoter and an enhancer was reported *(59)*. Another example of controlling expression in vivo has been used in the HSV-TK/ganciclovir (GCV) system expression in vivo with the use of the glucose-regulated protein (*grp-78*)-inducible promoter coupled with photodynamic therapy *(60)*.

The efficiency of a GDEPT system can be measured in vitro, on a given cell line, as the differential of the cytotoxicity of the prodrug in the same non-enzyme-expressing cells vs its cytotoxicity in the enzyme-expressing cells ($\Delta = IC_{50}$ in nonexpressing cells/IC_{50} in expressing cells). The efficiency of each GDEPT system may be different in various cell lines. To make valid comparisons of GDEPT systems, two additional parameters have been introduced. These are the potential of activation of a given system and its degree of activation. The first is defined as the ratio of IC_{50} of the prodrug/IC_{50} of the released drug in a control non-enzyme-expressing cell system. It represents the maximum possible efficiency of a given enzyme/prodrug system in a cell line. The degree of activation is defined as the ratio of the IC_{50} of the prodrug in the non-enzyme-expressing cell line to the IC_{50} of the prodrug in the enzyme-expressing cell line and demonstrates the efficiency of the system in the considered cell line. In other words, the potential of activation is the maximum possible degree of activation of a GDEPT system in a given cell line *(47)*.

2.2. Enzyme Kinetics

The concentration of the drug and the rate at which it is released at the activation site depends on the kinetic parameters of the enzyme/prodrug system. The Km is an expression of the amount of substrate needed to reach half of the maximal velocity V_{max}. It describes the enzyme–substrate interaction, with a lower Km associated with tighter fit between the two entities. It is difficult to compare enzyme/prodrug systems solely on this basis. It has been hypothesized that a low Km and high V_{max} (or high k_{cat}) are associated with more effective systems. This is the case, for instance, when yeast CD is com-pared with bacterial CD. The yeast enzyme, which proved to be more effective than its bacterial counterpart in GDEPT models, has a lower Km and a higher V_{max} (*see* Table 3) *(61)*.

As V_{max} is often determined under different experimental conditions for the various GDEPT systems, a direct comparison of the systems is impossible. However, it appears, that prodrugs such as 4-[(2-mesyloxyethyl)(2-chloroethyl)amino]-benzoyl-L-glutamic acid (CMDA), GCV, and irinotecan (CPT-11) approach the requirements for an "ideal" substrate more closely than, for example, 5-FC or 5'-deoxy-5-fluorouridine because the 5'-deoxy-5-fluorouridine results in higher K_ms and lower V_{max}s (*see* Table 3).

The turnover number k_{cat} or V_{max} supplies additional information about the activation rate because they are terms to express the rate of drug release. It is not yet known if a fast "bolus" release of the active drug is better than a slow "infusion." We can infer that, for drugs acting on quiescent and proliferating cells, the former is an appropriate choice. By contrast, for drugs acting only on proliferating cells, the second alternative may be preferable.

Structure–activity studies have been performed to determine the optimal structure of a prodrug for a given enzyme. One of the criteria of assessment is the kinetics of activation. The effect of the substitution on the aromatic ring of prodrugs for CPG2 on the kinetics has been investigated. It was found that both steric and electronic effects play a role in the kinetics *(62,63)*.

An alternative approach to alter the kinetics of activation is to use self-immolative linkers (*vide infra*). Whereas the direct carbamate linker between the α-galactosyl and doxorubicin was poorly cleaved by α-galactosidase, the insertion of a 4-aminobenzyl linker afforded good substrates for the enzyme *(64)*. The rationale for this effect is probably the increased distance between the cleavage site and the drug, releasing the steric hindrance around the site of activation. Increasing the distance between the drug and the cleavage point even further using multiple cascade linkers improved the kinetics even further, as demonstrated for a series of self-immolative prodrugs for plasmin *(65)*. The substituents on the aromatic ring included in the linker structure also influence the fragmentation of the self-immolative prodrugs *(66–68)*.

Table 3
Quantitative Data on GDEPT Systems[a]

No.	Enzyme/prodrug system	Potency, IC_{50} (μM) Prodrug	Drug	K_M ($S_{0.5}$) (μ_M)	V_{max} (nM/mg.min)
1	CA/CPT-11	1.6–8.1	SN-38 0.003–0.011	23–52.9	1.43[b]
2	CD/5-FC	26,000	5-FU 4–23.5	17,900[c], 800[d]	11.7[c,e], 68[d,e]
3	CPG2/CMDA, CJS278[f]	CMDA 1700–3125; CJS278 0.256	CMBA 8–65; Doxorubicin 0.012	CMDA 3.4	CMDA 583[g]
	CPG2/ZD2767P	47.2	0.34	2.0	29.5[g]
4	Cyt-450/CP, IF, ipomeanol, 2-AA	CP, IF ~4000	ND[h]	CP 300; IF 480	CP 39.1; IF 17.8
5	dCK/ara-C	0.3–0.6	NA[i]	25.6	NA[i]
6	β-Glu/HMR1826	350–720[j]	15[j]	1300	635[k]
	β-Glu/Dox-GA3	530[j]	15[j]	1100	25[k]
7	HSV-TK/GCV, ACV	GCV 200–600	GCVTP[i]	GCV 11–47.6; ACV 305–417	GCV 0.1[g]; ACV 1.5.10[-2g]
8	NR/CB1954	>1000	0.02[l]	900	6.0[g]
9	PNP/6-MePdR	>200	3.7	14–23[m]	422–638[k,m]
10	TP/5-FUdR	17	5-FUdR 0.0023	325–433	0.17–2.28
11	VZK-TK/ara-M	>2000	Ara-MTP <1[n]	56	680[o]
12	XGPRT/6-TX, 6-TG	6-TX >50; 6-TG 0.5	NA[i]	NA[i]	NA[i]

2-AA, 2-aminoanthracene; ACV, acyclovir; ara-M, 6-methoxypurine arabinonucleoside; CA, carboxylesterase; CB 1954, 5-aziridinyl-2,4-dinitrobenzamide; CD, cytosine deaminase; HSV-TK, herpes simplex virus–thymidine kinase; VZV-tk, varicella zoster virus thymidine kinase; CMBA, 4[*N,N*-(2-chloroethyl)(2-mesyloxyethyl)]aminobenzoic acid; CMDA , 4[*N,N*-(2-chloroethyl) (2-mesyloxyethyl)]aminobenzoyl-L-glutamic acid; CP, cyclophosphamide; CPG2, carboxypeptidase G2; CPT-11, irinotecan; Cyt-450, cytochrome P-450; Dox-GA3, *N*[4-(glucuron-4-yl-oxycarbonyl-amino-phenyl)-methylene-oxycarbonyl]-doxorubicin; 5-FUdR, 5-fluoro-deoxyuridine; 5-FC, 5-fluorocytosine; 5-FU, 5-fluorouracil; GCV, ganciclovir; GCVTP, ganciclovir triphosphate; β-Glu, β-glucuronidase; HMR-1286, *N*[4-(glucuron-1-yl-oxy-phenyl)-methylene-oxycarbonyl]-doxorubicin; IF, ifosfamide; 6-MePdR, 6-methylpurine-2'-deoxyribonucleoside; 6-MeP, 6-methylpurine; NR, nitroreductase; PNP, purine nucleoside phosphorylase; SN-38, 7-ethyl-10-hydroxy-camptothecine; 6-TG, 6-thioguanine; 6-TX, 6-thioxanthine; TP, thymidine phosphorylase; XGPRT, xanthine-guanine phosphorybosyl transferase; ZD2767P, 4-[*N,N*-bis(2-iodoethyl)amino]-phenyl-oxycarbonyl-L-glutamic acid.

[a]In alphabetical order.
[b]pmol/mg.min.
[c]Bacterial origin.
[d]Yeast origin.
[e]μM/min.μg.
[f]*N*-[4-(L-Glutamylcarbonylamino)benzyloxycarbonyl]doxorubicin.
[g]s^{-1}.
[h]Not determined in the same system.
[i]No data were obtainable.
[j]Maximum tolerated dose in mice.
[k]μM/min.mg
[l]For 5-(aziridin-1-yl)-2-nitro-4-hydroxylamino-benzamide in V79 cells.
[m]For inosine, adenine, and guanine nucleosides.
[n]Inferred from in vitro experiment.
[o]Relative maximal velocity.

However, in some cases, introduction of a linker can make the kinetics worse *(69)*. This can be explained by the fact that the smaller prodrug sat better in the catalytic pocket of the enzyme, whereas the larger self-immolative prodrug was oversized for the pocket and clashed sterically with other residues of the enzyme. For self-immolative prodrugs, the kinetics of activation is also complicated by the fact that there are two steps: enzymatic reaction and fragmentation. The rate-determining step is usually the former.

In some cases, obtaining the optimal activity profile does not mean increasing the rate of activation. A drop in the kinetic performance of prodrugs for an enzyme is acceptable if the advantages obtained by modifying the structure more than compensate the loss in enzyme activity. For instance, the best substrates for CPG2 were based on benzoic acid derivatives coupled to glutamic acid as amides *(62)*. Benzoic acid mustards, as exemplified by CMDA, possess an excellent turnover (k_{cat} = 583 s^{-1}) and showed a 19-fold differential in the breast carcinoma MDA MB361 cell line expressing CPG2. The self-immolative compounds derived from anthracyclin antibiotics were cleavable by CPG2 *(70)* and exhibited poorer kinetics; an accurate k_{cat} is difficult to measure. However, a similar differential of 11-fold was obtained in the MDA MB361 CPG2-expressing cells, with an additional advantage that the released doxorubicin is 4000-fold more potent than the nitrogen mustard released by CMDA.

A second example refers to prodrugs for which the drug is coupled to glutamic acid as a urea or carbamates rather than an amide *(71)*. In this case, aniline or phenol nitrogen mustards, respectively, are released after the cleavage by CPG2. Despite a lower k_{cat} of 20-fold *(46,62)*, the lead prodrug had greater cytotoxicity differentials and had improved performance because of the differences in the potency of the released drugs *(72)* (*vide infra*).

2.3. Improving the Enzymes

New techniques are available to increase the efficacy of enzymes to activate prodrugs for GDEPT *(45)*. There are three ways of improving the efficacy of enzymes: (1) using the discovery of ortho-logous enzymes or enzymes with similar profiles of activity from different species; (2) crystallo-graphic investigation of the active site of the GDEPT enzyme allows the rational synthesis of better substrates using molecular modeling and computer-aided techniques; and (3) modification of the active site of the enzyme by site-directed mutagenesis to increase its catalytic efficiency toward a given substrate or to allow the location of modified substrates better adapted to GDEPT.

Enzymes from different origins can have very different kinetics with the same substrate. The rat DT-d is an improved activating enzyme compared to the human DT-d for 5-aziridinyl-2,4-dinitroben-zamide (CB1954), with a sevenfold higher k_{cat}. The *Escherichia coli* NR exhibits a k_{cat} that is much higher (360 min^{-1} compared to 4.1 for the rat and 0.64 min^{-1} for the human enzyme) for the reduction of the nitro group, making it the enzyme of choice for GDEPT CB1954 *(73)*. The rabbit carboxylesterase is 100- to 1000-fold more efficient in activating the prodrug CPT-11 than the human homolog *(74)*. The yeast CD is also more effective in activating the 5-FC prodrug compared to the bacterial CD *(61)*.

Crystallographic data are now available for a number of GDEPT enzymes: HRP *(51)*, CYP2C *(75)*, HSV-TK complex, CPA, and nitroreductase, which aids in the design of better substrates and guiding mutagenesis assays.

Another way to modify the enzyme is by protein engineering and site-directed mutagenesis. An example was the engineering of HSV-TK producing mutants with increased sensitivity to both GCV and acyclovir (ACV). This enhancement is explained by improvement in kinetic factors. Compared to wild type, the Km was slightly higher for GCV and ACV in the mutant, but much higher (35-fold) for the endogenous thymidine substrate competing for the same site. The k_{cat} for thymidine was significantly reduced (88-fold) compared to the k_{cat} for GCV and ACV (six- and eightfold, respectively). As a consequence, the specificity constant (k_{cat}/Km) for thymidine was 3000-fold lower in mutant than in wild type, whereas the reduction of this constant for GCV was only 40-fold. The mutant displayed greatly reduced competition for the active site and better selectivity for the prodrug substrates than for endogenous thymidine *(76)*.

Further progress was achieved by introducing a restricted set of semirandom sequences in the active site of HSV-1-TK enzyme. Three mutants were selected that conferred a substantial increase in IC_{50} of GCV and ACV (of 39- to 294-fold and 3- to 182-fold, respectively) with respect to the wild-type enzyme *(77,78)*. The efficacy of the mutant SR39 was investigated in vivo on xenograft models in nude mice. At a GCV dose of 5 mg/kg, the growth of the xenograft expressing the SR39 mutant enzyme was completely prevented, but the tumors expressing the wild-type TK grew *(77)*.

Other modifications to the active site (the mutant A167Y) allowed the design of a different nucleoside for the HSV-TK enzyme. The replacement of the alanine with tyrosine in the active site was assumed to block the pyrimidine phosphorylation site in the enzyme and maintain its purine nucleoside phosphorylation capacity. The efficiency of conversion of ACV, GCV, lobucavir, penciclovir, and A5021 to their phosphorylated forms by the A167Y mutant was greater than for the wild type. It was demonstrated that a single mutation in the active site was able to change HSV-1-TK from a pyrimidine nucleoside kinase to a purine (guanine) nucleotide kinase *(79)*. A further example is the site-directed mutagenesis of carboxypeptidase A, which allows the design of modified and more specific substrates less prone to interfere with the human carboxypeptidase A *(79a)*.

2.4. Prodrugs

The prodrugs for GDEPT should be considerably less cytotoxic than their corresponding active drugs and should be suitable substrates for the activating enzyme under physiological conditions. They should be chemically stable under physiological conditions, be highly diffusible in the tumor interstitium, and have good pharmacological and pharmacokinetic properties.

The prodrug must be able to cross the tumor cell membrane if activation occurs intracellularly. If the enzyme is expressed on the surface of cells, then the prodrug will be cleaved extracellularly, and its corresponding drug must cross the cell membrane for cytotoxicity. The cytotoxicity differential between the prodrug and its corresponding drug should be as high as possible, and the active drug should be highly diffusible or be actively taken up or exported by cells.

Scanning various substrate prodrugs for an enzyme, altering the linkage between drug and the cleavage site, and looking for structure–activity correlations between substitution patterns and linker kinetics have been instrumental in obtaining substrates with favorable kinetic profiles for GDEPT.

Most of the prodrugs, like cyclophosphamide (CP), isofosfamide (IF), 5-FC, ACV, GCV, mitomycin C, or the released drugs (5-fluorouracil [5-FU], 7-ethyl-10-hydroxycamptothecin [SN-38], nitrogen mustards, anthracyclins, etoposide) used in suicide gene therapy are clinically licensed drugs. An additional advantage is that the pharmacological, pharmacokinetic, dosage, and safety parameters of these compounds are known. However, it is likely that the next generation of prodrugs will be especially tailored for GDEPT.

The design of the prodrugs tailored for GDEPT is an easier task than the design of drugs intrinsically specific for cancer cells. Usually, the enzymes used in GDEPT systems have been well investigated; in many cases, crystallographic data are available (*see* Section 2.3.). On this basis, substrates releasing cytotoxic agents after activation could be rationally designed. Another advantage of such an approach is that the potency (IC_{50}) of the designed compounds toward the enzyme can be accurately measured in vitro, contributing to an early selection of leads.

An important factor in designing prodrugs for GDEPT is the potency of the released drug. The lead compound for the design of prodrugs for the GDEPT system based on CPG2 was CMDA, which reached clinical phase I trial in ADEPT *(80)*. The prodrug was characterized by good kinetics (k_{cat} = 583 s^{-1}), and the IC_{50} of the released nitrogen mustard was in the range of 50–65 µM in various cell lines. Differentials of 19- and 32-fold were measured between CPG2-expressing and non-expressing MDA MB361 and WiDr cell lines, respectively. However, the $t_{1/2}$ of the released drug of 48 minutes was long enough to allow it to leak back from the tumor and elicit side effects.

A more potent drug is released from the prodrug 4-[*bis*-(2-iodoethyl)amino]phenyl-oxycarbonyl-L-glutamic acid *(62)*. The released phenol mustard drug (4-[*N,N*-4-*bis*-(2-iodoethyl)amino]phenol)

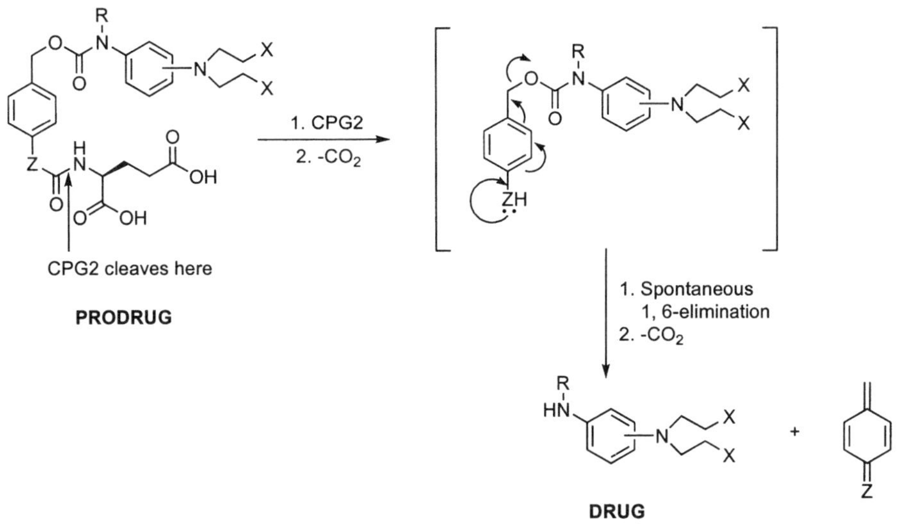

Fig. 2. Mechanism of activation of self-immolative prodrugs cleavable by CPG2.

has an IC_{50} of 0.3–0.7 μM and a much shorter $t_{1/2}$ of less than 1 minute. Despite poorer kinetics (k_{cat} = 29.5 s^{-1}), the differentials obtained for MDA MB361 and WiDr were 249- and 450-fold, respectively *(72)*. The highest BE is not associated always with the highest activity. In optimization of the prodrugs in BE terms, the potency of the released drug and the kinetics of activation remain important parameters *(72)*.

Sixty compounds were assessed as substrates for *E. coli* PNP, and the prodrugs with the best kinetics that also fulfilled several other criteria were chosen for further evaluation *(81)*. Several bioreductive prodrugs were assessed with NR for GDEPT *(82,83)*. In addition to CB1954, nitrofurazone had reasonable cytotoxicity differentials, and the rate of reduction was 10 times faster than for CB1954 *(83)*. New tricyclic analogs of ACV and GCV, as effective substrates for HSV-TK, were designed and synthesized. The new derivatives were also fluorescent, which allows simple and sensitive monitoring of their concentration in biological fluids. They also possess increased lipophilicity compared to GCV and ACV, which enables them to cross the blood–brain barrier. *(84)*

An alternative way to extend the range of prodrugs specially tailored for GDEPT is the design of self-immolative prodrugs. A self-immolative prodrug can be defined as a compound generating an unstable intermediate that, following the activation process, will extrude the active drug in a number of subsequent steps. The following elements are important in defining the concept: The activation process is generally enzymatic and is distinct from the extrusion step; the drug is generated by an extrusion process following the fragmentation of the prodrug, and the site of activation will normally be separated from the site of extrusion. Potential advantages of self-immolative prodrugs are the possibility of altering the lipophilicity of the prodrugs with minimal effects on the activation kinetics and the improvement of unfavorable kinetics of activation because of unsuitable electronic or steric features of the active drug. The range of drugs that can be converted to prodrugs is greatly extended and is unrestricted by the structural substrate requirements for a given enzyme.

A number of self-immolative prodrugs have been specially designed for use in GDEPT systems. Self-immolative prodrugs derived from alkylating agents and anthracyclins have been synthesized for activation by CPG2 *(46,69,70)*. Following the activation step, these prodrugs release the corresponding drug by a 1,6-elimination mechanism *(see* Fig. 2*)*.

Based on similar concepts, *seco*-cyclopropylindolines and ene-diyne prodrugs have been synthesized for use with NR *(44,85)*.

There are further means to increase the efficacy of a GDEPT system in terms of prodrugs. One is to increase the available intracellular concentration of the prodrug. An improved uptake of the prodrug is important for the efficacy of the intracellularly expressed enzyme in GDEPT systems. The concomitant expression of *E. coli* CD and uracil phosphoribosyl transferase (UPRT) significantly improved the cytotoxicity of 5-FC. It was shown that the combination of the two enzymes facilitated the uptake of 5-FC by direct channeling of 5-FU (the product of 5-FC activation) to 5-fluoro-uridine-monophosphate by the second enzyme in the cascade, UPRT *(86)*.

Modifying the lipophilicity of the prodrug is another possibility, especially when passive diffusion is involved in prodrug uptake. A drawback may result in a concomitant increase in prodrug cytotoxicity. A lipophilic derivative of GCV, ganciclovir elaidic acid ester (E-GCV) was evaluated for its cytotoxicity in vitro in HSV-TK transfected cells and proved to be superior to GCV. Metabolic studies revealed that E-GCV was converted to the mono-, di-, and triphosphate derivative of GCV, and these metabolites were retained longer in E-GCV-treated cells *(87)*.

Ideally, for GDEPT systems in which the enzyme is tethered to the outer cell membrane, the prodrug should be prevented from crossing the cell membrane, in contrast to the released drug, which should be membrane permeable. By manipulating the lipophilicities of both prodrug and drug, this goal could be achieved for passive diffusion situations.

An alternate target for manipulation is the use of prodrugs that release drugs effective against both quiescent and proliferating cells. Examples are in the use of CMDA, 4-[*N*,*N*-bis(2-iodoethyl)amino]-phenyl-oxycarbonyl-L-glutamic acid) (ZD2767P), 6-methylpurine deoxyribonucleoside, flutarabine, and CB1954.

Ultimately, an enzyme prodrug system should be designed with as large as possible activation potential. To improve the activation potential, prodrugs with lower cytotoxicity should be designed that release very cytotoxic drugs. Some highly cytotoxic compounds (with an IC_{50} in the nanomolar range), such as enediynes, cyclopropylindolines, taxoids, or epothilones, are now available, but generally their structures are complicated, and more efficient ways to convert them into low-cytotoxicity prodrugs need to be developed. A quantitative structure–activity relationship (QSAR) based on nitrogen mustard self-immolative prodrugs showed a direct correlation between the potency of the released prodrugs and the logarithm of differential in a GDEPT system with CPG2 *(87a)*.

The properties of prodrugs determined in vitro do not always correlate with in vivo results because of pharmacological factors such as biodistribution, metabolism, retention time, excretion, and so on. Also of importance are the physicochemical properties, such as water solubility and lipophilicity, which also influence cellular uptake and metabolism.

The biodistribution of prodrugs of clinical use was determined for several GDEPT systems. Delivery systems may be adapted to compensate for poor biological distribution. Uptake of cyclophosphamide in lung tumors is very variable *(88)*. An option to improve the tumor concentration of prodrug and achieve a more sustained concentration is to use a polymer-based implant containing CP, which has been demonstrated to be activated by virally transfected CYP2B1 *(89)*.

2.5. Potentiation of Drug Effects

An alternative strategy to increase the efficiency of GDEPT systems was developed based on an understanding of the activation step and of the mechanisms of action of the released drugs by using synergistic or additive effects of drug combinations. Ponicidin (a diterpenoid isolated from *Rabdosia ternifolia*) was found preferentially to activate the HSV-1-TK kinase, but not the cellular enzymes. The compound showed a synergistic antiviral effect with both GCV and ACV. When ponicidin was combined with GCV or ACV at a concentration devoid of antiviral activity (0.2 µ*M*/L), the cytotoxicities of both prodrugs in TK-transfected cells were increased by 3- to 87-fold and 5- to 52-fold, respectively, as compared with prodrug alone *(90)*.

In an attempt to enhance the cytotoxicity of the HSV-TK/GCV system, another prodrug, E-5-(2-bromovinyl)-2'-deoxyuridine, was coadministrated with GCV in a number of cell lines. In 8 of 12 cell lines, addition of the E-5-(2-bromovinyl)-2'-deoxyuridine at noncytotoxic concentrations enhanced GCV-mediated cell killing by up to an order of magnitude. In cocultures of both enzyme-expressing and non-enzyme-expressing cells, a strongly increased BE was also observed *(91)*.

Four compounds with apoptosis-inducing properties (butyrate, camptothecin, taxol, and 7-hydroxy-staurosporine) were assayed in conjunction with the HSV-TK/GCV system. It was found that GCV plus butyrate and GCV plus 7-hydroxystaurosporine combinations resulted in increased Bak and decreased Bcl-X_L protein levels; the combinations of GCV plus camptothecin and GCV plus taxol increased the level of both proteins. These results may be useful in increasing cell apoptosis in colon cancers using HSV-TK/GCV *(92)*.

Finally, hydroxyurea (HU) was suggested as a possible combination with GCV in the HSV-TK/GCV system because HU is able to reduce the level of deoxy-guanine triphosphate (dGTP), which is the endogenous competitor of GCV-TP for DNA incorporation *(93)*. Isobologram analysis demonstrated that the combination GCV plus HU is additive in HSV-TK-transfected cell cultures and synergistic in HSV-TK bystander mixtures *(94)*. The study was extended in vivo, and SW620 human colon carcinoma xenografts in nude mice were treated with a combination of GCV (100 mg/kg) and HU (1500 mg/kg). Tumor regressions were observed in both 1:1 and 1:10 HSV-TK enzyme-expressing vs nonenzyme-expressing cell mixtures *(95)*.

A similar rationale was applied to enhance the capabilities of the CYP2B1/CP system. A strategy aimed at minimizing the hepatic toxicity without diminishing the antitumoral potency was devised by using a CP-methimazole (MMI) combination. MMI is an antithyroid drug that reduces P450-reductase gene expression in the liver and reduces the nicotinamide adenine dinucleotide phosphate-dependent P450-reductase activity by 28%. MMI did not affect the activity of P450-reductase in 9L glioma cells growing in vivo. The combination CP plus MMI increased the therapeutic index of CP in CYP2B1/CP models in vivo *(96)*. Another five inhibitors of the CYP450s were investigated for their potential to enhance the efficacy of the CYP450/CP GDEPT system. All proved useful in reducing CP hepatic activation, showing little impact on the *in situ* activation of CP within the tumor transduced with CYP450 genes *(97)*.

Also a bioreductive drug, tirapazamine was able to increase the efficacy of CYP2B6/CP under hypoxic conditions (1% O_2) after transfection of 9L glioma cells *(98)*.

The feasibility of combining gene therapy with chemotherapy effectively is also under investigation. A synergy was found when combining GCV and temozolomide in human U87MG glioblastoma cells expressing HSV-TK enzyme. A higher sensitivity to temozolomide (8.6-fold increase) was observed in U87MG glioblastoma cells transfected with the HSV-TK gene *(99)*.

The optimization of administration schedules as a means of improving the efficacy of suicide gene therapy is an alternative approach. It was reported that repeated transfections of hemagglutinating virus of Japan (HJV) liposomes combined with repeated injections of 5-FC elicited improved results in vivo compared to single transfections *(100)*. A CYP2B1-P450-reductase/CP system showed that daily injections (6 days) of a moderate dose (140 mg/kg) significantly improved the efficacy of the system *(101)*.

3. COMBINATION SUICIDE THERAPY

A different strategy to develop more efficient suicide gene therapy systems uses transgenes with more than one gene. Several different approaches based either on transfection of multiple suicide genes or on a combination of suicide genes with cytokine or other genes have been reported. A typical example is the combination of HSV-TK and endostatin (angiogenesis inhibitor) genes followed by treatment with GCV, which is capable of eradicating orthotopic human renal cell carcinomas (Caki-1) in nude mice *(102)*.

3.1. Two or Three Suicide Gene Therapies

Several reports indicated that a double gene transfer is able to enhance the efficacy of a GDEPT system. By transfecting target cells with two different suicide genes, the expressed enzymes are able to activate two distinct types of prodrug-releasing anticancer drugs with different mechanisms of action, therefore making the system more effective.

The first attempt concerned the association between CD and TK genes, followed by 5-FC and GCV administration. The rationale behind this is that the permeable toxic metabolites resulting from the CD/5-FC system will enhance the overall BE, and therefore a synergistic antitumoral effect can be achieved *(103–105)*. Examples were reported in which cells were infected with CYP plus CD or TK plus CD genes. In each case, the double suicide gene systems proved more effective both in vitro and in vivo compared to each single system alone *(106,107)*.

If a metabolic cascade is to be considered in the activation of a prodrug that requires more than one enzyme (for example, in the activation of GCV to GCVTP), then the cotransfection of genes expressing the enzymes catalyzing each intermediate step of this pathway is expected to increase the overall yield of the desired final cytotoxic metabolite. The enhancement of GCV and ACV activation using the simultaneous transfection of HSV-TK, guanylate kinase, and nucleoside diphosphate kinase responsible for the mono-, di-, and triphosphorylation of these substrates has been claimed. This allows more than 90% of the GCV to be converted to GCV-TP *(108)*. An attempt was made to overcome resistance to 5-FU by modification of 5-FU phosphorylation. A recombinant adenovirus containing both the uracil phosphoribosyl transferase and HSV-TK was engineered, and the dual system was assayed on esophageal carcinoma cells. Significantly enhanced antitumor activity was reported *(109)*.

Another approach combining CD with TP/5-FC in 9L gliosarcoma cells showed that the addition of TP was beneficial, increasing the efficacy of the system *(110)*.

The same strategy was applied to the CD/5-FC system, which showed poor results in cancer cell lines (such as breast and pancreatic carcinoma cell lines) resistant to 5-FU because of defects in the downstream metabolism of 5-FU. Transduction of a bicistronic fusion gene encoding CD and uracil phosphotransferase was superior to the CD system alone both in vitro and in vivo *(111)*.

Another example was the cotransfection of cyt-P450 gene with the P450 reductase, which resulted in a significant increase in the conversion of CP to its toxic metabolites and therefore in the overall increase of the efficiency of the cyt-P450/CP system. Quantitation of the degree of enhancement indicated up to a 10-fold increase in cell kill following treatment with CP *(75,112)*.

An alternative approach consisted of the transduction of two (or more) copies of the same gene in the target cells. It was demonstrated that the UMSCC29 and T98G human cancer cell lines containing two copies of the TK gene led to more effective metabolism of GCV and therefore exhibited enhanced sensitivity to the prodrug *(113)*.

However, a recent report investigating the double suicide gene therapy system CD plus HSV-TK in a 9L glioma model found no advantage and concluded that single suicide gene systems employing CD or HSV-TK may be preferable over combinations of two systems *(114)*.

3.2. Combination With Cytokine Gene Therapy

Enhancing the immune response can increase the effectiveness of a GDEPT system (*vide infra*), which may be done by cotransfecting a suicide gene with one or more cytokine genes. The role of interleukin 2 (IL-2) in these systems has been investigated. Cells grown as xenografts in BALB/c syngeneic mice were injected with an adenoviral vector containing the HSV-TK gene or the IL-2 gene, followed by treatment with GCV *(115)* While the tumors continued to grow in the animals injected with a control vector or the vector carrying the IL-2 gene, those treated with HSV-TK with or without coadministration of the IL-2 exhibited tumor necrosis and regressions. However, only animals treated with both HSV-TK and the IL-2 genes developed effective systemic antitumor immunity against tumorigenic rechallenges. The antitumor immunity was associated with the presence of tumor-specific cytolytic CD8[+] T lymphocytes. To enhance and prolong the antitumor immunity, a third vector containing the mouse granulocyte-macrophage colony stimulating factor gene was employed. The animals treated simultaneously with HSV-TK plus IL-2 plus mouse granulocyte-macrophage colony stimulating factor vectors followed by administration of GCV developed long-term antitumor immunity and survived for longer than 4 months without recurrence *(115)*.

IL-12 also plays a multifunctional role in controlling the immune system, augmenting the proliferation of T and natural killer cells. In a suicide gene strategy, both HSV-TK and IL-12 genes were incorporated in replication-defective vectors. Following CT26 murine colon adenocarcinoma infection, treatment with GCV was significantly more effective than in gene therapy using IL-12 or HSV-TK alone *(116)*. The combined treatment with adenovirus constructs AdHSV-TK/GCV and AdmIL-12 also resulted in enhanced tumor inhibition and improved antimetastatic activity *(117)*.

3.3. *Combinations With Radiosensitizing Genes*

Radiotherapy is a valuable adjunct to chemotherapy with or without surgery in cancer treatment. Therefore, its combination with suicide gene therapy has been proposed as an advantage. HSV-TK gene transfection was used to increase the radiosensitivity of various cell lines. Specific incorporation of halogenated pyrimidine radiosensitizers such as 5-bromo-2'-deoxycytidine and 5-bromo-2'-deoxyuridine was demonstrated in transfected cells, increasing their sensitization ratio 1.4–2.3 times compared with control β-Gal-transfected cells *(118)*. The effect was confirmed in vivo using RT2 glioma cells in Fisher 344 rats, and it was proposed that HSV-TK transfection followed by 5-bromo-2'-deoxycytidine administration and radiation may be a useful clinical treatment for glioma *(118)*.

A similar strategy of radiosensitization was proposed with the HSV-TK/ACV system. Using a mutant of the wild-type enzyme (HSV-TK-75, which is more effective in metabolizing ACV), an enhanced sensitizing effect was shown in RT2 glioma cells. The cells become more sensitive to low doses of radiation (2–4 Gy), suggesting that this combination could improve glioma treatment *(119,120)*.

Radiation-inducible promoters have been proposed to control the expression of transgenes in cancer cells *(121)* and in *Clostridium* bacteria *(39,122)*.

4. IMAGING THE THERAPEUTIC GENES

The development of noninvasive techniques to monitor the delivery and the distribution of therapeutic transgenes in vivo will be an advantage for monitoring the efficacy of GDEPT. There are now a number of technologies employed to analyze quantitatively the gene expression and the protein functions in vitro and in vivo. These are the optical reporters (fluorescent and bioluminescent proteins used for bioluminescent imaging [BLI]). Positron emission tomography (PET), magnetic resonance imaging, and radiolabeling are all important for imaging tumors.

The emerging field of cellular and molecular imaging using optical reporters enables continuous measurement of gene expression in vitro and in vivo. For gene transfer analysis in vitro, enhanced green fluorescent protein has been useful. This technique has been applied to the HSV-TK and rabbit cytochrome P450/ipomeanol systems *(123)*.

Bioluminescence imaging is a new imaging strategy that can be applied to a variety of models using small animals. This procedure, employing luciferase enzyme as optical reporters (which can emit light by oxidation), is sensitive, reliable, and accessible *(124)*. An application using an adenoviral vector containing both a therapeutic gene (yeast CD) and the optical reporter gene (luciferase) was used to localize the enzyme in an orthotopic 9L glioma rat model. The in vivo BLI showed a decrease of luciferase expression during treatment with 5-FC, providing a marker for monitoring the expression of the CD gene *(125)*.

One possible approach to the imaging of gene expression in animals utilizes PET with PET reporter genes and PET reporter probes. This technology was used for imaging the HSV-TK/GCV system *(126–128)*. 2'-Fluoro-2'-deoxy-1-β-D-arabinofuranosyl-5-iodouracil ([$^{124/125}$I]FIAU) was proposed as an effective PET reporter probe for imaging of HSV-TK expression in vivo *(129)*. The expression of the double suicide gene therapy system CD plus HSV-TK was also monitored using [^{124}I]FIAU and PET *(130)*.

In vitro ^{19}F-NMR was used to study the release of a fluorinated nitrogen mustard from its corresponding glucuronide prodrug using β-Gluc *(131)*. Magnetic resonance spectroscopy (MRS) is another way of tackling the imaging problem. Many studies have demonstrated a correlation between different cancer treatment in patients and modification of the MRS of the corresponding tumors. It has been reported that the efficacy of the treatment with the HSV-TK/GCV system could be monitored in vivo using ^{31}P-MRS *(10)*.

Radiolabeled [^{14}C]FIAU was used to demonstrate its localization in mouse tumors pretreated with *Salmonella typhimurium* expressing HSV-TK. A 30-fold accumulation of [^{14}C]FIAU in the tumor was demonstrated as compared with muscle tissue *(132)*.

5. THE BE AND ITS MECHANISMS

The BE can be defined as the tumor regression that takes place in a GDEPT model after prodrug administration, when only a fraction of the tumor mass is genetically modified with foreign enzyme or the effect of the treatment on nongenetically modified cells *(133)*. The successes described in GDEPT would not be possible without the existence of such an effect. Some tumor xenografts require only 1–2% of cells to be genetically modified to obtain therapeutically significant results *(133,134)*.

It is difficult to compare the BE obtained in different experimental conditions because of the different methodologies employed by the various investigators. However, because of its importance in achieving therapeutic benefit, the mechanisms of BE have been investigated. Important differences were reported between in vitro and in vivo BE experiments. The in vitro models are probably more relevant in BE mechanistic terms because a "pure" BE is investigated without the interference of the immune system, which is characteristic to some in vivo models.

The activation of the prodrugs used in GDEPT can generate cell membrane-permeable or -impermeable active drugs. In the former, cell-to-cell contact is not required for BE killing. In the latter, cell-to-cell contact is needed to achieve this effect.

Toxic metabolites are formed following prodrug activation. The permeable ones are released by efflux from dead and dying genetically modified cells. This mechanism is postulated for 5-FU formed from 5-FC; for the metabolites of CP or IF, aldophosphamide, phosphoramidic mustards, or acrolein; for benzoic acid mustard released from CMDA; and for 6-methylpurine and 2-fluoroadenine formed from the corresponding deoxynucleoside. The transport of toxic metabolites from transgenes to target cells is mainly based on diffusion. This assumption is supported by the fact that no cell-to-cell contact is required to obtain a BE in these systems, and that toxic metabolites were detected in the medium.

For purine or pyrimidine nucleosides for which the toxic metabolites, because they are phosphorylated, are not diffusible across cell membranes, a direct cell-to-cell contact is required to achieve a BE.

More than one mechanism has been postulated for this BE, depending on how the toxic metabolites can be transported into target cells via gap junctional intercellular communications (GJIC), by phagocytosis of the apoptotic bodies, or by release of the cytostatic metabolites.

The transfer of cytotoxic GCV metabolites from HSV-TK-transfected cells to wild-type tumor cells via gap junctions has been proposed as the main mechanism of the BE for this type of system *(48,50, 135)*. A number of data support this assumption. First, the extent of BE usually parallels the level of GJIC independent of the origin of the cancer cell *(48,50)*.

Second, the transfection of connexin genes in cancer cells that poorly express GJIC enhances significantly the BE *(136)*. The expression of the Cx43 is essential for the expression of BE in glioma and colon cancer cells *(137–139)*. Other connexin genes (Cx26, Cx37) were also transfected with positive effect for the expression of the BE in recipient cells *(50,140)*. It was also reported that the BE depends not only on the level of GJIC expression, but also on the type of connexins expressed on the cell surface *(141)*.

Third, GJIC function was evaluated with a dye transfer technique. Tumor cells resistant to BE did not show dye transfer from cell to cell, but BE-sensitive tumor cells did *(135)*.

Fourth, the BE can be manipulated pharmacologically based on the GJIC mechanism. Dieldrin, a drug known to decrease gap junction communications, diminished the dye transfer and inhibited the BE. It was suggested that the enhancement of the HSV-TK/GCV BE and the antitumor effect could be achieved by pharmacological manipulation of the gap junctions in vivo. Apigenin (a flavonoid) and lovastatin (an HMG-coenzyme A reductase inhibitor) were shown to upregulate GJIC function and dye transfer in tumor cells expressing this type of communication. On treatment with GCV of mice bearing tumors grown from a mixture of 90% wild-type cells and 10% HSV-TK adenocarcinoma cells, 30% become tumor free. Tumor-bearing mice were administered two or three injections of lovastatin or apigenin during GCV treatment and had double the antitumor response rate, with 60–70% of the mice achieving complete remissions *(135,142)*.

However, there are types of cells in which the BE is independent of the GJIC, suggesting that other mechanisms may be involved. In human lung tumor cell lines of different origins, the GJIC were measured using a double dye transfer assay. Significant cytotoxicity was obtained when cultured cells comprised only 10% of HSV-TK-expressing cells. Although GJIC were not observed by the rapid transfer of lucifer yellow, they were detected by the slow transfer of calcein-AM. However, neither an inhibitor (1-octanol) nor an enhancer (all-*trans* retinoic acid) of GJIC affected the extent of the BE. These data suggest that low levels of gap junctions may be enough to produce a BE, or that other mechanisms are involved *(143)*.

Despite the fact that SW60.TK cells were capable of transferring only 3% of the dye to the surrounding cells, they still can transfer GCV-TP, which was found in the neighboring cells and in the culture medium *(144,145)*. It was found that the BE depended on the concentration of the enzyme, the number of cells expressing HSV-TK, and the overall confluency of the cells by comparing the efficacy of the HSV-TK/GCV system in two human carcinoma cell lines following exposure to 10 μM GCV. However, the BE did not correlate with the GJIC, as determined by the lucifer yellow assay *(145)*.

Another suggestion was that the TK-enzyme is transported by apoptotic vesicles. Phagocytosis of material from dying TK-positive cells (e.g., hydrolases or other lytic enzymes) to bystander cells has also been suggested as a mechanism for the BE. Apoptosis was detected in bystander cells, and it was found that this event could be inhibited by BCL2 expression. However, during the apoptosis induction period, in bystander cells cocultured with HSV-TK-expressing cells, no phagocytosis was observed. It has also been suggested that killing of tumor cells by apoptosis could heighten the immune response to wild-type tumor cells by a priming effect *(146,147)*.

In experiments in which no cell-to-cell contact was necessary to mount a BE in an HSV-TK system, release of cytotoxic metabolites was proposed as an alternative mechanism *(144,148)*.

A quantitative expression of the BE was proposed using the NR/CB1954 system in a range of human tumor cell types. The IC_{50}'s of non-NR-expressing cells were measured in the presence of differing proportions of NR-expressing cells. The shift in IC_{50} was used to calculate a value for the BE, termed the transmission efficiency (TE), which is the decrease in IC_{50} caused by the BE as the percentage of the maximum decrease possible. The percentage of NR-expressing cells for which the TE was 50% (TE_{50}) is a single datum point for the BE. The TE_{50} in the cell lines ranged from 0.3 to approx 2% *(149)*. Three-dimensional cell cultures were developed and used for quantifying the BE. The model was validated for the NR/CB1954 system and allowed the identification of prodrugs with superior therapeutic activity and BE compared to CB1954 *(150)*.

The in vivo BE was first noticed by Culver *(151)* and then was demonstrated in a number of experiments. In vitro, 30% of cells expressing CD were enough to eradicate the whole cell population. This BE is more impressive in vivo; only 2% CD-positive tumor cells were sufficient to obtain tumor regressions in athymic mice. With 4% CD-positive cells, 66% of animals were cured of their xenografts *(133,152)*. When similar experiments were performed in immunocompetent animals, the results were even better because of an immune response.

It has been shown in vivo that a distant BE can be induced when the treatment of a tumor transfected with a suicide gene followed by the corresponding prodrug administration resulted in regression not only of the transfected tumor, but also of physically separated nontransfected tumors. This phenomenon was reported with the HSV-TK/GCV system for colorectal metastasis, myelomas, and mammary, prostate, head and neck, and ovarian cancers *(153,154)* and is explained by the in vivo contribution of additional immune mechanisms *(154)* (*see also* Section 6.).

6. IMMUNITY: FRIEND OR FOE?

Three main immunological aspects are involved in GDEPT: immunogenicity of the vectors, immunogenicity of the expressed enzyme, and immunity induction following the modifications or the killing of the cancer cells in response to GDEPT. Although the first two are detrimental by reducing the transfection efficiency and/or preventing repeat treatment, the last one is beneficial by increasing the BE and inducing a distant BE in some models (*vide infra*).

The immunogenicity of adenoviruses has been extensively studied, and it was shown that the attenuation of the gene expression results from three types of host immune response: innate, humoral, and cellular *(21)*. Most adults have low levels of neutralizing antibodies against adenoviruses of the serotype used in the more common vectors (Adenoviruses serotype 5). Nevertheless, systemic treatment with such vectors resulted in a relatively low level of circulating virus *(49)*.

Nonviral vectors may also induce immune effects. The most common mechanism of inactivation of lipoplexes in vivo seems to be mediated by complement activation. Opsonization by complement components leads to elimination of complexes from blood via uptake by reticuloendothelial system (RES) cells *(155,156)* This was dependent on cationic lipid type and charge *(156)*.

Apart from its detrimental effect in eliminating lipoplexes, the immune effect of the liposomes can exacerbate preexisting inflammatory processes *(157)*. Another clinical factor related to the immunogenicity of the liposomes is the effect on repeat dosing. Immunogenicity of lipoplexes might preclude repeat administration. However, the immunogenicity of liposome–DNA complexes is in general lower than for viral vectors, and repeated administration of interferon-β DNA has been demonstrated, provided that enough time (14 days) is left between the two consecutive dosages *(158)*.

There were early suggestions that the immune response following suicide gene therapy is a favorable event. Although data are available that show that the BE also occurs in immunocompromised animals, other findings suggest that the BE in vivo is mediated through the release of cytokines *(159)*. Coinjection of carcinoma cells and the HSV-TK-expressing retroviral packaging cells followed by injection of GCV resulted in almost total tumor ablation in immunocompetent BALB/c mice, but not in immunocompromised athymic BALB/c animals. In a similar experiment, the HSV-TK gene was transfected into cells grown as xenografts. It was shown that the activity of the HSV-TK inhibited tumor growth for up to 50 days in immunocompromised nude mice following GCV treatment, but was not sufficient to eliminate all the tumor cells in these animals (tumors regrew 40–50 days after cell implantation). By contrast, immunocompetent BALB/c mice developed a long-lasting immunity in response to HSV-TK transduction followed by GCV treatment *(160)*. Taken together, these studies imply that an intact immune system is important for long-term tumor suppression with TK in vivo.

7. CONCLUSIONS

Suicide gene therapy of cancer represents 8% of all 113 protocols for cancer gene therapy listed by the US Recombinant Advisory Committee *(49)*. Most of these used the HSV-TK/GCV system and are phase I/phase II trials *(161,162)*. One phase III trial using a retroviral vector has been completed and showed no benefit in terms of survival for the patients *(163)*. Using an adenoviral vector by direct intratumoral injection (in brain tumors) showed some improved survival *(164)*.

Phase I/II clinical trials were reported with CD/5-FC *(165)* and CYP450/CP or IF *(75)*. In the United Kingdom, a retroviral vector expressing CYP2B6 (MetXia) is undergoing testing in patients with advanced breast and ovarian cancers. In Germany, microencapsulated mammalian cells expressing CYP2B1 and IF were tested on 14 patients with inoperable pancreatic carcinoma. The follow-up 1-year survival was increased threefold *(166)*.

Suicide gene therapy proved to be safe; minor side effects were reported.

Some hurdles must be overcome before GDEPT will become a clinically efficient treatment for cancers. Major improvements are needed in the vector area with respect to both targeting and delivery of suicide genes. Multiple options are available, from nonviral vectors to more complex systems involving coexpression of suicide genes with immunological or tumor suppressor genes.

ACKNOWLEDGMENT

This work was funded by the Cancer Research Campaign (SP2330/0201 and SP2330/0102) and the Institute of Cancer Research.

REFERENCES

1. Workman, P. (2000) Editorial overview. Toward genomic cancer pharmacology: innovative drugs for the new millennium. *Curr. Opin. Oncol. Endocrine Metab. Investig. Drugs* **2,** 21–25.
2. Niculescu-Duvaz, I. and Springer, C. J. (1995) Antibody-directed enzyme prodrug therapy (ADEPT): a targeting strategy in cancer chemotherapy. *Curr. Med. Chem.* **2,** 687–706.
3. Melton, R. G. and Knox, R. (1999) *Enzyme-Prodrug Strategies for Cancer Therapy.* Kluwer Academic/Plenum, New York.
4. Roth, J. A. and Cristiano, R. G. (1997) Gene therapy for cancer: what have we done and where are we going? *J. Natl. Cancer Inst.* **89,** 21–30.
5. Niculescu-Duvaz, I., Spooner, R., Marais, R., and Springer, C. J. (1998) Gene-directed enzyme prodrug therapy. *Bioconj. Chem.* **9,** 4–22.
6. Springer, C. J. and Niculescu-Duvaz, I. (2001) Gene-directed enzyme prodrug therapy. In *Anticancer Drug Development* (Baguley, B., ed.), Academic Press, New York, pp. 137–135.
7. Marais, R., Spooner, R. A., Light, Y., Martin, J., and Springer, C. J. (1996) Gene-directed enzyme prodrug therapy with a mustard prodrug/carboxypeptidase G2 combination. *Cancer Res.* **56,** 4735–4742.
8. Bridgewater, G., Springer, C. J., Knox, R., Minton, N., Michael, P., and Collins, M. (1995) Expression of the bacterial nitroreductase enzyme in mammalian cells renders them selectively sensitive to killing by the prodrug CB1954. *Eur. J. Cancer* **31A,** 2362–2370.
9. Huber, B. E., Richards, C. A., and Austin, E. A. (1995) VDEPT; An enzyme/prodrug gene therapy approach for the treatment of metastatic colorectal cancer. *Adv. Drug Deliv. Rev.* **17,** 279–292.
10. Eaton, J. L., Perry, M. J. A., Todryk, S. M., et al. (2001) Genetic prodrug activation therapy (GPAT) in two rat prostate models generates an immune bystander effect and can be monitored by magnetic resonance techniques. *Gene Ther.* **8,** 557–567.
11. Zvelebil, M. (2000) STI-571, Novartis AG. *Curr. Opin. Oncol. Endocrine Metab. Investig. Drugs* **2,** 74–82.
12. Sedlacek, H. H., Seemann, G., Hoffmann, D., et al. (1992) *Antibodies as Carriers of Cytotoxicity.* Karger, Basel, Switzerland.
13. Bagshawe, K. D. (1989) Toward generating cytotoxic agents at cancer sites. *Br. J. Cancer* **60,** 275–281.
14. Senter, P. D. (1990) Activation of prodrugs by antibody-enzyme conjugates: a new approach to cancer therapy. *FASEB J.* **4,** 188–193.
15. Bagshawe, K. D., Rogers, G. T., Sharma, S. K., et al. (1990) In *Monoclonal Antibodies and Immunoconjugates* (Baldwin, R. W., Byers, V. S., and Mann, R. D., eds.), Parthenon, London, UK, pp. 95–102.
16. Marais, R., Spooner, R. A., Stribbling, S. M., Light, Y., Martin, J., and Springer, C. J. (1997) A cell surface tethered enzyme improves efficiency in gene-directed enzyme prodrug therapy. *Nat. Biotechnol.* **15,** 1373–1377.
17. Heine, D., Muller, R., and Brusselbach, S. (2001) Cell surface display of a lysosomal enzyme for extra-cellular gene-directed enzyme prodrug therapy. *Gene Ther.* **8,** 1005–1010.
18. Cowen, R. L., Williams, J. C., Emery, S., et al. (2002) Adenovirus vector-mediated delivery of the prodrug-converting enzyme carboxypeptidase G2 secreted or GPI-anchored form: High level expression of this active conditional cytotoxic enzyme at the plasma membrane. *Cancer Gene Ther.* **9,** 897–907.
19. Bilbao, G., Contreras, J. L., Gomez-Navarro, J., and Curiel, D. T. (1998) Improving adenoviral vectors for cancer gene therapy. *Tumor Targeting* **3,** 59–79.
20. Robbins, P. D. and Ghivizzani, S. C. (1998) Viral vectors for gene therapy. *Pharm. Ther.* **80,** 35–47.
21. Zhang, W. W. (1999) Development and application of adenoviral vectors for gene therapy of cancer. *Cancer Gene Ther.* **7,** 113–138.

22. Curiel, D. T., Gerritsen, W. R., and Krul, M. R. (2000) Progress in cancer gene therapy. *Cancer Gene Ther.* **7,** 1197–1199.
23. Ponnazhagan, S., Curiel, D. T., Shaw, D. R., Alvarez, R. D., and Siegal, G. P. (2001) Adeno-associated virus for cancer gene therapy. *Cancer Res.* **61,** 6313–6321.
24. Green, N. K. and Seymour, L. W. (2002) Adenoviral vectors: systemic delivery and tumor targeting. *Cancer Gene Ther.* **9,** 1036–1042.
25. King, I., Bermudes, D., Lin, S., et al. (2002) Tumor-targeted *Salmonella* expressing cytosine deaminase as an anti-cancer agent. *Hum. Gene Ther.* **13,** 1225–1233.
26. Theys, J., Landuyt, W., Nuyts, S., et al. (2001) Specific targeting of cytosine deaminase to solid tumors by engineered *Clostridium acetobutylicum. Cancer Gene Ther.* **8,** 294–297.
27. Hermiston, T. (2000) Gene-delivery from replication-selective viruses: arming guided missiles in the war against cancer. *J. Clin. Investig.* **105,** 1169–1172.
28. Martuza, R. L. (2000) Conditionally replicating herpes vector for gene therapy. *J. Clin. Investig.* **105,** 841–846.
29. Kirn, D. (2001) Clinical research results with dI 1520 (ONYX-015), a replication selective adenovirus for the treatment of cancer: what have we learned? *Gene Ther.* **8,** 89–98.
30. Hermiston, T. V. and Kuhn, I. (2002) Armed therapeutic viruses: strategies and challenges to arming oncolytic viruses with therapeutic genes. *Cancer Gene Ther.* **9,** 1022–1035.
31. Dachs, G. U., Dougherty, G. J., Stratford, I. J., and Chaplin, D. J. (1997) Targeting gene therapy for cancer. *Oncol. Res.* **9,** 313–325.
32. Spear, M. A. (1998) Gene therapy of gliomas: receptors and transcriptional targeting. *Anticancer Res.* **18,** 3223–3232.
33. Hayes, G. M., Carpenito, C., Davis, P. D., Dougherty, S. T., Dirks, G. F., and Dougherty, G. H. (2002) Alternative splicing as a novel means of regulating the expression of therapeutic genes. *Cancer Gene Ther.* **9,** 133–141.
34. De Fatta, R. J., Li, Y., and De Benedetti, A. (2002) Selective killing of cancer cells based on translational control of suicide gene therapy. *Cancer Gene Ther.* **9,** 573–578.
35. De Fatta, R. J., Chervenack, R. P., and De Benedetti, A. (2002) A cancer gene therapy approach through translational control of a suicide gene. *Cancer Gene Ther.* **9,** 502–505.
36. Pawelek, J. M., Low, K. B., and Bermudes, D. (1997) Tumor-targeted *Salmonella* as a novel anticancer vector. *Cancer Res.* **57,** 4537–4544.
37. Kirn, D. (2000) Replication-selective microbiological agents: fighting cancer with targeted germ warfare. *J. Clin. Investig.* **105,** 837–839.
38. Yazawa, K., Fujimori, M., Amano, J., Kano, Y., and Taniguchi, S. (2000) *Bifidobacterium longum* as a delivery system for cancer gene therapy: selective localization and growth in hypoxic tumors. *Cancer Gene Ther.* **7,** 269–274.
39. Nuyts, S., Van Mellaert, L., Theys, J., Landuyt, W., Lambin, P., and Anne, J. (2001) The use of radiation-induced bacterial promoters in anaerobic-conditions: a means to control gene expression in *Clostridium*-mediated gene therapy. *Radiat. Res.* **155,** 716–723.
40. Liu, S.-C., Minton, N. P., Giaccia, A. J., and Brown, J. M. (2002) Anticancer efficacy of systemically delivered anaerobic bacteria as gene therapy vectors targeting tumor hypoxia/necrosis. *Gene Ther.* **9,** 291–296.
41. Miller, A. D. (1998) Cationic liposomes for gene therapy. *Angew. Chem. Int. Ed. Engl.* **37,** 1768–1785.
42. Schatzlein, A. G. (2001) Non-viral vectors in cancer gene therapy: principles and progress. *Anti-Cancer Drug Des.* **12,** 275–304.
43. Ilies, M. A., Seitz, M. A., and Balaban, A. T. (2002) Cationic lipids in gene delivery: principles, vector design and therapeutical application. *Curr. Pharm. Des.* **8,** 2441–2474.
44. Denny, W. A. and Wilson, W. R. (1998) The design of selectively-activated anti-cancer prodrugs for use in antibody-directed and gene-directed enzyme prodrugs therapies. *J. Pharm. Pharmacol.* **50,** 387–394.
45. Encell, L. P., Landis, D. M., and Loeb, L. A. (1999) Improving enzymes for gene therapy. *Nat. Biotechnol.* **17,** 143–147.
46. Niculescu-Duvaz, I., Friedlos, F., Niculescu-Duvaz, D., Davies, L., and Springer, C. J. (1999) Prodrugs for antibody- and gene-directed enzyme prodrug therapies (ADEPT and GDEPT). *Anticancer Drug Des.* **14,** 517–538.
47. Springer, C. J. and Niculescu-Duvaz, I. (2000) Prodrug-activating systems in suicide gene therapy. *J. Clin. Investig.* **105,** 1161–1167.
48. Mesnil, M. and Yamasachi, H. (2000) Bystander effect in herpes simplex virus-thymidine kinase/ganciclovir cancer gene therapy: role of gap-junctional intercellular communications. *Cancer Res.* **60,** 3989–3999.
49. McCormick, F. (2001) Cancer gene therapy: fringe or cutting edge? *Nat. Rev. Cancer* **1,** 130–141.
50. Van Dillen, I. J., Mulder, N. H., Vaalburg, W., De Vries, E. F. J., and Hospers, G. A. P. (2002) Influence of the bystander effect on HSV-tk/GCV gene therapy. A review. *Curr. Gene Ther.* **2,** 307–322.
51. Wardman, P. (2002) Indole-3-acetic acid and horseradish peroxidase: a new prodrug/enzyme combination for targeted cancer therapy. *Curr. Pharm. Des.* **8,** 1363–1374.
52. Greco, O., Folkes, L. K., Wardman, P., Tozer, G. M., and Dachs, G. U. (2000) Development of a novel enzyme/prodrug combination for gene therapy of cancer: horseradish peroxidase/indole-3-acetic acid. *Cancer Gene Ther.* **7,** 1414–1420.

53. Patterson, A. V., Williams, K. J., Coven, R. L., et al. (2002) Oxygen-sensitive enzyme-prodrug gene therapy for the eradication of radiation-resistant solid tumors. *Gene Ther.* **9,** 946–954.
54. Miki, K., Xu, M., Gupta, A., et al. (2001) Methioninase cancer gene therapy with selenomethionine as suicide prodrug substrate. *Cancer Res.* **61,** 6805–6810.
55. Trudeau, C., Yuan, S., Galipeau, J., Benlimame, N., Alaoui-Jamali, M. A., and Batist, G. (2001) A novel parasite-derived suicide gene for cancer gene therapy with specificity for lung cancer cells. *Hum. Gene Ther.* **12,** 1673–1680.
56. Bernt, K. M., Steinwaerder, D. S., Ni, S., Li, Z.-Y., Roffler, S. R., and Lieber, A. (2002) Enzyme-activated prodrug therapy enhances tumor-specific replication of adenovirus vectors. *Cancer Res.* **62,** 6089–6098.
57. Misra, V., Klamut, H. J., and Rauth, A. M. (2002) Expression of the prodrug-activating enzyme DT-diaphorase via Ad5 delivery to human colon carcinoma cells in vitro. *Cancer Gene Ther.* **9,** 209–217.
58. Voeks, D., Martiniello-Wilks, R., Maden, V., et al. (2002) Gene therapy for prostate cancer delivered by ovine adenovirus and mediated by purine nucleoside phosphorylase and fludarabine in mouse models. *Gene Ther.* **9,** 759–768.
59. Nyati, M. K., Sreekumar, A., Li, S., et al. (2002) High and selective expression of yeast cytosine deaminase under a carcinoembryonic antigen promoter-enhancer. *Cancer Res.* **62,** 2337–2342.
60. Luna, M., Chen, X., Wong, S., et al. (2002) Enhanced photodynamic therapy efficacy with inducible suicide gene therapy controlled by the grp promoter. *Cancer Res.* **62,** 1458–1461.
61. Kievit, E., Bershad, E., Ng, E., et al. (1999) Superiority of yeast over bacterial cytosine deaminase for enzyme/prodrug gene therapy in colon cancer. *Cancer Res.* **59,** 1417–1421.
62. Springer, C. J., Dowell, R., Burke, P. J., et al. (1995) Optimization of alkylating agent prodrug derived from phenol and aniline mustards: a new clinical candidates prodrug (ZD2767) for antibody-directed prodrug therapy (ADEPT). *J. Med. Chem.* **38,** 5051–5065.
63. Springer, C. J. and Niculescu-Duvaz, I. (1995) Antibody-directed enzyme prodrug therapy (ADEPT) with mustard prodrugs. *Anticancer Drug Des.* **10,** 361–372.
64. Azoulay, M., Florent, J.-C., Monneret, C., et al. (1995) Prodrugs of anthracycline antibiotics suited for tumor specific activation. *Anticancer Drug Des.* **10,** 441–450.
65. De Groot, F. M. J., Loos, V. J., Koekkoek, R., et al. (2001) Elongated multiple electronic cascade and cyclization spacer systems in activatable anticancer prodrugs for enhanced drug release. *J. Org. Chem.* **66,** 8815–8830.
66. Gesson, J. P., Jacquesy, J. C., Mondon, M., et al. (1994) Prodrugs of anthracyclines for chemotherapy via enzyme-monoclonal antibody conjugates. *Anticancer Drug Des.* **9,** 409–423.
67. Leenders, R. C. G., Damen, E. W. P., Bijterveld, E. J. A., et al. (1999) Novel anthracycline-spacer-β-glucuronide, -β-glucoside and -β-galactoside prodrugs for application in selective chemotherapy. *Bioorg. Med. Chem.* **7,** 1597–1610.
68. Hay, M. P., Sykes, B. M., Denny, W. A., and O'Connor, C. J. (1999) Substituents effect of the kinetics of reductively-initiated fragmentation of nitrobenzylcarbamates designed as triggers for prodrugs. *J. Chem. Soc. Perkin Trans.* **1,** 2759–2770.
69. Niculescu-Duvaz, D., Niculescu-Duvaz, I., Friedlos, F., et al. (1998) Self-immolative nitrogen mustard prodrugs for suicide gene therapy. *J. Med. Chem.* **41,** 5297–5309.
70. Niculescu-Duvaz, I., Niculescu-Duvaz, D., Friedlos, F., et al. (1999) Self-immolative anthracycline prodrugs for suicide gene therapy. *J. Med. Chem.* **42,** 2485–2489.
71. Dowell, R. I., Springer, C. J., Davies, D. H., et al. (1996) New mustard prodrug for antibody-directed enzyme prodrug therapy: alternative to amide link. *J. Med. Chem.* **39,** 1100–1105.
72. Friedlos, F., Davies, L., Scanlon, I., et al. (2002) Three new prodrugs for suicide gene therapy using carboxypeptidase G2 elicit bystander efficacy in two xenograft models. *Cancer Res.* **62,** 1724–1729.
73. Grove, J. I., Searle, P. F., Weedon, S. J., Green, N. K., McNeish, I. A., and Kerr, D. J. (1999) Virus-directed enzyme prodrug therapy using CB1954. *Anticancer Drug Des.* **14,** 461–472.
74. Wierdl, M., Morton, C. L., Weeks, J. K., Danks, M. K., Harris, L. C., and Potter, P. M. (2001) Sensitization of human tumor cells to CPT-11 via adenoviral-mediated delivery of a rabbit liver carboxylesterase. *Cancer Res.* **61,** 5078–5082.
75. Chen, L. and Waxman, D. J. (2002) Cytochrome P-450 gene-directed enzyme prodrug therapy (GDEPT) for cancer. *Curr. Pharm. Des.* **8,** 1405–1416.
76. Kokoris, M. S., Sabo, P., Adman, E. T., and Black, M. E. (1999) Enhancement of tumor ablation by a selected HSV-1 thymidine kinase mutants. *Gene Ther.* **6,** 1415–1426.
77. Black, M., Kokoris, M. S., and Sabo, P. (2001) Herpes simplex virus-1 thymidine kinase mutants created by semi-random sequence mutagenesis improve prodrug-mediated tumor cell killing. *Cancer Res.* **61,** 3022–3026.
78. Kokoris, M. S. and Black, M. E. (2002) Characterization of herpes simplex virus type 1 kinase mutants engineered for improved ganciclovir and acyclovir activity. *Protein Sci.* **11,** 2267–2272.
79. Balzarini, J., Liekens, S., Esnouf, R., and De Clercq, E. (2002) The A167Y mutation converts the herpes simplex virus type 1 thymidine kinase into a guanosineanalogue kinase. *Biochemistry* **41,** 6517–6524.
79a. Smith, G. K., Banks, S., Blumenkopf, T. A., et al. (1997) Toward antibody-directed enzyme prodrug therapy with the T268G mutant of human carboxypeptidase A1 and novel in vivo stable prodrugs of methotrexate. *J. Biol. Chem.* **20,** 15,804–15,816.

80. Bagshawe, K. D., Sharma, S. K., Springer, C. J., et al. (1991) Antibody-directed enzyme prodrug therapy (ADEPT): clinical report. *Dis. Markers* **9**, 233–238.

81. Secrist, J. A. III, Parker, W. B., Allan, P. W., et al. (1999) Gene therapy of cancer: activation of nucleoside prodrugs with *E. coli* purine nucleoside phosphorylase. *Nucleosides Nucleotides* **18**, 745–757.

82. Friedlos, F., Denny, W. A., Palmer, B. D., and Springer, C. J. (1997) Mustard prodrugs for activation by *Escherichia coli* nitroreductase in gene-directed enzyme prodrug therapy. *J. Med. Chem.* **40**, 1270–1275.

83. Bailey, S. M., Knox, R. J., Hobbs, S. M., et al. (1996) Investigation of alternative prodrugs for use with *E. coli* nitroreductase in "suicide gene" approaches to cancer therapy. *Gene Ther.* **3**, 1143–1150.

84. Balzarini, J., Ostrowski, T., Goslinski, T., De Clercq, E., and Golankiewicz, B. (2002) Pronounced cytostatic activity and bystander effect of a novel series of fluorescent tricyclic acyclovir and ganciclovir derivatives in herpes simplex virus thymidine kinase gene-transduced tumor cell lines. *Gene Ther.* **9**, 1173–1182.

85. Denny, A. W. (2002) Nitroreductase-based GDEPT. *Curr. Pharm. Des.* **8**, 1349–1361.

86. Tiraby, M., Cazaux, C., Baron, M., Drocourt, D., Reynes, J.-P., and Tiraby, G. (1998) Concomitant expression of *E. coli* cytosine deaminase and uracil phosphoribosyltransferase improves the cytotoxicity of 5-fluorocytosine. *FEMS Microbiol. Lett.* **167**, 41–49.

87. Balzarini, G., Degreve, B., Andrei, G., et al. (1998) Superior cytostatic activity of the ganciclovir elaidic acid ester due to the prolonged intracellular retention of ganciclovir anabolites in herpes simplex virus type 1 thymidine kinase gene-transfected tumor cells. *Gene Ther.* **5**, 419–426.

87a. Niculescu-Duvaz, D., Niculescu-Duvaz, I., Friedlos, F., et al. (2003) Self-immolative nitrogen mustards prodrugs cleavable by carboxypeptidase G2 (CPG2) showing large cytotoxicity differentials in GDEPT. *J. Med. Chem.* **46**, 1690–1705.

88. Bohnenstengel, F., Friedel, G., Ritter, C. A., et al. (2000) Variability of cyclophosphamide uptake into human bronchial carcinoma: consequence for local bioactivation. *Cancer Chemother. Pharmacol.* **45**, 63–68.

89. Ichikawa, T., Petros, W. P., Ludeman, S. M., et al. (2001) Intraneoplastic polymer-based delivery of cyclophosphamide for intratumoral bioconversion by a replicating oncolytic viral vector. *Cancer Res.* **61**, 864–868.

90. Hayashi, K., Hayashi, T., Sun, H.-D., and Takeda, I. (2000) Potentiation of ganciclovir toxicity in the herpes simplex virus thymidine kinase/ganciclovir administration system by ponicidin. *Cancer Gene Ther.* **7**, 45–42.

91. Hamel, W., Zirkel, D., Mehdorn, H. M., Westphal, M., and Israel, M. A. (2001) E-5-(2-bromovinyl)-2'-deoxyuridine potentiates ganciclovir-mediated cytotoxicity on herpes simplex virus-thymidine kinase-expressing cells. *Cancer Gene Ther.* **8**, 388–396.

92. McMasters, R. A., Wilbert, T. N., Jones, K. E., et al. (2000) Two-drug combinations that increase apoptosis and modulate Bak and Bcl-X$_L$ expression in human colon tumor cell lines transduced with herpes simplex virus thymidine kinase. *Cancer Gene Ther.* **7**, 563–573.

93. Rubsam, L. Z., Davidson, L., and Shewach, D. S. (1998) Superior cytotoxicity with gancyclovir compared with acyclovir and 1-β-D-arabinofuranosylthymine in herpes simplex virus-thymidine kinase-expressing-cells: a novel paradigm for cell killing. *Cancer Res.* **58**, 3873–3882.

94. Boucher, P. D., Ostruszka, L. J., and Shewach, D. S. (2000) Synergistic enhancement of herpes simplex virus thymidine kinase/ganciclovir mediated cytotoxicity by hydroxyurea. *Cancer Res.* **60**, 1631–1636.

95. Boucher, P. D., Ostruszka, l. J., MKurphy, P. J. M., and Shewach, D. S. (2002) Hydroxyurea significantly enhances tumor growth delay in vivo with herpes simplex virus thymidine kinase/ganciclovir gene therapy. *Gene Ther.* **9**, 1023–1030.

96. Huang, Z., Raychowdhury, K., and Waxman, D. J. (2000) Impact of liver P450 reductase suppression on cyclophosphamide activation, pharmacokinetics and antitumoral activity in a cytochrome P450-based cancer gene therapy model. *Cancer Gene Ther.* **7**, 1034–1042.

97. Huang, Z. and Waxman, D. J. (2001) Modulation of cyclophosphamide-based cytochrome p450 gene therapy using liver P450 inhibitors. *Cancer Gene Ther.* **8**, 450–458.

98. Jounaidi, Y. and Waxman, D. J. (2000) Combination of the bioreductive drug tirapazamine with the chemotherapeutic prodrug cyclophosphamide for P450/P450-reductase-based cancer gene therapy. *Cancer Res.* **60**, 3761–3769.

99. Rainov, N. G., Fels, C., Droge, J. W., Schafer, C., Kramm, C. M., and Chou, T.-C. (2001) Temozolomide enhances herpes simplex virus thymidine kinase/ganciclovir therapy of malignant glioma. *Cancer Gene Ther.* **8**, 662–668.

100. Kanyama, H., Tomita, N., Yamano, T., et al. (2001) Usefulness of repeated intratumoral gene transfer using hemagglutinating virus of Japan-liposome method for cytosine deaminase suicide gene therapy. *Cancer Res.* **61**, 14–18.

101. Jounaidi, Y. and Waxman, D. J. (2001) Frequent, moderate dose cyclophosphamide administration improves the efficacy of cytochrome P-450/cytochrome P-450 reductase based cancer gene therapy. *Cancer Res.* **61**, 4437–4444.

102. Pulkanen, K. J., Laukanen, J. M., Fuxe, J., et al. (2002) The combination of HSV-tk and endostatin gene therapy eradicates orthotopic human renal cell carcinomas in nude mice. *Cancer Gene Ther.* **9**, 908–916.

103. Rogulski, K. R., Zhang, K., Kolozsvary, A., Kim, J. H., and Freitag, S. O. (1997) Pronounced antitumor effect and tumor radiosensitization of double suicide gene therapy. *Clin. Cancer Res.* **3**, 2081–2088.

104. Uckert, W., Kammertons, T., Haack, K., et al. (1998) Double suicide gene (cytosine deaminase and herpes simplex

virus thymidine kinase) but not single gene transfer allows reliable elimination of tumor cells in vivo. *Hum. Gene Ther.* **9**, 855–865.

105. Blackburn, R. V., Galoforo, S. S., Corry, P. M., and Lee, Y. J. (1998) Adenoviral-mediated transfer of a heat-inducible double suicide gene into prostate carcinoma cells. *Cancer Res.* **58**, 1358–1362.

106. Kammertoens, T., Gelbmann, W., Karle, P., et al. (2000) Combined chemotherapy of murine mammary tumors by local activation of the prodrug ifosfamide and 5-fluorocytosine. *Cancer Gene Ther.* **7**, 629–636.

107. Rogulski, K. R., Wing, M. S., Paielli, D. L., Gilbert, J. D., Kim, J. H., and Freytag, S. O. (2000) Double suicide gene therapy augments the antitumor activity of a replication-competent lytic adenovirus through enhanced cytotoxicity and radiosensitization. *Hum. Gene Ther.* **11**, 67–76.

108. Blanche, F., Cameron, B., Couder, M., and Crouzet, J. (1997) W09735024. Rhone-Poulenc Roerer, p. 61.

109. Shimizu, T., Shimada, H., Ochiai, T., and Hamada, H. (2001) Enhanced growth suppression in esophageal carcinoma cells using adenovirus-mediated fusion gene transfer uracil phosphoryl transferase and herpes simplex virus thymidine kinase. *Cancer Gene Ther.* **8**, 512–521.

110. Manome, Y., Watanabe, M., Abe, T., et al. (2001) Transduction of thymidine phosphorylase cDNA facilitates efficacy of cytosine deaminase/5-FC gene therapy for malignant brain tumors. *Anticancer Res.* **21**, 2265–2272.

111. Erbs, P., Regulier, E., Kintz, J., et al. (2000) In vivo cancer gene therapy by adenovirus-mediated transfer of a bifunctional yeast cytosine deaminase/uracil phosphoribosyltransferase fusion gene. *Cancer Res.* **60**, 3813–3822.

112. Chen, L., Yu, L. J., and Waxman, D. J. (1997) Potentiation of cytochrome P450/cyclophosphamide-based cancer gene therapy by coexpression of the P450 reductase gene. *Cancer Res.* **57**, 4830–4837.

113. Kim, Y. G., Bi, W., Feliciano, E. S., Drake, R. R., and Stambrook, P. J. (2000) Ganciclovir-mediated cell killing and bystander effect is enhanced in cells with two copies of the herpes simplex virus thymidine kinase. *Cancer Gene Ther.* **7**, 240–246.

114. Moriuchi, S., Wolfe, D., Tamura, M., et al. (2002) Double suicide gene therapy using a replication defective herpes simplex virus vector reveals reciprocal interference in a malignant glioma model. *Gene Ther.* **9**, 584–591.

115. Chen, S. H., Kosai, K., Xu, B., et al. (1996) Combination suicide and cytokine gene therapy for hepatic metastases of colon carcinoma: sustained antitumor immunity prolongs animal survival. *Cancer Res.* **56**, 3758–3762.

116. Toda, M., Martuza, R. L., and Rabkin, S. D. (2001) Combination suicide/cytokine gene therapy as adjuvants to a defective herpes simplex virus-based cancer vaccine. *Gene Ther.* **8**, 332–339.

117. Hall, S. J., Canfield, S. E., Yan, Y., Hassen, W., Selleck, W. A., and Chen, S.-H. (2002) A novel bystander effect involving tumor cell-derived Fas and FasL interactions following Ad.HSV-TK and Ad.mIL-12 gene therapies in experimental prostate cancer. *Gene Ther.* **9**, 511–517.

118. Brust, D., Feden, J., Farnsworth, J., Amir, C., Broaddus, W. C., and Valerie, K. (2000) Radiosensitization of rat glioma with bromodeoxycytidine and adenovirus expressing herpes simplex virus-thymidine kinase delivered by slow, rate-controlled positive pressure infusion. *Cancer Gene Ther.* **7**, 778–788.

119. Valerie, K., Brust, D., Farnsworth, J., et al. (2000) Improved radiosensitization of rat glioma cells with adenovirus-expressed mutant herpes simplex virus-thymidine kinase in combination with acyclovir. *Cancer Gene Ther.* **7**, 879–884.

120. Valerie, K., Hawkins, W., Farnsworth, J., et al. (2001) Substantially improved in vivo radiosensitization of rat glioma with mutant HSV-TK and acyclovir. *Cancer Gene Ther.* **8**, 3–8.

121. Kawashita, Y., Ohtsuru, A., Kaneda, Y., et al. (1999) Regression of hepatocellular carcinoma in vitro and in vivo by radiosensitising suicide gene therapy under the inducible and spatial control of radiation. *Hum. Gene Ther.* **10**, 1509–1519.

122. Nuyts, S., Theys, J., Landuyt, W., Van Mellaert, L., Lambin, P., and Anne, J. (2001) Increasing specificity of anti-tumour therapy: cytotoxic proteins delivery by non-pathogenic clostridia under regulation of radio-induced promoter. *Anticancer Res.* **21**, 857–862.

123. Steffens, S., Frank, S., Fisher, U., et al. (2000) Enhanced green fluorescent proteinfusion proteins of herpes simplex virus type 1 thymidine kinase and cytochrome P450 4B1: applications for prodrug-activating gene therapy. *Cancer Gene Ther.* **7**, 806–812.

124. O'Connell-Rodwell, C. E., Burns, S. M., Bachman, M. H., and Contag, C. H. (2002) Bioluminescent indicators for in vivo measurements of gene expression. *Trends Biotechnol.* **20**, S19–S23.

125. Rehemtulla, A., Hall, D. E., Stegman, L. D., et al. (2002) Molecular imaging of gene expression and efficacy following adenoviral-mediated brain tumor gene therapy. *Mol. Imaging* **1**, 43–55.

126. Tjuvajev, J. G., Finn, R., Watanabe, K., et al. (1996) Noninvasive imaging of herpes simplex virus thymidine kinase gene transfer and expression: a potential method for monitoring clinical gene therapy. *Cancer Res.* **56**, 4087–4095.

127. Tjuvajev, J. G., Avril, N., Oku, T., et al. (1998) Imaging herpes virus thymidine kinase gene transfer and expression by positron emission tomography. *Cancer Res.* **58**, 4333–4341.

128. Yagoubi, S. S., Wu, L., Liang, Q., et al. (2001) Direct correlation between positron emission tomographic images of two reporter genes delivered by two distinct adenoviral vectors. *Gene Ther.* **8**, 1072–1080.

129. Brust, P., Haubner, R., Friedrich, A., et al. (2001) Comparison of [18F]FHPG and [124/125I]FIAU for imaging herpes simplex virus type 1 thymidine kinase gene expression. *Eur. J. Nuclear Med.* **28**, 721–729.

130. Hackman, T., Dubrovin, M., Balatoni, J., et al. (2002) Imaging expression of cytosine deaminase-herpes virus thymidine kinase fusion gene (CD/TK) expression with [^{124}I]-FIAU and PET. *Mol. Imaging* **1,** 36–42.

131. Schmidt, F. and Monneret, C. (2002) In vitro fluorine-19 nuclear magnetic resonance study of the liberation of antitumor nitrogen mustard from prodrugs. *J. Chem. Soc. Perkin Trans.* **1,** 1302–1308.

132. Tjuvaev, J., Blasberg, R., Luo, X., Zheng, L. M., King, I., and Bermudes, D. (2001) *Salmonella*-based tumor-targeted cancer therapy: tumor amplified protein expression therapy (TAPET$^{™}$) for diagnostic imaging. *J. Controlled Release* **74,** 313–315.

133. Huber, B. E., Austin, E. A., Richards, C. A., Davis, S. T., and Good, S. S. (1994) Metabolism of 5-fluorocytidine to 5-fluorouracil in human colorectal tumor cells transduced with the cytosine deaminase gene: significant antitumor effects when only a small percentage of tumor cells express cytosine deaminase. *Proc. Natl. Acad. Sci. USA* **91,** 8302–8306.

134. Sorscher, E. J., Peng, S., Bebock, Z., Allan, P. W., Bennett, L. L. Jr., and Parker, W. B. (1994) Tumor cell bystander killing in colonic carcinoma utilizing the *Escherichia coli* deo-D gene to generate toxic purines. *Gene Ther.* **1,** 233–238.

135. Touraine, R. L., Ishii-Morita, H., Ramsey, W. J., and Blaese, R. M. (1998) The bystander effect in the HSVtk/ganciclovir system and its relation to gap junctional communication. *Gene Ther.* **5,** 1705–1711.

136. Mesnil, M., Piccoli, C., and Yamasaki, H. (1997) A tumor suppressor gene Cx26, also mediates the bystander in HeLa cells. *Cancer Res.* **57,** 2929–2932.

137. McMasters, R. A., Saylors, R. L., Jones, K. E., Hendrix, M. E., Moyers, M. P., and Drake, R. R. (1998) Lack of bystander killing in herpes virus thymidine kinase-transduced colon cell lines due to deficient connexin43 gap junction formation. *Hum. Gene Ther.* **9,** 2253–2261.

138. Namba, H., Iwadate, Y., Kawamura, K., Sakiyama, S., and Tagawa, M. (2001) Efficacy of the bystander effect in the herpes simplex virus thymidine kinase-mediated gene therapy is influenced by the expression of connexin43 in the target cells. *Cancer Gene Ther.* **8,** 414–420.

139. Sanson, M., Marcaud, V., Robin, E., Valery, C., Sturtz, F., and Zalc, B. (2002) Connexin-43-mediated bystander effect in two rat glioma cell models. *Cancer Gene Ther.* **9,** 149–155.

140. Tanaka, M., Fraizer, G. C., De La Cerda, J., Cristiano, R. J., Liebert, M., and Grossman, H. B. (2001) Connexin 26 enhances the bystander effect in HSVtk/GCV gene therapy for human bladder cancer by adenovirus/PLL/DNA gene delivery. *Gene Ther.* **8,** 138–148.

141. Andrade-Rosenthal, A. F., Rosental, R., Hopperstad, M. D., Wu, J. K., Vrionis, F. D., and Spray, D. C. (2000) Gap junctions: the "kiss of death" and the "kiss of life." *Brain Res. Rev.* **32,** 308–315.

142. Touraine, R. L., Vahanian, N., Ramsey, W. J., and Blaese, R. M. (1998) Enhancement of the herpes simplex virus thymidine kinase/ganciclovir bystander effect and its antitumor efficacy in vivo by pharmacologic manipulation of gap junctions. *Hum. Gene Ther.* **9,** 2385–2391.

143. Imaizumi, K., Hasegawa, Y., Kawabe, T., et al. (1998) Bystander tumoricidal effect and gap junctional communication in lung cancer cells. *Am. J. Respir. Cell Mol. Biol.* **18,** 205–212.

144. Drake, R. R., Pitlyk, K., McMasters, M. A., Mercer, K. E., Young, H., and Moyer, M. P. (2000) Connexin-independent ganciclovir mediated killing conferred on bystander effect-resistant cell lines by a herpes simplex virus-thymidine kinase-expressing colon cell line. *Mol. Ther.* **2,** 515–523.

145. Boucher, P. D., Ruch, R. J., and Shewach, D. S. (1998) Differential ganciclovir-mediated cytotoxicity and bystander killing in human colon carcinoma cell lines expressing herpes simplex virus thymidine kinase. *Hum. Gene Ther.* **9,** 801–814.

146. Kaneko, Y. and Tsukamoto, A. (1995) Gene therapy of hepatoma: bystander effects and non-apoptotic cell death induced by thymidine kinase and ganciclovir. *Cancer Lett.* **96,** 105–110.

147. Grignet-Debrus, C., Cool, V., Baudson, N., Velu, T., and Calberg-Bacq, C.-M. (2000) The role of cellular- and prodrug-associated factors in the bystander effect induced by the *Varicella zoster* and *Herpes simplex* viral thymidine kinases in suicide gene therapy. *Cancer Gene Ther.* **7,** 1456–1468.

148. Bai, S., Du, L., Liu, W., Whittle, I. R., and He, L. (1999) Tentative novel mechanism of the bystander effect in glioma gene therapy with HSV-TK/GCV system. *Biochem. Biophys. Res. Commun.* **259,** 455–459.

149. Friedlos, F., Court, S., Ford, M., Denny, W. A., and Springer, C. J. (1998) Gene-directed enzyme prodrug therapy: quantitative bystander cytotoxicity and DNA damage induced by CB1954 in cells expressing bacterial nitroreductase. *Gene Ther.* **5,** 105–112.

150. Wilson, R. W., Pullen, S. M., Hogg, A., Helsby, N. A., Hichs, K. O., and Denny, W. A. (2002) Quantitation of the bystander effects in nitroreductase suicide gene therapy using three-dimensional cell cultures. *Cancer Res.* **62,** 1425–1432.

151. Culver, K. W., Ram, Z., Wallbridge, S., Oldfield, H. E. H., and Blaese, M. R. (1992) In vivo gene transfer with retroviral vector-producer cells for treatment of experimental brain tumors. *Science* **256,** 1550–1552.

152. Trinh, Q. T., Austin, E. A., Murray, D. M., Knick, V. C., and Huber, B. E. (1995) Enzyme/prodrug gene therapy: comparison of cytosine deaminase/5-fluoro cytosine versus thymidine kinase/ganciclovir enzyme/prodrug system in a human colorectal carcinoma cell line. *Cancer Res.* **55,** 4808–4812.

153. Agard, C., Ligeza, C., Dupas, B., et al. (2001) Immune-dependent distant bystander effect after adenovirus-mediated suicide gene transfer in a rat model of liver colorectal metastasis. *Cancer Gene Ther.* **8,** 128–136.
154. Engelman, C., Heslan, J.-M., Fabre, M., Lagarde, J.-P., Klatzmann, D., and Panis, Y. (2002) Importance, mechanisms and limitation of the distant bystander effect in cancer gene therapy of experimental liver tumors. *Cancer Lett.* **179,** 59–69.
155. Smith, J. G., Walzem, R. L., and German, J. B. (1993) Liposomes as agents of DNA transfer. *Biochim. Biophys. Acta* **1154,** 327–340.
156. Plank, C., Mechtler, K., Szoka, F. C. Jr., and Wagner, E. (1996) Activation of the complement system for synthetic DNA complexes: a potential barrier for intravenous gene delivery. *Hum. Gene Ther.* **7,** 1437–1446.
157. Norman, J., Denham, W., Denham, D., et al. (2000) Liposome-mediated, non-viral gene transfer induces a systemic inflammatory response which can exacerbate pre-existing inflammation. *Gene Ther.* **7,** 1425–1430.
158. Meyer, O., Shughart, K., Pavirani, A., and Kolbe, H. V. J. (2000) Multiple systemic expression of human interferon-β in mice can be achieved upon repeated administration of optimized pcTG90-lipoplex. *Gene Ther.* **7,** 1606–1611.
159. Ramesh, R., Marrogi, A. J., Munshi, A., Abboud, C. N., and Freeman, S. M. (1996) In vivo analysis of the "bystander effect": a cytokine cascade. *Exp. Hematol.* **24,** 829–838.
160. Pavlovic, J., Nawrath, M., Tu, R., Heinicke, T., and Moelling, K. (1996) Anti-tumor immunity is involved in the thymidine kinase-mediated killing of tumors induced by activated Ki-ras (G12V). *Gene Ther.* **3,** 635–643.
161. Ganly, I. (1999) Phase II trial of intratumoral infection with an E1B deleted adenovirus in patients with recurrent refractory head and neck cancers. *Hum. Gene Ther.* **10,** 844.
162. Sunk, M. W., Yeh, H. C., Thung, S. N., et al. (2001) Intratumoral adenovirus-mediated suicide gene transfer for hepatic metastasis from colorectal carcinoma: results of a phase I clinical trial. *Mol. Ther.* **4,** 182–191.
163. Rainov, N. G. (2000) A phase III clinical evaluation of herpes simplex virus type 1 thymidine kinase and ganciclovir gene therapy as an adjuvant to surgical resection and radiation in adults with previously untreated glioblastoma multiforme. *Hum. Gene Ther.* **11,** 2389–2401.
164. Sandmair, A. M. (2000) Thymidine kinase gene therapy for human malignant glioma, using replication deficient retroviruses and adenoviruses. *Hum. Gene Ther.* **11,** 2197–2205.
165. Pandha, H. S., Martin, L.-A., Rigg, A., et al. (1999) Genetic prodrug activation therapy for breast cancer: a phase I clinical trial of erbB-2-directed suicide gene expression. *J. Clin. Oncol.* **17,** 2180–2189.
166. Lohr, M., Hoffmeyer, A., Kroeger, J., et al. (2001) Microencapsulated cell-mediated treatment of inoperable pancreatic carcinoma. *Lancet* **357,** 1591–1592.

8

Molecular Chemotherapy Approaches

Daniel H. Palmer and David J. Kerr

1. INTRODUCTION

Although many cytotoxic drugs can induce 100% tumor cell kill in vitro, their efficacy in vivo is generally restricted by dose-limiting systemic toxicity. The therapeutic index of these drugs may be improved by regional delivery to the tumor site. This may be achieved by intraarterial, intraperitoneal, intrapleural, intravesical, intrathecal, or intratumoral administration.

Similarly, gene-directed enzyme prodrug therapy (GDEPT) aims to maximize local tumor cell kill while minimizing systemic side effects by delivering an enzyme that converts an inactive prodrug to a cytotoxic metabolite specifically at the tumor site. Clearly, this relies on extremely well-regulated mechanisms to control the accuracy of gene delivery and expression.

To date, approx 600 gene therapy clinical trial protocols have been opened in the United States, 60% of which pertain to cancer gene therapy. Nearly 3500 patients have been treated within these protocols, of which about 2400 are patients with cancer (1). Similarly in the United Kingdom, of approx 70 gene therapy protocols, 70% relate to cancer gene therapy (2). The majority of these trials have been phase I dose-finding and toxicity studies, with less than 1% phase III randomized studies against current best practice.

This chapter provides an overview of the rationale behind regional chemotherapy as a basis for GDEPT within the context of the objectives governing phase I clinical trials, including clinical observation, pharmacokinetics, and pharmacodynamics. It then summarizes the clinical trials for each enzyme/prodrug system reported to date. Finally, speculation is made as to the future direction of GDEPT.

2. RATIONALE FOR REGIONAL CHEMOTHERAPY

Certain tumors stay confined to organs or body compartments for significant periods of their natural history. Approximately 20% of patients who have undergone apparently curative resection of colorectal cancer relapse with disease macroscopically confined to the liver, which could lend itself to hepatic arterial chemotherapy. The peritoneal cavity is a common site of metastases for ovarian cancer, and a third of colorectal cancer patients have recurrences at this site. The premise underlying regional chemotherapy is pharmacokinetic and depends on differential drug clearance from the regional compartment compared to systemic drug clearance. In addition, there have been significant technical improvements in catheters that allow prolonged access to the hepatic artery and peritoneal and pleural cavities.

Usually, regional advantage is assessed by estimation of the concentration of the therapeutic agent in venous blood following regional and systemic administration. This is reflected in the ratio [AUC(IP)]/[AUC(IV)], where AUC is the area under the concentration–time curve for the drug or virus. A regional

From: *Contemporary Cancer Research*
Cancer Gene Therapy
Edited by: D. T. Curiel and J. T. Douglas © Humana Press Inc., Totowa, NJ

advantage has been established for a range of conventional cytotoxic agents such as 5-fluorouracil (5-FU), cisplatin, mitomycin C, and doxorubicin when administered via the hepatic artery or into the peritoneal cavity *(3)*.

The pharmacokinetic gain can be large *(4–7)*. For example, the regional advantage for 5-FU in favor of the peritoneal cavity is in the range of 5000–10,000. This means that there is large potential to increase the concentration of drug or virus to which the tumor is exposed and therefore the extent of cell kill.

Hepatic arterial chemotherapy represents a special case because the liver has the capacity to extract large amounts of certain agents on first arterial pass *(8–12)*. This phenomenon depends on the concentration of the antineoplastic agent in the bloodstream, the surface area of the endothelium, and the rate of blood flow (slower flow resulting in higher extraction). Peritoneal administration of cytotoxics should be within a volume of at least 1 L to ensure homogeneous distribution throughout the peritoneal cavity. In both cases, it is possible to implant permanent catheters without laparotomy, which allows repeated access to the compartment harboring tumor bulk.

2.1. Intravesical Chemotherapy

Intravesical administration of cytotoxic drugs or bacillus Calmette Guérin (BCG) is employed in the treatment of superficial bladder cancer. High concentrations can be achieved with minimal systemic toxicity, achieving a reduction or delay in recurrent disease. This may be mediated by the cytotoxic effect of the drug or by excitation of local inflammatory responses *(13)*.

2.2. Intrathecal Chemotherapy

Because many drugs do not efficiently cross the blood–brain barrier, chemotherapy may be administered by direct intrathecal injection to achieve therapeutic concentrations in the central nervous system. Intrathecal methotrexate is commonly used in the prophylaxis and treatment of hematological malignancies involving the central nervous system and to a lesser extent in patients with breast cancer, small cell lung cancer, and melanoma *(14)*.

2.3. Intratumoral Chemotherapy

Because a strong pharmacokinetic advantage can be attained by regional delivery of chemotherapy, a logical extension of this is to deliver the drug by direct intratumoral injection with the aim of achieving still higher drug concentrations at selected sites. Further, a collagen matrix gel has been developed with the aim of maintaining a prolonged high concentration of drug within the tumor. Preclinical studies with this gel in combination with a number of cytotoxic drugs have confirmed the ability to achieve and maintain high intratumoral drug concentrations and induce cell death *(15)*.

An ongoing phase II trial of cisplatin in collagen gel and epinephrine given by direct intratumoral injection in patients with hepatocellular carcinoma has reported a response rate of 41% (12 of 29 patients) and a median survival already in excess of 15 months *(16)*. A separate pharmacokinetic study in similar patients has reported a prolonged t_{max} and initial half-life of cisplatin delivered in this mixture compared to free cisplatin, consistent with sustained retention of drug at the tumor site *(17)*. Similar studies have been undertaken with promising results in patients with head and neck cancer and skin cancers *(18,19)*.

2.4. Summary

In summary, there is a strong pharmacological rationale for the use of regional chemotherapy. Data from clinical trials using a range of approaches to increase drug concentration at the tumor site while minimizing systemic exposure have reported promising results with encouraging response rates, improvements in survival, and well-tolerated toxicities.

With the burgeoning knowledge in biotechnology underpinning the concept of gene therapy, a logical extension to the field of regional drug delivery is to utilize gene therapy to direct chemotherapeutic activity specifically to the tumor site. This forms the backbone of the GDEPT approach, in which a gene for a nontoxic enzyme is delivered specifically to tumor cells. At present, this approach shares the limitations of other regional delivery strategies in that it can target only localized areas of disease. However, gene therapy has the potential advantage that, as vector technology is improved, it may allow targeting of this approach to disseminated disease.

3. OBJECTIVES OF PHASE I CLINICAL TRIALS

Clinical trials are prospective studies designed to investigate the properties of a new drug, initially to define the pharmacokinetic profile, toxicity, and maximum tolerated dose (MTD) and ultimately to determine clinical utility of the drug and assess its role in standard practice.

3.1. Phase I Clinical Trials

The aim of phase I trials is to establish the appropriate dose of drug for use in subsequent studies. The drug dose is escalated to define its dose-limiting toxicity and MTD. This information is important because the steep dose–response curve of most cytotoxic drugs and their narrow therapeutic index suggest that a dose close to the MTD will maximize the response rate.

The starting dose is usually equal to 1/10 of the murine LD_{10} (lethal dose for 10% of mice). Typically, three patients are treated at each dose level; if no significant toxicity is seen, the dose is escalated according to a predetermined schedule in progressively decreasing increments. If one patient of three suffers significant toxicity, then an additional three are treated at the same dose. If no further toxicity is seen, then dose escalation continues. If toxicity is seen in more than one patient at that dose level, then dose-limiting toxicity is defined. The MTD is then usually defined as the dose level immediately below this.

Conventionally, the dose is not increased in individual patients receiving subsequent treatments because of the theoretical problem of inability to distinguish toxicity related to an individual dose level from cumulative toxicity of multiple doses. A potential drawback of this approach is that the majority of patients may be treated at a dose well below MTD and so are unlikely to benefit even if the drug ultimately shows antitumor activity. Further, such studies can be frustratingly slow to complete. For these reasons, there is now an increasing interest in designing phase I studies in which intrapatient dose escalation is permitted.

A further important aspect of phase I clinical trials is the investigation of pharmacokinetic and pharmacodynamic parameters. *Pharmacokinetic analysis* describes the change in plasma concentration over time and provides data about the distribution, metabolism, and excretion of the drug. This gives important information about the basis of drug toxicity. Further, this may facilitate more rational dose escalation guided by the approximate target pharmacokinetic parameters from preclinical studies and may aid optimum dose and scheduling in future studies. *Pharmacodynamics* describe the effect of a drug dose on the body, and in the phase I trial setting, end points generally relate to toxicity and how this may be influenced by variation in pharmacokinetics (for example, how nadir blood counts relate to plasma drug concentration), although the relationship between dose and antitumor effect may also be explored. Pharmacodynamic studies in phase I trials may be confounded by the wide range of doses used between patients, and in general, more information is gained from phase II studies in which a fixed dose is used.

With the increasing use of novel compounds such as biological response modifiers (e.g., interferon, tumor necrosis factor, angiogenesis inhibitors, cell signaling inhibitors), the classical phase I trial design may not be the most suitable for these agents. It may be more appropriate to design trials to establish the maximum effective dose (which may require a surrogate marker of activity) rather than MTD because these may not be the same.

3.2. Special Principles Applicable to Phase I Trials of Gene Therapy

Compared with standard phase I studies, clinical trials of gene therapy are subject to additional regulatory controls because of the potential hazards to people and the environment from the use of a genetically modified organism (GMO). Before embarking on such trials, an appropriate assessment of potential risks should be made based on the properties of the delivery vector and the transgene used. This allows classification of the GMO according to the level of risk posed so that appropriate precautions can be taken.

In general, pharmacy facilities should be used that can maintain stability of the GMO while ensuring safety of the operatives (usually by using a negative-pressure isolator in a clean air environment). Similarly, patients should be treated in a single-bed isolation facility with standard reverse barrier nursing care practiced until shedding of the GMO from the patient has ceased. This may necessitate the examination of patient samples for GMO at regular intervals until shedding of the GMO from the patient has ceased. Further, waste generated in the treatment process should be inactivated prior to disposal. This may require secure transport of waste materials in hermetically sealed containers before high-temperature incineration.

Such procedures require coordination of clinicians, scientists, pharmacists, nurses, other support/ancillary staff, and health and safety advisors to ensure that risks are minimized and there is adherence regarding legislation for the GMO. This requires clear communication and should provide a framework for audit to ensure ongoing compliance with regulations.

A further aspect unique to clinical trials involving enzyme/prodrug gene therapy is the potential for toxicity at three levels: prodrug alone, vector/transgene alone, and the combination. Therefore, clinical trials should be designed with this in mind. For example, it may first be necessary to undertake a phase I trial of prodrug to determine the dose that may be given safely while achieving sufficient plasma levels to allow a GDEPT approach to be feasible. Similarly, a separate trial to determine the safety of the vector and the extent of delivery and expression of the transgene should be undertaken before embarking on early phase studies using the vector/prodrug in combination.

Frequently, vectors used for gene delivery are modified viruses; their use may require special monitoring in the context of a clinical trial. This should include monitoring of local, regional, and systemic vector distribution within the host and assessment of host immune responses to the vector. Further, assays to detect replication-competent virus generated by genetic recombination, to screen for contaminating viruses, and to monitor for virus shedding from the patient should be employed.

The use of virus vectors may require specific eligibility criteria for patient selection. In particular, patients with known or perceived immunoincompetence (e.g., recent chemo- or radiotherapy, human immunodeficiency virus [HIV] positivity, concomitant corticosteroid use) may be excluded from such trials.

Finally, appropriate clinical end points to assess efficacy should be considered. Conventional radiological assessment of tumor volume may not accurately detect molecular changes in the tumor that may indicate treatment activity. Instead, more sophisticated biochemical or molecular markers and imaging techniques capable of assessing gene distribution and expression should be employed (*see* Chapter 27).

4. CLINICAL TRIALS UTILIZING GDEPT

GDEPT is a two-step process. The first step is to deliver a gene encoding a nonhuman enzyme specifically to tumor cells. Frequently, a modified virus is used as the vector for gene delivery; in this case the term virus-directed enzyme prodrug therapy (VDEPT) may be used. The second step is administration of prodrug, which is converted from a nontoxic form to a cytotoxic species by the enzyme. Therefore, the concentration of activated drug is higher at the tumor site than might be achieved by systemic administration, thus increasing the therapeutic index of the drug.

Table 1
Clinical Trials of GDEPT in Patients With Cancer

Enzyme/prodrug	Vector	Trial phase	Disease site	Patient no.	Reference
TK/GCV	Retrovirus	I	Brain	5	*38*
	Retrovirus	I	Brain	15	*39*
	Retrovirus	I/II	Brain	48	*40*
	Retrovirus	III	Brain	248	*41*
	Retrovirus	I / II	Brain	12	*42*
	RAd	I	Brain	13	*43*
	RAd vs retrovirus	I	Brain	14	*44*
	RAd	I	Prostate	18	*45*
	RAd	I	Prostate	4	*46*
	RAd	I	Prostate	52	*47*
	RAd	I/II	Prostate	36	*48*
	RAd	I	Colorectal	16	*50*
	RAd	I	Mesothelioma	21	*51*
TK/valacyclovir/acyclovir	RAd	I	Ovary	10	*52*
CD/5-FC	Plasmid DNA	I	Breast	12	*67*
	RAd	I	Colorectal	Ongoing	*68*
	Salmonella	I		Ongoing	*69*
NTR/CB1954	RAd	I	Liver 1° + 2°	Ongoing	*86*
	RAd	I	Prostate	Ongoing	
	RAd	I	SCC head/neck	Ongoing	
P450/ifosfamide	Allogeneic cells	I/II	Pancreas	14	*88*
P450/cyclophos	Retrovirus	I	Breast/melanoma	12	*89*

RAd, replication-defective adenovirus; SCC, squamous cell carcinoma.

An important facet of this system is the ability of the activated drug to pass from the cell in which it was generated into neighboring nontransduced cells to effect "bystander" killing. In this way, a marked antitumor effect can be achieved even when only a fraction of cells are transduced. This is particularly relevant as current vector technology generally facilitates transduction of only a small percentage of the target cell population.

The ideal enzyme/prodrug combination should possess certain characteristics. The enzyme should be a low molecular weight polypeptide that functions independently of posttranslational modification. Its catalytic activity and substrate specificity should be distinct from human enzymes. For this reason, viral or bacterial enzymes are often used. Further, the enzyme should have a low K_m and a high K_{cat} so that production of the active species is maximized. The half-life and tissue distribution of the active drug are important determinants of the extent of distribution through the tumor and therefore of the degree of bystander killing and systemic toxicity extent. Also important in optimizing the VDEPT approach is a high differential toxicity between the active drug and its prodrug.

In an attempt to achieve these ideals, a number of enzyme/prodrug combinations have been investigated in the laboratory. Promising results have been reported in in vitro and in vivo model systems (*see* Chapter 7) and several such combinations have now entered clinical trials (Table 1).

4.1. Vectors Used in GDEPT Clinical Trials

Clinical effectiveness of any gene therapy approach relies on an efficient vector to deliver the therapeutic gene specifically to tumor cells. Vectors can be broadly divided into viral and nonviral vectors

(20). Nonviral vectors include naked deoxyribonucleic acid (DNA) and DNA linked to cationic lipids or polymers. The advantages of such vectors include relative ease of production, unlimited gene insert size, and lack of immunogenicity. However, at present transfection efficiency in vivo remains disappointingly low, such that clinical trials have rarely been conducted using these vectors.

Of viral vectors, retroviruses and adenoviruses have been used most frequently in clinical trials *(21)*. As part of their life cycle, retroviral vectors integrate into the target cell genome and may therefore facilitate long-term transgene expression. However, long-term expression may not be necessary for a suicide gene therapy approach as the aim is to eliminate target cells. Further, there is a risk of insertional mutagenesis in transduced cells. Other disadvantages of current retrovirus vectors include their ability to infect only dividing cells, a narrow tissue tropism, and technical difficulties in growing to high titer in cell culture. Nevertheless, retrovirus vectors have been frequently used in GDEPT clinical trials. Further, with advances in retrovirus vector technology, such as improved stability allowing more concentrated formulations *(22)*, the use of lentiviruses to allow gene transfer into nondividing cells *(23,24)*, retargeting, and the use of replication-competent retroviruses, their use in clinical trials may be further refined.

Adenoviral vectors have wide tissue tropism and are able to infect both dividing and nondividing cells. They are easily manipulated in cell culture and can be grown to high titer. The adenovirus life cycle does not require integration into the host cell genome, so long-term transgene expression is not anticipated. However, for cancer gene therapy, the aim is to eradicate the target cell, so this may not represent a major limitation to successful therapy. A potential major disadvantage of adenoviral vectors is the elicitation of strong inflammatory and immune responses to the vector, which again may limit the duration of transgene expression. However, such a response, if localized to the tumor milieu, may actually enhance tumor cell killing. For these reasons, adenovirus vectors have been widely used in GDEPT cancer gene therapy clinical trials.

4.2. Thymidine Kinase/Ganciclovir

Thymidine kinase (TK) is a key enzyme in pyrimidine metabolism, catalyzing the phosphorylation of thymidine to thymidine monophosphate. Herpes simplex virus thymidine kinase (HSV-TK) has a wider substrate specificity than human TK, phosphorylating the purine analogue ganciclovir (GCV) up to 1000-fold more efficiently than the human enzyme. Phosphorylation of GCV generates GCV monophosphate. This is further phosphorylated by cellular kinases to the triphosphate, which competes with deoxyguanosine 5'-triphosphate to inhibit DNA synthesis and induce cell death.

These features make the combination of HSV-TK and GCV an attractive model for GDEPT. Indeed, sensitization of TK-expressing mouse tumor cells to GCV was first reported in 1986 *(25)*. Subsequent reports have confirmed in vitro and in vivo activity in a range of human tumors (e.g., breast, glioma, pancreas, mesothelioma, colon) using a variety of vectors (e.g., retrovirus, adenovirus, liposome-coated DNA, naked DNA) to deliver the gene *(26–33)*.

In a syngeneic murine model of colorectal cancer, the HSV-TK/GCV system achieved complete tumor regression when only 9% of tumor cells expressed TK *(34)*. A similar bystander effect was observed in vitro, but only when cells were plated out at high density, implying that direct cell–cell contact is required *(35)*. The lipid-insoluble GCV metabolite cannot diffuse into adjacent cells, suggesting that the bystander effect may be mediated by gap junctional transport. Indeed, cotransfection of connexins, major gap junction proteins, to gap junction-deficient cells in vitro dramatically enhanced bystander killing *(36)*.

Interestingly, there is evidence of a "vaccination effect" in that, in mice with TK-expressing tumors treated with GCV, tumor regression can occur following rechallenge with untransduced tumors, suggesting that the immune response may contribute to a bystander effect in vivo *(37)*. Further, in an in vivo model of colon cancer, better outcomes were observed in immunocompetent mice than in nude mice, again indicating that antitumor activity is enhanced by an intact immune system *(34)*.

4.2.1. TK/GCV and Brain Tumors

The TK/GCV system is the most widely studied GDEPT combination in clinical trials. Initial studies were undertaken in patients with primary brain tumors; murine fibroblast producer cells were modified to generate retroviruses encoding HSV-TK. Retroviruses were used for their capacity to infect and integrate only into dividing tumor cells and not the nondividing cells of the central nervous system.

In the first published study, virus producer cells (VPCs) were implanted stereotactically into locally recurrent brain tumors, followed by intravenous GCV 5 mg/kg twice daily for 14 days. Of the 5 patients treated, a single lesion in 1 patient showed a partial response, but all other treated lesions failed to respond *(38)*. In a similar study, 19 tumors in 15 patients with locally recurrent or metastatic brain tumors were injected with VPCs followed by intravenous GCV. In 1 patient, there were complete responses in two lesions; in a further 3 patients, partial responses were seen. All these lesions were of low volume (<2cc). In 2 patients, tumors were resected 7 days postinjection. *In situ* hybridization revealed TK-positive tumor cells, but only in small numbers *(39)*.

In a larger multicenter phase I/II single-arm feasibility and safety study, 48 patients undergoing surgical resection of recurrent glioblastoma multiforme were injected with TK-expressing retrovirus VPCs into the resection site and then treated with intravenous GCV. In 4 of 48 patients, there was some regression of postoperative residual enhancement on computerized tomographic scanning. However, median survival of 8.6 months was no better than that of historical controls. Interestingly, at postmortem 10 patients had TK-expressing tumor cells, indicating their survival despite treatment with GCV *(40)*.

A randomized phase III multicenter clinical trial of retrovirus-mediated HSV-TK/GCV was conducted in 248 patients with previously untreated malignant glioblastoma multiforme; this represents the largest randomized controlled trial in cancer gene therapy to date. Patients were treated either by conventional surgical resection and radiotherapy alone or with the addition of VPC injection into the tumor site followed by GCV treatment. Adjuvant gene therapy was feasible and safe in this setting. Disappointingly, median time to progression and 12-month survival were not significantly different in the two groups *(41)*.

Notably, these and other trials using VPCs to deliver HSV-TK-expressing retrovirus to brain tumors have demonstrated this approach is well tolerated with only modest toxicity, which usually resolved at the end of the treatment period *(39–42)*. However, efficacy in general had been disappointingly low. This failure is most probably a result of inadequate levels of gene delivery *(40,41)*. Because VPCs are nonmigrating fibroblasts, the distribution of cells and released virus is confined to the immediate vicinity of the needle track. It may also be because of poor penetration of GCV across the blood–brain barrier, so that only low concentrations of drug are achieved at the tumor site. Further, a high fraction of brain tumor cells are in the resting phase of cell cycle G_0 and so would not be susceptible to the S-phase-specific GCV. Finally, a paucity of gap junction interaction between adjacent brain tumor cells may limit local bystander killing.

In an attempt to improve on the limited level and extent of transgene expression achieved by TK-encoding retrovirus VPCs, other early phase trials have employed replication-deficient adenovirus vectors carrying the HSV-TK gene (RAd-HSV-TK). In a phase I dose escalation study, 13 patients with recurrent primary malignant brain tumors were treated with a single intratumoral injection of RAd-HSV-TK virus particles, followed by intravenous GCV. Doses up to and including 2×10^{11} virus particles were well tolerated. However, in 2 of 2 patients treated at the maximum dose of 2×10^{12} virus particles, dose-limiting neurotoxicity (confusion, seizures) was seen. Of 13 patients, 3 achieved survival in excess of 25 months. Although this is better than predicted from historical controls, clearly this may be because of other favorable prognosis factors rather than because of a response to gene therapy. Postmortem examination in these patients did show cavitation at the site of injection, foci of necrosis in the tumor, and tumor-infiltrating lymphocytes and macrophages not seen in the surrounding normal brain tissue *(43)*.

A further trial has directly compared TK-encoding retrovirus vector with RAd-HSV-TK in a small number of patients. Median survival in the two groups was 7.4 months and 15 months, respectively ($p < .012$). This study confirmed RAd-HSV-TK delivered by direct intratumoral injection is safe, well tolerated, and possibly superior to a retrovirus vector, although further, larger studies are warranted *(44)*.

4.2.2. TK/GCV and Prostate Cancer

The HSV-TK/GCV system has also been extensively investigated in patients with prostate cancer. A phase I dose-escalating study utilized RAd-HSV-TK injected directly into locally recurrent prostate cancer at a dose of 1×10^8 to 1×10^{11} plaque-forming units (pfu) followed by intravenous GCV. At the maximum dose, 1 patient experienced transient grade 4 thrombocytopenia and another had self-limiting grade 3 hepatotoxicity. Of 18 patients, 3 demonstrated an objective response with a greater than 50% reduction in serum prostate-specific antigen (PSA) lasting between 6 weeks and 12 months *(45)*. This was the first report of objective responses in a prostate cancer gene therapy trial.

A smaller trial treated four patients with RAd-HSV-TK/GCV prior to prostatectomy. Morphological studies of the resected glands showed evidence of tumor necrosis and tumor infiltration by CD8+ T lymphocytes, suggesting generation of an immune response to HSV-TK/GCV-mediated tumor cell killing *(46)*.

A further study in patients with locally recurrent prostate cancer examined the feasibility of multiple and/or repeated intratumoral injection of a RAd-HSV-TK vector with the aim of improving the quantity and distribution of transgene expression. There were 52 patients treated with a total of 76 cycles of RAd-HSV-TK/GCV; 29 patients received multiple vector injections in a single treatment, 20 patients received two consecutive injections, and 4 patients were injected on three separate occasions. Toxicity was mild in all patient groups, comprising grade 1–2 fever in 16 patients and grade I thrombocytopenia in 3 patients, which resolved with discontinuation of GCV. There was no hepatotoxicity and no evidence of additive or cumulative toxicity, confirming the safety of multiple and repeat injections with a replication-deficient adenovirus vector. Of 28 patients assessed for evidence of an antitumor response, a decrease in serum PSA of at least 44% was observed in 12, indicating promising clinical activity *(47)*.

An extended phase I/II study in patients with locally recurrent prostate cancer treated 36 patients with repeated cycles of RAd-HSV-TK intratumorally, followed by systemic GCV. In 28 of 36 patients, there was a 28% mean reduction in PSA after the first cycle of treatment. Repeat cycles led to further decreases in PSA level. There was also a statistically significant increase in the mean percentage of CD8+ T lymphocytes displaying markers of activation in patient serum following treatment. Biopsy of treated glands demonstrated a correlation between the presence of apoptotic tumor cells and tumor-infiltrating CD8+ T cells in the biopsy specimen, again suggesting that HSV-TK/GCV-induced cell death may mediate a cytotoxic cellular immune response, and that multiple treatments are feasible and well tolerated *(48)*.

4.2.3. TK/GCV and Colorectal Cancer

Preclinical studies of the HSV-TK/GCV systems have shown promising results in murine models of colorectal cancer, with marked bystander killing even when less than 10% of tumor cells express TK *(34)*. Further, a number of colorectal tumor-associated antigens have been identified that may serve as potential targets for immune-mediated bystander effect *(49)*.

A phase I clinical trial using an adenovirus vector to deliver HSV-TK via ultrasound-guided direct intratumoral injection has been performed in patients with hepatic metastatic colorectal cancer *(50)*. There were 16 patients treated, with virus dose escalating from 1×10^{10} to 1×10^{13} particles, followed by a fixed dose of GCV. Treatment was well tolerated, with no dose-limiting toxicity reported, confirming the safety of the adenovirus vector when delivered by the intratumoral route. Toxicity was mild and in line with that seen in other trials using intratumoral injection of replication-deficient adenovirus vectors, largely comprising low-grade fever (12 patients), grade 1 hepatotoxicity (3 patients), and grade 2–3 bone marrow toxicity (4 patients). The early occurrence of these toxicities suggested that it was related to the virus vector rather than GCV, which might be expected to occur later. In the 15 evaluable patients, no objective responses were seen, although 11 patients had disease stability 4 weeks posttreatment.

Notably, other locally ablative techniques used in the treatment of liver cancers are reported to induce pathological necrosis without apparent reductions in tumor size on cross-sectional imaging, highlighting the potential limitations of current techniques of response assessment. In this study, 6 patients underwent tumor biopsy before and after treatment. In 1 patient, there was extensive necrosis (but also residual viable tumor) 11 weeks after treatment. There was no necrosis in biopsies from the other 5 patients, although these were taken at a later time *(50)*.

4.2.4. Intracavitary Use of TK/GCV

Malignant mesothelioma and ovarian carcinoma present models of localized malignancy such that regional delivery of treatment may provide a potential pharmacokinetic advantage (*see* Section 2.). Similarly, intracavitary gene delivery may achieve extensive transduction of tumor cells. To this end, clinical trials using adenovirus vectors encoding the HSV-TK gene delivered by intrapleural and intraperitoneal instillation have been conducted.

In a phase I trial, 21 patients with malignant mesothelioma were treated with RAd-HSV-TK at 1×10^9 to 1×10^{12} pfu into the pleural space, followed by intravenous GCV. Toxicity was minimal, with fever, anemia, and transient elevation of liver transaminases. A strong intrapleural and intratumoral inflammatory infiltrate was reported. Evidence of HSV-TK gene transfer was seen in 11 of 20 evaluable patients on pleural biopsy, increasing in a dose-dependent manner, although this was confined to superficial layers of tumor. No formal assessment of objective responses was made *(51)*.

A further trial examined the safety and feasibility of intraperitoneal instillation of an RAd-HSV-TK vector in patients with recurrent ovarian cancer. Ten patients, having undergone debulking surgery, were given the vector at 2×10^{10} to 2×10^{13} virus particles, followed by valacyclovir or acylovir and intravenous topotecan. The treatment was well tolerated with no dose-limiting toxicity reported. Myelosuppression occurred commonly, but was independent of virus dose and most likely chemotherapy related *(52)*.

4.2.5. Summary

In summary, the HSV-TK/GCV combination has been widely investigated in clinical trials using both retrovirus and adenovirus vectors administered by direct intratumoral or intracavitary routes in a variety of tumor types. These trials confirmed the safety of the reagents. However, significant therapeutic benefit has yet to be demonstrated. This is most likely limited by inefficient gene delivery. Other limiting factors may include development of GCV resistance in transduced cells, poor bystander effects between cells lacking gap junction communication, the high fraction of tumor cells in the G_0 phase of the cell cycle, and difficulty in achieving effective concentrations of GCV at the tumor site without prodrug-related systemic toxicity.

Promising preclinical developments are being made to overcome some of these obstacles. For example, cotransfection of gap junctional proteins dramatically increases local bystander killing in vitro *(53,54)*. Further, gap junctions can be upregulated by lovastatin and other drugs *(55)*.

Other studies have demonstrated that activated GCV induces mostly apoptotic cell death, which may not be optimal in generating immune responses to tumor-associated antigens. So, immune-mediated bystander killing may be enhanced by combining TK/GCV with immunostimulatory molecules.

Other groups have attempted to improve the enzymic activity of TK. This may be done by utilizing the TK gene from other herpes viruses, for example, from equine HSV or human herpes virus 8, which are reported to catalyze the phosphorylation of GCV more rapidly than HSV-TK *(56,57)*. Alternatively, attempts to improve the catalytic activity of HSV-TK by random and site-directed mutagenesis have generated mutants with markedly increased activity compared to the wild-type enzyme *(58,59)*.

Improvements in enzymic activity may allow the use of lower, less-toxic doses of GCV or the use of other prodrugs such as acyclovir or famcyclovir. Because these drugs can be administered orally, this may allow more prolonged treatment than is possible with GCV so that a greater proportion of tumor cells may enter the S phase and therefore be sensitive to the activated drug.

Other future directions for the development of the HSV-TK system include its use in combination with other enzyme/prodrug combinations and with conventional therapies such as chemotherapy and radiotherapy.

4.3. Cytosine Deaminase/5-Fluorocytosine

The cytosine deaminase/5-fluorocytosine (CD/5-FC) system, like TK/GCV, is based on the production of a toxic nucleoside analogue. The CD enzyme is found in certain bacteria and fungi, but not in mammalian cells. CD catalyses the hydrolytic deamination of cytosine to uracil. Thus, the nontoxic antifungal drug 5-FC is converted to 5-FU by CD. 5-FU is widely used in the treatment of gastrointestinal and other malignancies.

5-FU is further metabolized in a series of reactions to 5-fluoro-2'-deoxyiridine-5'-monophosphate, which inhibits the enzyme thymidylate synthase to inhibit DNA and ribonucleic acid (RNA) synthesis in an S-phase-specific manner. This presents a potential limitation to the success of CD/5-FC given that only a fraction of tumor cells are in the appropriate phase of the cell cycle at a certain time.

In vitro studies demonstrated that expression of the CD gene via transfection or retroviral transduction results in up to 2000-fold sensitization to 5-FC in a range of cell lines compared to the parental cells *(60,61)*. Further, in vivo studies have demonstrated activity in several animal models, including carcinomas, fibrosarcoma, and glioma *(61–64)*.

Significantly, a profound bystander effect is seen both in vitro and in vivo. In vitro, this effect is independent of cell–cell contact, suggesting an ability of 5-FU to diffuse out of and into cells. Indeed, significant concentrations of 5-FU can be detected in the supernatant of CD-expressing cells treated with 5-FC *(62)*. Further, a bystander effect is observed in cell lines lacking gap junctions *(65)*. In murine xenograft models, significant tumor regression is observed when only 2% of cells express CD, and very high intratumoral concentrations of 5-FU (>400 μM) are generated with few systemic side effects. This compares to no tumor shrinkage in response to MTDs of systemic 5-FU in similar models *(62)*. Further, an immune-mediated distant bystander effect is observed; immunocompetent mice pretreated with CD/5-FC demonstrated significant resistance to rechallenge with wild-type tumor *(63,66)*.

Several clinical trial protocols utilizing CD/5-FC have been approved. The first reported study utilized direct injection of plasmid DNA encoding the *Escherichia coli* CD gene under the control of the c-erbB-2 promoter into cutaneous recurrent c-erbB-2-positive breast cancer nodules. In the study, 12 women received CD-plasmid DNA into one nodule along with control plasmid DNA and mock injection into two further nodules, followed (in 8 cases) by systemic 5-FC. Treated nodules were biopsied 1 and 7 days later and analyzed for CD expression by immunohistochemistry and messenger RNA *in situ* hybridization. The treatment was safe and well tolerated. Specifically, there was no evidence of anti-DNA antibody formation. Tumor-selective CD expression was detected in 11 of 12 patients. In all cases, this was restricted to tumor cells with no detectable expression in surrounding stroma, lymphocytes, or endothelium. Four patients showed evidence of tumor shrinkage. In 1 of these patients, this was restricted to the CD-injected lesion and followed 5-FC treatment. In another, there was regression also in the control lesions. In 2 patients, there was regression in the CD-injected lesions even without exposure to 5-FC. These responses may reflect the immunogenicity of CD itself. However, because spontaneous regression of cutaneous breast cancer nodules is not uncommon, interpretation must be made with caution *(67)*.

A phase I trial of a replication-defective adenovirus carrying the *E. coli* CD gene (Ad-GVCD-10) given intratumorally followed by oral 5-FC to patients with hepatic metastatic colorectal cancer is under way. Dose escalation to a maximum of 2×10^9 pfu is planned. The trial has two arms, one of which is treated with vector and prodrug only; in the other, the tumor is excised after treatment so that histological and molecular analyses can be undertaken. Results are awaited *(68)*.

A genetically modified *Salmonella typhimurium* with deletions of msbB and purI genes, altering the bacterial lipopolysaccharide to attenuate its pathogenicity can preferentially colonize, replicate in, and lyse tumor cells up to 1000-fold more readily than in normal tissue. A phase I trial with this bacterium (VNP20009) delivered by direct intratumoral or intravenous injection demonstrated it is safe and well tolerated. A further modification has been made to VNP20009 with the insertion of the *E. coli* CD gene so that it acts as a prodrug-activating gene therapy vector. Preclinical studies have verified that this vector (TAPET-CD) is safe and can result in generation of high levels of 5-FU exclusively in the tumor following 5-FC treatment. A phase I trial is under way *(69)*.

In summary, the efficacy of the CD/5-FC combination, with a profound bystander effect, has been confirmed in vitro and in vivo. Early phase clinical trials are in progress, although as yet most remain unreported.

In common with TK/GCV, CD/5-FC generates an immune-mediated distant bystander effect, suggesting a potential role for combining this system with immunotherapy. Indeed, the combined use of adenovirus-delivered CD and granulocyte-macrophage colony-stimulating factor in immunocompetent mouse tumor models is reported to result in enhanced tumor shrinkage and greater immunity to tumor rechallenge than from adenovirus-delivered CD alone *(70)*.

Conventional 5-FU chemotherapy is frequently used as a radiosensitizing agent. In vitro and in vivo studies suggested that CD/5-FC may have a similar favorable interaction with radiotherapy, and this may present a fruitful combination in future clinical trials *(71,72)*. Similarly, additive or even synergistic interactions with conventional chemotherapy or other enzyme-prodrug systems may be seen *(73)*. Combination of the pyrimidine salvage pathway enzyme uracil phosphoribosyl transferase with CD has been shown to enhance the antitumoral effect in vitro, probably by increasing the turnover of 5-FU to 5-fluoro-2'-deoxyiridine-5'-monophosphate, thereby accelerating a rate-limiting step in the conversion of 5-FU to its cytotoxic metabolite. An adenovirus vector encoding a CD/uracil phosphoribosyl transferase fusion gene has been constructed and may aid the clinical development of the CD/5-FC system *(74)*.

Although the use of direct intratumoral gene transfer to well-defined hepatic colorectal metastases provides a useful demonstration of in vivo gene transfer, its clinical utility is limited. A more useful scenario might be in the adjuvant setting and the treatment of hepatic micrometastases. This requires regional delivery of the CD gene via the hepatic blood supply so that 5-FC is converted to 5-FU at high concentration in the liver, where it can diffuse locally to suppress the growth of cancer cells. Because 5-FU is cell cycle specific, toxicity to noncycling hepatocytes should be minimal. The safety and feasibility of this approach have been demonstrated in preclinical studies using adenovirus-delivered CD, so clinical trials are warranted *(75)*.

4.4. Nitroreductase/CB1954

CB1954 [5-(aziridin-1-yl)-2,4-dinitrobenzamide] first stimulated interest when it was found to be highly active against Walker rat 256 tumor xenografts, mediated by DT-diaphorase, which is able to convert CB1954 from a weak monofunctional alkylating agent to a highly potent bifunctional cytotoxic agent that is up to 100,000 times more potent than the prodrug *(76)*. Further, CB1954 is a poor substrate for human DT-diaphorase, which differs from its rat counterpart with a glycine for tyrosine substitution at residue 104, so it is not converted to the active species in human tissues *(77)*. Subsequent studies have demonstrated that the enzyme nitroreductase (NTR), encoded by the *nfsB* gene of *E. coli* B, can perform this bioreduction 100-fold more efficiently than rat DT-diaphorase *(78)*. These properties make the combination of NTR/CB1954 exploitable by a VDEPT gene therapy approach.

A replication-defective adenovirus vector encoding the bacterial *ntr* gene under the control of the strong CMV immediate early promoter (CTL102) has been constructed. Preclinical studies have shown that adenoviral delivery of NTR to a range of human cancer cell lines sensitizes them to CB1954 by 500- to 2000-fold compared to the parental cell line *(79)*. Further, in an in vivo xenograft model of peritoneal pancreatic cancer (Suit-2), a doubling in median survival was seen in mice treated with virus and CB1954 compared to controls ($p < 0.0001$).

In vitro cell-mixing experiments using unmodified and NTR-expressing tumor cell lines have demonstrated significant sensitization of the total cell population to CB1954 when only 5% of cells express NTR *(80)*. Similarly, in vivo murine xenograft models show a significant antitumor effect and prolonged survival in which only 5% of cells express NTR, confirming a significant bystander effect *(81)*. Unlike GCV, activated CB1954 transfers to adjacent cells via a gap junction-independent mechanism. This may be clinically relevant because human tumors frequently lack functional gap junctions.

Activated CB1954 forms a relatively high proportion of interstrand DNA crosslinks compared to other alkylating agents *(82)*. This lesion is reported to be a unique C8–O6 DNA crosslink that is poorly repaired, which may explain the marked toxicity of CB1954 and its lack of cross-resistance with other cytotoxic agents *(83)*.

Unlike the active species generated by TK/GCV and CD/5-FC systems, which are both antimetabolites and are therefore cell cycle specific, activated CB1954 has the potential advantage of being non-phase specific and can kill noncycling cells *(84)*. Further, conversion of CB1954 to the active species relies on an intracellular cofactor NADH (nicotinamide adenine dinucleotide phosphate), increasing safety because no extracellular activation can occur.

The use of the prodrugs GCV and 5-FC is well characterized from their extensive use as antiviral and antifungal drugs, respectively. This is not the case for the prodrug CB1954. Because VDEPT has three potential sources of toxicity (prodrug alone, vector alone, and prodrug-vector combination), a phase I and pharmacokinetic study of CB1954 has been undertaken. Dose-limiting toxicity consisted of asymptomatic transaminitis and diarrhea. However, a dose of 24 mg/m^2 could be administered intravenously without significant side effects. The mean peak serum concentration of CB1954 at this dose was 6.3 μM. Preclinical data have demonstrated IC_{50}'s for CB1954 in the range 0.5–5 μM, suggesting that delivery of prodrug should not be the dose-limiting component of this system *(85)*.

A further study addressed the safety and feasibility of intratumoral administration of the adenovirus-NTR vector CTL102. In this phase I dose escalation study, patients with primary or secondary (hepatic metastatic colorectal) liver cancer were treated with CTL102 prior to surgical resection so that efficiency of transgene expression could be assessed in the entire resected tumor *(86)*.

A single dose of 1×10^8 to 5×10^{11} virus particles was given to 18 patients. Grade 1 pyrexia (<38.5°C) was observed in 4 patients between 4 and 8 hours postinoculation, unrelated to dose received. No dose-limiting toxicity was observed. In common with similar trials using replication-defective adenoviruses, vector DNA was detectable only transiently in patient blood, and robust antivector antibody responses were mounted. Immunohistochemical staining for NTR in resected tumors confirmed transgene expression increasing in a dose-dependent manner. NTR was clearly present in tumor cells, and fibroblasts and lymphoid cells within the tumor mass. Staining for the coxsackie and adenovirus receptor (CAR) showed that expression was high throughout the tumor, so that uptake of virus was unlikely to be limited by a lack of primary virus receptor. The high level of tumoral NTR expression seen in this study has prompted further studies in patients with nonresectable tumors, who will receive CTL102 followed by intravenous CB1954 to look for evidence of antitumor efficacy. Identical studies are under way in patients with prostate cancer and head and neck cancer.

It is widely reported that other VDEPT systems (TK/GCV and CD/5-FC) can generate an immune-mediated bystander effect. Data suggest that the same may occur in response to NTR/CB1954. The use of an adenovirus vector encoding NTR and granulocyte-macrophage colony-stimulating factor in a murine colorectal cancer model showed an improved antitumor response compared to either modality alone, suggesting this is a potentially useful approach for future clinical trials *(87)*. Further, in vitro data showed a potentially synergistic interaction between CB1954 and 5-FU, so that the combination of NTR/CB1954 with CD/5-FC or with conventional chemotherapy may be clinically useful *(87a)*.

4.5. Other Enzyme/Prodrug Combinations

Ongoing research on other enzyme/prodrug systems is still in the preclinical stage, including cytochrome P450/cyclophosphamide, carboxypeptidase G2/4-[(2-mesyloxyethyl)(2-chloroethyl)amino]-benzoyl-L-glutamic acid, and carboxylesterase/irinotecan. These are reviewed in detail in Chapter 7.

A phase I/II clinical trial in patients with inoperable pancreatic cancer used modified allogeneic cells expressing a cytochrome P450 enzyme delivered angiographically to the tumor vasculature to activate systemically administered ifosfamide. In 4 of 14 patients, there was evidence of tumor regression; in the other 10 patients, disease was stabilized. Median survival was doubled compared to historical controls. Based on these results, further studies are warranted *(88)*.

Another study utilized a retroviral vector encoding cytochrome P450 injected directly into cutaneous metastatic nodules of breast cancer or melanoma to activate systemically administered cyclophosphamide. There were 12 patients treated with vector 5×10^5 to 5×10^7 pfu/mL. Treatment was safe and well tolerated. Gene transfer was detected in biopsies at all dose levels. One patient had a partial response, and 2 patients achieved disease stability *(89)*.

5. THE USE OF ENZYME/PRODRUG THERAPY IN OTHER SETTINGS

As well as extensive investigation of enzyme/prodrug therapy in the treatment of a variety of human cancers, the attributes of this system may also be exploited for benefit in other clinical settings.

5.1. Prevention of Graft-vs-Host Disease in Allogeneic Bone Marrow Transplant

A common complication of allogeneic bone marrow transplantation (BMT) is graft-vs-host disease (GVHD) mediated by alloreactive T cells in the donor marrow. However, depletion of donor T cells results in immune impairment and loss of graft-vs-leukemia effect.

In a model in which transgenic mice express HSV-TK in T cells, it has been shown that GCV can selectively eliminate dividing T cells. Immediately post-BMT, most activated T cells are alloreactive and, because they are dividing, should be susceptible to cell cycle-specific activated GCV. TK expression in donor T cells, followed by early, transient treatment with GCV may therefore allow elimination of T cells mediating GVHD while preserving an otherwise normal T-cell pool *(90)*.

This approach has been investigated in clinical trials. For example, eight recipients of T-cell-depleted BMT were then treated with donor T cells transduced ex vivo to express HSV-TK. Significant graft-vs-leukemia effect was seen in five patients, indicating functional T cells. Three patients developed GVHD, which was successfully controlled by GCV *(91)*.

5.2. Purging Bone Marrow of Tumor Cells Prior to Autologous BMT

Contaminating tumor cells in hemopoietic cell preparations contribute to the failure of autologous stem cell rescue in patients with neuroblastoma. Preclinical studies using an adenovirus vector to deliver the carboxylesterase gene to a mixed cell population demonstrated sensitization of the neuroblastoma cells to the prodrug irinotecan with sparing of hemopoietic progenitor cells. Interestingly, no bystander killing of these progenitors was observed. This method may therefore offer a novel protocol for purging tumor cells prior to bone marrow autograft *(92,93)*. Assessment of purging efficacy in bone marrow samples from patients with neuroblastoma is under way.

5.3. Treatment of HIV Infection

In vitro studies demonstrate that CD4-positive T cells expressing HSV-TK under control of HIV-1 long terminal repeat (LTR) are protected from HIV in the presence of acyclovir because active metabolites inhibit HIV reverse transcriptase and mediate cell death. There may be scope, therefore, for application of this treatment for HIV-limiting therapy *(94)*.

5.4. Treatment of Vascular Pathology

Arterial injury, such as following angioplasty, may be complicated by vascular proliferative disorders mediated by accumulation of vascular smooth muscle cells, resulting in restenosis. Studies have shown that infection of smooth muscle cells by a recombinant adenovirus encoding the TK gene can sensitize them to GCV. Porcine studies have shown this to be a safe and feasible treatment capable of reducing intimal hyperplasia in response to vascular injury *(95)*.

Similarly encouraging results have been reported with the use of adenovirus-delivered cytosine deaminase, followed by exposure to 5-FC *(96)*.

6. FUTURE DIRECTIONS FOR ENZYME/PRODRUG THERAPY

Clinical experience in the use of enzyme/prodrug gene therapy is expanding. Several enzyme/prodrug combinations have been investigated using a variety of gene delivery vectors. In general, these studies have confirmed the safety of this approach, although evidence of antitumor responses is, so far, sparse. Current strategies require further refinement to achieve clinically significant efficacy. This may be achieved by several means.

6.1. Improving the Low Efficiency of Gene Transfer

The major limitation of current enzyme/prodrug strategies is the low level of transgene expression achieved using current vector technology. Genetically modified oncolytic viruses, including adenoviruses, herpes simplex virus, and reovirus, have been developed and tested. These viruses require key tumorigenic pathways to be mutated for viral replication and hence can selectively replicate in and lyse tumor cells while sparing normal cells. Clinical trials are under way. These vectors are described more fully in Chapters 13–16. Replicating virus vectors may have the potential to improve on the disappointingly low gene transfer efficiency seen in clinical trials to date given their potential to infect a greater proportion of tumor cells. It is attractive, therefore, to combine such viruses with prodrug-activating enzymes by inserting the appropriate complementary DNA into the vector.

Preclinical studies using the combination of a replicating HSV vector encoding the *TK* gene have been performed. In a colorectal cancer model, the addition of GCV actually reduced the cytotoxic effect of the oncolytic vector, probably because of the antiviral activity of the activated drug *(97)*.

More encouraging results have been reported with E1B-attenuated adenovirus vectors encoding a combination of CD and *TK*. Data showed that the vector alone was cytotoxic, but the addition of both 5-FC and GCV did further enhance cell killing *(98)*. Similar data are emerging with the combination of a replicating adenovirus vector and NTR/CB1954 (Ming-Jen Chen, 2003, personal communication).

Future clinical studies will address the optimum combination of replicating vector and prodrug-activating gene insert to maximize therapeutic potential.

6.2. Improving the Potency of Antitumor Effect

One of the approaches to improve the potency of antitumor effect is to combine enzyme/prodrug therapy with conventional chemotherapy and radiotherapy. A synergistic antitumor effect has been reported between HV-TK/GCV and the topoisomerase I inhibitor topotecan. Similarly, oncolytic adenovirus encoding prodrug-activating enzymes used in conjunction with radiotherapy show a synergistic interaction, with evidence that radiotherapy may enhance viral replication within tumors *(99)*.

Another way to augment the antitumor effect is to enhance the bystander killing. This may be done using measures to increase cell–cell communications or to provoke cell-mediated immunity to tumor cells *(100)*.

6.3. Specific Gene Expression at the Tumor Site to Avoid Toxicity to Normal Tissue

To limit specific enzyme expression to the tumor site, tumor- or tissue-specific promoters such as carcinoembryonic antigen, prostate-specific antigen, or α-fetoprotein can be used. Also, the use of replicating virus vectors, which exploit differences in tumor cell biology for their selective replication, may facilitate gene delivery to the tumor.

6.4. Systemic Targeting of Gene Transfer to Multiple Tumor Sites

Virus vectors may be retargeted to specific tumor receptors to allow systemic targeting of gene transfer. Adenovirus fiber may be modified to block its interaction with CAR and to introduce a novel receptor interaction. For example, a bispecific antibody that at one end binds to and blocks fiber and at the other end interacts with cell surface folate receptor has been shown to retarget adenovirus to a range of tumor cell lines that overexpress this receptor. Importantly, because the folate receptor is internalized following ligation, virus internalization is maintained *(101,102)*. This approach is currently limited by rapid sequestration by the reticuloendothelial system before vectors reach their targets. A further problem is that viral vectors can be immunogenic, which may prevent their repeated administration. A novel way to circumvent these problems is to coat adenovirus with an inert polymer such as *N*-(2-hydroxypropyl)methacrylamide. As well as reducing antiadenovirus immune responses, the polymer coat prevents interaction with CAR, thus inhibiting virus infection. The incorporation of specific ligands into the polymer could then facilitate retargeting to specific tumor receptors *(103)*.

6.5. Safety of Viral Vectors: Avoiding Overwhelming Virus Infection

Safety of gene therapy vectors remains a concern, especially when viral vectors are used. For adenovirus, viral clearance is dependent on the immune system. Therefore, in screening patients for these clinical trials, those who are immunocompromised should be excluded. Safety may potentially be improved by the development of "gutless" or helper-dependent virus *(104)*, chimeric virus *(105)*, minivirus *(106)*, or complementary oncolytic virus *(107)*.

6.6. Noninvasive Monitoring of Transgene Expression

It is critical that noninvasive imaging systems are developed that can detect transgene expression in vivo and evaluate the pharmacokinetics of gene therapy vectors to allow thorough pharmacological studies. Through such analysis, gene therapy efficacy may be better quantified and evaluated *(108)* (*see* Chapter 27).

7. CONCLUSIONS

Although preclinical results of enzyme/prodrug gene therapy have been promising, obstacles remain in the path of its clinical development. To fulfill its potential, there are several innovative developments that will improve results.

It is likely that gene therapy will be integrated with existing treatment modalities. The envisaged future practice for cancer treatment may involve a multimodality approach, integrating curative or debulking resection, followed by adjuvant therapies, including concurrent or sequential gene therapy, chemotherapy, and radiotherapy.

REFERENCES

1. Journal Gene Medicine website. http://www.wiley.co.uk/genmed/clinical. Date accessed: 04/22/2003.
2. Gene Therapy Advisory Committee. Website available at http://www.doh.gov.uk/genetics/gtac/. Date accessed: 04/22/2003.

3. Collins, J. M. (1984) Pharmacologic rationale for regional drug delivery. *J. Clin. Oncol.* **2**, 498–504.

4. McClay, E. F. and Howell, S. B. (1990) A review: intraperitoneal cisplatin in the management of patients with ovarian cancer. *Gynecol. Oncol.* **36**, 1–6.

5. Markman, M., Rowinsky, E., Hakes, T., et al. (1992) Phase I trial of intraperitoneal taxol: a Gynecologic Oncology Group study. *J. Clin. Oncol.* **10**, 1485–1491.

6. Reichman, B., Markman, M., Hakes, T., et al. (1989) Intraperitoneal cisplatin and etoposide in the treatment of refractory/recurrent ovarian carcinoma. *J. Clin. Oncol.* **7**, 1327–1332.

7. Alberts, D. S., Liu, P. Y., Hannigan, E. V., et al. (1995) Phase III study of intraperitoneal (IP) cisplatin (CDDP)/intravenous (IV) cyclophosphamide (CPA) versus IV CDDP/IV CPA in patients (PTS) with optimal disease stage III ovarian cancer: a SWOG-GOG-ECOG intergroup study [abstract 760]. (INT 0051). *Proc. Am. Soc. Clin. Oncol.* **14**, 273.

8. Ensminger, W. D., Rosowsky, A., Raso, V., et al. (1978) A clinical-pharmacological evaluation of hepatic arterial infusions of 5-fluoro-2'-deoxyuridine and 5-fluorouracil. *Cancer Res.* **38(11, Pt. 1)**, 3784–3792.

9. Kemeny, N., Daly, J., Reichman, B., Geller, N., Botet, J., and Oderman, P. (1987) Intrahepatic or systemic fluorodeoxyuridine in patients with liver metastases from colorectal carcinoma. *Ann. Intern. Med.* **107**, 459.

10. Kerr, D. J., Ledermann, J. A., McArdle, C. S., et al. (1995) Phase I clinical and pharmacokinetic study of leucovorin and infusional hepatic arterial fluorouracil. *J. Clin. Oncol.* **13**, 2968–2972.

11. Court, W. S., Order, S. E., Siegel, J. A., et al. (2002) Remission and survival following monthly intraarterial cisplatinum in nonresectable hepatoma. *Cancer Invest.* **20**, 613–625.

12. Okuda, K., Tanaka, M., Shibata, J., et al. (1999) Hepatic arterial infusion chemotherapy with continuous low dose administration of cisplatin and 5-fluorouracil for multiple recurrence of hepatocellular carcinoma after surgical treatment. *Oncol. Rep.* **6**, 587–591.

13. Lamm, D. L. and Griffith, J. G. (1992) Intravesical therapy: does it affect the natural history of superficial bladder cancer? *Semin. Urol.* **10**, 39–44.

14. Tubergen, D. G., Gilchrist, G. S., O'Brien, R. T., et al. (1993) Prevention of CNS disease in intermediate-risk acute lymphoblastic leukemia: comparison of cranial radiation and intrathecal methotrexate and the importance of systemic therapy: a Children's Cancer Group report. *J. Clin. Oncol.* **11**, 520–526.

15. Curley, S. A., Fuhrman, G. M., Siddik, Z. H., Davidson, B. S., Cleary, K. R., and Cromeens, D. M. (1995) Direct intratumoral injection of a novel collagen matrix gel and cisplatin effectively controls experimental liver tumors. *Cancer Res. Ther. Con.* **4**, 247–254.

16. Johnson, P. J., Leung, T. W., Vogel, T. J., et al. (2000) Percutaneous administration of cisplatin/epinephrine injectable gel for treatment of intrahepatic lesions of hepatocellular carcinoma [abstract]. *Proc. Am. Soc. Clin. Oncol.* **35**, 1201.

17. Mok, T. S., Kanekal, S., Lin, X. R., et al. (2001) Pharmacokinetic study of intralesional cisplatin for the treatment of hepatocellular carcinoma. *Cancer* **91**, 2369–2377.

18. Wenig, B. L., Werner, J. A., Castro, D. J., et al. (2002) The role of intratumoral therapy with cisplatin/epinephrine injectable gel in the management of advanced squamous cell carcinoma of the head and neck. *Arch. Otolaryngol. Head Neck Surg.* **128**, 880–885.

19. Kraus, S., Miller, B. H., Swinehart, J. M., et al. (1998) Intratumoral chemotherapy with fluorouracil/epinephrine injectable gel: a nonsurgical treatment of cutaneous squamous cell carcinoma. *J. Am. Acad. Dermatol.* **38**, 438–442.

20. Romano, G., Pacilio, C., and Giordano, A. (1999) Gene transfer technology in therapy: current applications and future goals. *Stem Cells* **17**, 191–202.

21. Dyer, M. R. and Herring, P. L. (2000) Progress and potential for gene-based medicine. *Mol. Ther.* **1**, 213–224.

22. Tamura, K., Tamura, M., Ikenaka, K., et al. (2001) Eradication of murine brain tumors by direct inoculation of concentrated high titer-recombinant retrovirus harboring the herpes simplex virus thymidine kinase gene. *Gene Ther.* **8**, 215–222.

23. Naldini, L., Blomer, U., Gallay, P., et al. (1996) In vivo gene delivery and stable transduction of nondividing cells by a lentiviral vector. *Science* **272**, 263–267.

24. Akkina, R. K., Walton, R. M., Chen, M. L., Li, Q. X., Planelles, V., and Chen, I. S. (1996) High-efficiency gene transfer into CD34$^+$ cells with a human immunodeficiency virus type 1-based retroviral vector pseudotyped with vesicular stomatitis virus envelope glycoprotein G. *J. Virol.* **70**, 2581–2585.

25. Moolten, F. L. (1986) Tumor chemosensitivity conferred by inserted herpes thymidine kinase genes: paradigm for a prospective cancer control strategy. *Cancer Res.* **46**, 5276–5281.

26. Sacco, M. G., Mangiarini, L., Villa, A., et al. (1995) Local regression of breast tumors following intramammary ganciclovir administration in double transgenic mice expressing neu oncogene and herpes simplex virus thymidine kinase. *Gene Ther.* **2**, 493–497.

27. Chen, S. H., Shine, H. D., Goodman, J. C., Grossman, R. G., and Woo, S. L. (1994) Gene therapy for brain tumors: regression of experimental gliomas by adenovirus-mediated gene transfer in vivo. *Proc. Natl. Acad. Sci. USA* **91**, 3054–3057.

28. DiMaio, J. M., Clary, B. M., Via, D. F., Coveney, E., Pappas, T. N., and Lyerly, H. K. (1994) Directed enzyme prodrug gene therapy for pancreatic cancer in vivo. *Surgery* **116**, 205–213.

29. Chen, S. H., Chen, X. H., Wang, Y., et al. (1995) Combination gene therapy for liver metastasis of colon carcinoma in vivo. *Proc. Natl. Acad. Sci. USA* **92,** 2577–2581.
30. Culver, K. W., Ram, Z., Wallbridge, S., Ishii, H., Oldfield, E. H., and Blaese, R. M. (1992) In vivo gene transfer with retroviral vector-producer cells for treatment of experimental brain tumors. *Science* **256,** 1550–1552.
31. O'Malley, B. W. Jr., Chen, S. H., Schwartz, M. R., and Woo, S. L. (1995) Adenovirus-mediated gene therapy for human head and neck squamous cell cancer in a nude mouse model. *Cancer Res.* **55,** 1080–1085.
32. Fife, K., Bower, M., Cooper, R. G., et al. (1998) Endothelial cell transfection with cationic liposomes and herpes simplex-thymidine kinase mediated killing. *Gene Ther.* **5,** 614–620.
33. Vile, R. G. and Hart, I. R. (1993) In vitro and in vivo targeting of gene expression to melanoma cells. *Cancer Res.* **53,** 962–967.
34. Link, C. J. Jr., Levy, J. P., McCann, L. Z., and Moorman, D. W. (1997) Gene therapy for colon cancer with the herpes simplex thymidine kinase gene. *J. Surg. Oncol.* **64,** 289–294.
35. Samejima, Y. and Meruelo, D. (1995) "Bystander killing" induces apoptosis and is inhibited by forskolin. *Gene Ther.* **2,** 50–58.
36. Mesnil, M., Piccoli, C., Tiraby, G., Willecke, K., and Yamasaki, H. (1996) Bystander killing of cancer cells by herpes simplex virus thymidine kinase gene is mediated by connexins. *Proc. Natl. Acad. Sci. USA* **93,** 1831–1835.
37. Vile, R. G., Nelson, J. A., Castleden, S., Chong, H., and Hart, I. R. (1994) Systemic gene therapy of murine melanoma using tissue specific expression of the HSVtk gene involves an immune component. *Cancer Res.* **54,** 6228–6234.
38. Izquierdo, M., Martin, V., de Felipe, P., et al. (1996) Human malignant brain tumor response to herpes simplex thymidine kinase (HSVtk)/ganciclovir gene therapy. *Gene Ther.* **3,** 491–495.
39. Ram, Z., Culver, K. W., Oshiro, E. M., et al. (1997) Therapy of malignant brain tumors by intratumoral implantation of retroviral vector-producing cells. *Nat. Med.* **3,** 1354–1361.
40. Shand, N., Weber, F., Mariani, L., et al. (1999) A phase 1–2 clinical trial of gene therapy for recurrent glioblastoma multiforme by tumor transduction with the herpes simplex thymidine kinase gene followed by ganciclovir. GLI328 European-Canadian Study Group. *Hum. Gene Ther.* **10,** 2325–2335.
41. Rainov, N. G. (2000) A phase III clinical evaluation of herpes simplex virus type 1 thymidine kinase and ganciclovir gene therapy as an adjuvant to surgical resection and radiation in adults with previously untreated glioblastoma multiforme. *Hum. Gene Ther.* **11,** 2389–2401.
42. Klatzmann, D., Valery, C. A., Bensimon, G., et al. (1998) A phase I/II study of herpes simplex virus type 1 thymidine kinase "suicide" gene therapy for recurrent glioblastoma. Study Group on Gene Therapy for Glioblastoma. *Hum. Gene Ther.* **9,** 2595–2604.
43. Trask, T. W., Trask, R. P., Aguilar-Cordova, E., et al. (2000) Phase I study of adenoviral delivery of the HSV-tk gene and ganciclovir administration in patients with current malignant brain tumors. *Mol. Ther.* **1,** 195–203.
44. Sandmair, A. M., Loimas, S., Puranen, P., et al. (2000) Thymidine kinase gene therapy for human malignant glioma, using replication-deficient retroviruses or adenoviruses. *Hum. Gene Ther.* **11,** 2197–2205.
45. Herman, J. R., Adler, H. L., Aguilar-Cordova, E., et al. (1999) *In situ* gene therapy for adenocarcinoma of the prostate: a phase I clinical trial. *Hum Gene Ther.* **10,** 1239–1249.
46. Ayala, G., Wheeler, T. M., Shalev, M., et al. (2000) Cytopathic effect of *in situ* gene therapy in prostate cancer. *Hum. Pathol.* **31,** 866–870.
47. Shalev, M., Kadmon, D., Teh, B. S., et al. (2000) Suicide gene therapy toxicity after multiple and repeat injections in patients with localized prostate cancer. *J. Urol.* **163,** 1747–1750.
48. Miles, B. J., Shalev, M., Aguilar-Cordova, E., et al. (2001) Prostate-specific antigen response and systemic T cell activation after *in situ* gene therapy in prostate cancer patients failing radiotherapy. *Hum. Gene Ther.* **12,** 1955–1967.
49. Todryk, S., Melcher, A., Bottley, G., Gough, M., and Vile, R. (2001) Cell death associated with genetic prodrug activation therapy of colorectal cancer. *Cancer Lett.* **174,** 25–33.
50. Sung, M. W., Yeh, H. C., Thung, S. N., et al. (2001) Intratumoral adenovirus-mediated suicide gene transfer for hepatic metastases from colorectal adenocarcinoma: results of a phase I clinical trial. *Mol. Ther.* **4,** 182–191.
51. Sterman, D. H., Treat, J., Litzky, L. A., et al. (1998) Adenovirus-mediated herpes simplex virus thymidine kinase/ganciclovir gene therapy in patients with localized malignancy: results of a phase I clinical trial in malignant mesothelioma. *Hum. Gene Ther.* **9,** 1083–1092.
52. Hasenburg, A., Tong, X. W., Rojas-Martinez, A., et al. (2000) Thymidine kinase gene therapy with concomitant topotecan chemotherapy for recurrent ovarian cancer. *Cancer Gene Ther.* **7,** 839–844.
53. Mesnil, M., Piccoli, C., Tiraby, G., Willecke, K., and Yamasaki, H. (1996) Bystander killing of cancer cells by herpes simplex virus thymidine kinase gene is mediated by connexins. *Proc. Natl. Acad. Sci. USA* **93,** 1831–1835.
54. Elshami, A. A., Saavedra, A., Zhang, H., et al. (1996) Gap junctions play a role in the "bystander effect" of the herpes simplex virus thymidine kinase/ganciclovir system in vitro. *Gene Ther.* **3,** 85–92.
55. Touraine, R. L., Vahanian, N., Ramsey, W. J., and Blaese, R. M. (1998) Enhancement of the herpes simplex virus thymidine kinase/ganciclovir bystander effect and its antitumor efficacy in vivo by pharmacologic manipulation of gap junctions. *Hum. Gene Ther.* **9,** 2385–2391.

56. Loubiere, L., Tiraby, M., Cazaux, C., et al. (1999) The equine herpes virus 4 thymidine kinase is a better suicide gene than the human herpes virus 1 thymidine kinase. *Gene Ther.* **6,** 1638–1642.

57. Cannon, J. S., Hamzeh, F., Moore, S., Nicholas, J., and Ambinder, R. F. (1999) Human herpesvirus 8-encoded thymidine kinase and phosphotransferase homologues confer sensitivity to ganciclovir. *J. Virol.* **73,** 4786–4793.

58. Black, M. E., Kokoris, M. S., and Sabo, P. (2001) Herpes simplex virus-1 thymidine kinase mutants created by semirandom sequence mutagenesis improve prodrug-mediated tumor cell killing. *Cancer Res.* **61,** 3022–3026.

59. Pantuck, A. J., Matherly, J., Zisman, A., et al. (2002) Optimizing prostate cancer suicide gene therapy using herpes simplex virus thymidine kinase active site variants. *Hum. Gene Ther.* **13,** 777–789.

60. Mullen, C. A., Kilstrup, M., and Blaese, R. M. (1992) Transfer of the bacterial gene for cytosine deaminase to mammalian cells confers lethal sensitivity to 5-fluorocytosine: a negative selection system. *Proc. Natl. Acad. Sci. USA* **89,** 33–37.

61. Huber, B. E., Austin, E. A., Good, S. S., Knick, V. C., Tibbels, S., and Richards, C. A. (1993) In vivo antitumor activity of 5-fluorocytosine on human colorectal carcinoma cells genetically modified to express cytosine deaminase. *Cancer Res.* **53,** 4619–4626.

62. Huber, B. E., Austin, E. A., Richards, C. A., Davis, S. T., and Good, S. S. (1994) Metabolism of 5-fluorocytosine to 5-fluorouracil in human colorectal tumor cells transduced with the cytosine deaminase gene: significant antitumor effects when only a small percentage of tumor cells express cytosine deaminase. *Proc. Natl. Acad. Sci. USA* **91,** 8302–8306.

63. Mullen, C. A., Coale, M. M., Lowe, R., and Blaese, R. M. (1994) Tumors expressing the cytosine deaminase suicide gene can be eliminated in vivo with 5-fluorocytosine and induce protective immunity to wild type tumor. *Cancer Res.* **54,** 1503–1506.

64. Ge, K., Xu, L., Zheng, Z., Xu, D., Sun, L., and Liu, X. (1997) Transduction of cytosine deaminase gene makes rat glioma cells highly sensitive to 5-fluorocytosine. *Int. J. Cancer* **71,** 675–679.

65. Lawrence, T. S., Rehemtulla, A., Ng, E. Y., Wilson, M., Trosko, J. E., and Stetson, P. L. (1998) Preferential cytotoxicity of cells transduced with cytosine deaminase compared to bystander cells after treatment with 5-flucytosine. *Cancer Res.* **58,** 2588–2593.

66. Pierrefite-Carle, V., Baque, P., Gavelli, A., et al. (2002) Subcutaneous or intrahepatic injection of suicide gene modified tumour cells induces a systemic antitumour response in a metastatic model of colon carcinoma in rats. *Gut* **50,** 387–391.

67. Pandha, H. S., Martin, L. A., Rigg, A., et al. (1999) Genetic prodrug activation therapy for breast cancer: a phase I clinical trial of erbB-2-directed suicide gene expression. *J. Clin. Oncol.* **17,** 2180–2189.

68. Crystal, R. G., Hirschowitz, E., Lieberman, M., et al. (1997) Phase I study of direct administration of a replication deficient adenovirus vector containing the E. coli cytosine deaminase gene to metastatic colon carcinoma of the liver in association with the oral administration of the pro-drug 5-fluorocytosine. *Hum. Gene Ther.* **8,** 985–1001.

69. Cunningham, C. and Nemunaitis, J. (2001) A phase I trial of genetically modified *Salmonella typhimurium* expressing cytosine deaminase (TAPET-CD, VNP20029) administered by intratumoral injection in combination with 5-fluorocytosine for patients with advanced or metastatic cancer. Protocol no: CL-017. Version: April 9, 2001. *Hum. Gene Ther.* **12,** 1594–1596.

70. Cao, X., Ju, D. W., Tao, Q., et al. (1998) Adenovirus-mediated GM-CSF gene and cytosine deaminase gene transfer followed by 5-fluorocytosine administration elicit more potent antitumor response in tumor-bearing mice. *Gene Ther.* **5,** 1130–1136.

71. Khil, M. S., Kim, J. H., Mullen, C. A., Kim, S. H., and Freytag, S. O. (1996) Radiosensitization by 5-fluorocytosine of human colorectal carcinoma cells in culture transduced with cytosine deaminase gene. *Clin. Cancer Res.* **2,** 53–57.

72. Hanna, N. N., Mauceri, H. J., Wayne, J. D., Hallahan, D. E., Kufe, D. W., and Weichselbaum, R. R. (1997) Virally directed cytosine deaminase/5-fluorocytosine gene therapy enhances radiation response in human cancer xenografts. *Cancer Res.* **57,** 4205–4209.

73. Uckert, W., Kammertons, T., Haack, K., et al. (1998) Double suicide gene (cytosine deaminase and herpes simplex virus thymidine kinase) but not single gene transfer allows reliable elimination of tumor cells in vivo. *Hum. Gene Ther.* **9,** 855–865.

74. Chung-Faye, G. A., Chen, M. J., Green, N. K., et al. (2001) In vivo gene therapy for colon cancer using adenovirus-mediated, transfer of the fusion gene cytosine deaminase and uracil phosphoribosyltransferase. *Gene Ther.* **8,** 1547–1554.

75. Ohwada, A., Hirschowitz, E. A., and Crystal, R. G. (1996) Regional delivery of an adenovirus vector containing the *Escherichia coli* cytosine deaminase gene to provide local activation of 5-fluorocytosine to suppress the growth of colon carcinoma metastatic to liver. *Hum. Gene Ther.* **7,** 1567–1576.

76. Knox, R. J., Boland, M. P., Friedlos, F., Coles, B., Southan, C., and Roberts, J. J. (1988) The nitroreductase enzyme in Walker cells that activates 5-(aziridin-1-yl)-2,4-dinitrobenzamide (CB 1954) to 5-(aziridin-1-yl)-4-hydroxylamino-2-nitrobenzamide is a form of NAD(P)H dehydrogenase (quinone) (EC 1.6.99.2). *Biochem. Pharmacol.* **37,** 4671–4677.

77. Chen, S., Knox, R., Wu, K., et al. (1997) Molecular basis of the catalytic differences among DT-diaphorase of human, rat, and mouse. *J. Biol. Chem.* **272,** 1437–1439.

78. Knox, R. J., Friedlos, F., Sherwood, R. F., Melton, R. G., and Anlezark, G. M. (1992) The bioactivation of 5-(aziridin-1-yl)-2,4-dinitrobenzamide (CB1954)—II. A comparison of an *Escherichia coli* nitroreductase and Walker DT diaphorase. *Biochem. Pharmacol.* **44,** 2297–2301.

79. Weedon, S. J., Green, N. K., McNeish, I. A., et al. (2000) Sensitisation of human carcinoma cells to the prodrug CB1954 by adenovirus vector-mediated expression of *E. coli* nitroreductase. *Int. J. Cancer* **86,** 848–854.

80. McNeish, I. A., Green, N. K., Gilligan, M. G., et al. (1998) Virus directed enzyme prodrug therapy for ovarian and pancreatic cancer using retrovirally delivered *E. coli* nitroreductase and CB1954. *Gene Ther.* **5,** 1061–1069.

81. Djeha, A. H., Hulme, A., Dexter, M. T., et al. (2000) Expression of *Escherichia coli* B nitroreductase in established human tumor xenografts in mice results in potent antitumoral and bystander effects upon systemic administration of the prodrug CB1954. *Cancer Gene Ther.* **7,** 721–731.

82. Friedlos, F., Quinn, J., Knox, R. J., and Roberts, J. J. (1992) The properties of total adducts and interstrand crosslinks in the DNA of cells treated with CB 1954. Exceptional frequency and stability of the crosslink. *Biochem. Pharmacol.* **43,** 1249–1254.

83. Knox, R. J. (ed.). (1998) *Targeted Anti-cancer Therapies: Are They ADEPT or INEPT?* University of Greenwich Inaugural Lecture Series, Greenwich, UK.

84. Bridgewater, J. A., Springer, C. J., Knox, R. J., Minton, N. P., Michael, N. P., and Collins, M. K. (1995) Expression of the bacterial nitroreductase enzyme in mammalian cells renders them selectively sensitive to killing by the prodrug CB1954. *Eur. J. Cancer* **31A,** 2362–2370.

85. Chung-Faye, G., Palmer, D., Anderson, D., et al. (2001) Virus-directed, enzyme prodrug therapy with nitroimidazole reductase: a phase I and pharmacokinetic study of its prodrug, CB1954. *Clin. Cancer Res.* **7,** 2662–2668.

86. Palmer, D. H., Mautner, V., Mirza, D., et al. (2004) Virus-directed enzyme prodrug therapy: intratumoral administration of a replication-deficient adenovirus encoding nitroreductase to patients with resectable liver cancer. *J. Clin. Oncol.* **22,** 1546–1552.

87. Green, N. K., McNeish, I. A., Doshi, R., Searle, P. F., Kerr, D. J., and Young, L. S. (2003) Immune enhancement of nitroreductase-induced cytotoxicity: studies using a bicistronic adenovirus vector. *Int. J. Cancer* **104,** 104–112.

87a. Palmer, D. H., Milner, A.E., Kerr, D. J., and Young, L. S. (2003) Mechanism of cell death induced by the novel enzyme-prodrug combination, nitroreductase/CB1954, and identification of synergism with 5-fluorouracil. *Br. J. Cancer* **89,** 944–509.

88. Lohr, M., Hoffmeyer, A., Kroger, J., et al. (2001) Microencapsulated cell-mediated treatment of inoperable pancreatic carcinoma. *Lancet* **357,** 1591–1592.

89. Braybrooke, J. P., Slade, A., Gibson, R., et al. (2002) Phase one study of MetXia-P450 gene therapy for patients with advanced breast cancer or melanoma [abstract]. *Proc. Am. Soc. Clin. Oncol.* Abstract no. 84.

90. Cohen, J. L., Boyer, O., Salomon, B., et al. (1997) Prevention of graft-versus-host disease in mice using a suicide gene expressed in T lymphocytes. *Blood* **89,** 4636–4645.

91. Bonini, C., Ferrari, G., Verzeletti, S., et al. (1997) HSV-TK gene transfer into donor lymphocytes for control of allogeneic graft-vs-leukemia. *Science* **276,** 1719–1724.

92. Meck, M. M., Wierdl, M., Wagner, L. M., et al. (2001) A virus-directed enzyme prodrug therapy approach to purging neuroblastoma cells from hematopoietic cells using adenovirus encoding rabbit carboxylesterase and CPT-11. *Cancer Res.* **61,** 5083–5089.

93. Wagner, L. M., Guichard, S. M., Burger, R. A., et al. (2002) Efficacy and toxicity of a virus-directed enzyme prodrug therapy purging method: preclinical assessment and application to bone marrow samples from neuroblastoma patients. *Cancer Res.* **62,** 5001–5007.

94. Caruso, M., Salomon, B., Zhang, S., et al. (1995) Expression of a Tat-inducible herpes simplex virus-thymidine kinase gene protects acyclovir-treated CD4 cells from HIV-1 spread by conditional suicide and inhibition of reverse transcription. *Virology* **206,** 495–503.

95. Ohno, T., Gordon, D., San, H., et al. (1994) Gene therapy for vascular smooth muscle cell proliferation after arterial injury. *Science* **265,** 781–784.

96. Harrell, R. L., Rajanayagam, S., Doanes, A. M., et al. (1997) Inhibition of vascular smooth muscle cell proliferation and neointimal accumulation by adenovirus-mediated gene transfer of cytosine deaminase. *Circulation* **96,** 621–627.

97. Carroll, N. M., Chase, M., Chiocca, E. A., and Tanabe, K. K. (1997) The effect of ganciclovir on herpes simplex virus-mediated oncolysis. *J. Surg. Res.* **69,** 413–417.

98. Rogulski, K. R., Wing, M. S., Paielli, D. L., Gilbert, J. D., Kim, J. H., and Freytag, S. O. (2000) Double suicide gene therapy augments the antitumor activity of a replication-competent lytic adenovirus through enhanced cytotoxicity and radiosensitization. *Hum. Gene Ther.* **11,** 67–76.

99. Advani, S. J., Sibley, G. S., Song, P. Y., et al. (1998) Enhancement of replication of genetically engineered herpes simplex viruses by ionizing radiation: a new paradigm for destruction of therapeutically intractable tumors. *Gene Ther.* **5,** 160–165.

100. Vile, R. G., Russell, S. J., and Lemoine, N. R. (2000) Cancer gene therapy: hard lessons and new courses. *Gene Ther.* **7,** 2–8.

101. Douglas, J. T., Rogers, B. E., Rosenfeld, M. E., Michael, S. I., Feng, M., and Curiel, D. T. (1996) Targeted gene delivery by tropism-modified adenoviral vectors. *Nat. Biotechnol.* **14,** 1574–1578.
102. Weitman, S. D., Lark, R. H., Coney, L. R., et al. (1992) Distribution of the folate receptor GP38 in normal and malignant cell lines and tissues. *Cancer Res.* **52,** 3396–3401.
103. Fisher, K. D., Stallwood, Y., Green, N. K., Ulbrich, K., Mautner, V., and Seymour, L. W. (2001) Polymer-coated adenovirus permits efficient retargeting and evades neutralising antibodies. *Gene Ther.* **8,** 341–348.
104. Hardy, S., Kitamura, M., Harris-Stansil, T., Dai, Y., and Phipps, M. L. (1997) Construction of adenovirus vectors through Cre-lox recombination. *J. Virol.* **71,** 1842–1849.
105. Reynolds, P. N., Feng, M., and Curiel, D. T. (1999) Chimeric viral vectors—the best of both worlds? *Mol. Med. Today* **5,** 25–31.
106. Zhang, W. W. (1999) Development and application of adenoviral vectors for gene therapy of cancer. *Cancer Gene Ther.* **6,** 113–138.
107. Alemany, R., Lai, S., Lou, Y. C., Jan, H. Y., Fang, X., and Zhang, W. W. (1999) Complementary adenoviral vectors for oncolysis. *Cancer Gene Ther.* **6,** 21–25.
108. Bartlett, J. S. and Samulski, R. J. (1998) Fluorescent viral vectors: a new technique for the pharmacological analysis of gene therapy. *Nat. Med.* **4,** 635–637.

9

Genetic Immunotherapy Approaches

Denise R. Shaw and Albert F. LoBuglio

1. INTRODUCTION

The idea of exploiting the immune system to treat tumors (*cancer immunotherapy*) is at least a century old. Immunotherapy is generally classified into two functional approaches: *Passive immunotherapy* administers preformed elements of the immune system (tumor-reactive antibodies, antitumor cytokines, or tumoricidal effector cells) to patients with the intent that these agents will directly attack the cancer cells. *Active immunotherapy* (including tumor vaccines and immunostimulatory cytokines) is intended to stimulate the patients' immune system to generate effective antitumor immunity. Both passive and active immunotherapies are integral parts of modern medical practice for problems as diverse as the treatment of snakebites and the prevention of infectious diseases. Yet, for cancer, the role of the immune system and immunotherapy has been a topic of spirited debate for the last 50 years [1]. Major points of contention have been whether tumor cells are immunogenic in their host of origin and whether the immune system is capable of controlling or eradicating malignant cells.

At present, the argument seems to have swung in favor of cancer immunotherapy, partly because of better understanding of tumor biology as well as the mechanisms operating to regulate effective antitumor immune responses [2]. Indeed, it has been proposed that the immune system exerts a selective pressure that shapes the characteristics of tumors that "evolve" into clinical problems in much the same way that host immune responses are believed to influence evolution of microbial pathogens [1,3,4]. If cancer cells are susceptible to control by the immune system, then the success of cancer immunotherapy may simply be a matter of getting a jump on tumor "escape" from immunosurveillance.

Credit for the first active immunotherapy trial is generally given to Coley [5], who injected tumors with killed bacteria in the late 19th and early 20th centuries. Later trials injected tumors with other agents that induce general inflammatory responses (such as the BCG strain of *Mycobacterium bovis* or viruses) or vaccinated cancer patients with whole-tumor cell preparations [6]. Although some patients appeared to benefit from these early immunotherapies, overall success rates were disappointing.

Following the development of B-cell hybridoma and monoclonal antibody technology in the late 1970s, patients were treated by passive immunotherapy with purified mouse monoclonal antibodies reactive with defined tumor antigens. About the same time, the immunostimulatory lymphokine interleukin-2 (IL-2) was cloned, leading to the first clinical trials of immunotherapy with a recombinant cytokine [7]. Recombinant deoxyribonucleic acid (DNA) technology led rapidly to trials of other cytokines that promote immune antitumor activity or mediate direct antitumor effects [6]. The same technology led to the production of recombinant tumor antigen proteins for tumor-specific vaccines. Yet, despite the increasing sophistication of immunotherapy strategies based on administration of recombinant proteins, successes as judged by tumor control are relatively few. More important, administration of some recombinant cytokines in clinical trials has been accompanied by severe, even life-threatening, toxicities [8].

From: *Contemporary Cancer Research*
Cancer Gene Therapy
Edited by: D. T. Curiel and J. T. Douglas © Humana Press Inc., Totowa, NJ

Table 1
Examples of Clinical Trials Using Genetic Immunotherapy in Cancer Patients

Nonspecific immune stimulation	
Immune stimulatory cytokines	Intratumoral injection of the gene encoding IL-12
Immune costimulatory receptors/ligands	Intralesional recombinant fowlpox encoding costimulatory molecules ICAM-1, LFA-3, and B7.1
Genetic vaccines	
Vector-encoded tumor antigen genes	Recombinant vaccinia virus expressing HPV 16 and 18 E6 and E7 genes
Gene-modified dendritic cell vaccines	Autologous DCs transduced with adenovirus expressing MART-1
Gene-modified whole-tumor cell vaccines	Autologous tumor cells modified with the CD80 (B7.1) costimulatory molecule gene
Modified immune effector cells	
Gene-modified T cells	Allogeneic lymphocytes transduced with gene encoding a chimeric TCR reactive with folate-binding protein

Trials listed on the NCI Clinical Trials PDQ® website (http://www.cancer.gov/clinicaltrials/) on December 6, 2002.

Gene therapy has the potential to deliver immunotherapeutic modalities in both a more effective and a less-dangerous manner. The administration of genes encoding therapeutic proteins can allow for more "natural" sustained protein levels in vivo, reducing problems with cytokines that are toxic at high concentrations but exhibit short circulating half-lives. Genetic immunotherapy also circumvents the need to produce and purify large amounts of recombinant proteins, a process that can impede initiation of human trials. For tumor vaccines, genetic delivery also can result in immune recognition of antigens in a manner more conducive for initiating the effective antitumor immune responses. These are some of the reasons that gene therapy approaches have been enthusiastically embraced in the development of contemporary immunotherapy strategies.

This chapter provides an overview of the immune system as it relates to cancer and then briefly introduces some of the genetic immunotherapy approaches investigated in animal models and human trials to date. Table 1 presents a few examples of genetic immunotherapy in contemporary human clinical trials. Other chapters in this book provide more detailed discussions of the vectors and specific therapeutic strategies developed and tested to date.

2. TUMOR IMMUNOLOGY

2.1. Immune Effector Mechanisms

Elements of the immune response are classified in two basic ways: innate and adaptive (acquired). In simplified terms, adaptive immune responses result from antigen "education" of the immune system, whereas for innate responses the knowledge is "inherited." In innate immune responses, effector activity is triggered via ligation of receptors encoded by germline genes. Adaptive immune responses depend on the diverse variable antigen receptors expressed by T and B cells, which are assembled by somatic recombination of germline gene elements. The innate immune response can be envisioned as a frontline immune defense mechanism that has evolved by "profiling" suspect antigens, whereas acquired immunity is a delayed response tailored to a particular encountered antigen. Both innate and adaptive arms of the immune responses have been implicated in cancer immunosurveillance. Furthermore, each may influence the response of the other arm *(1)*. Table 2 lists the effectors of each type thought to be involved in tumor immunity.

Table 2
Effectors of Antitumor Immune Responses

Innate immunity
    NK cells
    LAK cells
    NKT cells
    γδ-T cells
    Monocytes/macrophages
    Neutrophils/granulocytes
    Cytokines
Adaptive immunity
    B cells
    αβ-T cells
    Cytokines

2.1.1. Innate Immunity

The innate immune response has had a somewhat controversial history with respect to effective antitumor immunity. Natural killer (NK) cells were first described as lymphoidlike cells that mediate killing of some tumor cells in a major histocompatibility complex (MHC)-unrestricted manner (meaning that classical T-cell receptors [TCRs] were not implicated in the cytotoxicity). NK cell cultures treated with the immunostimulatory cytokine IL-2 (termed lymphokine-activated killer cells, LAK) generated cytolytic effector cells capable of killing an even wider variety of tumor cell targets, again in an MHC-unrestricted manner.

There are at least three classifications of lymphoid cells that have been shown to be capable of MHC-unrestricted tumor cell killing in various experimental systems: NK cells, which do not express TCR; natural killer T (NKT) cells, which express restricted repertoires of αβ-TCRs; and the relatively rare γδ-TCR lymphocytes *(1,2,9,10)*. Each of these lymphoid effectors can be distinguished by cell surface phenotypes, mechanisms of tumor cell recognition and killing, and phenotypes of tumor cell targets susceptible to attack. In addition to innate tumor cytolytic activity mediated by direct cell–cell interactions, these lymphoid innate immune effectors may affect tumor growth by secretion of cytokines (such as interferon-γ) that either directly inhibit tumor cell proliferation or modulate tumor cell MHC and antigen expression to enhance adaptive immune responses.

Immune cells of the myeloid lineage, monocytes/macrophages and neutrophils/granulocytes, also have a long history of study as mediators of tumor control and tumor cell killing. Both of these effector cell types express receptors for immunoglobulin G and are capable of mediating antibody-dependent cellular cytotoxicity against tumor cells opsonized with antibodies *(see* Section 2.1.2.). However, some experiments suggest that these myeloid effector cells can also mediate "innate" antitumor suppressive activities, either by direct cell–cell contact-dependent cytolytic mechanisms or by secretion of tumor-suppressive factors *(10)*. On the other hand, there is evidence that tumor-associated macrophages may suppress the development of adaptive antitumor immune responses.

As discussed above, one aspect of the innate immune response to tumors is the induction of tumor-suppressive cytokines. For example, interferons (IFNs) of both type I (IFN-α and IFN-β) and type II (IFN-γ) can directly inhibit tumor cell growth in experimental models *(6)*, and specific interferon therapies have been approved by the Food and Drug Administration for some malignancies (Roferon®, Intron®). But, perhaps more important is the induction of cytokines and chemokines that promote the activation of adaptive immune responses to tumors *(1)*.

2.1.2. Adaptive Immunity

Adaptive (or acquired) immune responses are dependent on αβT- and B-cell antigen receptors (αβ-TCRs and BCRs, respectively). TCRs and BCRs are generated by somatic recombination of multiple possible germline gene elements (V, D, J, C). Diversity of antigen specificity is provided by the large numbers of receptor variable region gene elements available for recombination and by somatic mutations and joining region degeneracy, which create additional unique receptor sequences. The adaptive response is established by antigen-driven clonal selection of cells expressing receptors with appropriate affinity for antigen, by costimulation with necessary second signals, and usually by the generation of memory B or T cells.

The BCR is a membrane-bound form of the secreted antibody, which is the effector arm of the B-cell adaptive response. Antibodies can mediate at least three types of effector activity against tumor cells. Complement-dependent cytolysis (CDC) is effected by activation of the complement cascade by antibody bound to the target cell surface. The role of CDC in tumor immunity is controversial; although tumor CDC can be demonstrated by in vitro experiments, it is less certain that effective CDC operates in vivo, and most cells (including tumor cells) express membrane regulators of complement that inhibit efficient complement lysis *(10)*. Antibody-dependent cell-mediated cytolysis is mediated by immune effector cells that express receptors for the Fc portion of immunoglobulin G antibodies (FcγR), including NK cells, macrophages/monocytes, and granulocytes. Antibodies to certain tumor cell antigens may also directly mediate antitumor effects in the absence of complement or FcγR effector cells. This has been demonstrated for certain antibodies specific for receptors involved in growth or proliferation or cell survival, including the Her2/neu/erbB2 epidermal growth factor family receptor expressed by several solid tumors *(11)* and the CD20 molecule expressed by many B-cell lymphomas *(12)*.

The αβ-TCR participates in multiple pathways of the adaptive immune response *(13)*. CD4+ T-helper cells, which recognize peptide antigens presented in the context of MHC class II molecules, are important in the amplification and regulation of antigen-specific immune responses initiated by antigen-presenting cells. The nature of the T-helper cell response modulates the relative response of B cells (antibody production) and cytotoxic T lymphocytes (CTLs) to a given antigen. Classical CTLs are CD8+ CD3+ T cells that recognize antigen peptides in the context of MHC class I. Tumor cells frequently express MHC class I, but not class II; however, participation of appropriate MHC class II-recognizing T-helper cells may be necessary to generate a robust CTL antitumor response *(10)*.

The balance between MHC class I and class II presentation to αβ-T cells in part directs the balance between antibody and CTL responses to a given antigen. This is influenced by the manner in which T or B lymphocytes interact with the antigen-presenting cell (APC). APCs in which the antigen is endogenously expressed (such as tumor cells expressing their own antigens) favor MHC class I peptide presentation, which in turn can promote activation of antigen-specific CTLs. APCs in which the antigen is exogenously taken up (such as by macrophage phagocytosis) favor MHC class II peptide presentation, which in turn favors activation of antigen-specific CD4+ T cells, which may promote antigen-specific B-cell antibody responses, CTLs, or even immune suppressor T cells.

The final outcome of either BCR or αβ-TCR antigen recognition depends in part on ancillary stimuli, including cytokines and costimulatory molecule engagement between APCs and the responding B or T cells. It is experimentally suggested that certain strategies for tumor antigen immunization promote B-cell antibody responses to the detriment of CTL responses and vice versa. Genetic immunotherapy allows for latitude in tumor antigen expression mechanisms to investigate such differences and to translate them into clinical trials for effective tumor immunity.

2.1.3. Dendritic Cells

Dendritic cells (DCs) are potent regulators of both innate and adaptive immune responses *(14–16)*. In the adaptive immune response, DCs represent the most effective type of APC for MHC class I and class II peptide antigen presentation to lymphocytes. In the innate immune system, DCs respond directly to microbial products and other inflammatory stimuli to secrete immune-enhancing cytokines and to activate effectors such as NK and NKT cells. Although DCs have been most studied as initiators of immune responses, there is also accumulated evidence that these cells can directly participate in the induction of immune tolerance, which should be avoided for most cancer immunotherapies, but may be desirable for immunotherapies directed at autoimmune syndromes or allergies.

2.2. Tumor Antigens

There is much accumulated evidence that most tumors are immunogenic. In animal models, this can be readily demonstrated by the development of tumor-specific immunity to syngeneic experimental tumors. In humans, cancer patients frequently develop spontaneous immunity to their own tumors *(17)*. This immunogenicity has facilitated the identification of tumor antigens that may be suitable for targeted immunotherapy.

2.2.1. Self- vs Non-Self-Antigens

Although the majority of tumor antigens identified to date are "self-antigens," some malignancies are known to express antigens that should be recognized as "foreign" by the host *(18,19)*. One category of foreign antigens expressed by cancer cells is viral antigens. These are frequently the products of agents thought to initiate malignant transformation, such as Epstein-Barr virus in some B-cell lymphomas, human papilloma virus (HPV) in cervical carcinoma, and hepatitis C virus in hepatocellular carcinoma. Other virus-derived tumor antigens are products of endogenous retroviruses such as murine leukemia virus (MuLV) in mice *(20)* and human endogenous retrovirus (HERV)-K10 in humans *(21,22)*, although it is debatable that these represent true "foreign" antigens considering that the proviral sequences have been present in the host genomes for millions of years.

A second category of non-self-antigens includes neoantigens created by acquired point mutations or chromosomal translocations in tumor cells *(18,19)*. Common examples include mutations in the tumor suppressor p53 or the proto-oncogene *RAS*, which frequently occur in multiple types of cancer, and the oncogenic fusion protein created by the *BCR/ABL* translocation, which is characteristic of chronic myeloid leukemia.

However, most tumor antigens are products of unmutated host genes (self-antigens), and their utility as immunotherapy targets resides primarily in the fact that they are aberrantly expressed by tumor cells. For some antigens, aberrant expression has been shown to provide a growth advantage for the malignant cells, such as Her2/neu/erbB-2 overexpression in breast, ovarian, and other carcinomas *(11)*. For other antigens, biological advantages of expression are less clear, but nonetheless distinct from that of normal tissues. Carcinoembryonic antigen is an example of an oncofetal antigen normally expressed during fetal development and by a restricted set of normal adult cells, but overexpressed by many adenocarcinomas *(23)*. Similarly, differentiation or lineage-restricted antigens are expressed by normal terminally differentiated cells, but aberrantly expressed by tumors, such as the MART-1 and gp100 antigens in normal melanocytes as well as malignant melanoma *(18)*. A recently recognized type of unmutated tumor antigen is the cancer-testis antigen, which has expression that is normally restricted to the testis or sperm, but like the NY-ESO-1 antigen in melanoma, is expressed by malignancies of seemingly unrelated lineages *(18)*.

The distinction between self- and non-self-antigens has significance for the design of tumor vaccines (active specific immunotherapy) as well as passive immunotherapies. First, immune responses to non-self- (foreign) antigens like viral products or mutated proteins are generally easier to elicit. However, the delineation between self- and non-self-antigen is not absolute, as evidenced by the common expression of spontaneous immune responses to unmutated "self" tumor antigens in cancer patients. Second, the induction of robust immune responses to tumor antigens expressed by normal tissues can potentially lead to pathological autoimmunity. For example, some melanoma vaccine trials have resulted in vitiligo, the autoimmune destruction of normal melanocytes *(18)*. To date, serious autoimmune reactions have not been reported in cancer vaccine trials, but severe toxicities to nontargeted normal tissues have been observed in passive immunotherapy trials using tumor antigen-specific monoclonal antibodies conjugated to toxins or radiochemicals *(24)*.

2.2.2. B-Cell vs T-Cell Antigens

Another way to classify tumor antigens is based on the type of adaptive immune responses elicited, that is, either antibodies (produced by B cells) or CTLs. Antibodies recognize a wide variety of antigens and epitopes, including both contiguous and noncontiguous peptide domains, carbohydrates, gangliosides, and modified peptides such as phosphorylated amino acids. By contrast, classical CTLs recognize linear peptides (8–12 residues) generated by proteolytic processing of antigens. This fundamental difference is explained by the nature of antigen receptors expressed by B cells and T cells. The BCR is a membrane-bound version of the antibody that can bind to and respond to unprocessed antigens of almost any chemical composition. In contrast, classical $\alpha\beta$-TCRs recognize antigens as processed peptides presented in association with MHC class I or II molecules on the surface of APCs and ultimately the target tumor cells. Whereas the repertoire of potential tumor antigen targets for antibodies is much larger than that for CTLs, the antitumor activity of CTL responses is generally regarded as more potent for cancer control than antibody.

2.3. Tumor Escape Mechanisms

It is evident that tumors develop and expand even in the presence of measurable host antitumor immune responses. Multiple mechanisms have been implicated in the ability of tumors to escape or evade what might otherwise be effective immunity *(1,2,4,10,25)*. One is the loss of MHC class I antigen expression, which would preclude antitumor CTL activity. Another is loss of tumor antigen expression, which would circumvent both antibody and CTL arms of the adaptive immune response. Many tumors have also been shown to produce cytokines and other mediators that are immunosuppressive (including IL-4, IL-10, transforming growth factor-β, vascular endothelial growth factor, gangliosides) and could either prevent initiation of the antitumor immune response or thwart an established response. Tumors have also been reported to acquire resistance to apoptosis through defective death receptor signaling, as well as to induce apoptosis of tumor antigen-activated T cells. Design of novel cancer immunotherapy strategies must take these tumor escape mechanisms into account.

3. GENETIC IMMUNOTHERAPY BY NONSPECIFIC IMMUNE STIMULATION

The term *nonspecific immunotherapy* is frequently applied to strategies that do not employ a predefined tumor antigen target. The goals are to provide immune factors that directly affect tumor cell survival or promote host immunity. The latter goal is particularly relevant with respect to host immunosuppression or immunodeficiency associated with malignant diseases *(26)*. Such "nonspecific" therapies often promote antigen-specific adaptive immune responses to tumors, similar to true vaccines. However, nonspecific immunotherapy has several advantages over conventional vaccines: (1) It is not limited by the requirement for prior identification and characterization of tumor antigens, and (2) it may enhance both adaptive and innate arms of the antitumor immune response.

3.1. Immune-Stimulatory Cytokines and Chemokines

Many soluble factors have been described with properties of enhancing immune responses in general, and more specifically to tumor cells, and are under exploration as targets for genetic immunotherapy. Cancer patients are generally described as exhibiting immunosuppression of some degree, including abnormal patterns of immune cytokine production *(26)*, that might be offset by immunotherapy with the deficient factors. For factors that can function systemically by activating immune effector cells, such as interferons and certain interleukins (IL-2, IL-12), gene transfer to any convenient tissue may be effective as long as sufficient concentrations of the circulating cytokine activate sufficient numbers of immune effector cells *(6,8,26,27)*.

However, in most cases to date, gene delivery has been directly into tumors, a route particularly preferred for chemokines and cytokines such as granulocyte-macrophage colony-stimulating factor (GM-CSF) that are chemotactic for specific immune cell types. The choice of vectors for these applications should take into consideration the duration of transgene expression desired (either prolonged or brief, depending on the specific cytokine or chemokine) and the types of host cells targeted for transduction.

A major limitation is that intratumoral gene vector injection is not possible for many types of cancer and cancer patients. However, recent attempts to design retargeted gene vectors that selectively transduce specific types of host immune or malignant cells or that will be selectively expressed in restricted cell types because of the engineering of lineage-restricted transgene promoters have the potential to obviate requirements for intratumoral injection of gene vectors.

3.2. Immune Costimulatory Receptors/Ligands

One general mechanism by which tumors may evade immune control is the lack of tumor cell expression of MHC molecules, costimulatory molecules, and other ligands required to induce and sustain an effective immune response. Thus, gene therapy has been used to introduce such deficient receptors and ligands into tumors to enhance host immune system recognition and antitumor activity. In addition to MHC molecules, a variety of molecules involved in both innate and adaptive immune effector cell recognition have been tested for sensitization of tumor cells to immune effectors, including CD54 (ICAM-1), CD58 (LFA-3), CD80 (B7.1), and CD40 *(28)*.

The intent is to render some tumor cells susceptible to immune recognition and attack and thereby amplify a more generalized immune response to unmodified tumor cells. Vectors for gene delivery should be selected for the ability to transduce tumor cells efficiently, and both short- and long-term transgene expression may be effective. As mentioned in Section 3.1., the types of cancer patients in whom direct intratumoral injection of gene vectors is applicable are limited, but cell-targeted genetic vectors have the potential to overcome this limitation as well as restrictions of the native vector's cell tropism.

4. GENETIC VACCINES (ACTIVE SPECIFIC IMMUNOTHERAPY)

Tumor vaccines of various types have been extensively studied in animal models, and many have been used in clinical trials for cancer treatment and prevention *(6)*. A clinical trial of an HPV type 16 viruslike particle vaccine to prevent HPV-associated cervical cancer *(29)* ranks as one of the most encouraging accomplishments in the field of tumor vaccines. This and multiple other completed tumor vaccine trials use inoculation with the antigen itself, often in combination with immune adjuvants. Genetic vaccines have the advantage over these types of vaccines in that the antigens themselves do not have to be prepared, purified, and formulated—only genes are required. Another advantage is that immune adjuvants may not be required because of the nature of the vector and host cell expression of the transgene; alternatively, adjuvants can be coadministered by genetic transfer of immunostimulatory factors.

Considerations in the design of both genetic and conventional (nongenetic) tumor vaccines are similar: (1) an appropriate tumor antigen target; (2) duration and extent of host immune system exposure to tumor antigen, dependent on dose and schedule of inoculations for nongenetic vaccines, but in part determined by the choice of vector for genetic vaccines; (3) host cell types encountering or expressing the antigen; and (4) incorporation of immune adjuvants. An additional consideration specific for genetic vaccines is whether the encoded antigen will be primarily secreted or cell associated.

Each of these considerations can affect the overall nature of the immune response, including the balance between innate and adaptive responses and that between antibody and CTL adaptive immunity. For example, a vaccine that elicits predominantly antibody responses is applicable to tumor antigens expressed on the tumor cell surface (such as Her2/neu/erbB2), in contrast to a vaccine targeting an intracellular antigen (such as mutated p53), which should elicit strong MHC class I restricted CTL responses. Design considerations also affect the ability of the vaccine to break immunologic tolerance, which is less of a factor for preventive vaccines targeting viral proteins (such as HPV) compared to unmutated self-antigens (such as Her2/neu/erbB2 and the majority of identified tumor antigens).

In general, genetic vaccines offer greater flexibility and ease in the construction of formulations with the desired characteristics of antigen delivery and the elicited immune responses compared to conventional vaccines. The following sections outline strategies most frequently exploited for genetic cancer vaccine development; most of these subjects are covered in greater detail in other chapters of this book.

4.1. Vector-Encoded Tumor Antigen Genes

The simplest approach to genetic vaccines is to inoculate patients directly with a recombinant vector that encodes a tumor antigen. The intent is to induce host cells to express the tumor antigen transgene (with or without immune costimulatory factors), which in theory should promote effective tumor-specific adaptive immune responses similar to the robust immunity elicited by host infection with common viral or bacterial pathogens. A major advantage is that host cells will express the vector-encoded genes, thus promoting MHC class I receptor presentation of transgene products favorable for development of CTL responses believed important for effective antitumor immunity. These approaches facilitate efficient utilization of recombinant DNA technology to create artificial genes encoding defined immunogenic portions of tumor antigens, immunogenic variants of the tumor antigen, tumor antigen fusions with highly immunogenic peptides from other proteins, or tumor antigen fusions with ligands targeting them to receptor-specific uptake by host antigen-presenting cells *(30)*. In addition, each of the vaccine approaches described below has potential intrinsic adjuvant activity because of the host's innate immune response to the gene delivery vector.

4.1.1. Polynucleotide Vectors

Since the initial report of polynucleotide vaccination *(31)*, innumerable published studies have demonstrated the vaccine efficacy of plasmid DNA, messenger ribonucleic acid (mRNA), or viral DNA/ RNA genomes encoding target antigens in animal models following polynucleotide injection via intramuscular, intradermal, and subcutaneous routes, as well as following mucosal surface (nasal, gastrointestinal, vaginal) administration *(30)*. Safety of polynucleotide vaccination has been documented by several reported clinical trials *(32–34)*. Polynucleotide vectors may exhibit additional intrinsic immune adjuvant activities, such as the toll-like receptor recognition of bacterial plasmid unmethylated CpG motifs and the innate cellular responses to viral RNA transcription. Furthermore, the immune potency of "naked" polynucleotide vaccines may be enhanced by polynucleotide encapsulation or conjugation using a variety of biocompatible polymers. The inherent simplicity of constructing polynucleotide vaccines has promoted their use as vectors in preclinical and clinical studies of genetic tumor vaccines, especially for those employing antigens altered by genetic manipulations to enhance immunity.

4.1.2. Viral Vectors

Attenuated live virus vaccines have proven successful for infectious diseases such as smallpox, polio, and influenza. A major factor in efficacy of live attenuated virus vaccines is that they mimic actual viral infections. Virus uptake and gene expression by host cells elicits both innate and adaptive immune responses, including antigen-specific antibodies and MHC class I-restricted CTLs. These properties make recombinant viruses highly attractive as genetic vectors for tumor vaccines, and multiple viruses expressing tumor antigens have been tested in preclinical models as well as in a more limited number of clinical trials.

A major consideration for viral vectors used as genetic vaccines is that they have minimal intrinsic pathogenicity; that is, the viral vector should not be capable of causing significant disease in the vaccinated host, and the virus should not be capable of infectious spread to other individuals. These conditions are most commonly accomplished by ensuring that the virus strain used for vaccine construction is severely "crippled" (defective) in its ability to produce progeny virus in normal human cells. Safety may also be provided by robust virus-neutralizing immune responses in "healthy" humans, with the caveat that patients with advanced cancer are frequently immunocompromised. Viruses that have been pursued as genetic vectors for vaccines include poxviruses (cowpox and fowlpox strains), adenovirus, adeno-associated virus, and influenza virus *(28,35–38)*.

Vaccinia (the cowpox virus used in smallpox vaccines) has a fairly good safety record and was one of the first viral vectors used in clinical trials for tumor vaccines *(39)*. Routine smallpox vaccinations were discontinued in most developed countries in the 1970s and 1980s, primarily because of eradication of smallpox as a natural infection in major parts of the world and secondarily because of the risks of vaccinia pathogenicity revealed by universal smallpox vaccination. In early 2003, large numbers of previously unvaccinated military and health care personnel in the United States received the smallpox vaccine, and cases of vaccinia pathogenicity, including person-to-person transmission of symptomatic vaccinia infections, were documented *(40)*. This example serves as a cautionary tale for plans to exploit presumed "nonpathogenic" viruses as gene vectors for tumor vaccines.

Beyond issues of safety, viral vectors considered for use as genetic vaccines should be evaluated for several additional criteria. First, the virus should efficiently infect host cells that potently promote the desired immune response (e.g., professional APCs). If the virus does not exhibit natural tropism for APCs, this can sometimes be overcome by appropriate selection of the route, dose, and schedule of virus vaccine administration. In other cases, modifications of recombinant virus particles can "retarget" the genetic vector to the desired APC.

Second, preexisting virus-neutralizing antibodies and T-cell responses, including the reactivation of memory immune responses, against viruses must be considered. This is most important with vectors based on common human infectious viruses (e.g., wild-type adenovirus serotype 5), but may also present problems for any viral vector that elicits strong primary host immune responses because effective tumor vaccines are currently thought to require a schedule of repeated administration for antitumor efficacy *(28,37,41,42)*. If host immune responses are sufficient to prevent primary viral vector infection of host cells or to rapidly eliminate host cells expressing early viral gene products, then vaccine efficacy may be severely compromised. Again, careful selection of vaccine dose and schedule may circumvent some of these concerns.

Third, time-course and duration of virally encoded transgene expression by transduced host cells can influence the strength and the nature of the immune response (antibody vs CTL vs suppressor) to virally encoded tumor antigens. Although current evidence suggests that sustained expression of virus transgene expression may be most beneficial for eliciting effective antitumor immunity, definitive conclusions await additional experimental data.

4.2. Gene-Modified DC Vaccines

Another approach for genetic vaccines is to directly modify potent antigen-presenting cells (especially DCs) by genetic modification in vitro and then to administer modified APCs or DCs as a vaccine. The ability to generate both immature and mature DCs of different phenotypes from readily accessible progenitors in human subjects or experimental animals has promoted numerous studies of genetically altered DCs as tumor vaccines *(6,15,18,43)*. Cultured DCs can be modified to present tumor antigens by nongenetic approaches, including in vitro "pulsing" with tumor proteins or cellular fusions between DCs and tumor cells, but a common approach has been to genetically modify the APCs or DCs in vitro using polynucleotide transfection or viral transduction. Advantages of this approach include the ability to deliver tumor antigen genes efficiently to DCs in vitro and the potential to further modify activation status of the cultured DC prior to vaccination. Disadvantages include the need to harvest, culture, and modify cells from patients prior to delivery of the tumor vaccine, which limits widespread clinical application of this approach to patient treatment centers with approved ex vivo culture facilities.

4.3. Gene-Modified Whole-Tumor Cell Vaccines

Autologous or homologous tumor cell preparations comprised some of the earliest tumor vaccines tested in clinical trials. Similarly, cultured tumor cells genetically modified in vitro to express immune-activating cytokines were among the first genetic vaccines tested experimentally *(6)*. More recently, cultured tumor cells genetically modified to express GM-CSF as immune adjuvant have exhibited encouraging antitumor vaccine activity in clinical trials *(44)*. One advantage of this approach is that whole-tumor cell vaccines target the immune response to a cell that resembles the patient's tumor using genetic manipulation to enhance immune activation and potentially counteract tumor cell "immune escape" mechanisms exhibited by the endogenous tumor. A disadvantage is that the approach requires in vitro culture and gene modification of the vaccine tumor cells, with the same limitations mentioned for conduct of clinical trials.

4.4. Combination Vaccine Strategies

An increasing number of experimental active immunotherapies utilize combination strategies. In some cases, these combine "conventional" with "genetic" approaches, as with viral vectors encoding tumor antigen administered with recombinant GM-CSF protein as an immune adjuvant *(45)*. In other cases, different genetic approaches may be combined, such as in diversified prime-boost vaccine strategies using plasmid DNA as primary immunizations and recombinant adenovirus as the boosting immunization *(35,36,46)*. The intent in the combination protocols is to take full advantage of the desirable properties of each component and to devise a schedule of combined administration that efficiently promotes the desired effective immune response. Combination approaches will probably require longer times for development and testing because of the increased number of variables (timing of coadministration), but seem likely to constitute a continuing strategy for novel genetic vaccine research.

5. MODIFIED IMMUNE EFFECTOR CELLS (ADOPTIVE SPECIFIC IMMUNOTHERAPY)

5.1. Gene-Modified T Cells

CTLs (MHC class I-restricted αβ-T cells) have long been considered the most potent immune effectors for tumor control. Gene therapy provides the opportunity to redirect CTL activity by providing "artificial" TCRs that directly target tumor cells. The artificial TCRs may be conventional TCRs specific for tumor antigen peptides presented classically in MHC class I molecules. But, more powerfully, they may also be "chimeric" receptors that recognize tumor cells in an MHC-unrestricted manner. Thus, genetic constructs encoding chimeric receptors with antibody-binding domains as the antigen-binding portion of the TCR have been generated and shown experimentally to redirect transfected T-cell cytotoxicity to tumor cells expressing the cognate antigen on their cell surface *(47–50)*. The potential of this general approach for adoptive immunotherapy is limited only by the state of current knowledge regarding the precise mechanisms of CTL recognition and killing of tumor cells.

5.2. Gene-Modified NK/NKT Cells

Similar to CTLs, the ever-expanding understanding of molecular recognition and signaling events that lead to NK and NKT cell killing of tumor cells provides opportunities for ex vivo genetic modifications of these effectors for more efficient tumor cytotoxicity. The potential in vivo longevity and proliferative capacity of adoptively transferred NK cells support future applications of gene-modified NK or NKT cells in cancer immunotherapy *(51,52)*. Also, for these cell types, it may be possible to design gene vectors for in vivo modulation of NK cell antitumor activity.

6. FUTURE DIRECTIONS

The scope and nature of genetic immunotherapy approaches are continuously expanding in response to (1) new knowledge about the effector mechanisms and regulating factors in tumor immunity and (2) advances in the development of novel gene therapy vectors. Thus, the future should show new cytokines, chemokines, costimulatory receptors, and even intracellular signaling molecules incorporated into genetic immunotherapy. Identification of novel tumor antigens as well as better delineation of the nature of antigens and antigenic determinants that elicit the most effective antitumor immune responses will particularly impact the development of genetic vaccines. In addition, novel recombinant genetic vectors with targeted host cell infectivity or with selective transgene expression can be exploited to enhance the effectiveness of genetic immunotherapy.

Another area likely to be investigated intensely in the coming years is the combination of genetic immunotherapy with established "conventional" tumor therapies, such as chemotherapy or radiation. Experiments in animals as well as clinical trials have suggested beneficial results from combining some chemotherapy regimens with immunotherapy *(53–56)*, and the intrinsic advantages of genetic immunotherapy ensure that it will be used in increasing numbers and types of combination regimens.

REFERENCES

1. Dunn, G. P., Bruce, A. T., Ikeda, H., Old, L. J., and Schreiber, R. D. (2002) Cancer immunoediting: from immunosurveillance to tumor escape. *Nat. Immunol.* **3,** 991–998.
2. Smyth, M. J., Godfrey, D. I., and Trapani, J. A. (2001) A fresh look at tumor immunosurveillance and immunotherapy. *Nat. Immunol.* **2,** 293–299.
3. Phillips, R. E. (2002) Immunology taught by Darwin. *Nat. Immunol.* **3,** 987–989.
4. Khong, H. T. and Restifo, N. P. (2002) Natural selection of tumor variants in the generation of "tumor escape" phenotypes. *Nat. Immunol.* **3,** 999–1005.
5. Coley, W. B. (1893) The treatment of malignant tumors by repeated inoculations of erysipelas. With a report of 10 original cases. *Clin. Orthop.* **262,** 3–11.
6. Mocelin, S., Rossi, C. R., Lise, M., and Marincola, F. M. (2002) Adjuvant immunotherapy for solid tumors: from promise to clinical application. *Cancer Immunol. Immunother.* **51,** 583–595.
7. Rosenberg, S. A., Lotze, M. T., Muul, L. M., et al. (1985) Observations on the systemic administration of autologous lymphokine-activated killer cells and recombinant interleukin-2 to patients with metastatic cancer. *N. Engl. J. Med.* **313,** 1485–1492.
8. Portielje, J. E. A., Gratama, J. W., van Ojik, H. H., Stoter, G., and Kruit, W. H. J. (2003) IL-12: a promising adjuvant for cancer vaccination. *Cancer Immunol. Immunother.* **52,** 133–144.
9. Smyth, M. J., Crowe, N. Y., Hayakawa, Y., Takeda, K., Yagita, H., and Godfrey, D. I. (2002) NKT cells—conductors of tumor immunity? *Curr. Opin. Immunol.* **14,** 165–171.
10. Mitra, R., Singh, S., and Khar, A. (2003) Antitumor immune responses. *Exp. Rev. Mol. Med.* 5; Date accessed: 01/28/2003; available at http://www.expertreviews.org/03005623h.htm.
11. Yip, Y. L. and Ward, R. L. (2002) Anti-erbB-2 monoclonal antibodies and ErbB-2-directed vaccines. *Cancer Immunol. Immunother.* **50,** 569–587.
12. Shan, D., Ledbetter, J. A., and Press, O. W. (2000) Signaling events involved in anti-CD20-induced apoptosis of malignant human B cells. *Cancer Immunol. Immunother.* **48,** 673–683.
13. Kaech, S. M., Wherry, E. J., and Ahmed, R. (2002) Effector and memory T-cell differentiation: implications for vaccine development. *Nat. Rev. Immunol.* **2,** 251–262.
14. Steinman, R. M., Hawiger, D., and Nussenzweig, M. C. (2002) Tolerigenic dendritic cells. *Annu. Rev. Immunol.* **21,** 685–711.
15. Schuler, G., Schuler-Thurner, B., and Steinman, R. M. (2003) The use of dendritic cells in cancer immunotherapy. *Curr. Opin. Immunol.* **15,** 138–147.
16. Woltman, A. M. and van Kooten, C. (2003) Functional modulation of dendritic cells to suppress adaptive immune responses. *J. Leukoc. Biol.* **73,** 428–441.
17. Dranoff, G. (2002) Tumor immunology: immune recognition and tumor protection. *Curr. Opin. Immunol.* **14,** 161–164.
18. Jäger, E., Jäger, D., and Knuth, A. (2002) Clinical cancer vaccine trials. *Curr. Opin. Immunol.* **14,** 178–182.
19. Meese, E. and Comtesse, N. (2002) Cancer genetics and tumor antigens: time for a combined view? *Genes Chromosomes Cancer* **33,** 107–113.
20. Huang, A. Y., Gulden, P. H., Woods, A. S., et al. (1996) The immunodominant major histocompatibility complex class I-restricted antigen of a murine colon tumor derives from an endogenous retroviral gene product. *Proc. Natl. Acad. Sci. USA* **93,** 9730–9735.

21. Schiavetti, F., Thonnard, J., Colau, D., Boon, T., and Coulie, P. G. (2002) A human endogenous retroviral sequence encoding and antigen recognized on melanoma by cytolytic T lymphocytes. *Cancer Res.* **62,** 5510–5516.

22. Lower, R., Lower, J., and Kurth, R. (1996) The viruses in all of us: characteristics and biological significance of human endogenous retrovirus sequences. *Proc. Natl. Acad. Sci. USA* **93,** 5177–5184.

23. Hörig, H., Medina, F. A., Conkright, W. A., and Kaufman, H. L. (2000) Strategies for cancer therapy using carcino-embryonic antigen vaccines. *Exp. Rev. Mol. Med.* Date accessed: 04/19/2003; available at: http://www-ermm.cbcu.cam.ac.uk/0000168Xh.htm.

24. Carter, P. (2001) Improving the efficacy of antibody-based cancer therapies. *Nat. Rev. Cancer* **1,** 118–129.

25. McKallip, R., Li, R., and Ladisch, S. (1999) Tumor gangliosides inhibit the tumor-specific immune response. *J. Immunol.* **163,** 3718–3726.

26. Waller, E. K. and Ernstoff, M. S. (2003) Modulation of antitumor immune responses by hematopoietic cytokines. *Cancer* **97,** 1797–1809.

27. Paul, S., Regulier, E., Poitevin, Y., Hormann, H., and Acres, R. B. (2002) The combination of a chemokine, cytokine and TCR-based T cell stimulus for effective gene therapy of cancer. *Cancer Immunol. Immunother.* **51,** 645–654.

28. Hodge, J. W., Grosenback, D. W., and Schlom, J. (2002) Vector-based delivery of tumor-associated antigens and T-cell co-stimulatory molecules in the induction of immune responses and anti-tumor immunity. *Cancer Detect. Prev.* **26,** 275–291.

29. Koutsky L. A., Ault, K. A., Wheeler, C. M., et al. for the Proof of Principle Study Investigators. (2002) A controlled trial of a human papillomavirus type 16 vaccine. *N. Engl. J. Med.* **347,** 1645–1651.

30. Haupt, K., Roggendorf, M., and Mann, K. (2002) The potential of DNA vaccination against tumor-associated antigens for antitumor therapy. *Exp. Biol. Med.* **227,** 227–237.

31. Wolff, J. A., Malone, R. W., Williams, P., et al. (1990) Direct gene transfer into mouse muscle in vivo. *Science* **247,** 1465–1468.

32. Conry, R. M., Curiel, D. T., Strong, T. V., et al. (2002) Safety and immunogenicity of a DNA vaccine encoding carcinoembryonic antigen and hepatitis B surface antigen in colorectal carcinoma patients. *Clin. Cancer Res.* **8,** 2782–2787.

33. MacGregor, R. R., Boyer, J. D., Ugen, K. E., et al. (1998) First human trial of a DNA based vaccine for treatment of human immunodeficiency virus type 1 infection: safety and host response. *J. Inf. Dis.* **178,** 92–100.

34. Sheets, E. E., Urban, R. G., Crum, C. P., et al. (2003) Immunotherapy of human cervical high-grade cervical intra-epithelial neoplasia with microparticle-delivered human papillomavirus 16 E7 DNA. *Am. J. Obstet. Gynecol.* **188,** 916–926.

35. Meng, W. S., Butterfield, L. H., Ribas, A., et al. (2001) Alpha-fetoprotein-specific tumor immunity induced by plasmid prime-adenovirus boost genetic vaccination. *Cancer Res.* **61,** 8782–8786.

36. Ready, T. (2003) AIDSVAX flop leaves vaccine field unscathed. *Nat. Med.* **9,** 376.

37. Xiao, W., Chirmule, N., Schnell, M. A., Tazelaar, J., Hughes, J. V., and Wilson, J. M. (2000) Route of administration determines induction of T-cell-dependent humoral responses to adeno-associated virus vectors. *Mol. Ther.* **1,** 323–329.

38. Palese, P., Zavala, F., Muster, T., Nussenzweig, R. S., and Garcia-Sastre, A. (1997) Novel influenza virus vaccines and vectors. *J. Inf. Dis.* **176,** S45–S49.

39. Hamilton, J. M., Chen, A. P., and Nguyen, B. (1994) Phase I study of recombinant vaccinia virus (rV) that expresses human carcinoembryonic antigen (CEA) in adult patients with adenocarcinomas [abstract]. *Proc. Am. Soc. Clin. Oncol.* **13,** 961.

40. Smallpox vaccine adverse events among civilians—United States, March 4–10, 2003. (2003) *MMWR Morb. Mortal. Wkly Rep.* **52,** 201–203.

41. Blackwell, J. L., Li, H., Gomez-Navarro, J., et al. (2000) Using a tropism-modified adenoviral vector to circumvent inhibitory factors in ascites fluid. *Hum. Gene Ther.* **11,** 1657–1669.

42. Chirmule, N., Propert, K., Magosin, S., Qian, Y., Qian, R., and Wilson, J. (1999) Immune responses to adenovirus and adeno-associated virus in humans. *Gene Ther.* **6,** 1574–1583.

43. Gilboa, E., Nair, S. K., and Lyerly, H. K. (1998) Immunotherapy of cancer with dendritic-cell-based vaccines. *Cancer Immunol. Immunother.* **46,** 82–87.

44. Jaffee, E. M., Hruban, R. H., Biedrzycki, B., et al. (2001) Novel allogeneic granulocyte-macrophage colony-stimulating factor-secreting tumor vaccine for pancreatic cancer: a phase I trial of safety and immune activation. *J. Clin. Oncol.* **19,** 145–156.

45. Von Mehren, M., Arlen, P., Gulley, J., et al. (2001) The influence of granulocyte macrophage colony-stimulating factor and prior chemotherapy on the immunological response to a vaccine (ALVAC-CEA B7.1) in patients with metastatic carcinoma. *Clin. Cancer Res.* **7,** 1181–1191.

46. Marshall, J. L., Hoyer, R. J., Toomey, M. A., et al. (2000) Phase I study in advanced cancer patients of a diversified prime-and-boost vaccination protocol using recombinant vaccinia virus and recombinant nonreplicating avipox virus to elicit anti-carcinoembryonic antigen immune responses. *J. Clin. Oncol.* **18,** 3964–3973.

47. Willemsen, R. A., Debets, R., Chames, P., and Bolhuis, R. L. H. (2003) Genetic engineering of T cell specificity for immunotherapy of cancer. *Hum. Immunol.* **64,** 56–68.

48. Patel, S. D., Moskalenko, M., Tian, T., et al. (2000) T-cell killing of heterogeneous tumor or viral targets with bispecific chimeric immune receptors. *Cancer Gene Ther.* **7,** 1127–1134.
49. Hwu, P. and Freedman, R. S. (2002) The immunotherapy of patients with ovarian cancer. *J. Immunother.* **25,** 189–201.
50. Sheen, A. J., Sherlock, D. J., Irlam, J., Hawkins, R. E., and Gilham, D. E. (2003) T lymphocytes isolated from patients with advanced colorectal cancer are suitable for gene immunotherapy approaches. *Br. J. Cancer* **88,** 1119–1127.
51. Cooper, M. A., Bush, J. E., Fehniger, T. A., et al. (2002) In vivo evidence for a dependence on interleukin-15 for natural killer cell survival. *Blood* **100,** 3633–3638.
52. Smyth, M. J., Hayakawa, Y., Takeda, K., and Yagita, H. (2002) New aspects of natural-killer-cell surveillance and therapy of cancer. *Nat. Rev. Cancer* **2,** 850–861.
53. Berd, D., Maguire, H. C., and Mastrangelo, M. J. (1986) Induction of cell-mediated immunity to melanoma cells and regression of metastases after treatment with a melanoma cell vaccine preceded by cyclophosphamide. *Cancer Res.* **46,** 2572–2577.
54. Livingston, P. O., Cunningham-Rundles, S., Marfleet, G., et al. (1987) Inhibition of suppressor-cell activity by cyclophosphamide in patients with malignant melanoma. *J. Biol. Response Modif.* **6,** 392–403.
55. Nigam, A., Yacavone, R. F., Zahurak, M. L., et al. (1998) Immunomodulatory properties of antineoplastic drugs administered in conjunction with GM-CSF-secreting cancer cell vaccines. *Int. J. Cancer* **12,** 161–170.
56. Machiels, J. P., Reilly, R. T., Emens, L. A., et al. (2001) Cyclophosphamide, doxorubicin, and paclitaxel enhance the antitumor immune response of granulocyte/macrophage-colony stimulating factor-secreting whole-cell vaccines in HER-2/neu tolerized mice. *Cancer Res.* **61,** 3689–3697.

10

Immunotherapy of Cancer by Dendritic Cell-Targeted Gene Transfer

Tanja D. de Gruijl, Herbert M. Pinedo, and Rik J. Scheper

1. DENDRITIC CELLS AS THE BODY'S SENTINELS

Dendritic cells (DCs) have become the "bright new hope" of immunotherapists. DCs are the most powerful antigen-presenting cells (APCs) identified to date, with the unique ability to prime naïve T cells and thus initiate immune responses. Essentially, they provide the crucial link between the innate and the adaptive immune system and as such have proven to be operating at the most fundamental levels of regulation in numerous immune processes *(1,2)*.

DCs stem from a common CD34$^+$ bone marrow (BM)-derived precursor and can differentiate into various subsets, which can be myeloid or lymphoid in nature. From the blood, DC precursors seed peripheral tissues, where they develop into so-called immature or quiescent DCs. In truth, immature DCs are not so much quiescent as constantly active: They continuously sample their surroundings and monitor the well-being of the peripheral tissues through multiple contacts with adjacent cells. It is because of this need to maintain simultaneous contact with numerous cells that DCs adopt their characteristic dendritic morphology that lends them their name.

Excessive tissue damage or signs of microbial invasion can prompt maturation (i.e., terminal differentiation) and migration of the DCs to draining lymph nodes (LNs), where they can alert the immune system to any threatening situation. Thus, DCs have an important sentinel function and serve as the body's security system. Usually, this security system is very efficient and activates appropriate effector cells to combat bacterial or viral infections. DCs communicate with and regulate activation of a number of immune effector cells, such as T-helper (Th) cells, cytotoxic T lymphocytes (CTLs), B cells, natural killer (NK) cells, and natural killer T (NKT) cells *(1)*. Through a sophisticated system of precisely orchestrated expression patterns of cytokines, chemokines (and their respective receptors), as well as costimulatory and adhesion molecules and, ultimately, immune effector molecules (e.g., antibodies, granzymes, cytokines, FasL), DCs, and the various effector cells activated by them can take appropriate measures to handle any outside threats to the body. Clearly, the ability to harness the capacity of the DCs for immune regulation is a very attractive proposition in the fight against any disease with an immunological basis. It is therefore not surprising that tremendous effort has gone into exploring ways to target DCs for gene therapeutic modulation of their functions.

1.1. Generating Cancer Immunity: Triggering Through Trickery

"Danger" is an important concept in DC biology. Indeed, since Polly Matzinger proposed her danger model a number of years ago, danger has become a fashionable and much used designation for the force generally driving the activation of DCs *(3)*. Whereas T-cell immunity was previously believed

From: *Contemporary Cancer Research*
Cancer Gene Therapy
Edited by: D. T. Curiel and J. T. Douglas © Humana Press Inc., Totowa, NJ

determined by the distinction between self and nonself, the danger model suggested that signals in peripheral tissues were the determining factor in T-cell activation: proinflammatory signals associated with microbial infections would lead to DC activation, empowering the DCs to migrate to LNs and activate specific T cells. In contrast, in steady-state conditions, a lack of DC activation (i.e., maturation) would maintain a state of peripheral tolerance. Much evidence has been gathered to support this model, and tumor immunologists in particular have been much encouraged by it.

In general, the tumor milieu lacks danger signals: The immune system does not perceive the tumor as a possible threat *(4)*. Instead, the microenvironment of burgeoning tumors for the most part resembles a steady-state situation in which DCs are not activated. At later stages of tumor development, DC differentiation and activation may even be suppressed. As a result, peripheral T-cell tolerance is maintained.

As tumor-associated antigens (TAAs) often are self-antigens, the generation of antitumor immunity in essence requires the induction of autoimmunity. Inherent to the danger concept is the possibility to break peripheral tolerance to self-antigens through the delivery of sufficient danger signals. In other words, if the immune system could be tricked into perceiving tumors as an outside microbial threat rather than a part of the self, intratumoral DCs might become activated and stimulate T-cell immunity. The validity of this concept has now been confirmed by a large and ever-growing number of tumor rejection studies in mouse models and holds great promise for the future of cancer immunotherapy.

1.2. Targeting DCs for the Immunogene Therapy of Cancer

The identification of an ever-growing number of TAAs opens the door to the targeted immunotherapy of cancer *(5)*. TAA genes can be divided into different categories, such as mutated oncogenes (e.g., *ras*) or tumor-suppressor genes (e.g., *p53*), deregulated developmental or embryonic genes (e.g., carcinoembryonic antigen), growth factor (receptor) genes (e.g., *ErbB2*), tissue-specific genes (e.g., *tyrosinase*), cancer-testis genes (e.g., *mage*), or oncovirus-derived genes (e.g., HPV-16 E7).

To be suitable candidates for vaccination, TAAs should only be expressed in tumor tissue or at least be overexpressed there to allow for a window in which T-cell-mediated tumor eradication can occur without concomitant destruction of normal tissue. Ideally, TAAs are essential to the oncogenic process, so they are a permanent fixture of the malignant phenotype. This will prevent the outgrowth of CTL-escape variants through the downregulation of the targeted TAA.

Numerous clinical trials are under way to study the effect of DC-based vaccination with specific TAAs. A common strategy is the ex vivo generation of autologous DCs from blood-derived DC precursors, which are then loaded with TAA proteins or TAA-derived peptides, carrying known CTL and/or Th epitopes, and subsequently readministered to the patient *(6)*. Alternatively, TAA-encoding genes can be transferred to DCs.

Genetic modification of DCs for immunotherapy may carry certain advantages *(7)*. In contrast to the use of proteins, a genetic TAA vaccine provides a long-lived continuous source of antigen and will lead to relatively protracted presentation of TAA by the transduced DCs. Moreover, endogenous TAA expression resulting from gene transfer ensures access to the major histocompatibility complex (MHC) class I processing pathway, which is essential for subsequent activation of specific CTLs. With the wide array of molecular recombinant techniques and a rapidly growing knowledge of DC biology, it has now become possible to modify vaccines genetically to target them specifically to DCs in vivo and at the same time achieve DC activation. Not only is this an intellectually satisfying vaccination strategy, it may ultimately obviate the need for costly, time-consuming, and laborious approaches involving the generation and loading of autologous DCs ex vivo.

In this chapter, an overview is given of current knowledge concerning the phenotypic and functional state of DCs in tumor-conditioned environments and ways in which DCs residing in tumor milieus can be modulated and targeted by immunogene therapy to raise the chances of clinical success. Currently applied ex vivo approaches are contrasted with possible in vivo approaches.

2. DC ORIGINS AND SUBSETS

Various DC subsets can be discerned, each of which may have specialized regulatory immune functions. Clearly, if DC-targeted therapies are to be effective, it is important to know which of these subsets to target. Below, a brief overview is given of the major human DC precursors and subsets identified to date. It is important to realize that, in many cases, it is not absolutely clear if these are actual distinct subsets or merely DCs from the same subset with different phenotypes dictated by microenvironmental factors. Study of this matter is ongoing, but is complicated by the extremely low numbers of DCs in vivo.

2.1. DC Precursor Cells

In this section a brief overview is given of the different DC precursor cells (identified either in vitro or in vivo) for a better understanding of their possible significance and uses in therapeutic settings.

2.1.1. Monocytes

$CD14^+$ blood-derived monocytes are the most commonly used precursors to generate DCs in vitro, both for research and for clinical uses *(1,6)*. Relatively large numbers of monocytes can be isolated from peripheral blood (e.g., by plastic adherence) and differentiated into $CD1a^+CD14^-$ immature DCs over the course of 5–7 days through culture in the presence of granulocyte-macrophage colony-stimulating factor (GM-CSF) and interleukin 4 (IL-4). DC cells like Langerhans cells (LCs, which are the specialized DCs of the epidermis; *see* Section 2.2.1), characterized by the expression of the lectin langerin, can also be generated from monocytes by the inclusion of transforming growth factor-β (TGF-β) or IL-15 in the DC cultures *(8,9)*. These monocyte-derived DCs (MoDCs) can be further matured in the presence of commonly used maturation-inducing agents such as tumor necrosis factor-α (TNF-α), lipopolysaccharides (LPS), or monocyte-conditioned medium.

On maturation, MoDCs express CD83, a member of the immunoglobulin family and the hallmark of DC maturation, and can readily be used to activate tumor-specific CTLs *(1,10)*. Monocytes represent a heterogeneous precursor population from which both DCs and macrophages can develop. $CD2^+$ monocytes were previously identified as a monocyte subset from which MoDCs preferentially differentiate *(11)*.

Monocytes were also shown to differentiate into fully mature DCs through the process of reverse transmigration over endothelial cell layers *(12)*. This interesting observation suggests that monocytes or macrophages in peripheral tissues, in the presence of appropriate danger signals (phagocytosis has also been implicated in this process), may migrate into lymphatic vessels (from the basal to the apical side; i.e., reverse transmigration) and instantly mature into T-cell-stimulatory DCs. Targeting $CD14^+$ monocytes/macrophages in vivo may thus be an interesting option for cancer immunotherapy, on the condition that their subsequent reverse transmigration into lymph vessels and maturation to DCs can somehow be enforced.

2.1.2. CD34$^+$ Stem Cells

$CD1a^+$ DCs can be differentiated from BM-derived proliferative $CD34^+$ stem cells recirculating in peripheral blood by in vitro culture for 2–3 weeks in the presence of GM-CSF, IL-4, and TNF-α (hereafter referred to as CD34-DCs) *(13)*. Addition of TGF-β to these cultures will result in the generation of langerin$^+$ LCs. The resulting DCs can be further matured and used for T-cell activation *(14)*. Indeed, there is evidence to suggest that CD34-DCs may be more efficient in CTL priming than MoDCs *(15)*.

However, despite their proliferative potential, the extremely low frequencies at which $CD34^+$ cells are found in peripheral blood (typically <0.1%) are prohibitive for clinical use and would require their enhanced mobilization to the blood through prior systemic treatment with hematopoietic growth factors, such as granulocyte colony-stimulating factor (G-CSF), GM-CSF, or Fms-like tyrosine kinase 3 ligand (FLT3L) *(1)*. Alternatively, isolated $CD34^+$ cells can be expanded in vitro by cytokine cocktails comprising FLT3L, stem cell factor, IL-3, thrombopoietin, and IL-6 prior to their differentiation into functional DCs *(16)*.

2.1.3. CD11c+ Myeloid Peripheral Blood DCs

A subset of CD11c^{hi}CD14^{lo}CD33$^+$ cells has been identified as direct precursors of myeloid DCs *(17–21)*. Through short-term in vitro culture (1–2 days) with or without DC-differentiating cytokines, these peripheral blood DC precursors *(PBDCs)* can be turned into fully differentiated DCs, express-ing costimulatory molecules, high levels of HLA-DR, and the DC-specific markers CMRF-56 and CMRF-44 *(17,19,22)*. PBDCs are believed to derive from earlier CD34$^+$ precursors and generally make up less than 1% of the total PBMC population.

Different subsets within this myeloid PBDC population can now be identified by differential expres-sion of the markers CD1c, BDCA-3, and M-DC8 (i.e., 6-sulfo LacNac, a carbohydrate modification of the P-selectin glycoprotein ligand-1) *(21,23–25)*. It is still unclear which particular tissue DC equivalents may derive from the CD1c$^+$ and BDCA-3$^+$ PBDC subsets, but it has been suggested that LCs may differentiate from the CD1c$^+$ PBDC subset *(21)*.

M-DC8$^+$CD16$^+$CD14^{lo} PBDCs were identified as a preferential migratory DC population in a skin equivalent model and were suggested to represent a proinflammatory DC subset that can be rapidly recruited to sites of infection through their expression of FcγR III (CD16) and complement receptors (C5aR and C3aR) *(25,26)*. CD11c$^+$ PBDCs, once activated in vitro, are superior T-cell stimulators with the ability to prime allogeneic T cells and specific CTLs *(23,27)*. This indicates their utility for the generation of autologous DCs for vaccination purposes in the treatment of cancer *(28)*. However, this may not be feasible because of their reduced frequency and impaired phenotypic and functional activation state in cancer patients. Tumor-derived suppressive factors (e.g., vascular endothelial growth factor [VEGF]) have been implicated in this phenomenon of cancer-associated DC suppression (*see also* Section 4).

2.1.4. CD11c− Plasmacytoid PBDCs

A novel PBDC subset has been identified and is characterized by a lack of CD11c expression and high expression levels of the IL-3 receptor CD123 *(17,21,29)*. Based on their morphological appear-ance, these cells were designated plasmacytoid DCs (PDCs). Unlike their CD11c$^+$ counterparts, plas-macytoid PBDCs display certain lymphoid characteristics, such as the expression of CD4 and the messenger ribonucleic acid (mRNA) for germline immunoglobulin K and the pre-T-cell receptor *(30,31)*. Plasmacytoid PBDCs home directly to LNs through L-selectin, in which they may serve a sentinel function similar to myeloid DCs in peripheral tissues *(29,32)*. Beside their characteristic CD123^{hi}CD11c$^-$phenotype, plasmacytoid PBDCs can be further discerned and easily isolated by their expression of BDCA-2 (recently identified as a C-type lectin *(33)* and BDCA-4 (neutropilin). On culture in IL-3, plasmacytoid PBDCs terminally differentiate into PDCs with the ability to skew T cells to a type 2 response or, on CD40L and/or viral stimulation, to boost NK cell and CTL immu-nity *(29,32,34,35)*.

2.1.5. Leukemic DC Precursors and DC Precursor Cell Lines

A special kind of DC precursor that deserves mention here is the myeloid leukemia cell, derived from either chronic or acute myeloid leukemia *(36–38)*. These leukemic cells can be regarded as pluri-potent myeloid precursor cells. On culture with GM-CSF and IL-4, with or without TNF-α, they acquire phenotypic and functional DC characteristics. Because these acute myeloid leukemia- or chronic myeloid leukemia-derived DCs still express TAA (most notably the bcr-abl fusion oncoprotein), they make a convenient and suitable autologous tumor vaccine.

Finally, some cell lines derived from these malignancies have been reported to have maintained the ability to differentiate into immature DCs in a cytokine-dependent manner *(38,39)*. These imma-ture DCs could be loaded with immunogenic proteins or peptides or infected by antigen-encoding adenoviral vectors and on maturation were shown to activate T cells in an antigen-specific manner.

These cell lines may provide an attractive research tool as a constant and easy supply of DC precursors as well as prove useful in (semi)allogeneic vaccine approaches. Moreover, stable transfectants of DC cell lines may provide ready-made tools for a variety of immunogene therapy approaches.

2.2. DC Subsets

The main DC subsets and their possible roles in the generation and regulation of specific T-cell responses are discussed in this section as well as the possibility to target each specifically for therapeutic manipulation. There has been much debate whether each subset has a specialized regulatory function or whether the various subsets all have similar regulatory functions that largely depend on the state of DC maturation *(31)*. Most likely, the final immunological outcome is intimately linked to the maturation state of each of these subsets, but their different anatomical localizations will translate into certain specialized functions.

2.2.1. Langerhans Cells

LCs are the DCs of the epidermis and were the first DCs described. They are still regarded as the prototype DC and as such are the subject of intense study *(40)*. LCs are found in the basal and suprabasal layers of the epidermis and in the immature state are characterized by high expression levels of CD1a and the C-type lectin langerin.

Langerin is involved in antigen capture and has been shown to induce the formation and to be an integral part of the LC-specific cytoplasmic Birbeck granules *(41)*. Birbeck granules are membrane-bound, tubule-shaped organelles believed to constitute a specialized intracellular compartment for the channeling of antigens into specific processing pathways. Immature LCs and their precursors are further characterized by their expression of cutaneous leukocyte antigen and E-cadherin, both adhesion molecules involved in the respective homing to the skin and the epidermis *(31)*.

Its localization in the outer reaches of the body means that, in many instances, the dense and widely branched network of LCs in the epidermis forms the first line of defense against any outside threats. There is evidence to suggest that, on their activation and migration to LNs, LCs preferentially bind and activate T cells (as opposed to B cells). As a consequence, they would be responsible for the initiation of type 1 cell-mediated immunity rather than type 2 humoral immunity *(30)*. In keeping with this, LC-like cells generated from monocytes were shown to be superior CTL activators *(9)*. As cell-mediated immunity is generally believed to be crucial in tumor eradication, it may be beneficial to specifically target LCs and their precursors for tumor immunotherapy *(42)*; their specific expression of E-cadherin, langerin, and high levels of CD1a may allow for this.

2.2.2. Interstitial or Dermal DCs

In contrast to LCs, dermal DCs (DDCs) do not express langerin and only intermediate-to-low levels of CD1a. Instead, DDCs express an alternative set of lectins, including the mannose receptor (MR), DEC-205, and DC-SIGN, as well as factor XIIIa and CD68 *(43)*. Myeloid DCs in nonepithelial tissues throughout the body resemble DDCs in phenotype and are also known as interstitial DCs. The differential expression pattern of antigen capture receptors between LCs and DDCs should enable the specific targeting of each subset.

Unlike LCs, DDCs have been shown to produce IL-10 and to be able to direct the generation of type 2 antibody responses *(30)*. However, the T-cell skewing abilities of interstitial DCs/DDCs are not fixed, but rather dictated by a balance of factors in the microenvironment. The presence of LPS, interferon-γ (IFN-γ), IL-15, or IL-4 may increase the propensity of DDCs to release IL-12 on CD40L stimulation and thus stimulate the activation of Th1 cells and CTL; TNF-α, IL-10, and PGE2 stimulate production of IL-10, resulting in the suppression of cell-mediated immunity, the activation of Th2 cells, and the generation of humoral responses *(44–47)*.

The ability to modulate this balance may be crucially important for the successful immunotherapy of cancer. As MoDCs phenotypically resemble interstitial DCs/DDCs, they provide an easily accessible in vitro model to study and fine-tune these processes, although ultimately the wide variety of stromal and extracellular matrix elements present in vivo are bound to be of influence and should also be taken into account.

2.2.3. Plasmacytoid DCs

Although originally believed to contribute to skewing of immunity toward type 2 humoral responses, PDCs were recently described to release large amounts of IFN-α on stimulation by CD40L and viruses and thereby to boost NK cell and CTL responses *(32,34,35)*. The last characteristic may be harnessed to enhance the efficacy of tumor vaccination. PDCs seed LNs, straight from the blood, through L-selectin-mediated homing. They may reside in LNs in the steady state, constantly screening the surroundings for signs of bacterial or viral infection. Alternatively, they may be recruited to LNs, draining a site of inflammation, through CXCR3 *(35)*. CXCR3 is expressed on the surface of the PDCs and binds the effector cell-attracting chemokines IP-10 and Mig.

PDCs "sense" the presence of microbes through specific receptors, such as the toll-like receptor 9 (TLR9). TLR9 binds unmethylated CpG sequences derived from bacterial deoxyribonucleic acid (DNA) and subsequently activates the PDC, which then releases IFN-α and possibly IL-12 *(48)*. CD40L stimulation may also induce PDCs to release IL-12 *(32,35,48)*. The combined action of IL-12 and IFN-α will result in the activation of CTL and NK cells; IFN-α will also promote the maturation of neighboring myeloid DCs and thus further stimulate T-cell activation *(49)*.

The use of CpG DNA as an adjuvant for tumor vaccination is under investigation. CpG has a strong type 1 T-cell-skewing ability, which in murine studies was shown to be of great benefit for tumor rejection *(49)*. Ongoing studies will show whether this is also the case in humans and how PDCs may be involved.

A distinct pattern of TLR expression was reported on PDCs and myeloid DCs: TLR9 expression in humans appears to be PDC specific, whereas the expression of the LPS-binding TLR4 is restricted to myeloid DCs *(50)*. Differential TLR expression may thus allow for the specific targeting and activation of PDCs and myeloid DCs for immunotherapy.

3. DCs IN THE REGULATION OF IMMUNE ACTIVATION AND TOLERIZATION

Appropriate T-cell priming and activation is needed for a successful antitumor effector response, and DCs play a crucial role in this process. Insufficient immune activation in cancer may be overcome by improving DC functions in both the afferent and the efferent phases of the immune response.

3.1. Danger: T-Cell Activation

Immature DCs are in intimate contact with their surrounding cells and are constantly on the lookout for danger in their immediate vicinity. Potentially dangerous situations that can be recognized by DCs are microbial invasion and tissue stress or damage, resulting in abnormal cell death. DCs express an impressive arsenal of receptors to aid them in this function: Fc receptors (FcRs), microbial pattern recognition receptors (e.g., lectins and TLR), heat shock protein receptors (e.g., CD91), and scavenger receptors that can bind necrotic or apoptotic bodies (e.g., CD36 and $\alpha_v\beta_3$- and $\alpha_v\beta_5$-integrins) *(1,2)*. On engagement of these receptors and antigen uptake, DCs become activated, release their hold on their surroundings, and start to migrate out of the peripheral tissue. Local factors important in the induction of this process are TNF-α, IL-1β, GM-CSF, IL-18, and PGE2, and they are released at elevated levels under proinflammatory conditions by tissue-resident cells as well as by DCs themselves *(51,52)*.

Activated DCs downregulate molecules involved in antigen capture, upregulate MHC molecules, and start to express maturation markers (CD83, CMRF-44) and adhesion and costimulatory molecules needed for the optimal activation of T cells (CD40, CD54, CD80, CD86, 4-1BBL) *(1,2)*. Properly activated DCs downregulate expression of CCR5 and CCR6 (chemokine receptors involved in homing to peripheral nonlymphoid tissues) and instead upregulate expression of CCR7, which binds the LN-derived chemokines CCL19 and CCL21 and facilitates homing through afferent lymph to the paracortical T-cell areas inside LNs *(53)*. There, the DCs can interact with a constantly recirculating pool of naïve and memory Th cells and CTLs.

DCs have the unique capacity to take up antigens and process them not only for MHC class II-mediated presentation, but also for presentation to CD8$^+$ CTLs in the context of MHC class I. This process of exogenous antigen uptake and processing for specific CTL activation is known as cross-priming *(54)*. DCs will activate T cells on antigen-specific recognition, which further enforces the DC/T-cell binding.

CD40L on T cells "superactivates" the DCs and enables further upregulation of CD86 and the production of IL-12, which are essential conditions for the optimal activation of CTLs. Migration to the LNs is optimal by day 2, and DCs inside LNs have a reported turnover rate of 3–5 days *(55)*. DCs do not leave the LNs, but are believed to undergo apoptosis, triggered by interactions with CTLs or NK cells. Activated effector CTLs leave the LNs via efferent vessels and home to and infiltrate sites of inflammation to eradicate infected cells or tumor cells, as the case may be.

DCs are believed to also play a role in the efferent phase of the immune response by interacting with effector T cells to sustain their activation and prevent their premature apoptosis. In tumor situations, this may be particularly pertinent. Whereas T cells are sensitive to Fas-mediated apoptosis (induced by FasL expressed on tumor cells, a process known as *counterattack*), DCs are resistant and can even become activated through engagement of Fas on their cell surface, thus facilitating their T-cell-protective function *(56,57)*.

Various DC-targeted approaches of cancer gene therapy can be envisioned to modulate DC functions at every stage of the antitumor immune response. Therapeutic genetic modification of DCs (or their neighboring cells) should aim to increase antigen uptake, DC maturation, DC migration and LN homing, the strength and duration of DC/T-cell interactions, T-cell activation, and DC infiltration of the tumor (effector) site.

3.2. Cancer: Tolerance, Suppression, and Ignorance

Tumor-specific immune responses are often not detectable until advanced disease stages have set in, and by then they are usually powerless to control tumor growth because of the high tumor burden: Tumor proliferation is out of control, and immune effector cells simply cannot catch up. Moreover, high systemic levels of tumor-derived suppressive cytokines, usually associated with advanced cancer, will downmodulate immune effector functions and effectively suppress antitumor immunity. Why do the DCs not behave properly and alert the immune system to the tumor danger in time for it to act? A number of possible causes may exist:

1. The tumor tissue does not provide the necessary danger signals and is merely perceived by DCs as a normal steady-state tissue against which the usual self-tolerance needs to be maintained *(4)*. Only when tumors reach a certain size, at which angiogenic processes become inadequate and ensuing hypoxia may eventually result in increased (abnormal) levels of apoptosis and necrosis, may scavenging DCs finally sense danger and become activated. Unfortunately, by that time it may be too late for immune effector cells to keep up with the rapidly proliferating tumor cells.

2. Another explanation may be provided by a phenomenon known as *immunological ignorance*. Many solid tumors are encapsulated and resist infiltration by DCs. DCs may thus not have access to shed TAA or to any tumor-associated danger signals and are consequently unable to transport TAA to tumor-draining LNs to start an immune response. The immune system is kept in a state of ignorance regarding the tumor until its boundary is broken, and metastasis occurs *(58)*. Again, by this time, it may be too late for the immune system to take effective action.

3. Finally, DC maturation may be actively suppressed by tumor-derived factors, and proper T-cell activation is consequently sabotaged. High levels of IL-10, usually associated with tumor milieus, may be the principal culprit. IL-10-conditioned immature DCs were previously shown to be stinted in their maturation and to secrete IL-10 rather than IL-12. The upshot of these characteristics is the induction of antigen-specific

T-cell anergy. IL-10 was also shown to interfere with proper DC migration to the LNs through downregulation of CCR7 and the induction of CCR5 and CCR6 *(59)*. Finally, contact with IL-10-modulated DCs has also been reported to interfere with T-cell effector functions *(60)*. In tumor environments, all these processes may act in concert to support immune suppression and tumor progression.

To be effective, immunogene therapy will have to force contact between tumor and the immune system in a proinflammatory context to ensure proper DC- and TAA-specific T-cell activation. Moreover, the immunosuppressive effects of tumor-derived factors will have to be counteracted.

4. DCs IN CANCER

Hampered DC differentiation and maturation has been reported in many tumors, and decreased tumor infiltration by DCs has been identified as a generally poor prognostic factor (reviewed in ref. *61)*. Faulty DC development and functioning should be remedied before in vivo DC-targeted cancer therapies can succeed. In this section, the various mechanisms are discussed by which tumors interfere with DC differentiation and maturation.

4.1. Disturbed DC Differentiation

Reduced frequencies of PBDCs with decreased levels of costimulatory molecules have been reported in patients with advanced breast cancer *(62,63)*. Moreover, the remaining PBDCs were shown to be functionally impaired, with poor T-cell stimulatory abilities *(62)*. In a group of patients with head and neck tumors, non-small cell lung cancer, or breast cancer, an increase was observed in the number of immature CD11c− myeloid PBDC precursors, suggesting inhibited myeloid DC differentiation in early stages of development *(64)*. Different tumor-derived factors have been implicated in inhibited DC differentiation:

VEGF: Both in vitro CD34- DC differentiation models and in vivo tumor models have shown VEGF to block DC differentiation in early stages of development *(65,66)*. Increased numbers of immature CD11c− PBDCs were shown to correlate to increased plasma levels of VEGF *(67)*. A study suggested that the underlying molecular mechanism of VEGF-induced inhibition of DC differentiation might be the inhibition of the NF-κB-dependent expression of H1° histones *(68)*. H1° histones appear to be specifically involved in the transcriptional regulation of DC differentiation-related genes. H1° transcription could be blocked in differentiating DCs by supernatants derived from tumor cell lines.

IL-6: The differentiation of CD34-DCs, but not of MoDCs, could be inhibited in vitro by IL-6 present in supernatants derived either from tumor cell lines or from primary tumors *(33,69)*. IL-4 was shown to counteract this suppressive effect of IL-6 and might therefore be an attractive cytokine to use in immunotherapeutic protocols aiming at the improvement of DC functions in tumor environments *(70)*.

M-CSF: Macrophage colony-stimulating factor (M-CSF) was also shown to inhibit DC differentiation. Indeed, at least part of the IL-6-induced DC suppressive effect observed for tumor cell line-derived supernatants was ascribed to secondarily induced expression of M-CSF *(71)*. IL-4 could counteract this suppressive effect, which in part may explain the inability of IL-6 and M-CSF to inhibit MoDC differentiation because this process is absolutely dependent on IL-4 *(70)*.

Gangliosides: Gangliosides are neuron-derived lipids. They were reported to be released at high levels from neuroblastoma cells. Neuroblastoma cell line-derived gangliosides were shown to inhibit DC differentiation from CD34+ progenitor cells *(72)*.

IL-10: Both in vitro and in vivo IL-10 have been reported to seriously hamper DC differentiation *(73,74)*. Impaired DC differentiation with reduced CD40 expression was demonstrated in a murine tumor model *(74)*. These suppressed DCs released significantly reduced amounts of IL-12 on CD40L stimulation. The tumor-induced inhibition of DC functions and phenotype could be reversed by systemic treatment with anti-IL-10 antibodies or with FLT3L and/or CD40L.

Prostaglandins: Cyclooxygenase-2-regulated prostaglandins were reported to be the major DC differentiation inhibitory factor in 24-hour supernatants of primary melanoma, colon, breast, and renal cell cancer cultures *(69)*. Tumor-derived prostaglandins were solely responsible for the observed tumor-induced inhibition of MoDC differentiation and, together with IL-6, for the inhibition of CD34- DC differentiation. Besides frustrating their differentiation, tumor-derived prostaglandins skewed the DCs toward the preferential release of IL-10 (rather than IL-12) on CD40L stimulation. Treatment with specific cyclooxygenase-2 inhibitors, currently intensively studied for their antitumor and antiangiogenic effects, may be expected to alleviate these DC differentiation-inhibitory effects of prostaglandins.

4.2. Disturbed DC Maturation

In breast tumors CD83$^+$ mature DCs were found to surround and immature CD1a$^+$ DCs were found to infiltrate the tumor fields *(75)*. This strongly suggests a tumor-mediated inhibition of DC maturation. In line with this, DCs isolated from melanoma metastases were reported to display an immature DC phenotype and to induce T-cell tolerance *(76)*. DCs in tumor-draining LNs were similarly reported to display immature characteristics *(77,78)*. IL-10 seems to be the most likely tumor-derived perpetrator of this maturation inhibition *(79)*. Although PGE2 can induce expression of IL-10 and so affect DC maturation, it does not directly block DC maturation *(80)*. In fact, PGE2 can enhance the effects of other DC-maturing agents and lead to the upregulation of CD83 and CD86, although it may skew thus matured DCs toward an IL-10-producing and T-cell-tolerizing phenotype *(81)*. The overall effects of tumor-derived soluble factors on DC maturation may thus be dominated by IL-10, inhibiting the expression of CD83 and costimulatory markers, disturbing migration to LNs, decreasing IL-12 and increasing IL-10 release, and eventually leading to the induction of T-cell anergy or the activation of regulatory T cells. These IL-10-mediated effects may be counteracted by CD40L and/or GM-CSF administration *(74)*.

4.3. Tumor-Induced DC Apoptosis

DCs will eventually undergo apoptosis in LNs after they have presented antigens in the paracortical T-cell zones. Indeed, DCs may undergo apoptosis induced by the actual CTL they activate *(82,83)*. Thus, apoptosis is a natural part of the DC life cycle. However, premature apoptosis of DCs may interfere with proper T-cell activation. Indeed, a certain minimal duration of the DC/T-cell interaction is required for the generation of optimal effector CTL responses *(84,85)*. Although DCs have a natural resistance to Fas-induced apoptosis, soluble tumor-derived factors such as ceramides and cyclopentenone prostaglandins can induce premature apoptosis in DCs and thus interfere with their T-cell-activating functions *(56,86,87)*.

Apoptosis resistance can be enhanced by treatment of DCs with GM-CSF, CD40L, TNF-α, or LPS, which upregulate bcl-2 or blc-X(L) *(88–90)*. CD40L and LPS can also enhance expression of caspase inhibitors, known to confer resistance to granzyme-induced apoptosis (serpins; e.g., murine SPI-6 or human PI-9) *(84)*. Alternatively, DCs could be genetically modified to induce the expression of apoptosis resistance molecules and thus prolong and enhance their T-cell-stimulatory functions.

5. IMMUNOTHERAPY OF CANCER
THROUGH GENETIC MODULATION OF DC FUNCTIONS

In this section, different strategies are discussed to target DCs and modulate their immune functions for the immunogene therapy of cancer.

5.1. DC-Stimulatory Cytokines: Improving the Odds

Cytokine (gene) therapy may aid in counteracting the DC-suppressive effects of tumors by increasing (systemic or intratumoral) DC numbers, their differentiation and activation, and their overall functioning. In doing so, cytokine therapy may effectively convert cross-priming events in tumors from T-cell tolerization to activation. In an adjuvant setting, it will improve the odds on the success of any form of cancer immunotherapy and of in vivo DC-targeted approaches in particular. By administering cytokine genes rather than proteins, the desired DC-stimulatory effects may be maintained in vivo over protracted periods of time and in some instances have been shown to be more effective.

Cytokines can affect different stages in the differentiation and maturation process of DCs. FLT3L, IL-3, G-CSF, and GM-CSF can act as growth factors, increasing the overall numbers of DC precursors. Whereas FLT3L, IL-3, and G-CSF increase the numbers of both myeloid DCs and PDC precursors, GM-CSF may specifically promote the proliferation of myeloid DC precursors *(34,91–93)*. Importantly, G-CSF-mobilized DC precursors have been reported to differentiate into DCs that preferentially enhance type 2 immunity, whereas GM-CSF-mobilized DC precursors differentiate into DCs that enhance type 1 cell-mediated immunity *(34)*. GM-CSF, IL-4, IFN-α, IFN-β, TGF-β, and IL-3 can further advance the differentiation of DCs, with different combinations of these cytokines resulting in the differentiation of functionally and phenotypically different DC subsets *(14,94–96)*. GM-CSF, IL-4, IFN-α, IFN-β, IFN-γ, TNF-α, IL-1β, and IL-18 can all enhance DC maturation in vivo and facilitate migration of mature DCs to secondary lymphoid organs *(97,98)*.

The route of administration and dosing of cytokines is highly dependent on the targeted stage of DC development: Relatively high doses at sites that provide access to the circulation will be required for systemic effects on the proliferation and differentiation of DC precursors; local administration of lower doses may be more appropriate for the maturation of DCs and the stimulation of T-cell activation in the direct vicinity of tumors or at vaccination sites. For the treatment of cancer in preclinical in vivo models and in clinical settings, DC-stimulatory cytokine genes have been transferred using naked DNA plasmids or viral vectors, most commonly adenovirus or vaccinia virus (VV).

To enhance DC functions and stimulate tumor-specific T-cell immunity, vectors carrying cytokine genes have been injected directly into tumors or have been transferred to autologous tumor cells or allogeneic tumor cell lines in vitro and (re)administered as a biologically enhanced tumor vaccine. Alternatively, autologous DCs generated in vitro have been transduced with cytokine genes (often in combination with TAA genes) and injected either distant from the tumor (usually intradermally) or straight into the tumor.

GM-CSF: GM-CSF is the most commonly used cytokine to boost antitumor immunity. It is known to stimulate DCs at virtually all stages of their development and activation by mobilizing DC precursors to the blood and differentiated DCs to the site of administration by activating them, by stimulating their migration to LNs, and by endowing them with an increased resistance to apoptosis *(99)*. Vectors carrying the GM-CSF gene have been used to transduce tumor cells and DCs for adoptive transfer, but have also been directly injected (with or without TAA genes) in vivo. All these approaches resulted in effective and powerful antitumor immunity in murine models *(100–105)*. GM-CSF can act as a danger signal and is frequently used as an adjuvant in tumor vaccination protocols *(99)*. Combinations with other cytokines (e.g., IL-4 and FLT3L) or maturational agents (e.g., CD40L) can further enhance its efficacy as an immune adjuvant.

IL-4: IL-4-transduced tumor cell lines or autologous fibroblasts have been fused or admixed with autologous DCs to achieve enhanced antitumor immunity *(106,107)*. IL-4 coadministered with granulocyte-macrophage colony-stimulating factor (GM-CSF) has been shown to confer additional DC maturation both systemically and locally *(108,109)*. In addition, IL-4 can protect DC differentiation from the detrimental effects of tumor-derived IL-6 and/or M-CSF *(70)*.

TNF-α: TNF-α is a potent DC maturation inducer and a critical mediator of DC migration. Cotransduction of DCs with adenoviruses encoding Her-2/*neu* and TNF-α resulted in their enhanced maturation and a more efficient induction of antitumor immunity subsequent to subcutaneous administration in a murine colon tumor mode *(110)*.

IFN-α: IFN-α is up and coming as a candidate cytokine for adjuvant use in cancer immunotherapy *(111)*. It has strong DC-maturing effects, both in vitro and in vivo, and enhances DC migration from skin *(97)*. Vaccination with IFN-α-transduced tumor cells resulted in increased DC infiltration and the rejection of established tumors in a murine colon cancer model *(112)*.

IL-18: To stimulate effective cell-mediated antitumor immunity, DCs are often transduced by genes encoding Th1/CTL-stimulating cytokines such as IL-12, IL-15, and IL-18 *(113)*. In a mouse sarcoma model, adenovirus-mediated transfer of IL-18 was shown to enhance DC maturation specifically and, after single peptide vaccination, to induce a wider effective T-cell repertoire through the DC-driven process of epitope spreading *(114)*.

CCL21: An exciting development in the immunogene therapy of cancer is the transduction of autologous DCs with the CCR7-ligand CCL21/SLC. Intratumoral injection of CCL21-transduced DCs resulted in the recruitment of both T cells and DCs and in subsequent CTL-mediated tumor rejection *(115)*. In effect, the CCL21 provides the DCs with a suitable microenvironment to generate an antitumor immune response extranodally, with ready access to TAA and the activation of effector CTLs in the exact place they need to be *(116)*.

5.2. Genetic Modification of DCs to Express TAA

Instead of improving the likelihood of successful DC-mediated antitumor CTL cross-priming by the in vivo transfer of stimulatory cytokine genes, DCs can be directly transduced to express TAA. For successful CTL activation by TAA-transduced DCs, at least two conditions need to be met: (1) sufficient numbers of DCs with high enough expression levels of the targeted TAA antigen (i.e., adequate DC transduction efficiency) and (2) appropriate and sufficient activation (maturation) of the transduced DCs.

5.2.1. Choosing Vectors

The choice of vector for the transduction of DCs is crucial: Some (viral) vectors can influence DC activation either by inhibiting it or by stimulating it, and transducibility of DCs (precursors) can vary. Characteristics of the various viral and nonviral vectors pertinent to effective DC transduction for subsequent immune activation are listed in Table 1.

The youngest generations of attenuated viral vectors designed for gene therapeutic purposes are replication deficient and less immunogenic because of the deletion of structural proteins *(117,118)*. Infection of DCs with viral vectors yields considerably higher DC transduction efficiencies compared to transfection with naked DNA or RNA. This makes viruses very attractive gene transfer vehicles for DCs *(117)*. Major drawbacks of the use of viral vectors are preexistent immunity, which might interfere with infection efficiency and longevity of the transduced DC, and the possibility that viruses have developed ways to sabotage DC functions by way of immune escape. In contrast, naked DNA and RNA vaccines will not interfere with DC maturation, are not immunogenic in themselves, and are very easy and cheap to produce. Results obtained so far for DC transduction with the different available vector systems are discussed next.

5.2.1.1. DNA VIRUSES

Adenovirus: One of the most commonly used gene transfer vectors for DCs is the adenovirus type 5 (Ad5). Adenoviruses are easily grown to high titers and are highly efficient in gene transfer independent of host cell replication. This is important because fully differentiated DCs and their direct precursors have lost their proliferative potential. In addition, DCs infected by TAA-encoding Ad5 vectors have been used successfully to generate antitumor T-cell responses, both in vitro and in vivo, and vaccination with Ad-transduced DCs has been shown to lead to tumor rejection in mouse models *(119–127)*.

Despite these advantages, DCs show a relative resistance to Ad5 infection. In vitro studies with MoDCs have shown varying, but generally low to intermediate, Ad5 transduction efficiencies (20–30% at multiplicity of infection [MOI] 100) *(128–131)*. This is likely because of the absence of the primary Ad5 receptor coxsackie and adenovirus receptor (CAR) on the DC surface, although integrins needed for endocytosis of the virus are expressed *(129,130)*.

Table 1
Characteristics of Viral and Nonviral Vectors for Gene Transfer to DCs

	Adenovirus	Adeno-associated virus	Vaccinia virus	Herpes simplex virus amplicon	Retrovirus	Lentivirus	Alpha virus replicon	DNA	RNA
Transduction efficiency[a] (%)	15–80, MOI 100	2–50, MOI 100	80–100, MOI 2.5	25–100, MOI 1	20–70	25–90, MOI 100	80	<20[b]	60[c]
In vitro use	+	+	+	+	+	+	+	+	+
In vivo use	+	ND	+	+	+	ND	+	+	+
DC cytopathic	+	–	+	–	–	–	+	–[d]	–[d]
Cell division dependent	–	–	–	–	+	–	–	–	–
Integrating	–	+	–	+	+	+	–	ND	–
DC activating	+[e]	+[f]	–	+	–	–	+	–[g]	–
DC activation inhibiting	–[h]	–	+	–[i]	–	–	–	–	–
CD4+ T-cell activating	+	+	+	ND	+	ND	ND	–	+
CD8+ T cell activating	+	+	+	+	+	+	+	+	+
Cross-priming	+	+	+	+	ND	ND	+	+	+
Tumor protection	+	ND	+	+	+	ND	+	+	+
Reference	119–135,210	136–140, 211,212	141–150, 213	151–156	157–163	164–171	172–178	179–189	190–199

ND, not determined.

[a] A range or the highest reported transduction efficiencies are indicated, as are the corresponding multiplicities of infection (MOIs), if provided.

[b] Achieved either by liposome- or cationic peptide-mediated transfection or by electroporation.

[c] By square-wave electroporation.

[d] Target cell viability can be reduced by electroporation.

[e] Conflicting reports exist, but MHC class II and CD86 upregulation are commonly found.

[f] CD80 and CD83 upregulation are reported, but accompanied by CD86 downregulation.

[g] Can activate certain DC subsets when immunogenic CpG sequences are included.

[h] One study reported reduced allogeneic T-cell stimulation after adenoviral infection of MoDCs.

[i] HSV has strong DC suppressive capacity; this is abrogated by using its amplicon.

Only at extremely high virus titers (MOI > 1000; i.e., 1000 plaque-forming units [pfu] per cell), by protracted in vitro infection periods (>1 hour), or in combination with liposomes, this relative resistance to Ad5 infection can be overcome *(129,131,132)*. Replacement of the Ad5 fiber knob by the Ad35 fiber knob (the receptor of which does appear to be expressed on DCs) significantly increased DC transduction efficiency, as did the incorporation of Arg-Gly-Asp (RGD) sequences (which can bind $\alpha_v\beta_3$ and $\alpha_v\beta_5$ integrins expressed on immature DCs) into the HI loop of the Ad5 fiber knob *(122, 133)*. Retargeting of Ad5 to CD40 using a bispecific antibody conjugate, binding both the Ad5 fiber knob and CD40 on the DC surface, increased the DC transduction efficiency to 95% at MOI 100 *(130)*.

Conflicting reports exist regarding the ability of adenovirus vectors to activate immature DCs. Some have reported a full maturation induction (upregulated costimulatory molecules, induction of IL-12 production); some observed partial phenotypic maturation (upregulation of HLA-DR and CD86); others did not observe any effects *(124,128–130,132,134)*. Finally, one group reported an immuno-suppressive effect of adenovirus transduction on mature DCs *(135)*. These different observations may be explained by differences in adenovirus types, infection methods, and sources of the DCs used.

Adeno-associated virus (AAV): AAVs are small, nonpathogenic parvoviruses that are dependent on larger helper viruses such as adenoviruses for their replication. They can integrate into the host genome, but do not depend on replication for infection *(136,137)*. AAVs infect DCs at a transduction rate of about 50% at MOI 100, rising to 90% at MOI 300 *(137,138)*. AAV infection does not interfere with T-cell-stimulatory abilities of DCs and does not prevent subsequent maturation induction *(137, 139)*. AAV infection has been reported to enhance CD80 and CD83 expression, but to inhibit CD86 expression *(137)*. AAV-transduced DCs can induce antigen-specific Th and CTL responses, but their in vivo tumor therapeutic effect remains to be demonstrated *(137,138,140)*.

VV: VV is a member of the orthopox virus family. VV can infect DCs very efficiently at low MOIs (60% transduction efficiency of mature DCs at MOI 2.5) *(117,141)*. VVs are lytic viruses, which makes them relatively safe for in vivo use, and VV-based tumor vaccination is currently under clinical investigation. VV-transduced DCs can induce both TAA-specific Th and CTL responses, leading to in vivo tumor rejection *(142–147)*. However, VV infection interferes with proper DC maturation, downmodulating CD83 and various costimulatory molecules and hampering T-cell stimulation *(147–150)*. To circumvent this problem, DCs are matured prior to their in vitro transduction with VVs. To facilitate postmaturational MHC class II processing and presentation of the transgene, VV vectors have been designed to express the transgene in conjunction with the lysosomal-associated membrane protein-1 targeting sequence *(147)*. Mature DCs infected with these vectors were shown to activate both Th cells and CTL efficiently.

Herpes simplex virus (HSV): HSVs are large, linear DNA viruses, of which HSV type 1 (HSV-1) can infect DCs with intermediate to high efficiency *(118,151)*. Replication-defective HSVs or HSVs that can undergo one additional infectious cycle (recombinant disabled infectious single-cycle HSV-1) are cytopathic and interfere with DC maturation, leading to downregulated CD83 and CD86 expression and hampered DC migration *(151–153)*. Moreover, helperviruses that can contaminate such HSV stocks can also have considerable immunosuppressive effects *(118)*. HSV amplicons are plasmid-based viral vectors, packaged into HSV-1 capsids, that are generated in helpervirus-free systems and therefore preferred for DC infection.

HSV-1 amplicons transduce mature DCs at high efficiencies (70–90% at MOI 1), are noncytopathic, and enhance CD80, CD86, and CD40 levels on immature DCs *(154)*. DCs transduced by HSV amplicons induce tumor-specific CTLs and mediate tumor rejection in vivo *(155,156)*. In addition, the large HSV genome allows for the inclusion of multiple genes that can further modulate immunity (e.g., CD40L, GM-CSF, and CCL21) *(155,156)*.

5.2.1.2. RNA Viruses

Retroviruses: Retroviruses commonly used for DC transduction are recombinant replication-defective murine leukemia viruses *(117)*. The major disadvantage of these vectors is their inability to transduce nondividing cells. This makes them unsuitable for the transduction of MoDCs, but they can infect proliferating CD34⁺ DC precursors, which can subsequently be differentiated to DCs *(157–159)*. Relatively low DC transduction efficiencies of 10–20% have thus been achieved *(157–159)*. Improved protocols, including the use of retronectin, centrifuging, and repeated infection cycles, have raised transduction efficiencies to 70% *(160)*. Retroviral transduction of DCs does not interfere with subsequent maturation and can lead to the activation of both Th and CTL responses *(157,160, 161)*. Adoptive transfer of DCs, transduced by TAA-encoding retroviruses, can induce tumor rejection in vivo *(160,162,163)*.

Lentiviruses: DCs are natural targets for the lentiviruses human immunodeficiency virus and simian immunodeficiency virus. Naturally, safety concerns are a major issue in the development of lentiviral vectors for immunogene therapy, but third-generation minimal and self-inactivating lentiviral vectors meet clinical safety constraints and transduce DCs at high efficiencies (85–90% at MOI < 10) *(164–168)*. Lentiviruses can transduce nondividing cells; therefore, they are suitable for MoDC transduction and do not inhibit DC maturation *(164,167)*. Lentivirally transduced DCs can efficiently activate CTLs, but as yet no in vivo tumor rejection studies have been performed to show their therapeutic efficacy *(169–171)*.

Alpha viruses: Alpha viruses are a group of single-stranded RNA viruses comprising, among others, Semliki Forest virus (SFV), Venezuelan equine encephalitis virus, and Sindbis virus. Alpha virus-derived vectors for gene transfer do not encode structural proteins and undergo only one round of infection. They do encode the viral RNA replicase, which allows for cytoplasmic amplification of the RNA vector, thus enhancing transgene expression. These vectors are known as RNA replicons or self-replicating RNA vaccines and are very effective in the induction of CTL-mediated tumor rejection in vivo *(172–175)*. They can be used as naked RNA or complementary DNA, or they can be incorporated into viral capsids. Alpha virus replicon particles can infect nondividing cells, their RNA replicons cannot be integrated into the host genome, and they are lytic, allowing for further cross-priming *(172–174)*. SFV replicons can efficiently transduce DCs (at a reported transduction efficiency of 80%) and have been shown to induce LC maturation with upregulated expression levels of MHC class I and II, CD54, and CD80 *(176,177)*. Interestingly, Venezuelan equine encephalitis virus replicons seem able to target LCs specifically in vivo *(178)*.

5.2.1.3. NAKED DNA AND RNA

DNA: DCs are transfected by naked DNA at extremely low rates in vitro. Electroporation, complexation with cationic peptides, and liposome-mediated transfer can increase transfection efficiencies up to 10–20%, usually at the expense of DC viability *(179,180)*. DNA is not DC activating of itself, but the inclusion of unmethylated CpG sequences can enhance the immunogenicity of DNA vaccines, possibly by the activation of PDCs and LCs in vivo *(181,182)*. Mechanical stress, associated with DNA administration via the ballistic gene gun method, has also been shown to induce DC maturation *(183)*.

DNA vaccination has been reported to lead to TAA-specific CTL activation in vivo *(184–187)*. Additional Th activation after in vivo DNA vaccination is most likely because of cross-priming events *(188)*. The transfection of very low numbers of DCs in vivo (intradermally or intramuscularly) has been sufficient for CTL-mediated tumor rejection *(183,189)*.

RNA: TAA-encoding mRNA can be used to transfect DCs in vitro. In combination with square-wave electroporation, high transfection efficiencies (50–60%) of MoDCs and CD34-DCs have been reported *(190,191)*. Immunogenic sequences may be incorporated into RNA vaccines to enhance immune activation *(192–194)*. RNA-transduced DCs can efficiently prime TAA-specific CTLs in vitro; administered in vivo, they can induce tumor rejection *(195)*.

Based on these encouraging results and in view of the relative safety inherent with the use of RNA, clinical trials with autologous MoDCs transfected with TAA-encoding RNA are under way *(196)*. Another attractive approach may be the amplification of total tumor mRNA and its use to transfect

autologous DC. In vivo studies revealed total tumor mRNA-transfected DCs to constitute an efficacious cancer vaccine *(197–199)*.

5.2.2. The Need for Danger

Numerous studies have pointed to the importance of proper DC activation to obtain long-lasting
CTL memory responsiveness in vivo. As outlined in Section 3.1, optimal activation of DCs is absolutely essential for the generation of an effective antitumor T-cell response. If the employed vector
for gene transfer to DCs does not achieve this by itself, additional danger signals will be required.

Ligation of CD40 molecules on the surface of DCs has been identified as a critical signal for the
effective priming of CTLs and the generation of protective antitumor immunity. CD40 triggering
induces phenotypic and functional maturation of DCs and renders them capable of activating CTLs,
in effect providing the CTLs with "a license to kill" *(200,201)*. The importance of this phenomenon
for efficient tumor rejection has been confirmed by in vivo studies and was shown to depend in large
part on the production of IL-12 and on the upregulation of a broad range of costimulatory molecules
(e.g., CD86) *(56)*. CD40L is therefore an important candidate to include as a DC-maturational agent
in any tumor vaccination approach involving genetically modified DCs.

Other agents that alone or in combination with CD40L have been shown to induce adequate DC
maturation for subsequent antitumor CTL activation are CpG, GM-CSF, IL-4, double-stranded RNA
poly(I:C), LPS, IFN-α, and TNF-α *(1,202)*. Combinations of danger signals often have additive or
synergistic effects on the efficacy of tumor vaccines in murine tumor rejection models. Multiple
danger signals should therefore be considered for application in genetic vaccine formulations. Their
genes could be included in the employed TAA-encoding vector. This would guarantee coexpression
of TAA and danger signals, both in time and localization.

6. DC-BASED VACCINATION: AN IMMUNOTHERAPEUTIC BYPASS

The DC-inhibitory effects of tumors frustrate effective immune activation, but may be bypassed
by vaccine formulations involving autologous, fully mature DCs, which can present relevant TAA
and activate tumor-specific T cells. Two possible approaches can be taken to achieve this: (1) the ex
vivo generation, TAA loading, and maturation of autologous DCs, followed by readministration; and
(2) the in vivo targeting, TAA loading, and activation of tissue-resident DCs. The advantages and
disadvantages of both approaches in TAA gene-based DC vaccination are discussed in this section.

6.1. Ex Vivo or In Vivo: The Case for In Vivo DC-Targeted Genetic Vaccines

The most common approach to DC-based tumor vaccination is the generation of autologous DCs
in vitro, usually from monocytes; this can be followed by in vitro TAA gene transduction, maturation
induction, and adoptive transfer (*see* Fig. 1A). The ex vivo approach has certain advantages: It allows
for the control of the transduction efficiency and the maturation state of the DCs before they are
administered, benefiting qualitative uniformity of the vaccines. In vitro transduction may also be a
way to circumvent any preexisting antibody responses that in vivo might interfere with infection of
DCs by viral vectors.

On the down side, ex vivo generation of DC-based vaccines for clinical application is an extremely laborious and costly affair. Good manufacturing practices need to be observed, which often
proves prohibitive for rapid clinical implementation. The culture of autologous DCs should ideally
be performed in serum-free media to avoid infectious risks and the possibility of anaphylactic reactions to bovine serum components *(203)*. Serum-free generation of DCs often results in less-than-
optimal DC differentiation characterized by a lack of CD1a expression, which is associated with
reduced T-cell stimulatory capacity. In addition, because 1–10 million DCs usually are administered
per vaccination and multiple vaccinations are required for the generation and boosting of effective
immunity, large numbers of autologous DCs need to be cultured.

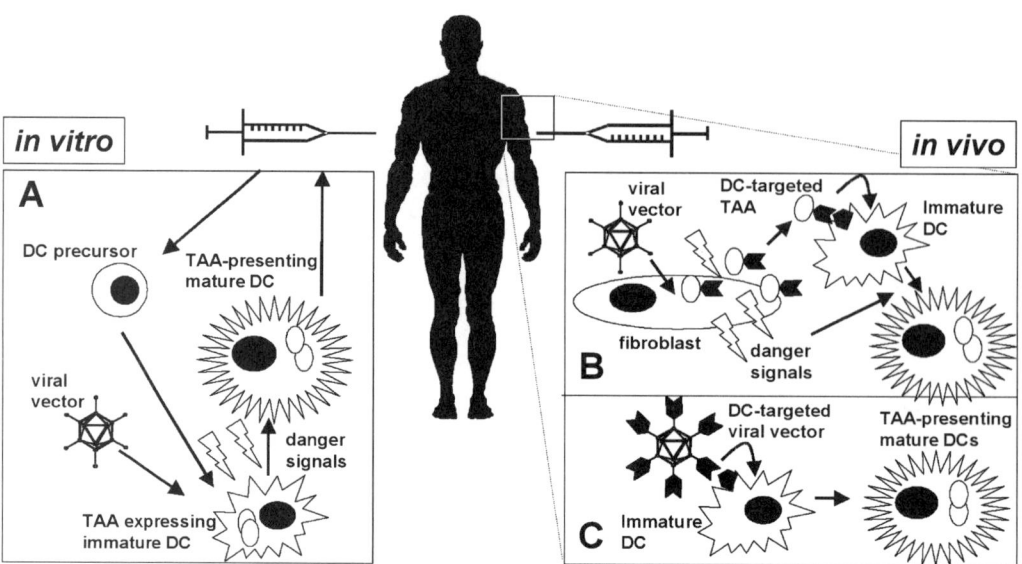

Fig. 1. Theory of dendritic cell (DC)-targeted gene transfer for tumor vaccination. Tumor-associated antigens (TAAs) are encoded by a viral vector (the presented schemes can also be applied to nonviral vectors), which can deliver TAA to DCs **(A)** in vitro or **(B)** and **(C)** in vivo. (A) In vitro DC transduction: DC precursors (e.g., CD14+ monocytes) are isolated from peripheral blood and cultured to DCs. DCs are infected by a TAA-encoding viral vector and subsequently matured by addition of danger signals. The resulting mature and TAA-presenting DCs are readministered to the patient. (B) In vivo DC targeting through cross-priming: TAA-encoding, untargeted viral vectors are intradermally injected and will mosly infect skin-resident fibroblasts. Transduced fibroblasts release TAA, fused to a DC-targeting motif, and danger-signaling proteins (i.e., virally encoded transgene products). Immature DCs selectively take up the targeted TAA and, under influence of the danger signals, start to mature. (C) Direct DC targeting in vivo: Alternatively, molecularly altered viral vectors, directly targeting DC, are intradermally injected and selectively transduce immature DCs. The virus–target molecule interaction may be selected to lead to immediate maturation of the bound DCs without addition of further danger signals. TAA-presenting, mature DCs will migrate to draining lymph nodes and activate TAA-specific cytotoxic T lymphocytes.

A less-laborious and more easily applicable alternative would be the direct in vivo immunization of patients with TAA-encoding viral or nonviral vectors. The feasibility of this approach has been demonstrated by in vivo tumor rejection studies in mice *(145,183–185,204)*. Vaccines based on tissue-resident DCs exploit the physiological processes already in place to facilitate DC activation, migration, LN homing, and subsequent T-cell activation. To home to draining LNs and subsequently activate specific T cells, DCs have to reach the correct level of activation and display the correct set of chemokine receptors, expression of which should be precisely orchestrated, both spatially and chronologically. DCs generated and readministered in vitro may not fulfill all these requirements. How these DCs are to be activated for optimal results is still a matter of debate and largely unknown.

The route of administration should also be carefully considered. Intradermal injection may be the most optimal route for DC transfer, but even then very low numbers of injected DCs (typically <1%) actually reach the draining LNs *(205,206)*. By targeting and triggering DCs *in situ*, their physiological characteristics are exploited to carry out their natural functions (i.e., homing to the LNs to meet and activate specific T cells and enhance antitumor immunity through the additional recruitment of other effector cells of the innate immune system). Direct in vivo administration of TAA-encoding vectors may thus present a more attractive and standardized "off-the-shelf" alternative for tumor vaccination.

6.2. Selective Transduction of DCs In Vivo

The efficacy of in vivo genetic immunization depends on DC-mediated activation of CTLs. Theoretically, this can result both from the direct transduction of DCs or from cross-priming after transduction of myocytes, keratinocytes, or fibroblasts. Both mechanisms have been shown to occur subsequent to genetic vaccination, but there is evidence to suggest that the directly transduced DCs are mainly responsible for CTL priming *(183,204,207,208)*. Massive uptake of the injected TAA-encoding vectors by tissue-resident cells other than DCs, which is usually the case, will interfere with DC transduction efficiency and effective CTL activation. Moreover, cross-priming under steady-state tumor conditions would result in T-cell tolerance induction, with detrimental effects on the vaccination efficacy.

It is therefore desirable to develop methods to target DCs selectively in vivo, which will reduce any cytopathic effects on bystander cells and allow increased control over the type of response that will result from vaccination. There are a number of approaches to achieve DC-targeted TAA expression:

1. TAA genes in the employed transfer vectors may be placed under the control of DC-specific promoters or enhancers, ensuring selective transcription in DCs. An example of this is the use of the dectin-2 promoter for LC-targeted gene therapy *(209)*. Although this approach will favor DC-specific transgene expression, it will not enhance the *in situ* transduction efficiency of DCs.
2. Vectors can be designed to encode TAA fused to natural ligands of DC-specific receptors. This would significantly enhance TAA uptake by DCs for cross-priming (outlined in Fig. 1B). The choice of vector for this particular application should take into account the facilitation of cross-priming *(143,210–213; see* Table 1). In taking this approach, it is essential that the vaccine formulation also provide danger signals to avoid cross tolerization. This may be achieved through simultaneous, but separate, administration of proinflammatory agents or by the inclusion of danger genes (e.g., CD40L or GM-CSF) in the vector. Antigens have previously been fused to CTLA-4, CCL21, Fc fragments, or mannosylated residues to target them to receptors on DCs *(214–216)*. DNA plasmids encoding antigens fused to CTLA-4 or FLT3L and CD40L were described to enhance antibody- and CTL-mediated immunity *(216–218)*.
3. Alternatively, DC-targeted vectors may be employed, which will increase direct DC transduction efficiency *in situ*. Some viral vectors (e.g., lentiviral vectors or SFV) have a natural DC-targeting ability, but most do not and will have to be either genetically altered or complexed to (immuno)conjugates to achieve selective DC targeting (Fig. 1C). Targeting can be mediated by natural ligands of DC-associated receptors or by DC-specific antibodies. Both viral and nonviral vectors may be targeted to DCs by complexation with antibody or mannose polyethylenimine conjugates *(109,134,219,220)*. Immunotargeting of protein antigens to APCs without further need for adjuvants to induce humoral immune responses in vivo was described using such targeting molecules as MHC-II and FcR *(214,221,222)*. Targeting to more DC-restricted markers (e.g., CD11c) was shown to induce even stronger responses *(223,224)*.

   It is important to keep in mind that DC targeting alone may not be enough; additional activation may be required. Hawiger et al. showed that targeting of a model antigen to the DEC-205 receptor on murine DCs led to specific T-cell unresponsiveness within 7 days after immunization. This unresponsiveness was only overcome after the coinjection of a CD40 agonistic antibody *(225)*. Adenovirus vectors were successfully retargeted to DCs through a CD40-binding immunoconjugate, resulting in enhanced and selective transduction of cutaneous DCs *in situ* and simultaneous maturation induction *(109)*. Such targeting strategies may ensure both DC-specific transduction and appropriate DC activation for the priming of antitumor immunity (Fig. 1C).

6.3. Target Molecules for In Situ *DC Transduction and Activation*

Which molecules are viable targets for DC-specific gene transfer? The answer to this question is closely related to the subset, the maturation state, and the anatomical location of the DCs to be targeted. A number of possible candidates are listed here. The most attractive targets would (1) be only expressed on DCs, (2) be rapidly internalized on binding, (3) route internalized antigens into MHC class I and II processing pathways, and (4) induce DC maturation and migration on binding to allow for optimal CTL activation.

1. Pattern recognition and antigen capture receptors are attractive targets because it is their natural function to internalize antigens and mediate their routing to antigen-processing pathways. In addition, their differential expression on different DC subsets may allow for subset-specific targeting, such as the following: LCs to Langerin; DDCs to MR, DEC-205, TLR2, TLR4, DC-SIGN; PDCs to BDCA-2, TLR7, and TLR9 *(31,43,50)*. Antigens internalized by MR, DEC-205, and DC-SIGN have been shown to be presented to CD4$^+$ T cells in the context of MHC class II molecules *(226–229)*. β2-Defensin, a peptide ligand of TLR4, was successfully fused to antigens to target DCs and elicit enhanced type-1 T cell immunity *(215,230)*.

2. CD1 molecules, involved in the antigen presentation of glycolipids, may also be suitable targets for specific targeting to LCs (CD1a) or DDCs (CD1b and CD1d) because of their differential expression in these subsets *(231,232)*.

3. Although their expression is not DC restricted, FcR make interesting candidates because they can efficiently channel antigens to both MHC class I and II processing pathways *(233,234)*. FcR expression can differ between DC subsets and maturation states *(233,235)*. FcR-mediated DC maturation has been reported and may further benefit vaccine efficacy *(234,235)*.

4. Members of the TNF and TNFR superfamilies are particularly attractive DC-targeting candidates. By agonistic binding and crosslinking, they can activate intracellular signaling pathways in DCs, leading to NF-κB-dependent maturation induction (e.g., CD40, Fas, Decoy rector-3 [i.e., LIGHT ligand], and 4-1BB) *(236–239)*, migration to LNs (CD40L and RANK) *(232,240)*, and increased survival (RANK) *(241)*. Fas-mediated TAA uptake from FasL$^+$ tumors was suggested, and CD40-mediated adenovirus transduction was shown to result in enhanced DC maturation and transgene-specific CTL activation *(109,242)*. Although the expression of TNF and TNFR superfamily members is not restricted to DCs, in peripheral nonlymphoid tissues their expression on DCs can be sufficiently high and specific to allow DC transduction with increased selectivity *(109)*.

5. HSP receptors (CD91) and receptors binding apoptotic fragments ($\alpha_v\beta_3$ and $\alpha_v\beta_5$ integrins) may also be useful targeting motifs with DC activational potential *(122,243)*. Indeed, RGD motifs targeting Ad vectors to $\alpha_v\beta_3$ and $\alpha_v\beta_5$ integrins enhanced DC activation; apoptotic bodies were identified as suitable antigen vehicles for the targeting of DCs in vivo *(122,244)*.

6. CD72, the ligand for the semaphorin CD100, may also serve as an antigen-targeting motif with DC-activational properties because soluble CD100 can induce DC maturation and enhance subsequent DC-mediated T-cell priming *(245)*.

7. CD83, CCR7, and CMRF-44 may provide motifs to specifically target mature DCs. However, vector internalization may be impaired in fully mature DC as well as their ability to process antigens for presentation to T cells *(215)*.

8. Because of their disturbed differentiation in cancer, DCs may be most efficiently in vivo targeted for tumor immunotherapy through precursor markers such as CD14, CD1c, BDCA-3, and CD11c *(21,23)*. An integral part of this particular approach should then be the inclusion of cytokines (or vectors carrying their genetic codes) to stimulate differentiation and maturation of the transduced DC precursors.

Expression of these targeting molecules on DCs may differ between subsets, developmental stages, tissue types, and disease states, but may be modulated by cytokine treatment. For instance, CD40-targeted adenovirus delivery to cutaneous DCs *in situ* required prior maturation induction by intradermal injection of GM-CSF and/or interleukin *(109)*. Care should be taken that such modulation of the DC activation state will not interfere with the ability of the DCs to take up and process antigens for subsequent T-cell activation. The kinetics of vector binding, uptake, TAA expression and processing, and DC activation and migration need to be timed carefully to allow for the optimal generation of TAA-specific T-cell responses *(215)*.

7. CLINICAL ADVANCES: SMALL STEPS

In vitro-generated autologous MoDCs, loaded with TAA-derived peptides, proteins, or tumor lysates, have been successfully used in clinical trials and shown to be safe. No toxicities or severe side effects were observed, and some clinical responses were reported in selected vaccinated patients in advanced stages of cancer *(246)*. Phase III trials to firmly demonstrate clinical efficacy of these DC-based vaccine strategies are being planned, but approaches with genetically modified DCs are lagging. Increased efficacy over protein-loaded DCs will have to be demonstrated, and safety issues will have to be resolved before DC-based immunogene therapy of cancer can move forward into the clinic.

7.1. Clinical Trials Past and Present

Reports on clinical trials involving the use of genetically modified DCs with cancer patients are rare. Although a number of phase I/II trials have been carried out exploring VV-based TAA vaccination, this has always been through direct in vivo administration of VV through skin scarification or intradermal, subcutaneous, or intramuscular injection and never through the in vitro transduction of autologous DCs. Patients with advanced cancer have thus been vaccinated with VV or avipox vectors (sometimes with both in a prime/boost protocol) encoding carcinoembryonic antigen, mucin 1, prostate-specific antigen (PSA), or HPV E6 and E7 *(247–252)*. Although no serious toxicity or safety issues emerged, the effects on TAA-specific antibody and CTL responses were very weak or absent, and no objective clinical responses were observed. This may be because of either strong tolerance or preexistent antibody responses to VV (which, incidentally, were clearly boosted by the vaccination) *(247)*. Inclusion of GM-CSF and B7.1 in the vaccine formulation could only slightly increase TAA-specific immune reactivity *(253,254)*.

An elegant confocal microscopy in vivo imaging system showed infected DCs were responsible for CTL priming in draining LNs subsequent to VV administration *(255)*. However, because VVs are known to interfere with DC maturation, this may not be very effective *(148–150)*. The induction of DC maturation prior to transduction (either in vivo or in vitro) may improve the efficacy of VV-based tumor vaccines *(147)*.

Clinical studies of the vaccination of patients with metastatic cancer with adenovirus vectors encoding p53, MART-1, or GP100 failed to induce specific immune responses or clinical responses *(256, 257)*. Again, prohibitive neutralizing antibody responses were offered as an explanation for the poor vaccine efficacy *(256)*. Clinical trials are currently under way to study the efficacy of vaccination with autologous adenovirus-infected MoDCs.

Although DNA vaccination should not be impeded by preexistent immunity, it was found to be equally ineffective in generating antigen-specific immunity, possibly because of poor in vivo transduction efficiency of DCs *(258,259)*. However, an increased CTL and delayed-type hypersensitivity reactivity was reported following vaccination with MoDCs that were in vitro transfected with MUC1 encoding complementary DNA *(260)*.

A most promising report came from Heiser et al., which showed consistently increased specific T-cell responsiveness after vaccination with autologous DCs transfected with mRNA encoding PSA *(261)*. Antitumor efficacy was strongly suggested by a decrease in the rate at which plasma PSA levels rose and a temporary decline in molecularly detected circulating tumor cells. The same group is currently testing the use of total tumor RNA for DC transfection and subsequent vaccination of renal cell cancer (RCC) patients with metastatic disease. Promising first data indicated the postvaccination generation of T-cell responses against various TAAs *(262)*.

Considerably more clinical trials have investigated the possibility of vaccinating cancer patients with autologous or allogeneic tumor cells expressing DC-stimulatory cytokines, such as IL-4 *(263)* and, most commonly, GM-CSF. Cells from autologous melanoma, prostate cancer, RCC, or pancreas tumors were transduced by viral vectors (adeno- or retroviral) or transfected by DNA plasmids to express GM-CSF prior to their (re)administration to cancer patients *(264–268)*. This approach was shown in some isolated cases to increase tumor-specific CTL and delayed-type hypersensitivity responses and disease-free survival and to result in partial clinical responses *(264–266)*. Similar observations for allogeneic GM-CSF-transduced tumor vaccines point to a major role for cross-priming by (autologous) DCs in the effectiveness of this approach *(265)*. These encouraging data from phase I/II trials certainly warrant further clinical studies.

7.2. Remaining Issues and Future Directions

Although vaccination with TAA-gene-modified DCs holds great promise, certain hurdles will need to be overcome before this therapeutic approach can be widely applied in the clinic. Considering obvious safety issues, the use of genetically modified DCs will have to be justified by proving its superior efficacy over the use of protein-pulsed DCs. Direct comparisons between different DC vaccination methodologies will have to be performed more rigorously in a preclinical setting before the most promising methods can be tested in clinical trials.

Similarly, the candidate viral vectors for DC transduction should be more carefully compared in vitro and in vivo in terms of their ability to induce antitumor T-cell responses and tumor rejection. The problem of preexistent, immunodominant responses against viral vectors, which may interfere with viral infection and the efficient priming of TAA-specific immunity, will need to be solved, either by advanced-generation, poorly immunogenic vectors or by optimized prime/boost protocols with different vector systems.

Another important question that is being addressed is which TAA genes to select for transfer to DCs. To avoid outgrowth of tumor escape variants, multiple TAA genes should be targeted. Ideally, a standard panel of common TAAs, expressed by a vast majority of tumors but not by normal tissues, should eventually be developed for genetic DC-based vaccination.

If TAA gene transfer is to be achieved by in vivo targeting, many more issues deserve careful consideration, such as which DC subsets to target and in which body compartment, which targeting molecules to select and which additional immunoadjuvants, which antigen processing routes to target, and the optimal timing of DC activation and vector delivery for efficient CTL activation. Finally, there is a general consensus that, for immunotherapy to be effective, it will have to be applied in an adjuvant setting. Optimized treatment protocols are needed to ensure that the traits of immunogene therapy and other therapeutic approaches combine to achieve synergistic antitumor effects.

The major item that remains on the immuno(gene) therapist's troubleshooting list, and that in one way or another relates to all the above-listed items, is how to break the strong tumor-related immune tolerance; in other words, how best to deploy DCs in the struggle against cancer so that they can serve as the definitive wake-up call to all the required components, both innate and adaptive, for a concerted and effective antitumor immune response. At the moment, all seem to agree, DCs may be our best shot.

REFERENCES

1. Guermonprez, P., Valladeau, J., Zitvogel, L., Thery, C., and Amigorena, S. (2002) Antigen presentation and T cell stimulation by dendritic cells. *Annu. Rev. Immunol.* **20,** 621–667.
2. Bhardwaj, N. (2001) Processing and presentation of antigens by dendritic cells: implications for vaccines. *Trends Mol. Med.* **7,** 388–394.
3. Matzinger, P. (1998) An innate sense of danger. *Semin. Immunol.* **10,** 399–415.
4. Fuchs, E. J. and Matzinger, P. (1996) Is cancer dangerous to the immune system? *Semin. Immunol.* **8,** 271–280.
5. Kawakami, Y. and Rosenberg, S. A. (1997) Human tumor antigens recognized by T-cells. *Immunol. Res.* **16,** 313–339.
6. Banchereau, J., Schuler-Thurner, B., Palucka, A. K., and Schuler, G. (2001) Dendritic cells as vectors for therapy. *Cell* **106,** 271–274.
7. Rea, D., Johnson, M. E., Havenga, M. J., Melief, C. J., and Offringa, R. (2001) Strategies for improved antigen delivery into dendritic cells. *Trends Mol. Med.* **7,** 91–94.
8. Geissmann, F., Prost, C., Monnet, J. P., Dy, M., Brousse, N., and Hermine, O. (1998) Transforming growth factor beta1, in the presence of granulocyte/macrophage colony-stimulating factor and interleukin 4, induces differentiation of human peripheral blood monocytes into dendritic Langerhans cells. *J. Exp. Med.* **187,** 961–966.
9. Mohamadzadeh, M., Berard, F., Essert, G., et al. (2001) Interleukin 15 skews monocyte differentiation into dendritic cells with features of Langerhans cells. *J. Exp. Med.* **194,** 1013–1020.
10. Nestle, F. O., Banchereau, J., and Hart, D. (2001) Dendritic cells: on the move from bench to bedside. *Nat. Med.* **7,** 761–765.
11. Crawford, K., Gabuzda, D., Pantazopoulos,V., et al. (1999) Circulating CD2$^+$ monocytes are dendritic cells. *J. Immunol.* **163,** 5920–5928.
12. Randolph, G. J., Beaulieu, S., Lebecque, S., Steinman, R. M., and Muller, W. A. (1998) Differentiation of monocytes into dendritic cells in a model of transendothelial trafficking. *Science* **282,** 480–483.
13. Caux, C., Vanbervliet, B., Massacrier, C., et al. (1996) CD34$^+$ hematopoietic progenitors from human cord blood differentiate along two independent dendritic cell pathways in response to GM-CSF$^+$TNF alpha. *J. Exp. Med.* **184,** 695–706.

14. Strobl, H., Riedl, E., Bello-Fernandez, C., and Knapp, W. (1998) Epidermal Langerhans cell development and differentiation. *Immunobiology* **198**, 588–605.

15. Mortarini, R., Anichini, A., Di Nicola, M., et al. (1997) Autologous dendritic cells derived from CD34$^+$ progenitors and from monocytes are not functionally equivalent antigen-presenting cells in the induction of melan-A/Mart-1(27-35)-specific CTLs from peripheral blood lymphocytes of melanoma patients with low frequency of CTL precursors. *Cancer Res.* **57**, 5534–5541.

16. Bontkes, H. J., de Gruijl, T. D., Schuurhuis, G. J., Scheper, R. J., Meijer, C. J., and Hooijberg, E. (2002) Expansion of dendritic cell precursors from human CD34(+) progenitor cells isolated from healthy donor blood; growth factor combination determines proliferation rate and functional outcome. *J. Leukoc. Biol.* **72**, 321–329.

17. Robinson, S. P., Patterson, S., English, N., Davies, D., Knight, S. C., and Reid, C. D. (1999) Human peripheral blood contains two distinct lineages of dendritic cells. *Eur. J. Immunol.* **29**, 2769–2778.

18. Thomas, R. and Lipsky, P. E. (1994) Human peripheral blood dendritic cell subsets. Isolation and characterization of precursor and mature antigen-presenting cells. *J. Immunol.* **153**, 4016–4028.

19. Fearnley, D. B., Whyte, L. F., Carnoutsos, S. A., Cook, A. H., and Hart, D. N. (1999) Monitoring human blood dendritic cell numbers in normal individuals and in stem cell transplantation. *Blood* **93**, 728–736.

20. MacDonald, K. P., Munster, D. J., Clark, G. J., Dzionek, A., Schmitz, J., and Hart, D. N. (2002) Characterization of human blood dendritic cell subsets. *Blood* **100**, 4512–4520.

21. Dzionek, A., Fuchs, A., Schmidt, P., et al. (2000) BDCA-2, BDCA-3, and BDCA-4: three markers for distinct subsets of dendritic cells in human peripheral blood. *J. Immunol.* **165**, 6037–6046.

22. Ho, C. S., Munster, D., Pyke, C. M., Hart, D. N., and Lopez, J. A. (2002) Spontaneous generation and survival of blood dendritic cells in mononuclear cell culture without exogenous cytokines. *Blood* **99**, 2897–2904.

23. de Baey, A., Mende, I., Riethmueller, G., and Baeuerle, P. A. (2001) Phenotype and function of human dendritic cells derived from M-DC8(+) monocytes. *Eur. J. Immunol.* **31**, 1646–1655.

24. Schakel, K., Mayer, E., Federle, C., Schmitz, M., Riethmuller, G., and Rieber, E. P. (1998) A novel dendritic cell population in human blood: one-step immunomagnetic isolation by a specific mAb (M-DC8) and in vitro priming of cytotoxic T lymphocytes. *Eur. J. Immunol.* **28**, 4084–4093.

25. Schakel, K., Kannagi, R., Kniep, B., et al. (2002) 6-Sulfo LacNAc, a novel carbohydrate modification of PSGL-1, defines an inflammatory type of human dendritic cells. *Immunity* **17**, 289–301.

26. Randolph, G. J., Sanchez-Schmitz, G., Liebman, R. M., and Schakel, K. (2002) The CD16(+) (FcgammaRIII(+)) subset of human monocytes preferentially becomes migratory dendritic cells in a model tissue setting. *J. Exp. Med.* **196**, 517–527.

27. Osugi, Y., Vuckovic, S., and Hart, D. N. (2002) Myeloid blood CD11c(+) dendritic cells and monocyte-derived dendritic cells differ in their ability to stimulate T lymphocytes. *Blood* **100**, 2858–2866.

28. Alejandro, L. J., Crosbie, G., Kelly, C., et al. (2002) Monitoring and isolation of blood dendritic cells from apheresis products in healthy individuals: a platform for cancer immunotherapy. *J. Immunol. Methods* **267**, 199–212.

29. Cella, M., Jarrossay, D., Facchetti, F., et al. (1999) Plasmacytoid monocytes migrate to inflamed lymph nodes and produce large amounts of type I interferon. *Nat. Med.* **5**, 919–923.

30. Liu, Y. J. (2001) Dendritic cell subsets and lineages, and their functions in innate and adaptive immunity. *Cell* **106**, 259–262.

31. Shortman, K. and Liu, Y. J. (2002) Mouse and human dendritic cell subtypes. *Nat. Rev. Immunol.* **2**, 151–161.

32. Patterson, S. (2000) Flexibility and cooperation among dendritic cells. *Nat. Immunol.* **1**, 273–274.

33. Dzionek, A., Sohma, Y., Nagafune, J., et al. (2001) BDCA-2, a novel plasmacytoid dendritic cell-specific type II C-type lectin, mediates antigen capture and is a potent inhibitor of interferon alpha/beta induction. *J. Exp. Med.* **194**, 1823–1834.

34. Arpinati, M., Green, C. L., Heimfeld, S., Heuser, J. E., and Anasetti, C. (2000) Granulocyte-colony stimulating factor mobilizes T helper 2-inducing dendritic cells. *Blood* **95**, 2484–2490.

35. Cella, M., Facchetti, F., Lanzavecchia, A., and Colonna, M. (2000) Plasmacytoid dendritic cells activated by influenza virus and CD40L drive a potent TH1 polarization. *Nat. Immunol.* **1**, 305–310.

36. Charbonnier, A., Gaugler, B., Sainty, D., Lafage-Pochitaloff, M., and Olive, D. (1999) Human acute myeloblastic leukemia cells differentiate in vitro into mature dendritic cells and induce the differentiation of cytotoxic T cells against autologous leukemias. *Eur. J. Immunol.* **29**, 2567–2578.

37. Padley, D. J., Dietz, A. B., Gastineau, D. A., and Vuk-Pavlovic, S. (2001) Mature myeloid dendritic cells for clinical use prepared from CD14$^+$ cells isolated by immunomagnetic adsorption. *J. Hematother. Stem Cell Res.* **10**, 427–429.

38. Fujii, N., Ikeda, T., Ikeda, K., et al. (2002) Differentiation of monoblastic cell line UG3 into leukemic dendritic cells. *Int. J. Oncol.* **21**, 617–620.

39. Masterson, A. J., Sombroek, C. C., de Gruijl, T. D., et al. (2002) MUTZ-3, a human cell line model for the cytokine-induced differentiation of dendritic cells from CD34$^+$ precursors. *Blood* **100**, 701–703.

40. Girolomoni, G., Caux, C., Lebecque, S., Dezutter-Dambuyant, C., and Ricciardi-Castagnoli, P. (2002) Langerhans cells: still a fundamental paradigm for studying the immunobiology of dendritic cells. *Trends Immunol.* **23**, 6–8.

41. Valladeau, J., Ravel, O., Dezutter-Dambuyant, C., et al. (2000) Langerin, a novel C-type lectin specific to Langer-hans cells, is an endocytic receptor that induces the formation of Birbeck granules. *Immunity* **12,** 71–81.
42. Kumamoto, T., Huang, E. K., Paek, H. J., et al. (2002) Induction of tumor-specific protective immunity by *in situ* Langerhans cell vaccine. *Nat. Biotechnol.* **20,** 64–69.
43. Larregina, A. T. and Falo, L. D. Jr. (2001) Dendritic cells in the context of skin immunity. In *Dendritic Cells— Biology and Clinical Applications* (Lotze, M. T. and Thomson, A. W., eds.), Academic Press, London, pp. 301–314.
44. Hochrein, H., O'Keeffe, M., Luft, T., et al. (2000) Interleukin (IL)-4 is a major regulatory cytokine governing bioactive IL-12 production by mouse and human dendritic cells. *J. Exp. Med.* **192,** 823–833.
45. Morelli, A. E., Zahorchak, A. F., Larregina, A. T., et al. (2001) Cytokine production by mouse myeloid dendritic cells in relation to differentiation and terminal maturation induced by lipopolysaccharide or CD40 ligation. *Blood* **98,** 1512–1523.
46. Lutz, M. and Schuler, G. (2002) Immature, semi-mature and fully mature dendritic cells: which signals induce toler-ance or immunity? *Trends Immunol.* **23,** 445.
47. Kalinski, P., Vieira, P. L., Schuitemaker, J. H., de Jong, E. C., and Kapsenberg, M. L. (2001) Prostaglandin E(2) is a selective inducer of interleukin-12 p40 (IL-12p40) production and an inhibitor of bioactive IL-12p70 heterodimer. *Blood* **97,** 3466–3469.
48. Krug, A., Towarowski, A., Britsch, S., et al. (2001) Toll-like receptor expression reveals CpG DNA as a unique microbial stimulus for plasmacytoid dendritic cells which synergizes with CD40 ligand to induce high amounts of IL-12. *Eur. J. Immunol.* **31,** 3026–3037.
49. Kawarada, Y., Ganss, R., Garbi, N., Sacher, T., Arnold, B., and Hammerling, G. J. (2001) NK- and CD8(+) T cell-mediated eradication of established tumors by peritumoral injection of CpG-containing oligodeoxynucleotides. *J. Immu-nol.* **167,** 5247–5253.
50. Kadowaki, N., Ho, S., Antonenko, S., et al. (2001) Subsets of human dendritic cell precursors express different toll-like receptors and respond to different microbial antigens. *J. Exp. Med.* **194,** 863–869.
51. Cumberbatch, M., Dearman, R. J., Antonopoulos, C., Groves, R. W., and Kimber, I. (2001) Interleukin (IL)-18 induces Langerhans cell migration by a tumour necrosis factor-alpha- and IL-1beta-dependent mechanism. *Immunol-ogy* **102,** 323–330.
52. Scandella, E., Men, Y., Gillessen, S., Forster, R., and Groettrup, M. (2002) Prostaglandin E2 is a key factor for CCR7 surface expression and migration of monocyte-derived dendritic cells. *Blood* **100,** 1354–1361.
53. Sallusto, F. and Lanzavecchia, A. (2000) Understanding dendritic cell and T-lymphocyte traffic through the analysis of chemokine receptor expression. *Immunol. Rev.* **177,** 134–140.
54. Brossart, P. and Bevan, M. J. (1997) Presentation of exogenous protein antigens on major histocompatibility com-plex class I molecules by dendritic cells: pathway of presentation and regulation by cytokines. *Blood* **90,** 1594–1599.
55. Ruedl, C., Koebel, P., Bachmann, M., Hess, M., and Karjalainen, K. (2000) Anatomical origin of dendritic cells determines their life span in peripheral lymph nodes. *J. Immunol.* **165,** 4910–4916.
56. Ashany, D., Savir, A., Bhardwaj, N., and Elkon, K. B. (1999) Dendritic cells are resistant to apoptosis through the Fas (CD95/APO-1) pathway. *J. Immunol.* **163,** 5303–5311.
57. Rescigno, M., Piguet, V., Valzasina, B., et al. (2000) Fas engagement induces the maturation of dendritic cells (DCs), the release of interleukin (IL)-1beta, and the production of interferon gamma in the absence of IL-12 during DC-T cell cognate interaction: a new role for Fas ligand in inflammatory responses. *J. Exp. Med.* **192,** 1661–1668.
58. Ochsenbein, A. F., Klenerman, P., Karrer, U., et al. (1999) Immune surveillance against a solid tumor fails because of immunological ignorance. *Proc. Natl. Acad. Sci. USA* **96,** 2233–2238.
59. Takayama, T., Morelli, A. E., Onai, N., et al. (2001) Mammalian and viral IL-10 enhance C-C chemokine receptor 5 but down-regulate C-C chemokine receptor 7 expression by myeloid dendritic cells: impact on chemotactic responses and in vivo homing ability. *J. Immunol.* **166,** 7136–7143.
60. Muller, G., Muller, A., Tuting, T., et al. (2002) Interleukin-10-treated dendritic cells modulate immune responses of naive and sensitized T cells in vivo. *J. Invest. Dermatol.* **119,** 836–841.
61. Lotze, M. T. and Jaffe, R. (2001) The identification of dendritic cells in cancer. In *Dendritic Cells; Biology and Clinical Applications* (Lotze, M. T. and Thomson, A. W., eds.), Academic Press, London, pp. 425–437.
62. Gabrilovich, D. I., Corak, J., Ciernik, I. F., Kavanaugh, D., and Carbone, D. P. (1997) Decreased antigen presentation by dendritic cells in patients with breast cancer. *Clin. Cancer Res.* **3,** 483–490.
63. Savary, C. A., Grazziutti, M. L., Melichar, B., et al. (1998) Multidimensional flow-cytometric analysis of dendritic cells in peripheral blood of normal donors and cancer patients. *Cancer Immunol. Immunother.* **45,** 234–240.
64. Almand, B., Clark, J. I., Nikitina, E., et al. (2001) Increased production of immature myeloid cells in cancer patients: a mechanism of immunosuppression in cancer. *J. Immunol.* **166,** 678–689.
65. Gabrilovich, D., Ishida, T., Oyama, T., et al. (1998) Vascular endothelial growth factor inhibits the development of dendri-tic cells and dramatically affects the differentiation of multiple hematopoietic lineages in vivo. *Blood* **92,** 4150–4166.
66. Oyama, T., Ran, S., Ishida, T., et al. (1998) Vascular endothelial growth factor affects dendritic cell matura-tion through the inhibition of nuclear factor-kappa B activation in hemopoietic progenitor cells. *J. Immunol.* **160,** 1224–1232.

67. Almand, B., Resser, J. R., Lindman, B., et al. (2000) Clinical significance of defective dendritic cell differentiation in cancer. *Clin. Cancer Res.* **6**, 1755–1766.

68. Gabrilovich, D. I., Cheng, P., Fan, Y. et al. (2002) H1(0) histone and differentiation of dendritic cells. A molecular target for tumor-derived factors. *J. Leukoc. Biol.* **72**, 285–296.

69. Sombroek, C. C., Stam, A. G., Masterson, A. J., et al. (2002) Prostanoids play a major role in the primary tumor-induced inhibition of dendritic cell differentiation. *J. Immunol.* **168**, 4333–4343.

70. Menetrier-Caux, C., Thomachot, M. C., Alberti, L., Montmain, G., and Blay, J. Y. (2001) IL-4 prevents the blockade of dendritic cell differentiation induced by tumor cells. *Cancer Res.* **61**, 3096–3104.

71. Menetrier-Caux, C., Montmain, G., Dieu, M. C., et al. (1998) Inhibition of the differentiation of dendritic cells from CD34(+) progenitors by tumor cells: role of interleukin-6 and macrophage colony-stimulating factor. *Blood* **92**, 4778–4791.

72. Shurin, G. V., Shurin, M. R., Bykovskaia, S., Shogan, J., Lotze, M. T., and Barksdale, E. M. Jr. (2001) Neuroblastoma-derived gangliosides inhibit dendritic cell generation and function. *Cancer Res.* **61**, 363–369.

73. Buelens, C., Verhasselt, V., De Groote, D., Thielemans, K., Goldman, M., and Willems, F. (1997) Interleukin-10 prevents the generation of dendritic cells from human peripheral blood mononuclear cells cultured with interleukin-4 and granulocyte/macrophage-colony-stimulating factor. *Eur. J. Immunol.* **27**, 756–762.

74. Shurin, M. R., Yurkovetsky, Z. R., Tourkova, I. L., Balkir, L., and Shurin, G. V. (2002) Inhibition of CD40 expression and CD40-mediated dendritic cell function by tumor-derived IL-10. *Int. J. Cancer* **101**, 61–68.

75. Bell, D., Chomarat, P., Broyles, D., et al. (1999) In breast carcinoma tissue, immature dendritic cells reside within the tumor, whereas mature dendritic cells are located in peritumoral areas. *J. Exp. Med.* **190**, 1417–1426.

76. Enk, A. H., Jonuleit, H., Saloga, J., and Knop, J. (1997) Dendritic cells as mediators of tumor-induced tolerance in metastatic melanoma. *Int. J. Cancer* **73**, 309–316.

77. Huang, R. R., Wen, D. R., Guo, J., et al. (2000) Selective modulation of paracortical dendritic cells and T-lymphocytes in breast cancer sentinel lymph nodes. *Breast J.* **6**, 225–232.

78. Lana, A. M., Wen, D. R., and Cochran, A. J. (2001) The morphology, immunophenotype and distribution of paracortical dendritic leucocytes in lymph nodes regional to cutaneous melanoma. *Melanoma Res.* **11**, 401–410.

79. Jonuleit, H., Schmitt, E., Steinbrink, K., and Enk, A. H. (2001) Dendritic cells as a tool to induce anergic and regulatory T cells. *Trends Immunol.* **22**, 394–400.

80. Harizi, H., Juzan, M., Pitard, V., Moreau, J. F., and Gualde, N. (2002) Cyclooxygenase-2-issued prostaglandin e (2) enhances the production of endogenous IL-10, which down-regulates dendritic cell functions. *J. Immunol.* **168**, 2255–2263.

81. Kalinski, P., Schuitemaker, J. H., Hilkens, C. M., and Kapsenberg, M. L. (1998) Prostaglandin E2 induces the final maturation of IL-12-deficient CD1a+CD83+ dendritic cells: the levels of IL-12 are determined during the final dendritic cell maturation and are resistant to further modulation. *J. Immunol.* **161**, 2804–2809.

82. Hermans, I. F., Ritchie, D. S., Yang, J., Roberts, J. M., and Ronchese, F. (2000) CD8+ T cell-dependent elimination of dendritic cells in vivo limits the induction of antitumor immunity. *J. Immunol.* **164**, 3095–3101.

83. Ronchese, F. and Hermans, I. F. (2001) Killing of dendritic cells: a life cut short or a purposeful death? *J. Exp. Med.* **194**, F23–F26.

84. Medema, J. P., Schuurhuis, D. H., Rea, D., et al. (2001) Expression of the serpin serine protease inhibitor 6 protects dendritic cells from cytotoxic T lymphocyte-induced apoptosis: differential modulation by T helper type 1 and type 2 cells. *J. Exp. Med.* **194**, 657–667.

85. Iezzi, G., Karjalainen, K., and Lanzavecchia, A. (1998) The duration of antigenic stimulation determines the fate of naive and effector T cells. *Immunity* **8**, 89–95.

86. Kanto, T., Kalinski, P., Hunter, O. C., Lotze, M. T., and Amoscato, A. A. (2001) Ceramide mediates tumor-induced dendritic cell apoptosis. *J. Immunol.* **167**, 3773–3784.

87. Nencioni, A., Lauber, K., Grunebach, F., et al. (2002) Cyclopentenone prostaglandins induce caspase activation and apoptosis in dendritic cells by a PPAR-gamma-independent mechanism: regulation by inflammatory and T cell-derived stimuli. *Exp. Hematol.* **30**, 1020–1028.

88. Rabinovich, G. A., Riera, C. M., and Iribarren, P. (1999) Granulocyte-macrophage colony-stimulating factor protects dendritic cells from liposome-encapsulated dichloromethylene diphosphonate-induced apoptosis through a Bcl-2-mediated pathway. *Eur. J. Immunol.* **29**, 563–570.

89. Bjorck, P., Banchereau, J., and Flores-Romo, L. (1997) CD40 ligation counteracts Fas-induced apoptosis of human dendritic cells. *Int. Immunol.* **9**, 365–372.

90. Lundqvist, A., Nagata, T., Kiessling, R., and Pisa, P. (2002) Mature dendritic cells are protected from Fas/CD95-mediated apoptosis by upregulation of Bcl-X(L). *Cancer Immunol. Immunother.* **51**, 139–144.

91. Gasparetto, C., Gasparetto, M., Morse, M., et al. (2002) Mobilization of dendritic cells from patients with breast cancer into peripheral blood stem cell leukapheresis samples using Flt-3-Ligand and G-CSF or GM-CSF. *Cytokine* **18**, 8–19.

92. Pulendran, B., Banchereau, J., Burkeholder, S., et al. (2000) Flt3-ligand and granulocyte colony-stimulating factor mobilize distinct human dendritic cell subsets in vivo. *J. Immunol.* **165**, 566–572.

93. Gilliet, M., Boonstra, A., Paturel, C., et al. (2002) The development of murine plasmacytoid dendritic cell precursors is differentially regulated by FLT3-ligand and granulocyte/macrophage colony-stimulating factor. *J. Exp. Med.* **195,** 953–958.

94. Ito, T., Amakawa, R., Inaba, M., Ikehara, S., Inaba, K., and Fukuhara, S. (2001) Differential regulation of human blood dendritic cell subsets by IFNs. *J. Immunol.* **166,** 2961–2969.

95. Ebner, S., Hofer, S., Nguyen, V. A., et al. (2002) A novel role for IL-3: human monocytes cultured in the presence of IL-3 and IL-4 differentiate into dendritic cells that produce less IL-12 and shift Th cell responses toward a Th2 cytokine pattern. *J. Immunol.* **168,** 6199–6207.

96. Buelens, C., Bartholome, E. J., Amraoui, Z., et al. (2002) Interleukin-3 and interferon beta cooperate to induce differentiation of monocytes into dendritic cells with potent helper T-cell stimulatory properties. *Blood* **99,** 993–998.

97. Grabbe, S., Bruvers, S., and Granstein, R. D. (1992) Effects of immunomodulatory cytokines on the presentation of tumor- associated antigens by epidermal Langerhans cells. *J. Invest. Dermatol.* **99,** 66S–68S.

98. Luft, T., Jefford, M., Luetjens, P., et al. (2002) IL-1 beta enhances CD40 ligand-mediated cytokine secretion by human dendritic cells (DC): a mechanism for T cell-independent DC activation. *J. Immunol.* **168,** 713–722.

99. Dranoff, G. (2002) GM-CSF-based cancer vaccines. *Immunol. Rev.* **188,** 147–154.

100. Dranoff, G., Jaffee, E., Lazenby, A., et al. (1993) Vaccination with irradiated tumor cells engineered to secrete murine granulocyte-macrophage colony-stimulating factor stimulates potent, specific, and long-lasting anti-tumor immunity. *Proc. Natl. Acad. Sci. USA* **90,** 3539–3543.

101. Ali, S. A., Lynam, J., McLean, C. S., et al. (2002) Tumor regression induced by intratumor therapy with a disabled infectious single cycle (DISC) herpes simplex virus (HSV) vector, DISC/HSV/murine granulocyte-macrophage colony-stimulating factor, correlates with antigen-specific adaptive immunity. *J. Immunol.* **168,** 3512–3519.

102. Sun, X., Hodge, L. M., Jones, H. P., Tabor, L., and Simecka, J. W. (2002) Co-expression of granulocyte-macrophage colony-stimulating factor with antigen enhances humoral and tumor immunity after DNA vaccination. *Vaccine* **20,** 1466–1474.

103. Kass, E., Panicali, D. L., Mazzara, G., Schlom, J., and Greiner, J. W. (2001) Granulocyte/macrophage-colony stimulating factor produced by recombinant avian poxviruses enriches the regional lymph nodes with antigen-presenting cells and acts as an immunoadjuvant. *Cancer Res.* **61,** 206–214.

104. Nakamura, M., Iwahashi, M., Nakamori, M., et al. (2002) Dendritic cells genetically engineered to simultaneously express endogenous tumor antigen and granulocyte macrophage colony-stimulating factor elicit potent therapeutic antitumor immunity. *Clin. Cancer Res.* **8,** 2742–2749.

105. Curiel-Lewandrowski, C., Mahnke, K., Labeur, M., et al. (1999) Transfection of immature murine bone marrow-derived dendritic cells with the granulocyte-macrophage colony-stimulating factor gene potently enhances their in vivo antigen-presenting capacity. *J. Immunol.* **163,** 174–183.

106. Liu, Y., Zhang, W., Chan, T., Saxena, A., and Xiang, J. (2002) Engineered fusion hybrid vaccine of IL-4 gene-modified myeloma and relative mature dendritic cells enhances antitumor immunity. *Leuk. Res.* **26,** 757–763.

107. Okada, H., Pollack, I. F., Lieberman, F., et al. (2001) Gene therapy of malignant gliomas: a pilot study of vaccination with irradiated autologous glioma and dendritic cells admixed with IL-4 transduced fibroblasts to elicit an immune response. *Hum. Gene Ther.* **12,** 575–595.

108. Roth, M. D., Gitlitz, B. J., Kiertscher, S. M., et al. (2000) Granulocyte macrophage colony-stimulating factor and interleukin 4 enhance the number and antigen-presenting activity of circulating CD14$^+$ and CD83$^+$ cells in cancer patients. *Cancer Res.* **60,** 1934–1941.

109. de Gruijl, T. D., Luykx-de Bakker, S. A., Tillman, B. W., et al. (2002) Prolonged maturation and enhanced transduction of dendritic cells migrated from human skin explants after *in situ* delivery of CD40-targeted adenoviral vectors. *J. Immunol.* **169,** 5322–5331.

110. Chen, Z., Huang, H., Chang, T., et al. (2002) Enhanced HER-2/neu-specific antitumor immunity by cotransduction of mouse dendritic cells with two genes encoding HER-2/neu and alpha tumor necrosis factor. *Cancer Gene Ther.* **9,** 778–786.

111. Rizza, P., Ferrantini, M., Capone, I., and Belardelli, F. (2002) Cytokines as natural adjuvants for vaccines: where are we now? *Trends Immunol.* **23,** 381–383.

112. Hiroishi, K., Tuting, T., Tahara, H., and Lotze, M. T. (1999) Interferon-alpha gene therapy in combination with CD80 transduction reduces tumorigenicity and growth of established tumor in poorly immunogenic tumor models. *Gene Ther.* **6,** 1988–1994.

113. Tang, Z. H., Qiu, W. H., Wu, G. S., Yang, X. P., Zou, S. Q., and Qiu, F. Z. (2002) The immunotherapeutic effect of dendritic cells vaccine modified with interleukin-18 gene and tumor cell lysate on mice with pancreatic carcinoma. *World J. Gastroenterol.* **8,** 908–912.

114. Tatsumi, T., Gambotto, A., Robbins, P. D., and Storkus, W. J. (2002) Interleukin 18 gene transfer expands the repertoire of antitumor Th1-type immunity elicited by dendritic cell-based vaccines in association with enhanced therapeutic efficacy. *Cancer Res.* **62,** 5853–5858.

115. Kirk, C. J., Hartigan-O'Connor, D., Nickoloff, B. J., et al. (2001) T cell-dependent antitumor immunity mediated by secondary lymphoid tissue chemokine: augmentation of dendritic cell-based immunotherapy. *Cancer Res.* **61,** 2062–2070.

116. Kirk, C. J., Hartigan-O'Connor, D., and Mule, J. J. (2001) The dynamics of the T-cell antitumor response: chemokine-secreting dendritic cells can prime tumor-reactive T cells extranodally. *Cancer Res.* **61**, 8794–8802.

117. Jenne, L., Schuler, G., and Steinkasserer, A. (2001) Viral vectors for dendritic cell-based immunotherapy. *Trends Immunol.* **22**, 102–107.

118. Gambotto, A., Cicinnati, V. R., and Robbins, P. D. (2001) Genetic engineering of dendritic cells. In *Dendritic Cells; Biology and Clinical Applications* (Lotze, M. T., and Thomson, A. W., eds.), Academic Press, London, pp. 609–625.

119. Philip, R., Alters, S. E., Brunette, E., et al. (2000) Dendritic cells loaded with MART-1 peptide or infected with adenoviral construct are functionally equivalent in the induction of tumor-specific cytotoxic T lymphocyte responses in patients with melanoma. *J. Immunother.* **23**, 168–176.

120. Wan, Y., Emtage, P., Zhu, Q., et al. (1999) Enhanced immune response to the melanoma antigen gp100 using recombinant adenovirus-transduced dendritic cells. *Cell Immunol.* **198**, 131–138.

121. Armstrong, A. C., Dermime, S., Allinson, C. G., et al. (2002) Immunization with a recombinant adenovirus encoding a lymphoma idiotype: induction of tumor-protective immunity and identification of an idiotype-specific T cell epitope. *J. Immunol.* **168**, 3983–3991.

122. Okada, N., Saito, T., Masunaga, Y., et al. (2001) Efficient antigen gene transduction using Arg-Gly-Asp fiber-mutant adenovirus vectors can potentiate antitumor vaccine efficacy and maturation of murine dendritic cells. *Cancer Res.* **61**, 7913–7919.

123. Herrera, O. B., Brett, S., and Lechler, R. I. (2002) Infection of mouse bone marrow-derived dendritic cells with recombinant adenovirus vectors leads to presentation of encoded antigen by both MHC class I and class II molecules-potential benefits in vaccine design. *Vaccine* **21**, 231–242.

124. Miller, G., Lahrs, S., Pillarisetty, V. G., Shah, A. B., and DeMatteo, R. P. (2002) Adenovirus infection enhances dendritic cell immunostimulatory properties and induces natural killer and T-cell-mediated tumor protection. *Cancer Res.* **62**, 5260–5266.

125. Song, W., Tong, Y., Carpenter, H., Kong, H. L., and Crystal, R. G. (2000) Persistent, antigen-specific, therapeutic antitumor immunity by dendritic cells genetically modified with an adenoviral vector to express a model tumor antigen. *Gene Ther.* **7**, 2080–2086.

126. Tillman, B. W., Hayes, T. L., DeGruijl, T. D., Douglas, J. T., and Curiel, D. T. (2000) Adenoviral vectors targeted to CD40 enhance the efficacy of dendritic cell-based vaccination against human papillomavirus 16-induced tumor cells in a murine model. *Cancer Res.* **60**, 5456–5463.

127. Song, W., Kong, H. L., Carpenter, H., et al. (1997) Dendritic cells genetically modified with an adenovirus vector encoding the cDNA for a model antigen induce protective and therapeutic antitumor immunity. *J. Exp. Med.* **186**, 1247–1256.

128. Rouard, H., Leon, A., Klonjkowski, B., et al. (2000) Adenoviral transduction of human "clinical grade" immature dendritic cells enhances costimulatory molecule expression and T-cell stimulatory capacity. *J. Immunol. Methods* **241**, 69–81.

129. Rea, D., Schagen, F. H., Hoeben, R. C., et al. (1999) Adenoviruses activate human dendritic cells without polarization toward a T-helper type 1-inducing subset. *J. Virol.* **73**, 10,245–10,253.

130. Tillman, B. W., de Gruijl, T. D., Luykx-de Bakker, S. A., et al. (1999) Maturation of dendritic cells accompanies high-efficiency gene transfer by a CD40-targeted adenoviral vector. *J. Immunol.* **162**, 6378–6383.

131. Dietz, A. B. and Vuk-Pavlovic, S. (1998) High efficiency adenovirus-mediated gene transfer to human dendritic cells. *Blood* **91**, 392–398.

132. Zhong, L., Granelli-Piperno, A., Choi, Y., and Steinman, R. M. (1999) Recombinant adenovirus is an efficient and non-perturbing genetic vector for human dendritic cells. *Eur. J. Immunol.* **29**, 964–972.

133. Rea, D., Havenga, M. J., van Den, A. M., et al. (2001) Highly efficient transduction of human monocyte-derived dendritic cells with subgroup B fiber-modified adenovirus vectors enhances transgene-encoded antigen presentation to cytotoxic T cells. *J. Immunol.* **166**, 5236–5244.

134. Diebold, S. S., Lehrmann, H., Kursa, M., Wagner, E., Cotten, M., and Zenke, M. (1999) Efficient gene delivery into human dendritic cells by adenovirus polyethylenimine and mannose polyethylenimine transfection. *Hum. Gene Ther.* **10**, 775–786.

135. Jonuleit, H., Tuting, T., Steitz, J., et al. (2000) Efficient transduction of mature CD83+ dendritic cells using recombinant adenovirus suppressed T cell stimulatory capacity. *Gene Ther.* **7**, 249–254.

136. Liu, Y., Santin, A. D., Mane, M., et al. (2000) Transduction and utility of the granulocyte-macrophage colony-stimulating factor gene into monocytes and dendritic cells by adeno-associated virus. *J. Interferon Cytokine Res.* **20**, 21–30.

137. Chiriva-Internati, M., Liu, Y., Salati, E., et al. (2002) Efficient generation of cytotoxic T lymphocytes against cervical cancer cells by adeno-associated virus/human papillomavirus type 16 E7 antigen gene transduction into dendritic cells. *Eur. J. Immunol.* **32**, 30–38.

138. Sun, J. Y., Krouse, R. S., Forman, S. J., et al. (2002) Immunogenicity of a p210(BCR-ABL) fusion domain candidate DNA vaccine targeted to dendritic cells by a recombinant adeno-associated virus vector in vitro. *Cancer Res.* **62**, 3175–3183.

139. Ponnazhagan, S., Mahendra, G., Curiel, D. T., and Shaw, D. R. (2001) Adeno-associated virus type 2-mediated transduction of human monocyte-derived dendritic cells: implications for ex vivo immunotherapy. *J. Virol.* **75,** 9493–9501.

140. Zhang, Y., Chirmule, N., Gao, G., and Wilson, J. (2000) CD40 ligand-dependent activation of cytotoxic T lymphocytes by adeno-associated virus vectors in vivo: role of immature dendritic cells. *J. Virol.* **74,** 8003–8010.

141. Brown, M., Zhang, Y., Dermine, S., et al. (2000) Dendritic cells infected with recombinant fowlpox virus vectors are potent and long-acting stimulators of transgene-specific class I restricted T lymphocyte activity. *Gene Ther.* **7,** 1680–1689.

142. Engelmayer, J., Larsson, M., Lee, A., et al. (2001) Mature dendritic cells infected with canarypox virus elicit strong anti- human immunodeficiency virus CD8+ and CD4+ T-cell responses from chronically infected individuals. *J. Virol.* **75,** 2142–2153.

143. Drexler, I., Antunes, E., Schmitz, M., et al. (1999) Modified vaccinia virus Ankara for delivery of human tyrosinase as melanoma-associated antigen: induction of tyrosinase- and melanoma-specific human leukocyte antigen A*0201-restricted cytotoxic T cells in vitro and in vivo. *Cancer Res.* **59,** 4955–4963.

144. Yang, S., Kittlesen, D., Slingluff, C. L. Jr., Vervaert, C. E., Seigler, H. F., and Darrow, T. L. (2000) Dendritic cells infected with a vaccinia vector carrying the human gp100 gene simultaneously present multiple specificities and elicit high-affinity T cells reactive to multiple epitopes and restricted by HLA-A2 and -A3. *J. Immunol.* **164,** 4204–4211.

145. Reilly, R. T., Gottlieb, M. B., Ercolini, A. M., et al. (2000) HER-2/neu is a tumor rejection target in tolerized HER-2/neu transgenic mice. *Cancer Res.* **60,** 3569–3576.

146. Irvine, K. R., McCabe, B. J., Rosenberg, S. A., and Restifo, N. P. (1995) Synthetic oligonucleotide expressed by a recombinant vaccinia virus elicits therapeutic CTL. *J. Immunol.* **154,** 4651–4657.

147. Bonini, C., Lee, S. P., Riddell, S. R., and Greenberg, P. D. (2001) Targeting antigen in mature dendritic cells for simultaneous stimulation of CD4+ and CD8+ T cells. *J. Immunol.* **166,** 5250–5257.

148. Engelmayer, J., Larsson, M., Subklewe, M., et al. (1999) Vaccinia virus inhibits the maturation of human dendritic cells: a novel mechanism of immune evasion. *J. Immunol.* **163,** 6762–6768.

149. Drillien, R., Spehner, D., Bohbot, A., and Hanau, D. (2000) Vaccinia virus-related events and phenotypic changes after infection of dendritic cells derived from human monocytes. *Virology* **268,** 471–481.

150. Jenne, L., Hauser, C., Arrighi, J. F., Saurat, J. H., and Hugin, A. W. (2000) Poxvirus as a vector to transduce human dendritic cells for immunotherapy: abortive infection but reduced APC function. *Gene Ther.* **7,** 1575–1583.

151. Mikloska, Z., Bosnjak, L., and Cunningham, A. L. (2001) Immature monocyte-derived dendritic cells are productively infected with herpes simplex virus type 1. *J. Virol.* **75,** 5958–5964.

152. Kruse, M., Rosorius, O., Kratzer, F., et al. (2000) Mature dendritic cells infected with herpes simplex virus type 1 exhibit inhibited T-cell stimulatory capacity. *J. Virol.* **74,** 7127–7136.

153. Salio, M., Cella, M., Suter, M., and Lanzavecchia, A. (1999) Inhibition of dendritic cell maturation by herpes simplex virus. *Eur. J. Immunol.* **29,** 3245–3253.

154. Willis, R. A., Bowers, W. J., Turner, M. J., et al. (2001) Dendritic cells transduced with HSV-1 amplicons expressing prostate-specific antigen generate antitumor immunity in mice. *Hum. Gene Ther.* **12,** 1867–1879.

155. Tolba, K. A., Bowers, W. J., Muller, J., et al. (2002) Herpes simplex virus (HSV) amplicon-mediated codelivery of secondary lymphoid tissue chemokine and CD40L results in augmented antitumor activity. *Cancer Res.* **62,** 6545–6551.

156. Toda, M., Martuza, R. L., and Rabkin, S. D. (2000) Tumor growth inhibition by intratumoral inoculation of defective herpes simplex virus vectors expressing granulocyte-macrophage colony-stimulating factor. *Mol. Ther.* **2,** 324–329.

157. Szabolcs, P., Gallardo, H. F., Ciocon, D. H., Sadelain, M., and Young, J. W. (1997) Retrovirally transduced human dendritic cells express a normal phenotype and potent T-cell stimulatory capacity. *Blood* **90,** 2160–2167.

158. Bello-Fernandez, C., Matyash, M., Strobl, H., et al. (1997) Efficient retrovirus-mediated gene transfer of dendritic cells generated from CD34+ cord blood cells under serum-free conditions. *Hum. Gene Ther.* **8,** 1651–1658.

159. Grignani, F., Kinsella, T., Mencarelli, A., et al. (1998) High-efficiency gene transfer and selection of human hematopoietic progenitor cells with a hybrid EBV/retroviral vector expressing the green fluorescence protein. *Cancer Res.* **58,** 14–19.

160. Specht, J. M., Wang, G., Do, M. T., et al. (1997) Dendritic cells retrovirally transduced with a model antigen gene are therapeutically effective against established pulmonary metastases. *J. Exp. Med.* **186,** 1213–1221.

161. zum Buschenfelde, C. M., Metzger, J., Hermann, C., Nicklisch, N., Peschel, C., and Bernhard, H. (2001) The generation of both T killer and Th cell clones specific for the tumor-associated antigen HER2 using retrovirally transduced dendritic cells. *J. Immunol.* **167,** 1712–1719.

162. Schnell, S., Young, J. W., Houghton, A. N., and Sadelain, M. (2000) Retrovirally transduced mouse dendritic cells require CD4+ T cell help to elicit antitumor immunity: implications for the clinical use of dendritic cells. *J. Immunol.* **164,** 1243–1250.

163. Reeves, M. E., Royal, R. E., Lam, J. S., Rosenberg, S. A., and Hwu, P. (1996) Retroviral transduction of human dendritic cells with a tumor- associated antigen gene. *Cancer Res.* **56,** 5672–5677.

164. Chinnasamy, N., Chinnasamy, D., Toso, J. F., et al. (2000) Efficient gene transfer to human peripheral blood mono-cyte-derived dendritic cells using human immunodeficiency virus type 1-based lentiviral vectors. *Hum. Gene Ther.* **11**, 1901–1909.

165. Mangeot, P. E., Negre, D., Dubois, B., et al. (2000) Development of minimal lentivirus vectors derived from sim-ian immunodeficiency virus (SIVmac251) and their use for gene transfer into human dendritic cells. *J. Virol.* **74**, 8307–8315.

166. Mangeot, P. E., Duperrier, K., Negre, D., et al. (2002) High levels of transduction of human dendritic cells with optimized SIV vectors. *Mol. Ther.* **5**, 283–290.

167. Salmon, P., Arrighi, J. F., Piguet, V., et al. (2001) Transduction of CD34+ cells with lentiviral vectors enables the pro-duction of large quantities of transgene-expressing immature and mature dendritic cells. *J. Gene Med.* **3**, 311–320.

168. Negre, D., Mangeot, P. E., Duisit, G., et al. (2000) Characterization of novel safe lentiviral vectors derived from simian immunodeficiency virus (SIVmac251) that efficiently transduce mature human dendritic cells. *Gene Ther.* **7**, 1613–1623.

169. Esslinger, C., Romero, P., and MacDonald, H. R. (2002) Efficient transduction of dendritic cells and induction of a T-cell response by third-generation lentivectors. *Hum. Gene Ther.* **13**, 1091–1100.

170. Dyall, J., Latouche, J. B., Schnell, S., and Sadelain, M. (2001) Lentivirus-transduced human monocyte-derived den-dritic cells efficiently stimulate antigen-specific cytotoxic T lymphocytes. *Blood* **97**, 114–121.

171. Firat, H., Zennou, V., Garcia-Pons, F., et al. (2002) Use of a lentiviral flap vector for induction of CTL immunity against melanoma. Perspectives for immunotherapy. *J. Gene Med.* **4**, 38–45.

172. Ying, H., Zaks, T. Z., Wang, R. F., et al. (1999) Cancer therapy using a self-replicating RNA vaccine. *Nat. Med.* **5**, 823–827.

173. Yamanaka, R., Zullo, S. A., Ramsey, J., et al. (2002) Marked enhancement of antitumor immune responses in mouse brain tumor models by genetically modified dendritic cells producing Semliki Forest virus-mediated interleukin-12. *J. Neurosurg.* **97**, 611–618.

174. Yamanaka, R., Zullo, S. A., Tanaka, R., Blaese, M., and Xanthopoulos, K. G. (2001) Enhancement of antitumor immune response in glioma models in mice by genetically modified dendritic cells pulsed with Semliki forest virus-mediated complementary DNA. *J. Neurosurg.* **94**, 474–481.

175. Cheng, W. F., Hung, C. F., Hsu, K. F., et al. (2001) Enhancement of Sindbis virus self-replicating RNA vaccine potency by targeting antigen to endosomal/lysosomal compartments. *Hum. Gene Ther.* **12**, 235–252.

176. Osterroth, F., Garbe, A., Fisch, P., and Veelken, H. (2000) Stimulation of cytotoxic T cells against idiotype immuno-globulin of malignant lymphoma with protein-pulsed or idiotype-transduced dendritic cells. *Blood* **95**, 1342–1349.

177. Johnston, L. J., Halliday, G. M., and King, N. J. (1996) Phenotypic changes in Langerhans' cells after infection with arboviruses: a role in the immune response to epidermally acquired viral infection? *J. Virol.* **70**, 4761–4766.

178. MacDonald, G. H. and Johnston, R. E. (2000) Role of dendritic cell targeting in Venezuelan equine encephalitis virus pathogenesis. *J. Virol.* **74**, 914–922.

179. Riedl, P., Buschle, M., Reimann, J., and Schirmbeck, R. (2002) Binding immune-stimulating oligonucleotides to cationic peptides from viral core antigen enhances their potency as adjuvants. *Eur. J. Immunol.* **32**, 1709–1716.

180. Strobel, I., Berchtold, S., Gotze, A., Schulze, U., Schuler, G., and Steinkasserer, A. (2000) Human dendritic cells transfected with either RNA or DNA encoding influenza matrix protein M1 differ in their ability to stimulate cyto-toxic T lymphocytes. *Gene Ther.* **7**, 2028–2035.

181. Klinman, D. M., Yamshchikov, G., and Ishigatsubo, Y. (1997) Contribution of CpG motifs to the immunogenicity of DNA vaccines. *J. Immunol.* **158**, 3635–3639.

182. Jakob, T., Walker, P. S., Krieg, A. M., Udey, M. C., and Vogel, J. C. (1998) Activation of cutaneous dendritic cells by CpG-containing oligodeoxynucleotides: a role for dendritic cells in the augmentation of Th1 responses by immunostimulatory DNA. *J. Immunol.* **161**, 3042–3049.

183. Porgador, A., Irvine, K. R., Iwasaki, A., Barber, B. H., Restifo, N. P., and Germain, R. N. (1998) Predominant role for directly transfected dendritic cells in antigen presentation to CD8+ T cells after gene gun immunization. *J. Exp. Med.* **188**, 1075–1082.

184. Mukai, K., Yasutomi, Y., Watanabe, M., et al. (2002) HER2 peptide-specific CD8(+) T cells are proportionally detectable long after multiple DNA vaccinations. *Gene Ther.* **9**, 879–888.

185. Piechocki, M. P., Pilon, S. A., and Wei, W. Z. (2001) Complementary antitumor immunity induced by plasmid DNA encoding secreted and cytoplasmic human ErbB-2. *J. Immunol.* **167**, 3367–3374.

186. Wolkers, M. C., Toebes, M., Okabe, M., Haanen, J. B., and Schumacher, T. N. (2002) Optimizing the efficacy of epitope-directed DNA vaccination. *J. Immunol.* **168**, 4998–5004.

187. Kalat, M., Kupcu, Z., Schuller, S., et al. (2002) In vivo plasmid electroporation induces tumor antigen-specific CD8+ T- cell responses and delays tumor growth in a syngeneic mouse melanoma model. *Cancer Res.* **62**, 5489–5494.

188. Mincheff, M., Altankova, I., Zoubak, S., et al. (2001) In vivo transfection and/or cross-priming of dendritic cells following DNA and adenoviral immunizations for immunotherapy of cancer—changes in peripheral mononuclear subsets and intracellular IL-4 and IFN-gamma lymphokine profile. *Crit. Rev. Oncol. Hematol.* **39**, 125–132.

189. Takashima, A. and Morita, A. (1999) Dendritic cells in genetic immunization. *J. Leukoc. Biol.* **66**, 350–356.

190. Lundqvist, A., Noffz, G., Pavlenko, M., et al. (2002) Nonviral and viral gene transfer into different subsets of human dendritic cells yield comparable efficiency of transfection. *J. Immunother.* **25**, 445–454.

191. Ponsaerts, P., Van den, B. G., Cools, N., et al. (2002) Messenger RNA electroporation of human monocytes, followed by rapid in vitro differentiation, leads to highly stimulatory antigen-loaded mature dendritic cells. *J. Immunol.* **169**, 1669–1675.

192. Saeboe-Larssen, S., Fossberg, E., and Gaudernack, G. (2002) mRNA-based electrotransfection of human dendritic cells and induction of cytotoxic T lymphocyte responses against the telomerase catalytic subunit (hTERT). *J. Immunol. Methods* **259**, 191–203.

193. Wang, L., Smith, D., Bot, S., Dellamary, L., Bloom, A., and Bot, A. (2002) Noncoding RNA danger motifs bridge innate and adaptive immunity and are potent adjuvants for vaccination. *J. Clin. Invest.* **110**, 1175–1184.

194. Gilboa, E., Nair, S. K., and Lyerly, H. K. (1998) Immunotherapy of cancer with dendritic-cell-based vaccines. *Cancer Immunol. Immunother.* **46**, 82–87.

195. Koido, S., Kashiwaba, M., Chen, D., Gendler, S., Kufe, D., and Gong, J. (2000) Induction of antitumor immunity by vaccination of dendritic cells transfected with MUC1 RNA. *J. Immunol.* **165**, 5713–5719.

196. Heiser, A., Coleman, D., Dannull, J., et al. (2002) Autologous dendritic cells transfected with prostate-specific antigen RNA stimulate CTL responses against metastatic prostate tumors. *J. Clin. Invest.* **109**, 409–417.

197. Ashley, D. M., Faiola, B., Nair, S., Hale, L. P., Bigner, D. D., and Gilboa, E. (1997) Bone marrow-generated dendritic cells pulsed with tumor extracts or tumor RNA induce antitumor immunity against central nervous system tumors. *J. Exp. Med.* **186**, 1177–1182.

198. Boczkowski, D., Nair, S. K., Nam, J. H., Lyerly, H. K., and Gilboa, E. (2000) Induction of tumor immunity and cytotoxic T lymphocyte responses using dendritic cells transfected with messenger RNA amplified from tumor cells. *Cancer Res.* **60**, 1028–1034.

199. Zhang, W., He, L., Yuan, Z., et al. (1999) Enhanced therapeutic efficacy of tumor RNA-pulsed dendritic cells after genetic modification with lymphotactin. *Hum. Gene Ther.* **10**, 1151–1161.

200. Bennett, S. R., Carbone, F. R., Karamalis, F., Flavell, R. A., Miller, J. F., and Heath, W. R. (1998) Help for cytotoxic-T-cell responses is mediated by CD40 signalling. *Nature* **393**, 478–480.

201. Schoenberger, S. P., Toes, R. E., van der Voort, E. I., Offringa, R., and Melief, C. J. (1998) T-cell help for cytotoxic T lymphocytes is mediated by CD40–CD40L interactions. *Nature* **393**, 480–483.

202. Fukao, T. (2002) Dendritic-cell-based anticancer vaccination: has it matured? *Trends Immunol.* **23**, 231–232.

203. Mackensen, A., Drager, R., Schlesier, M., Mertelsmann, R., and Lindemann, A. (2000) Presence of IgE antibodies to bovine serum albumin in a patient developing anaphylaxis after vaccination with human peptide-pulsed dendritic cells. *Cancer Immunol. Immunother.* **49**, 152–156.

204. Condon, C., Watkins, S. C., Celluzzi, C. M., Thompson, K., and Falo, L. D. Jr. (1996) DNA-based immunization by in vivo transfection of dendritic cells. *Nat. Med.* **2**, 1122–1128.

205. Eggert, A. A., Schreurs, M. W., Boerman, O. C., et al. (1999) Biodistribution and vaccine efficiency of murine dendritic cells are dependent on the route of administration. *Cancer Res.* **59**, 3340–3345.

206. De Vries I. J., Krooshoop, D. J., Scharenberg, N. M., et al. (2003) Effective migration of antigen-pulsed dendritic cells to lymph nodes in melanoma patients is determined by their maturation state. *Cancer Res.* **63**, 12–17.

207. Akbari, O., Panjwani, N., Garcia, S., Tascon, R., Lowrie, D., and Stockinger, B. (1999) DNA vaccination: transfection and activation of dendritic cells as key events for immunity. *J. Exp. Med.* **189**, 169–178.

208. Corr, M., von Damm, A., Lee, D. J., and Tighe, H. (1999) In vivo priming by DNA injection occurs predominantly by antigen transfer. *J. Immunol.* **163**, 4721–4727.

209. Morita, A., Ariizumi, K., Ritter, R. III, et al. (2001) Development of a Langerhans cell-targeted gene therapy format using a dendritic cell-specific promoter. *Gene Ther.* **8**, 1729–1737.

210. Mercier, S., Gahery-Segard, H., Monteil, M., et al. (2002) Distinct roles of adenovirus vector-transduced dendritic cells, myoblasts, and endothelial cells in mediating an immune response against a transgene product. *J. Virol.* **76**, 2899–2911.

211. Jooss, K., Yang, Y., Fisher, K. J., and Wilson, J. M. (1998) Transduction of dendritic cells by DNA viral vectors directs the immune response to transgene products in muscle fibers. *J. Virol.* **72**, 4212–4223.

212. Sarukhan, A., Soudais, C., Danos, O., and Jooss, K. (2001) Factors influencing cross-presentation of non-self antigens expressed from recombinant adeno-associated virus vectors. *J. Gene Med.* **3**, 260–270.

213. Larsson, M., Fonteneau, J. F., Somersan, S., et al. (2001) Efficiency of cross presentation of vaccinia virus-derived antigens by human dendritic cells. *Eur. J. Immunol.* **31**, 3432–3442.

214. Guyre, P. M., Graziano, R. F., Goldstein, J., et al. (1997) Increased potency of Fc-receptor-targeted antigens. *Cancer Immunol. Immunother.* **45**, 146–148.

215. Biragyn, A., Surenhu, M., Yang, D., et al. (2001) Mediators of innate immunity that target immature, but not mature, dendritic cells induce antitumor immunity when genetically fused with nonimmunogenic tumor antigens. *J. Immunol.* **167**, 6644–6653.

216. Foged, C., Sundblad, A., and Hovgaard, L. (2002) Targeting vaccines to dendritic cells. *Pharm. Res.* **19,** 229–238.

217. Xiang, R., Primus, F. J., Ruehlmann, J. M., et al. (2001) A dual-function DNA vaccine encoding carcinoembryonic antigen and CD40 ligand trimer induces T cell-mediated protective immunity against colon cancer in carcinoembryonic antigen-transgenic mice. *J. Immunol.* **167,** 4560–4565.

218. Hung, C. F., Hsu, K. F., Cheng, W. F., et al. (2001) Enhancement of DNA vaccine potency by linkage of antigen gene to a gene encoding the extracellular domain of Fms-like tyrosine kinase 3-ligand. *Cancer Res.* **61,** 1080–1088.

219. Deas, O., Angevin, E., Cherbonnier, C., et al. (2002) In vivo-targeted gene delivery using antibody-based nonviral vector. *Hum. Gene Ther.* **13,** 1101–1114.

220. Diebold, S. S., Kursa, M., Wagner, E., Cotten, M., and Zenke, M. (1999) Mannose polyethylenimine conjugates for targeted DNA delivery into dendritic cells. *J. Biol. Chem.* **274,** 19,087–19,094.

221. Berg, S. F., Mjaaland, S., and Fossum, S. (1994) Comparing macrophages and dendritic leukocytes as antigen-presenting cells for humoral responses in vivo by antigen targeting. *Eur. J. Immunol.* **24,** 1262–1268.

222. Carayanniotis, G. and Barber, B. H. (1990) Characterization of the adjuvant-free serological response to protein antigens coupled to antibodies specific for class II MHC determinants. *Vaccine* **8,** 137–144.

223. Skea, D. L. and Barber, B. H. (1993) Studies of the adjuvant-independent antibody response to immunotargeting. Target structure dependence, isotype distribution, and induction of long term memory. *J. Immunol.* **151,** 3557–3568.

224. Wang, H., Griffiths, M. N., Burton, D. R., and Ghazal, P. (2000) Rapid antibody responses by low-dose, single-step, dendritic cell- targeted immunization. *Proc. Natl. Acad. Sci. USA* **97,** 847–852.

225. Hawiger, D., Inaba, K., Dorsett, Y., et al. (2001) Dendritic cells induce peripheral T cell unresponsiveness under steady state conditions in vivo. *J. Exp. Med.* **194,** 769–779.

226. Tan, M. C., Mommaas, A. M., Drijfhout, J. W., et al. (1997) Mannose receptor-mediated uptake of antigens strongly enhances HLA class II-restricted antigen presentation by cultured dendritic cells. *Eur. J. Immunol.* **27,** 2426–2435.

227. Mahnke, K., Guo, M., Lee, S., et al. (2000) The dendritic cell receptor for endocytosis, DEC-205, can recycle and enhance antigen presentation via major histocompatibility complex class II-positive lysosomal compartments. *J. Cell Biol.* **151,** 673–684.

228. Schjetne, K. W., Thompson, K. M., Aarvak, T., Fleckenstein, B., Sollid, L. M., and Bogen, B. (2002) A mouse C(kappa)-specific T cell clone indicates that DC-SIGN is an efficient target for antibody-mediated delivery of T cell epitopes for MHC class II presentation. *Int. Immunol.* **14,** 1423–1430.

229. Engering, A., Geijtenbeek, T. B., van Vliet, S. J., et al. (2002) The dendritic cell-specific adhesion receptor DC-SIGN internalizes antigen for presentation to T cells. *J. Immunol.* **168,** 2118–2126.

230. Biragyn, A., Ruffini, P. A., Leifer, C. A., et al. (2002) Toll-like receptor 4-dependent activation of dendritic cells by beta-defensin 2. *Science* **298,** 1025–1029.

231. Salamero, J., Bausinger, H., Mommaas, A. M., et al. (2001) CD1a molecules traffic through the early recycling endosomal pathway in human Langerhans cells. *J. Invest. Dermatol.* **116,** 401–408.

232. Josien, R., Li, H. L., Ingulli, E., et al. (2000) TRANCE, a tumor necrosis factor family member, enhances the longevity and adjuvant properties of dendritic cells in vivo. *J. Exp. Med.* **191,** 495–502.

233. Regnault, A., Lankar, D., Lacabanne, V., et al. (1999) Fcgamma receptor-mediated induction of dendritic cell maturation and major histocompatibility complex class I-restricted antigen presentation after immune complex internalization. *J. Exp. Med.* **189,** 371–380.

234. Rafiq, K., Bergtold, A., and Clynes, R. (2002) Immune complex-mediated antigen presentation induces tumor immunity. *J. Clin. Invest.* **110,** 71–79.

235. Amigorena, S. (2002) Fc gamma receptors and cross-presentation in dendritic cells. *J. Exp. Med.* **195,** F1–F3.

236. Morel, Y., Truneh, A., Sweet, R. W., Olive, D., and Costello, R. T. (2001) The TNF superfamily members LIGHT and CD154 (CD40 ligand) costimulate induction of dendritic cell maturation and elicit specific CTL activity. *J. Immunol.* **167,** 2479–2486.

237. Rescigno, M., Piguet, V., Valzasina, B., et al. (2000) Fas engagement induces the maturation of dendritic cells (DCs), the release of interleukin (IL)-1beta, and the production of interferon gamma in the absence of IL-12 during DC-T cell cognate interaction: a new role for Fas ligand in inflammatory responses. *J. Exp. Med.* **192,** 1661–1668.

238. Hsu, T. L., Chang, Y. C., Chen, S. J., et al. (2002) Modulation of dendritic cell differentiation and maturation by decoy receptor 3. *J. Immunol.* **168,** 4846–4853.

239. Wilcox, R. A., Chapoval, A. I., Gorski, K. S., et al. (2002) Cutting edge: Expression of functional CD137 receptor by dendritic cells. *J. Immunol.* **168,** 4262–4267.

240. Moodycliffe, A. M., Shreedhar, V., Ullrich, S. E., et al. (2000) CD40-CD40 ligand interactions in vivo regulate migration of antigen- bearing dendritic cells from the skin to draining lymph nodes. *J. Exp. Med.* **191,** 2011–2020.

241. Cremer, I., Dieu-Nosjean, M. C., Marechal, S., et al. (2002) Long-lived immature dendritic cells mediated by TRANCE-RANK interaction. *Blood* **100,** 3646–3655.

242. Tada, Y., Wang, J., Takiguchi, Y., et al. (2002) Cutting edge: a novel role for Fas ligand in facilitating antigen acquisition by dendritic cells. *J. Immunol.* **169,** 2241–2245.

243. Castellino, F., Boucher, P. E., Eichelberg, K., et al. (2000) Receptor-mediated uptake of antigen/heat shock protein complexes results in major histocompatibility complex class I antigen presentation via two distinct processing pathways. *J. Exp. Med.* **191,** 1957–1964.

244. Chattergoon, M. A., Kim, J. J., Yang, J. S., et al. (2000) Targeted antigen delivery to antigen-presenting cells including dendritic cells by engineered Fas-mediated apoptosis. *Nat. Biotechnol.* **18,** 974–979.

245. Kumanogoh, A., Suzuki, K., Ch'ng, E., et al. (2002) Requirement for the lymphocyte semaphorin, CD100, in the induction of antigen-specific T cells and the maturation of dendritic cells. *J. Immunol.* **169,** 1175–1181.

246. Nestle, F. O., Banchereau, J., and Hart, D. (2001) Dendritic cells: On the move from bench to bedside. *Nat. Med.* **7,** 761–765.

247. Conry, R. M., Khazaeli, M. B., Saleh, M. N., et al. (1999) Phase I trial of a recombinant vaccinia virus encoding carcinoembryonic antigen in metastatic adenocarcinoma: comparison of intradermal vs subcutaneous administration. *Clin. Cancer Res.* **5,** 2330–2337.

248. Conry, R. M., Allen, K. O., Lee, S., Moore, S. E., Shaw, D. R., and LoBuglio, A. F. (2000) Human autoantibodies to carcinoembryonic antigen (CEA) induced by a vaccinia-CEA vaccine. *Clin. Cancer Res.* **6,** 34–41.

249. Gulley, J., Chen, A. P., Dahut, W., et al. (2002) Phase I study of a vaccine using recombinant vaccinia virus expressing PSA (rV-PSA) in patients with metastatic androgen-independent prostate cancer. *Prostate* **53,** 109–117.

250. Borysiewicz, L. K., Fiander, A., Nimako, M., et al. (1996) A recombinant vaccinia virus encoding human papillomavirus types 16 and 18, E6 and E7 proteins as immunotherapy for cervical cancer. *Lancet* **347,** 1523–1527.

251. Marshall, J. L., Hoyer, R. J., Toomey, M. A., et al. (2000) Phase I study in advanced cancer patients of a diversified prime-and- boost vaccination protocol using recombinant vaccinia virus and recombinant nonreplicating avipox virus to elicit anti-carcinoembryonic antigen immune responses. *J. Clin. Oncol.* **18,** 3964–3973.

252. Scholl, S. M., Balloul, J. M., Le Goc, G., et al. (2000) Recombinant vaccinia virus encoding human MUC1 and IL2 as immunotherapy in patients with breast cancer. *J. Immunother.* **23,** 570–580.

253. Horig, H., Lee, D. S., Conkright, W., et al. (2000) Phase I clinical trial of a recombinant canarypoxvirus (ALVAC) vaccine expressing human carcinoembryonic antigen and the B7.1 co-stimulatory molecule. *Cancer Immunol. Immunother.* **49,** 504–514.

254. von Mehren, M., Arlen, P., Gulley, J., et al. (2001) The influence of granulocyte macrophage colony-stimulating factor and prior chemotherapy on the immunological response to a vaccine (ALVAC- CEA B7.1) in patients with metastatic carcinoma. *Clin. Cancer Res.* **7,** 1181–1191.

255. Norbury, C. C., Malide, D., Gibbs, J. S., Bennink, J. R., and Yewdell, J. W. (2002) Visualizing priming of virus-specific CD8+ T cells by infected dendritic cells in vivo. *Nat. Immunol.* **3,** 265–271.

256. Rosenberg, S. A., Zhai, Y., Yang, J. C., et al. (1998) Immunizing patients with metastatic melanoma using recombinant adenoviruses encoding MART-1 or gp100 melanoma antigens. *J. Natl. Cancer Inst.* **90,** 1894–1900.

257. Kuball, J., Schuler, M., Antunes, F. E., et al. (2002) Generating p53-specific cytotoxic T lymphocytes by recombinant adenoviral vector-based vaccination in mice, but not man. *Gene Ther.* **9,** 833–843.

258. Conry, R. M., Curiel, D. T., Strong, T. V., et al. (2002) Safety and immunogenicity of a DNA vaccine encoding carcinoembryonic antigen and hepatitis B surface antigen in colorectal carcinoma patients. *Clin. Cancer Res.* **8,** 2782–2787.

259. Timmerman, J. M., Singh, G., Hermanson, G., et al. (2002) Immunogenicity of a plasmid DNA vaccine encoding chimeric idiotype in patients with B-cell lymphoma. *Cancer Res.* **62,** 5845–5852.

260. Pecher, G., Haring, A., Kaiser, L., and Thiel, E. (2002) Mucin gene (MUC1) transfected dendritic cells as vaccine: results of a phase I/II clinical trial. *Cancer Immunol. Immunother.* **51,** 669–673.

261. Heiser, A., Coleman, D., Dannull, J., et al. (2002) Autologous dendritic cells transfected with prostate-specific antigen RNA stimulate CTL responses against metastatic prostate tumors. *J. Clin. Invest.* **109,** 409–417.

262. Schmitz, M., Bornhauser, M., Ockert, D., and Rieber, E. P. (2002) Cancer immunotherapy: novel strategies and clinical experiences. *Trends Immunol.* **23,** 428–429.

263. Arienti, F., Belli, F., Napolitano, F., et al. (1999) Vaccination of melanoma patients with interleukin 4 gene-transduced allogeneic melanoma cells. *Hum. Gene Ther.* **10,** 2907–2916.

264. Kusumoto, M., Umeda, S., Ikubo, A., et al. (2001) Phase 1 clinical trial of irradiated autologous melanoma cells adenovirally transduced with human GM-CSF gene. *Cancer Immunol. Immunother.* **50,** 373–381.

265. Jaffee, E. M., Hruban, R. H., Biedrzycki, B., et al. (2001) Novel allogeneic granulocyte-macrophage colony-stimulating factor- secreting tumor vaccine for pancreatic cancer: a phase I trial of safety and immune activation. *J. Clin. Oncol.* **19,** 145–156.

266. Soiffer, R., Lynch, T., Mihm, M., et al. (1998) Vaccination with irradiated autologous melanoma cells engineered to secrete human granulocyte-macrophage colony-stimulating factor generates potent antitumor immunity in patients with metastatic melanoma. *Proc. Natl. Acad. Sci. USA* **95,** 13,141–13,146.

267. Simons, J. W., Mikhak, B., Chang, J. F., et al. (1999) Induction of immunity to prostate cancer antigens: results of a clinical trial of vaccination with irradiated autologous prostate tumor cells engineered to secrete granulocyte-macrophage colony-stimulating factor using ex vivo gene transfer. *Cancer Res.* **59,** 5160–5168.

268. Simons, J. W., Jaffee, E. M., Weber, C. E., et al. (1997) Bioactivity of autologous irradiated renal cell carcinoma vaccines generated by ex vivo granulocyte-macrophage colony-stimulating factor gene transfer. *Cancer Res.* **57,** 1537–1546.

11

Dendritic Cells

Weiping Zou, Shuang Wei, and Tyler J. Curiel

1. INTRODUCTION

Dendritic cells (DCs) are the principal immune cells priming naïve T lymphocytes to initiate adaptive immunity. DCs have been referred to as "nature's adjuvant" owing to their potency in igniting immune responses (1). They originate from proliferating hematopoietic progenitor cells in bone marrow and enter blood as nonproliferating precursor cells. These precursor cells then seed all tissues, in which they differentiate into immature DCs that sample the environment for "danger" or foreign antigens. If such is encountered, they migrate to locally draining lymph nodes, during which transit they undergo a process of maturation. In maturation, their capacity to acquire antigen is lost simultaneous with their acquisition of an enormous capacity to prime naïve T cells.

In the following sections, all major aspects of DCs are discussed in much greater detail, and issues of particular relevance to gene therapy are addressed.

2. HISTORICAL ASPECTS

Paul Langerhans originally described immune DCs in skin in 1868. He thought they were neural cells and failed to make the link between them and immune responses. Studies of DCs languished for almost a century until Ralph Steinman and his colleagues at the Rockefeller University rediscovered them in 1972. Links to immunity were quickly made, but progress in understanding the function of these cells was hampered by their scarcity in vivo and a lack of adequate means to propagate them in vitro. Progress in understanding the function of DCs was boosted tremendously by the discovery that bone marrow cells and blood monocytes differentiated into DCs in vitro when cultured with recombinant cytokines including granulocyte-macrophage colony-stimulating factor (GM-CSF), interleukin 4 (IL-4), or tumor necrosis factor-α (TNF-α). Details of these in vitro systems are described in Section 10.

3. DC DIFFERENTIATION

Bone marrow contains a population of proliferating CD34[+] progenitor cells that give rise to the cellular elements of blood, including DCs. As these progenitor cells differentiate, they exit marrow and enter blood as nonproliferating DC precursor cells (1). Two principal DC precursor cells circulate in human blood, giving rise to apparently distinct DC lineages. Myeloid DCs (MDCs) arise from lineage-negative precursor cells expressing human leukocyte antigen (HLA)-DR and CD11c, and plasmacytoid DCs (PDCs) arise from lineage-negative precursor cells expressing HLA-DR, but lacking CD11c (2,3). Figure 1 provides a graphic depiction. A hallmark of PDC precursor cells is their striking production of type I interferons following viral infection (3,4), which is used to confirm functional identity in vitro. Although there are clear functional differences between MDCs and PDCs, these lineage distinctions are still controversial and are likely to be modified as new data emerge.

From: *Contemporary Cancer Research*
Cancer Gene Therapy
Edited by: D. T. Curiel and J. T. Douglas © Humana Press Inc., Totowa, NJ

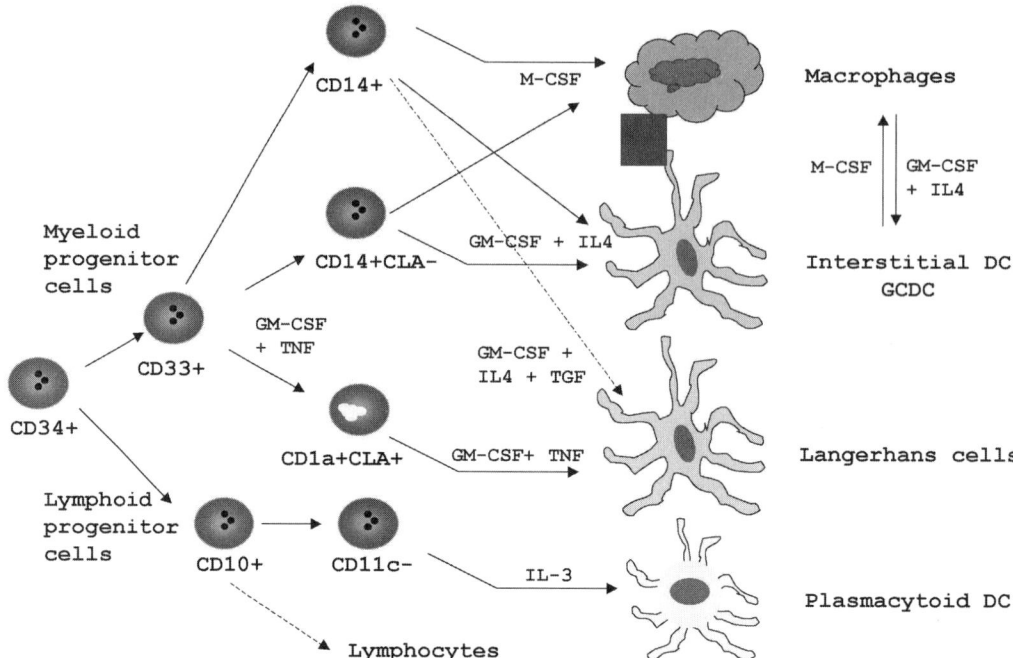

Fig. 1. Dendritic cells arise from proliferating CD34+ bone marrow progenitor cells. They seed blood as nonproliferating precursor cells that are categorized as CD11c+ (giving rise to MDCs and Langerhans DCs) or CD11c− (giving rise to PDCs). Various cytokines as indicated can be added to these cells to induce terminal differentiation of the various dendritic cell subsets.

4. DC MATURATION AND ACTIVATION

Nonproliferating DC precursor cells exit blood to seed essentially all lymphoid and nonlymphoid tissues, in which they remain in a nonmigratory, immature form, poised to sample the environment for signs of danger or foreign antigens. Proinflammatory signals such as interleukin (IL)-1β and TNF-α, viral and bacterial products such as CpG, and bacterial cell wall components such as lipopolysaccharide enhance DC maturation. For complete DC activation/maturation, a CD40 signal (usually delivered through T-cell CD40L) is also required. Following activation through CD40, DCs acquire a significant capacity to activate cytotoxic T lymphocytes (*5,6*).

Immature DCs are highly specialized to capture antigens, but are poor at priming naïve T cells. As DCs mature, they lose their capacity to capture antigen and simultaneously acquire an extraordinary capacity to prime naïve T cells. Mechanisms to capture antigen include pinocytosis, phagocytosis, and receptor-mediated mechanisms.

Immature DCs are highly migratory cells, although factors controlling their mobilization are poorly understood. Migration is dictated by expression of chemokine receptors, integrins, and selectins (*7,8*). Migration signals in human cancers may differ compared to homeostatic signals (*7*). DC migration likely also depends on the tissue origin of the DCs, local factors, and specific characteristics of the mobilizing/migratory signals. Figure 2 provides a depiction of critical events in DC migration.

5. DC MOBILIZATION

Granulocyte colony-stimulating factor (G-CSF), GM-CSF and Fms-like tyrosine kinase 3 ligand (FLT3L) are growth factors developed to help mobilize granulocytes and myeloid cells to combat infection in patients with low peripheral blood white cell counts, such as following cytotoxic chemo-

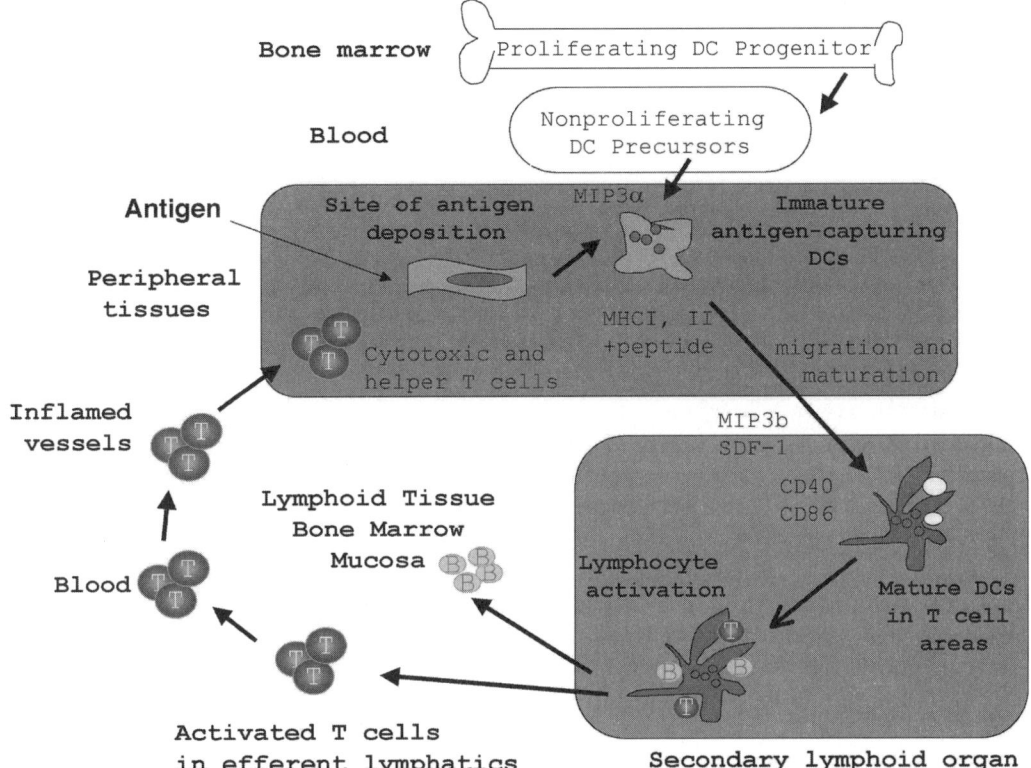

Fig. 2. Immature dendritic cells reside in peripheral tissue, in which they are attracted by local MIP3α expression. Immature dendritic cells are poised to capture antigen and continuously sample the environment. Following exposure to foreign antigens or proinflammatory danger signals, dendritic cells undergo a remarkable maturation process by which they exit into lymph channels to migrate to local draining lymph nodes. During maturation, antigen capture capacity is lost in place of strong T- or B-cell-stimulating capacity. In lymph nodes, these matured/activated dendritic cells instruct antigen-specific cells, which then exit and return to the original site of inflammation to execute their specific effector functions. Mature dendritic cells die by apoptosis in lymph nodes. M-CSF, macrophage colony-stimulating factor; MIP3α, macrophage inflammatory protein 3α; GCDC, germinal center dendritic cell.

therapy. Recent work demonstrated that these growth factors also mobilize circulating DCs. For example, G-CSF preferentially mobilizes CD11c⁻ PDC precursor cells (although it also mobilizes CD11c⁺ DC precursor cells). GM-CSF preferentially mobilizes CD11c⁺ MDCs and their precursor cells, whereas FLT3L mobilizes large numbers of both PDCs and MDCs in humans following exogenous administration (9).

6. MYELOID DC

MDCs appear as either interstitial DCs in the dermal layers of skin and most organs or as Langerhans DCs, which populate and survey the epidermal layer of skin (10). Interstitial DCs are equivalent to the well-known in vitro monocyte-derived DCs (1). Initiation of humoral responses might preferentially be regulated by interstitial DCs. Langerhans DCs are poor at pinocytosis and apoptotic body capture, but excellent in elicitation of cytotoxic T lymphocytes and induction of CD4⁺ and CD8⁺ T-cell proliferation. Interstitial DCs may preferentially elicit cellular immunity. Experimental evidence also suggests that Langerhans DCs are better than interstitial DCs in elicitation of cytotoxic T lymphocytes (11,12).

7. PLASMACYTOID DC

Human PDCs arise from circulating cells lacking lineage markers and CD11c, but expressing HLA-DR, and are further identified phenotypically by expression of CD123, the IL-3Rβ chain *(3)*. PDC precursor cells are the principal circulating cell of the PDC lineage and were identified as high type I interferon-producing cells following virus infection *(13)*. This type I interferon induces significant Th1 polarization *(14)*. When activated through CD40 or CpG motifs, PDCs may also induce T-cell interferon-γ through IL-12 secretion *(14,15)*. PDCs may also mediate antigen-specific tolerance *(16)*. The mouse equivalent of human PDCs was described *(17)*, which may help allow more detailed studies of this rare and little-known DC subset.

8. T-CELL ACTIVATION

Immature MDCs express few T-cell costimulatory molecules, such as CD40, CD54, CD80, CD86, major histocompatibility complex (MHC) classes I and II. Following maturation, through a variety of mechanisms, MDCs greatly increase all of these T-cell costimulatory molecules and also express CD83, a molecule with a function that is incompletely understood, but that is a hallmark of mature MDCs. PDCs express these molecules as well and upregulate them following maturation, but expression levels are generally lower in the immature and mature states compared to MDCs, and they are less potent in priming naïve T cells. The capacity of MDCs or PDCs to prime naïve T lymphocytes forms the basis of the standard mixed lymphocyte reaction.

Immature MDCs are poor at inducing naïve CD4+ T-cell proliferation and induce T-cell IL-4 and interferon-γ, but no significant T-cell IL-10. Following maturation, their capacity to induce T-cell interferon-γ increases substantially. Immature MDCs secrete little IL-12 and IL-10. Following maturation, they greatly increase IL-12 secretion, which is critical to their capacity to induce Th1 polarization and T-cell interferon-γ secretion, and increase IL-10 secretion, but to a much lesser degree. Mature MDCs also secrete a variety of other soluble factors, such as IL-6, IL-18, TNF-α, and chemokines. The immunobiological roles of all of these factors remain to be fully defined. The murine counterparts of human MDCs are similar in most of these important aspects.

Immature (precursor) PDCs secrete few type I interferons, but secrete enormous quantities following virus infection and other triggers, including CD40 ligation, immune complex engagement, and CpG motifs. These type I interferons induce Th1 polarization of T cells. Human PDCs do not generally secrete significant IL-12, although this may occur in virus infection through CpG stimulation *(15)*. The capacity of PDCs to secrete type I interferons following viral infections may be exploited in particular gene therapy strategies, although little published work in this regard exists. Mature PDCs also secrete the chemokines IP-10 and IL-8 and the cytokines TNF-α and IL-6. Murine PDCs are similar to human PDCs in many regards, but do express CD11c and, more important, do secrete significant IL-12 *(17,18)*.

9. ANTIGEN PROCESSING

DCs prime or activate a variety of antigen-specific immune cells through presentation of antigen in the context of both MHC class I and class II. Thus, DCs possess a variety of mechanisms by which antigen is introduced into the MHC class I or II pathways for eventual presentation to antigen-specific cells. DCs use classic antigen-processing pathways for processing exogenous antigen into MHC class II and endogenous antigen into class I. Further, they may capture apoptotic bodies through the surface receptors CD36 or $\alpha_v\beta_5$ integrins for processing and presentation in the MHC class I pathway *(19,20)*. Several DC-specific antigen capture receptors or processing mechanisms have been identified, including DC-LAMP *(21)* and DC-SIGN *(22)*. These relatively DC-specific molecules may make rational targets for DC-targeting gene therapy strategies.

The ultimate differentiation potential and effector function of MDCs or PDCs is dictated by micro-environmental conditions and signals. For example, MDCs differentiating and maturing under homeostatic conditions generally induce potent Th1 polarization. However, when matured in the presence of prostaglandins, they may induce Th2 polarization *(23)*. MDCs subjected to IL-10 may induce T-cell anergy or tolerance, which can impede tumor-specific immunity *(24,25)*. T cells repeatedly stimulated with immature, rather than mature, MDCs may induce IL-10-secreting regulatory T cells *(26)* and can induce antigen-specific tolerance in humans *(27)*.

Immature PDCs in blood may induce a Th0 phenotype characterized by T-cell secretion of both interferon-γ and IL-4. However, following activation by virus infection, they induce potent Th1 polarization through interferon-γ secretion. In tumors, PDCs may induce T-cell IL-10, contributing to tumor-mediated immune suppression *(7)*. The roles of PDCs in maintaining tolerance (16,28), mediating allergic airway disease *(29)*, and other functions remains poorly defined, but are under active investigation *(30)*.

10. IN VITRO GENERATION OF DCs

Study of DCs was hampered for decades by lack of sufficient numbers owing to their scarcity in vivo. It is now possible to generate large numbers of DCs in vitro using techniques that have revolutionized their study. Generally, the easiest way to generate DCs in vitro is to culture precursor cells in recombinant GM-SCF plus IL-4. R&D Systems (Minneapolis, MN) produces a variety of high-quality mouse and human cytokines for this purpose (we have no financial interest in this company). Different cytokine manufacturers may use different units to measure potency, so care should be taken to ensure that correct concentrations of cytokines are used if products are purchased from vendors with methods that differ from those cited in published methods.

DCs may routinely be cultured from human, mouse, or rhesus monkey cells *(31–34)*. DCs may also be cultivated from chimpanzees *(35–37)*, rats *(37,38)*, and pigs *(40)*, affording may potential applications in gene therapy studies. DC phenotype and function can be affected by the precursor cells from which they are derived, by any growth factors used to mobilize precursor cells, differentiation or maturation factors, or the anatomic location from which the DC or its precursor cell was recovered *(1)*. All these factors must be considered when choosing a DC system for a specific gene therapy (or other) application.

Monocytes can be induced to differentiate into DCs in the absence of exogenous cytokines. For example, mouse anti-CD40 agonist antibody induces monocytes to differentiate into DCs in a process augmented by addition of GM-CSF plus IL-4 *(41)*. Monocytes may differentiate into cells with many features of MDCs following exposure to specific calcium ionophores *(42)*. Monocytes reverse transmigrating across endothelial surfaces will differentiate into MDCs in the absence of exogenous cytokines *(43,44)*, which may be a mechanism by which DC precursor cells differentiate into DCs in vivo. Gene therapy vectors themselves have been reported to induce MDC differentiation in monocytes, which is addressed in detail in Section 11.

10.1. Cultivation of Mouse DCs

Inaba and associates *(45)* described a novel in vitro technique that has been modified over the years. Marrow cells are recovered from the femur and tibia, purified, and cultured with recombinant murine GM-CSF to induce DC differentiation. These DCs can be matured by lipopolysaccharide (LPS) or TNF-α treatment or other means. CD34$^+$ cells obtained from mouse bone marrow will also differentiate into DCs when cultured with GM-CSF plus FLT3L *(46)* or GM-CSF, TNF-α, and stem cell factor (SCF) *(47)*. Addition of transforming growth factor-β drives precursor cells down a Langerhans DC differentiation pathway *(48)*. Mouse skin is a significant source of Langerhans DCs (from epidermis) and interstitial DCs (from dermis) *(49)*. Macrophages of mouse *(50)* or human *(51)* origin also serve as DC precursor cells, with properties that may differ from typical monocyte-derived MDCs *(51)*. DCs may be isolated directly from mouse *(52,53)* or human *(7)* tumors for studies as desired. Several murine DC lines are available, some of which have many features typical of primary DCs *(54,55)*.

10.2. Cultivation of Human DCs

The best-studied human DCs are those monocyte-derived DCs (MDDCs) *(56–60)*. For most DC-generation purposes, monocytes may be isolated from peripheral blood mononuclear cells by simple plastic adherence. To produce immature MDDCs, monocytes are cultured with recombinant human GM-CSF plus IL-4 for 5 to 7 days. Reported amounts of GM-CSF and IL-4 used to differentiate MDDCs vary considerably. Some investigators use serum-free medium or autologous plasma instead of fetal calf serum as fetal calf serum may contain trace amounts of endotoxin, transforming growth factor-β, or other factors *(61)*. Maturation can be effected by an additional culture with *Escherichia coli* lipopolysaccharide or by a variety of other agents, well-described elsewhere, including TNF-α plus IL-1β, monocyte-conditioned medium, type I interferons, and more elaborate cocktails *(1,62,63)*.

Culture conditions other than GM-CSF plus IL-4 will also effect monocyte-to-MDDC differentiation. Advantages of one culture system over another may not always be clear, aside from cost considerations and from using what may not be considered "standard conditions." Investigators should give considerations to experimental conditions, desired results, and other factors when deciding on a specific DC culture method. Although Langerhans DCs may be derived from CD34+ precursor cells or monocytes, they were originally described following isolation from skin *(64)*.

DC progenitor cells differ from precursor cells in that they proliferate. Thus, DC yields can be increased if the progenitor pool is first expanded prior to differentiation into DCs. In this regard, CD34+ cells from leukopheresis or marrow serve as an excellent source of proliferating DC progenitor cells for DC generation. The yield of CD34+ cells in blood can be increased greatly by treating donors with factors such as FLT3L or G-CSF prior to leukopheresis. Umbilical cord blood contains many more CD34+ cells than normal adult blood. Cord blood CD34+ cells can be obtained using paramagnetic beads (Miltenyi or Dynal) with equivalent yields *(65–67)* or can be obtained by flow cytometry.

If human DCs grown ex vivo are to be transfused adoptively back into human subjects, special attention must be paid to the nature of the cell collection, culture conditions, differentiation agents, maturation agents, and antigens used. In the United States, the Food and Drug Administration closely scrutinizes human trials involving transfused, manipulated cells, particularly when gene therapy is involved, and usually must approve such trials before they can be effected. Cells and viruses must be cultivated and prepared in specialized good laboratory practice facilities, which are loosely defined and not as stringently controlled as good manufacturing process facilities used in manufacture of drugs and biologics by pharmaceutical and biotechnology companies.

11. DCs AND GENE THERAPY

DCs are highly efficient in priming naïve T lymphocytes. Thus, the majority of reported gene therapy studies involving DCs capitalize on this role and are designed to induce antigen-specific T cells for a variety of purposes. MDCs are transducible by standard retroviral and adenovirus *(68)* agents with variable degrees of success, although adenoviruses are probably superior in many instances *(69)*. Adenoviruses require coxsackie and adenovirus receptor for optimal transduction. Thus, MDC transfection may be improved using tropism-modified adenoviruses. Adenovirus genetically modified to express coxsackie and adenovirus receptor-binding motifs are improved in their capacity to transduce human and rhesus monkey MDCs *(70)*. CD40-conjugated adenovirus is more efficient in MDC transduction compared to parental virus and has the additional benefit of effecting MDC maturation through the CD40 signal *(71,72)*.

Other DC-targeting strategies for viral vectors have also been successful *(73)*. Bystander MDCs infused into animals treated with gene therapy agents to induce local TNF-α *(74,75)* or IL-18 *(74,75)* expression enhances tumor immunity. Repeated treatments with virus-transduced MDCs paradoxically may decrease protective antitumor immunity in some mouse strains *(76)*, although the implications for human trials remain unknown.

Because of the inherent difficulties in transducing DCs with lentiviral or retroviral vectors, improved vectors with enhanced DC gene transfer capacity have been proposed *(77,78)*, some with a claim of superiority to adenovirus vectors in DC transduction efficiency *(79)*. Murine leukemia virus (MLV), human immunodeficiency virus-based, and other retroviral or lentiviral vectors have also been used to improve DC transduction efficiency *(80–82)*. High tumor antigen expression and immunity may be achieved by fusion of DCs to live tumors *(83)*. A final variation on these themes of improved cell transduction and antigen presentation is to construct an artificial DC based on a cell type that is highly amenable to virus-driven gene expression, which has been done using engineered mouse fibroblasts *(84)*.

Mature CD83⁺ MDCs are also susceptible to adenovirus-mediated gene transfer, although such constructs may be immunosuppressive rather than stimulatory *(85)*. Adenoviruses may be encapsulated in liposomes further to enhance MDC transfection *(86)*. Adenovirus also transduces PDCs and induces secretion of PDC type I interferons in the process *(87)*, although specific gene therapy strategies in this regard have not been reported. Adeno-associated viruses also transduce DCs *(88)*. Nonvirologic methods to transduce DCs have also been successful *(89)*. Although DCs transduced with viral vectors may also induce immunity to the vector as well as the gene product, clinically significant tumor-specific immunity may nonetheless be effected *(90)*. Such approaches are discussed in much greater detail elsewhere in this textbook.

DCs can also be modified by gene therapy to mediate tolerance *(91,92)* or immune suppression *(93)* instead of active immunity, which may be clinically useful in a variety of settings, including transplant acceptance *(94)*.

Frustratingly, there are no single, DC-specific markers available for DC-targeted vector development. Nonetheless, DCs may be preferentially targeted through their high expression of class II molecules.

12. ADENOVIRUS-TRANSDUCED DCs IN HUMAN CLINICAL TRIALS

It is well established that adenoviruses can be modified to effect high-efficiency transfection of human DCs, and that this transduction induces DC maturation, augmenting T-cell-activating capacity *(72,86,95,96)*. Adenovirus-mediated gene transduction enhances vaccine-induced tumor immunity in mouse models *(68,71)*. Further, human DCs transduced with specific melanoma antigens using recombinant adenoviruses induce melanoma tumor antigen-specific CD8⁺ cytotoxic T lymphocytes in vitro *(97)*. Vaccination of melanoma patients with their autologous tumor cells engineered to secrete GM-CSF using recombinant adenovirus vectors induces specific antitumor immunity and measurable clinical responses. These responses may be caused in part by attraction of DCs to the tumor through expression of GM-CSF *(98,99)*.

13. MISCELLANEOUS DC GENE THERAPY CONSIDERATIONS

DCs can be genetically modified to enhance accumulation of bystander DCs to improve tumor-specific immunity *(100)*. GM-CSF-modified MDCs attracted abundant MDCs in vivo that were significantly more immunostimulatory compared to endogenous MDCs and had phenotypic and functional differences, suggesting that they were a distinct MDC subset *(101)*. The Th2-polarizing and humoral immune-inducing capacity of MDCs can be enhanced by transducing various factors, including macrophage-derived chemokines *(102)*. The trafficking patterns of DCs can be altered through gene therapy-mediated expression of chemokine receptors *(103)*.

Transduced DCs can be cryopreserved for later infusions *(104)*, which can increase efficiency of human clinical trials. Further, non-transduced MDCs can be cryopreserved and transduced with adenovirus at a later date, although at lower efficiency compared to MDCs not previously cryopreserved *(105)*. Adenovirus infection of monocytes is reported to induce MDC differentiation *(106)*. Modification of MDCs through gene therapy for use in antitumor immunity was reviewed *(107,108)*.

ACKNOWLEDGMENTS

We acknowledge the tremendous efforts of our colleagues, from whose work we have extracted summaries. We regret not mentioning the work of others owing to space limitations. This work was supported by National Institutes of Health grant AI39379, the Tulane Endowment, and Golfers Against Cancer to T. J. C. and National Institutes of Health grant CA092562, Department of Defense grant OC020173, the Louisiana Board of Regents, Concern Foundation, and Tulane Endowment to W. Z.

REFERENCES

1. Banchereau, J. and Steinman, R. M. (1998) Dendritic cells and the control of immunity. *Nature* **392,** 245–252.
2. Kohrgruber, N., Halanek, N., Groger, M., et al. (1999) Survival, maturation, and function of CD11c⁻ and CD11c⁺ peripheral blood dendritic cells are differentially regulated by cytokines. *J. Immunol.* **163,** 3250–3259.
3. Rissoan, M. C., Soumelis, V., Kadowaki, N., et al. (1999) Reciprocal control of T helper cell and dendritic cell differentiation. *Science* **283,** 1183–1186.
4. Cella, M., Jarrossay, D., Facchetti, F., et al. (1999) Plasmacytoid monocytes migrate to inflamed lymph nodes and produce large amounts of type I interferon. *Nat. Med.* **5,** 919–923.
5. Bennett, S. R., Carbone, F. R., Karamalis, F., Flavell, R. A., Miller, J. F., and Heath, W. R. (1998) Help for cytotoxic-T-cell responses is mediated by CD40 signalling. *Nature* **393,** 478–480.
6. Ridge, J. P., Di Rosa, F., and Matzinger, P. (1998) A conditioned dendritic cell can be a temporal bridge between a CD4⁺ T-helper and a T-killer cell. *Nature* **393,** 474–478.
7. Zou, W., Machelon, V., Coulomb-L'Hermin, A., et al. (2001) Stromal-derived factor-1 in human tumors recruits and alters the function of plasmacytoid precursor dendritic cells. *Nat. Med.* **7,** 1339–1346.
8. Sallusto, F., Schaerli, P., Loetscher, P., et al. (1998) Rapid and coordinated switch in chemokine receptor expression during dendritic cell maturation. *Eur. J. Immunol.* **28,** 2760–2769.
9. Pulendran, B., Smith, J. L., Caspary, G., et al. (1999) Distinct dendritic cell subsets differentially regulate the class of immune response in vivo. *Proc. Natl. Acad. Sci. USA* **96,** 1036–1041.
10. Mohamadzadeh, M., Berard, F., Essert, G., et al. (2001) Interleukin 15 skews monocyte differentiation into dendritic cells with features of Langerhans cells. *J. Exp. Med.* **194,** 1013–1020.
11. Caux, C., Massacrier, C., Dezutter-Dambuyant, C., et al. (1995) Human dendritic Langerhans cells generated in vitro from CD34⁺ progenitors can prime naive CD4⁺ T cells and process soluble antigen. *J. Immunol.* **155,** 5427–5435.
12. Caux, C., Durand, I., Moreau, I., Duvert, V., Saeland, S., and Banchereau, J. (1993) Tumor necrosis factor alpha cooperates with interleukin 3 in the recruitment of a primitive subset of human CD34⁺ progenitors. *J. Exp. Med.* **177,** 1815–1820.
13. Siegal, F. P., Kadowaki, N., Shodell, M., et al. (1999) The nature of the principal type 1 interferon-producing cells in human blood. *Science* **284,** 1835–1837.
14. Cella, M., Facchetti, F., Lanzavecchia, A., and Colonna, M. (2000) Plasmacytoid dendritic cells activated by influenza virus and CD40L drive a potent Th1 polarization. *Nat. Immunol.* **1,** 305–310.
15. Krug, A., Towarowski, A., Britsch, S., et al. (2001) Toll-like receptor expression reveals CpG DNA as a unique microbial stimulus for plasmacytoid dendritic cells which synergizes with CD40 ligand to induce high amounts of IL-12. *Eur. J. Immunol.* **31,** 3026–3037.
16. Kuwana, M., Kaburaki, J., Wright, T. M., Kawakami, Y., and Ikeda, Y. (2001) Induction of antigen-specific human CD4(+) T cell anergy by peripheral blood DC2 precursors. *Eur. J. Immunol.* **31,** 2547–2557.
17. Nakano, H., Yanagita, M., and Gunn, M. D. (2001) CD11c(+)B220(+)Gr-1(+) cells in mouse lymph nodes and spleen display characteristics of plasmacytoid dendritic cells. *J. Exp. Med.* **194,** 1171–1178.
18. Asselin-Paturel, C., Boonstra, A., Dalod, M., et al. (2001) Mouse type I IFN-producing cells are immature APCs with plasmacytoid morphology. *Nat. Immunol.* **2,** 1144–1150.
19. Albert, M. L., Sauter, B., and Bhardwaj, N. (1998) Dendritic cells acquire antigen from apoptotic cells and induce class I-restricted CTLs. *Nature* **392,** 86–89.
20. Albert, M. L., Pearce, S. F., Francisco, L. M., et al. (1998) Immature dendritic cells phagocytose apoptotic cells via alphavbeta5 and CD36, and cross-present antigens to cytotoxic T lymphocytes. *J. Exp. Med.* **188,** 1359–1368.
21. de Saint-Vis, B., Vincent, J., Vandenabeele, S., et al. (1998) A novel lysosome-associated membrane glycoprotein, DC-LAMP, induced upon DC maturation, is transiently expressed in MHC class II compartment. *Immunity* **9,** 325–336.
22. Geijtenbeek, B. H. T. (2000) DC-SIGN-ICAM-2 interaction mediates dendritic cell trafficking. *Nat. Immunol.* **1,** 353–357.
23. Kalinski, P., Hilkens, C. M., Snijders, A., Snijdewint, F. G., and Kapsenberg, M. L. (1997) IL-12-deficient dendritic cells, generated in the presence of prostaglandin E2, promote type 2 cytokine production in maturing human naïve T helper cells. *J. Immunol.* **159,** 28–35.
24. Enk, A. H., Jonuleit, H., Saloga, J., and Knop, J. (1997) Dendritic cells as mediators of tumor-induced tolerance in metastatic melanoma. *Int. J. Cancer* **73,** 309–316.

25. Steinbrink, K., Jonuleit, H., Muller, G., Schuler, G., Knop, J., and Enk, A. H. (1999) Interleukin-10-treated human dendritic cells induce a melanoma-antigen-specific anergy in CD8(+) T cells resulting in a failure to lyse tumor cells. *Blood* **93,** 1634–1642.

26. Jonuleit, H., Schmitt, E., Schuler, G., Knop, J., and Enk, A. H. (2000) Induction of interleukin 10-producing, non-proliferating CD4(+) T cells with regulatory properties by repetitive stimulation with allogeneic immature human dendritic cells. *J. Exp. Med.* **192,** 1213–1222.

27. Banchereau, J., Palucka, A. K., Dhodapkar, M., et al. (2001) Immune and clinical responses in patients with metastatic melanoma to CD34(+) progenitor-derived dendritic cell vaccine. *Cancer Res.* **61,** 6451–6458.

28. Gilliet, M. and Liu, Y. J. (2002) Generation of human CD8 T regulatory cells by CD40 ligand-activated plasmacytoid dendritic cells. *J. Exp. Med.* **195,** 695–704.

29. Jahnsen, F. L., Lund-Johansen, F., Dunne, J. F., Farkas, L., Haye, R., and Brandtzaeg, P. (2000) Experimentally induced recruitment of plasmacytoid (CD123high) dendritic cells in human nasal allergy. *J. Immunol.* **165,** 4062–4068.

30. Jarrossay, D., Napolitani, G., Colonna, M., Sallusto, F., and Lanzavecchia, A. (2001) Specialization and complementarity in microbial molecule recognition by human myeloid and plasmacytoid dendritic cells. *Eur. J. Immunol.* **31,** 3388–3393.

31. Pope, M. (1998) SIV replication and the dendritic cell. *AIDS Res. Hum. Retroviruses* **14(Suppl. 1),** S71–S73.

32. Messmer, D., Ignatius, R., Santisteban, C., Steinman, R. M., and Pope, M. (2000) The decreased replicative capacity of simian immunodeficiency virus SIVmac239Deltanef is manifest in cultures of immature dendritic cells and T cells. *J. Virol.* **74,** 2406–2413.

33. Stahl-Hennig, C., Steinman, R. M., Tenner-Racz, K., et al. (1999) Rapid infection of oral mucosal-associated lymphoid tissue with simian immunodeficiency virus. *Science* **285,** 1261–1265.

34. O'Doherty, U., Ignatius, R., Bhardwaj, N., and Pope, M. (1997) Generation of monocyte-derived dendritic cells from precursors in rhesus macaque blood. *J. Immunol. Methods* **207,** 185–194.

35. Barratt-Boyes, S. M., Kao, H., and Finn, O. J. (1998) Chimpanzee dendritic cells derived in vitro from blood monocytes and pulsed with antigen elicit specific immune responses in vivo. *J. Immunother.* **21,** 142–148.

36. Barratt-Boyes, S. M., Watkins, S. C., and Finn, O. J. (1997) In vivo migration of dendritic cells differentiated in vitro: a chimpanzee model. *J. Immunol.* **158,** 4543–4547.

37. Barratt-Boyes, S. M., Henderson, R. A., and Finn, O. J. (1996) Chimpanzee dendritic cells with potent immunostimulatory function can be propagated from peripheral blood. *Immunology* **87,** 528–534.

38. Kosco-Vilbois, M. H. and Imhof, B. A. (2000) In vivo veritas. *Immunol. Today* **21,** 64–65.

39. Stumbles, P. A., Thomas, J. A., Pimm, C. L., et al. (1998) Resting respiratory tract dendritic cells preferentially stimulate T helper cell type 2 (Th2) responses and require obligatory cytokine signals for induction of Th1 immunity. *J. Exp. Med.* **188,** 2019–2031.

40. West, K. A., al-Alwan, M. M., Colp, P. E., and Rowden, G. (1999) Characterization of porcine dendritic cells grown in vitro. *Transplant. Proc.* **31,** 666–667.

41. Zhou, Z. H., Wang, J. F., Wang, Y. D., et al. (1999) An agonist anti-human CD40 monoclonal antibody that induces dendritic cell formation and maturation and inhibits proliferation of a myeloma cell line. *Hybridoma* **18,** 471–478.

42. Czerniecki, B. J., Carter, C., Rivoltini, L., et al. (1997) Calcium ionophore-treated peripheral blood monocytes and dendritic cells rapidly display characteristics of activated dendritic cells. *J. Immunol.* **159,** 3823–3837.

43. Randolph, G. J., Beaulieu, S., Lebecque, S., Steinman, R. M., and Muller, W. A. (1998) Differentiation of monocytes into dendritic cells in a model of transendothelial trafficking. *Science* **282,** 480–483.

44. Randolph, G. J., Inaba, K., Robbiani, D. F., Steinman, R. M., and Muller, W. A. (1999) Differentiation of phagocytic monocytes into lymph node dendritic cells in vivo. *Immunity* **11,** 753–761.

45. Inaba, K., Inaba, M., Romani, N., et al. (1992) Generation of large numbers of dendritic cells from mouse bone marrow cultures supplemented with granulocyte/macrophage colony-stimulating factor. *J. Exp. Med.* **176,** 1693–1702.

46. Vecchi, A., Massimiliano, L., Ramponi, S., et al. (1999) Differential responsiveness to constitutive vs inducible chemokines of immature and mature mouse dendritic cells. *J. Leukoc. Biol.* **66,** 489–494.

47. Zhang, Y., Harada, A., Wang, J. B., et al. (1998) Bifurcated dendritic cell differentiation in vitro from murine lineage phenotype-negative c-kit⁺ bone marrow hematopoietic progenitor cells. *Blood* **92,** 118–128.

48. Zhang, Y., Zhang, Y. Y., Ogata, M., et al. (1999) Transforming growth factor-beta1 polarizes murine hematopoietic progenitor cells to generate Langerhans cell-like dendritic cells through a monocyte/macrophage differentiation pathway. *Blood* **93,** 1208–1220.

49. Schuler, G. and Steinman, R. M. (1985) Murine epidermal Langerhans cells mature into potent immunostimulatory dendritic cells in vitro. *J. Exp. Med.* **161,** 526–546.

50. Rezzani, R., Rodella, L., Zauli, G., Caimi, L., and Vitale, M. (1999) Mouse peritoneal cells as a reservoir of late dendritic cell progenitors. *Br. J. Haematol.* **104,** 111–118.

51. Zou, W., Borvak, J., Marches, F., et al. (2000) Macrophage-derived dendritic cells have strong Th1-polarizing potential mediated by beta-chemokines rather than IL-12. *J. Immunol.* **165,** 4388–4396.

52. Dembic, Z., Schenck, K., and Bogen, B. (2000) Dendritic cells purified from myeloma are primed with tumor-specific antigen (idiotype) and activate CD4⁺ T cells. *Proc. Natl. Acad. Sci. USA* **97,** 2697–2702.

53. Chiodoni, C., Paglia, P., Stoppacciaro, A., Rodolfo, M., Parenza, M., and Colombo, M. P. (1999) Dendritic cells infiltrating tumors cotransduced with granulocyte/macrophage colony-stimulating factor (GM-CSF) and CD40 ligand genes take up and present endogenous tumor-associated antigens, and prime naive mice for a cytotoxic T lymphocyte response. *J. Exp. Med.* **190,** 125–133.

54. Paglia, P., Girolomoni, G., Robbiati, F., Granucci, F., and Ricciardi-Castagnoli, P. (1993) Immortalized dendritic cell line fully competent in antigen presentation initiates primary T cell responses in vivo. *J. Exp. Med.* **178,** 1893–1901.

55. Yokota, K., Ariizumi, K., Kitajima, T., Bergstresser, P. R., Street, N. E., and Takashima, A. (1996) Cytokine-mediated communication between dendritic epidermal T cells and Langerhans cells. In vitro studies using cell lines. *J. Immunol.* **157,** 1529–1537.

56. Sallusto, F. and Lanzavecchia, A. (1994) Efficient presentation of soluble antigen by cultured human dendritic cells is maintained by granulocyte/macrophage colony-stimulating factor plus interleukin 4 and downregulated by tumor necrosis factor alpha. *J. Exp. Med.* **179,** 1109–1118.

57. Chapuis, F., Rosenzwajg, M., Yagello, M., Ekman, M., Biberfeld, P., and Gluckman, J. C. (1997) Differentiation of human dendritic cells from monocytes in vitro. *Eur. J. Immunol.* **27,** 431–441.

58. Bender, A., Sapp, M., Schuler, G., Steinman, R. M., and Bhardwaj, N. (1996) Improved methods for the generation of dendritic cells from nonproliferating progenitors in human blood. *J. Immunol. Methods* **196,** 121–135.

59. Kiertscher, S. M. and Roth, M. D. (1996) Human CD14+ leukocytes acquire the phenotype and function of antigen-presenting dendritic cells when cultured in GM-CSF and IL-4. *J. Leukoc. Biol.* **59,** 208–218.

60. Romani, N., Reider, D., Heuer, M., et al. (1996) Generation of mature dendritic cells from human blood. An improved method with special regard to clinical applicability. *J. Immunol. Methods* **196,** 137–151.

61. Strobl, H., Bello-Fernandez, C., Riedl, E., et al. (1997) FLT3 ligand in cooperation with transforming growth factor-beta1 potentiates in vitro development of Langerhans-type dendritic cells and allows single-cell dendritic cell cluster formation under serum-free conditions. *Blood* **90,** 1425–1434.

62. Bancheareau, J., Briere, F., Caux, C., et al. (2000) Immunobiology of dendritic cells. *Annu. Rev. Immunol.* **18,** 767–811.

63. Zou, W., Borvak, J., Marches, F., Wei, S., Isaeva, T., and Curiel, T. J. (2001) A guide to isolation, culture and propagation of dendritic cells. In *Dendritic Cells: Biology and Clinical Applications,* 2nd ed. (Lotze, M. T. and Thomson, A. W., eds.), Academic Press, London, UK, pp. 77–96.

64. Lenz, A., Heine, M., Schuler, G., and Romani, N. (1993) Human and murine dermis contain dendritic cells. Isolation by means of a novel method and phenotypical and functional characterization. *J. Clin. Invest.* **92,** 2587–2596.

65. Caux, C., Massacrier, C., Vanbervliet, B., et al. (1997) CD34+ hematopoietic progenitors from human cord blood differentiate along two independent dendritic cell pathways in response to granulocyte-macrophage colony-stimulating factor plus tumor necrosis factor alpha: II. Functional analysis. *Blood* **90,** 1458–1470.

66. Caux, C., Vanbervliet, B., Massacrier, C., et al. (1996) CD34+ hematopoietic progenitors from human cord blood differentiate along two independent dendritic cell pathways in response to GM-CSF+TNF alpha. *J. Exp. Med.* **184,** 695–706.

67. Arrighi, J. F., Hauser, C., Chapuis, B., Zubler, R. H., and Kindler, V. (1999) Long-term culture of human CD34(+) progenitors with FLT3-ligand, thrombopoietin, and stem cell factor induces extensive amplification of a CD34(−) CD14(−) and a CD34(−)CD14(+) dendritic cell precursor. *Blood* **93,** 2244–2252.

68. Song, W., Kong, H. L., Carpenter, H., et al. (1997) Dendritic cells genetically modified with an adenovirus vector encoding the cDNA for a model antigen induce protective and therapeutic antitumor immunity. *J. Exp. Med.* **186,** 1247–1256.

69. Lundqvist, A., Choudhury, A., Nagata, T., et al. (2002) Recombinant adenovirus vector activates and protects human monocyte-derived dendritic cells from apoptosis. *Hum. Gene Ther.* **13,** 1541–1549.

70. Pereboev, A. V., Asiedu, C. K., Kawakami, Y., et al. (2002) Coxsackievirus-adenovirus receptor genetically fused to anti-human CD40 scFv enhances adenoviral transduction of dendritic cells. *Gene Ther.* **9,** 1189–1193.

71. Tillman, B. W., Hayes, T. L., DeGruijl, T. D., Douglas, J. T., and Curiel, D. T. (2000) Adenoviral vectors targeted to CD40 enhance the efficacy of dendritic cell-based vaccination against human papillomavirus 16-induced tumor cells in a murine model. *Cancer Res.* **60,** 5456–5463.

72. Tillman, B. W., de Gruijl, T. D., Luykx-de Bakker, S. A., et al. (1999) Maturation of dendritic cells accompanies high-efficiency gene transfer by a CD40-targeted adenoviral vector. *J. Immunol.* **162,** 6378–6383.

73. Okada, N., Saito, T., Masunaga, Y., et al. (2001) Efficient antigen gene transduction using Arg-Gly-Asp fiber-mutant adenovirus vectors can potentiate antitumor vaccine efficacy and maturation of murine dendritic cells. *Cancer Res.* **61,** 7913–7919.

74. Kianmanesh, A., Hackett, N. R., Lee, J. M., Kikuchi, T., Korst, R. J., and Crystal, R. G. (2001) Intratumoral administration of low doses of an adenovirus vector encoding tumor necrosis factor alpha together with naive dendritic cells elicits significant suppression of tumor growth without toxicity. *Hum. Gene Ther.* **12,** 2035–2049.

75. Tanaka, F., Hashimoto, W., Robbins, P. D., Lotze, M. T., and Tahara, H. (2002) Therapeutic and specific antitumor immunity induced by co-administration of immature dendritic cells and adenoviral vector expressing biologically active IL-18. *Gene Ther.* **9,** 1480–1486.

76. Ribas, A., Butterfield, L. H., Hu, B., et al. (2000) Immune deviation and Fas-mediated deletion limit antitumor activity after multiple dendritic cell vaccinations in mice. *Cancer Res.* **60**, 2218–2224.
77. Sumimoto, H., Tsuji, T., Miyoshi, H., et al. (2002) Rapid and efficient generation of lentivirally gene-modified dendritic cells from DC progenitors with bone marrow stromal cells. *J. Immunol. Methods* **271**, 153–165.
78. Rouas, R., Uch, R., Cleuter, Y., et al. (2002) Lentiviral-mediated gene delivery in human monocyte-derived dendritic cells: optimized design and procedures for highly efficient transduction compatible with clinical constraints. *Cancer Gene Ther.* **9**, 715–724.
79. Esslinger, C., Romero, P., and MacDonald, H. R. (2002) Efficient transduction of dendritic cells and induction of a T-cell response by third-generation lentivectors. *Hum. Gene Ther.* **13**, 1091–1100.
80. Evans, J. T., Cravens, P., Gatlin, J., Kelly, P. F., Lipsky, P. E., and Garcia, J. V. (2001) Pre-clinical evaluation of an in vitro selection protocol for the enrichment of transduced CD34⁺ cell-derived human dendritic cells. *Gene Ther.* **8**, 1427–1435.
81. Gruber, A., Kan-Mitchell, J., Kuhen, K. L., Mukai, T., and Wong-Staal, F. (2000) Dendritic cells transduced by multiply deleted HIV-1 vectors exhibit normal phenotypes and functions and elicit an HIV-specific cytotoxic T-lymphocyte response in vitro. *Blood* **96**, 1327–1333.
82. Movassagh, M., Baillou, C., Cosset, F. L., Klatzmann, D., Guigon, M., and Lemoine, F. M. (1999) High level of retrovirus-mediated gene transfer into dendritic cells derived from cord blood and mobilized peripheral blood CD34⁺ cells. *Hum. Gene Ther.* **10**, 175–187.
83. Cao, X., Zhang, W., Wang, J., et al. (1999) Therapy of established tumour with a hybrid cellular vaccine generated by using granulocyte-macrophage colony-stimulating factor genetically modified dendritic cells. *Immunology* **97**, 616–625.
84. Latouche, J. B. and Sadelain, M. (2000) Induction of human cytotoxic T lymphocytes by artificial antigen-presenting cells. *Nat. Biotechnol.* **18**, 405–409.
85. Jonuleit, H., Tuting, T., Steitz, J., et al. (2000) Efficient transduction of mature CD83⁺ dendritic cells using recombinant adenovirus suppressed T cell stimulatory capacity. *Gene Ther.* **7**, 249–254.
86. Dietz, A. B. and Vuk-Pavlovic, S. (1998) High efficiency adenovirus-mediated gene transfer to human dendritic cells. *Blood* **91**, 392–398.
87. Zou, W., Borvak, J., Wei, S., Isaeva, T., Curiel, D. T., and Curiel, T. J. (2001) Reciprocal regulation of plasmacytoid dendritic cells and monocytes during viral infection. *Eur. J. Immunol.* **31**, 3833–3839.
88. Jooss, K., Yang, Y., Fisher, K. J., and Wilson, J. M. (1998) Transduction of dendritic cells by DNA viral vectors directs the immune response to transgene products in muscle fibers. *J. Virol.* **72**, 4212–4223.
89. Diebold, S. S., Cotten, M., Wagner, E., and Zenke, M. (1998) Gene-modified dendritic cells by receptor-mediated transfection. *Adv. Exp. Med. Biol.* **451**, 449–455.
90. Wan, Y., Emtage, P., Foley, R., Carter, R., and Gauldie, J. (1999) Murine dendritic cells transduced with an adenoviral vector expressing a defined tumor antigen can overcome anti-adenovirus neutralizing immunity and induce effective tumor regression. *Int. J. Oncol.* **14**, 771–776.
91. Lee, W. C., Wan, Y. H., Li, W., et al. (1999) Enhancement of dendritic cell tolerogenicity by genetic modification using adenoviral vectors encoding cDNA for TGF beta 1. *Transplant. Proc.* **31**, 1195.
92. Lu, L., Gambotto, A., Lee, W. C., et al. (1999) Adenoviral delivery of CTLA4Ig into myeloid dendritic cells promotes their in vitro tolerogenicity and survival in allogeneic recipients. *Gene Ther.* **6**, 554–563.
93. Lu, L., Lee, W. C., Takayama, T., et al. (1999) Genetic engineering of dendritic cells to express immunosuppressive molecules (viral IL-10, TGF-beta, and CTLA4Ig). *J. Leukoc. Biol.* **66**, 293–296.
94. Bonham, C. A., Peng, L., Liang, X., et al. (2002) Marked prolongation of cardiac allograft survival by dendritic cells genetically engineered with NF-kappa B oligodeoxyribonucleotide decoys and adenoviral vectors encoding CTLA4-Ig. *J. Immunol.* **169**, 3382–3391.
95. Rea, D., Schagen, F. H., Hoeben, R. C., et al. (1999) Adenoviruses activate human dendritic cells without polarization toward a T-helper type 1-inducing subset. *J. Virol.* **73**, 10,245–10,253.
96. Di Nicola, M., Siena, S., Bregni, M., et al. (1998) Gene transfer into human dendritic antigen-presenting cells by vaccinia virus and adenovirus vectors. *Cancer Gene Ther.* **5**, 350–356.
97. Philip, R., Alters, S. E., Brunette, E., et al. (2000) Dendritic cells loaded with MART-1 peptide or infected with adenoviral construct are functionally equivalent in the induction of tumor-specific cytotoxic T lymphocyte responses in patients with melanoma. *J. Immunother.* **23**, 168–176.
98. Kusumoto, M., Umeda, S., Ikubo, A., et al. (2001) Phase 1 clinical trial of irradiated autologous melanoma cells adenovirally transduced with human GM-CSF gene. *Cancer Immunol. Immunother.* **50**, 373–381.
99. Soiffer, R., Hodi, F. S., Haluska, F., et al. (2003) Vaccination with irradiated, autologous melanoma cells engineered to secrete granulocyte-macrophage colony-stimulating factor by adenoviral-mediated gene transfer augments antitumor immunity in patients with metastatic melanoma. *J. Clin. Oncol.* **21**, 3343–3350.
100. Kielian, T., Nagai, E., Ikubo, A., Rasmussen, C. A., and Suzuki, T. (1999) Granulocyte/macrophage-colony-stimulating factor released by adenovirally transduced CT26 cells leads to the local expression of macrophage inflammatory protein 1alpha and accumulation of dendritic cells at vaccination sites in vivo. *Cancer Immunol. Immunother.* **48**, 123–131.

101. Miller, G., Pillarisetty, V. G., Shah, A. B., Lahrs, S., Xing, Z., and DeMatteo, R. P. (2002) Endogenous granulocyte-macrophage colony-stimulating factor overexpression in vivo results in the long-term recruitment of a distinct dendritic cell population with enhanced immunostimulatory function. *J. Immunol.* **169,** 2875–2885.
102. Kikuchi, T. and Crystal, R. G. (2001) Antigen-pulsed dendritic cells expressing macrophage-derived chemokine elicit Th2 responses and promote specific humoral immunity. *J. Clin. Invest.* **108,** 917–927.
103. Wu, M. T. and Hwang, S. T. (2002) CXCR5-transduced bone marrow-derived dendritic cells traffic to B cell zones of lymph nodes and modify antigen-specific immune responses. *J. Immunol.* **168,** 5096–5102.
104. Di Nicola, M., Carlo-Stella, C., Milanesi, M., et al. (2000) Large-scale feasibility of gene transduction into human CD34+ cell-derived dendritic cells by adenoviral/polycation complex. *Br. J. Haematol.* **111,** 344–350.
105. John, J., Hutchinson, J., Dalgleish, A., and Pandha, H. (2003) Cryopreservation of immature monocyte-derived dendritic cells results in enhanced cell maturation but reduced endocytic activity and efficiency of adenoviral transduction. *J. Immunol. Methods* **272,** 35–48.
106. Lyakh, L. A., Koski, G. K., Young, H. A., Spence, S. E., Cohen, P. A., and Rice, N. R. (2002) Adenovirus type 5 vectors induce dendritic cell differentiation in human CD14(+) monocytes cultured under serum-free conditions. *Blood* **99,** 600–608.
107. Ribas, A., Butterfield, L. H., Glaspy, J. A., and Economou, J. S. (2002) Cancer immunotherapy using gene-modified dendritic cells. *Curr. Gene Ther.* **2,** 57–78.
108. Bubenik, J. (2001) Genetically engineered dendritic cell-based cancer vaccines (review). *Int. J. Oncol.* **18,** 475–478.

12

Polynucleotide Immunization for Cancer Therapy

Theresa V. Strong

1. INTRODUCTION

The limitations of conventional cancer therapy (surgery, radiation, and chemotherapy) combined with a better understanding of the molecular mechanisms regulating the immune system have led to increasing attention focused on the development of immunotherapies for cancer. Active immunotherapy approaches seek to eliminate tumor cells by eliciting immune responses directed against tumor-associated antigens. Gene transfer techniques have expanded the potential opportunities in this area by providing new methods for stimulating the immune response. Among the array of techniques under development for clinical application, nucleic acid or polynucleotide vaccines have emerged as a novel and effective method of inducing tumor antigen-specific immune responses.

Rather than immunizing with a protein, polynucleotide immunization (PNI) relies on delivery of deoxyribonucleic acid (DNA) or ribonucleic acid (RNA) molecules encoding an antigen of interest. There are several advantages to this mode of delivery. Perhaps most important, both antibody and cellular immune responses are elicited following PNI. The in vivo synthesis of the encoded antigen allows the protein to be processed for presentation on the major histocompatibility complex (MHC) class I complex, promoting the generation of class I-restricted cytotoxic T lymphocytes (CTLs). Because CTLs are known to be important mediators of the antitumor immune response, their activation against tumor antigens is critical to the success of cancer vaccine approaches. Furthermore, and in contrast to protein vaccines prepared in nonmammalian hosts, synthesis of the antigen in vivo allows appropriate folding and posttranslational modification of the protein.

DNA-based vaccines also direct antigen expression for extended periods, supporting persistent antitumor immune responses that should theoretically protect a patient from relapse. Additional factors favoring the development of plasmid DNA-based immunization strategies include the relative ease and inexpensive nature of vaccine preparation, as well as its stability. As discussed in more detail in Section 4, DNA vaccines prepared in bacterial hosts are inherently immunostimulatory because of the presence of unmethylated CpG dinucleotides. These sequences stimulate a nonspecific immune response that does not interfere with repeated delivery of the vaccine. This contrasts with viral-based vaccines, for which preexisting or vector-induced immune responses can strongly compromise the effectiveness of the vaccine (1,2). Safety considerations also favor polynucleotide vaccines compared to viral vaccines because there is no risk for recombination with wild-type viruses, and the risk of insertional mutagenesis is quite low. Finally, DNA and RNA vaccines have the potential to readily deliver multiple epitopes, and even multiple antigens, in a single injection, an important consideration given the propensity of tumors to escape immune detection by antigen loss variants (3).

Despite these potential advantages and encouraging preclinical studies, polynucleotide vaccines for cancer have thus far shown only minimal activity in the clinical setting. Many tumor antigens are not

From: *Contemporary Cancer Research*
Cancer Gene Therapy
Edited by: D. T. Curiel and J. T. Douglas © Humana Press Inc., Totowa, NJ

mutated, and therefore induction of an immune response to these antigens requires that the immune system be able to recognize and mount an effective response to a "self-antigen." Initial studies suggest that this will be difficult to achieve in the setting of human cancer. Therefore, improving the potency, and thereby the clinical efficacy, of polynucleotide vaccines has become the major focus of research in the field. This chapter delineates some of the approaches currently under evaluation in preclinical models designed to address this limitation.

The versatility of DNA- and RNA-based vaccines has led to the development of a number of delivery approaches to accomplish cancer immunotherapy. Whereas DNA or messenger RNA (mRNA) can be used to modify cells ex vivo, as in the case of transfected dendritic cells or irradiated tumor cells for vaccine therapy, this chapter focuses specifically on in vivo delivery of DNA or RNA for cancer immunotherapy.

2. GENE TRANSFER OF NUCLEIC ACIDS FOR IMMUNIZATION

The development of nucleic acid vaccines was sparked by the observation by Wolff and colleagues that intramuscular injection of naked DNA led to the expression of the encoded gene by myofiber cells (4). Subsequent studies demonstrated the general applicability of this approach for the expression of foreign genes in a variety of species, from fish (5) to nonhuman primates (6). Although an inefficient process, the transferred DNA appears to enter the myofibers via the myocyte caveolae and T tubules (7,8). The DNA is maintained in an extrachromosomal form in the nucleus, but expression can be detected for a prolonged period (9), depending on the immunogenicity of the encoded protein.

Ulmer and coworkers first demonstrated the ability of intramuscular delivery of DNA encoding a viral antigen to elicit a CD8[+] T cell, MHC class I-restricted immune response protective against infection, using a plasmid encoding the influenza protein nucleoprotein A (10). This study provided the rationale to develop polynucleotide vaccines for therapy of diseases, including cancer, previously not amenable to traditional vaccine approaches that rely primarily on humoral immune responses. Rather than preventing disease, therapeutic immunization against chronic disease became a possibility.

Induction of cellular and humoral immune responses following delivery of nucleic acids is not limited to intramuscular delivery. The skin is rich in antigen-presenting cells (APCs), such as immature Langerhans cells in the epidermis and mature dendritic cells (DCs) in the dermis. Tang and coworkers demonstrated the ability of DNA delivered to the skin to elicit a humoral immune response to the encoded gene (11). In this method, the DNA is delivered following precipitation onto gold microparticles (12). The gold particles are delivered to the skin under pressure by a ballistic delivery device. The process, commonly referred to as gene gun delivery, does not produce traumatic injury and requires much less DNA to achieve comparable humoral immune response to intramuscular delivery (13,14). Induction of effector CTLs capable of mediating tumor rejection was subsequently demonstrated in a mouse model of transplantable tumors (15).

Intradermal immunization can also be accomplished by injection of naked DNA or by a needle-free jet injection system delivering DNA-coated nanoparticles (16). Mucosal administration of DNA vaccines has also been explored primarily for immunization against infectious disease (17), but may also be applicable for cancer therapy (18).

In addition to naked DNA delivery to mucosal surfaces, plasmids can be delivered orally by employing bacteria as carriers, including attenuated *Salmonella (19–21)*, *Shigella (22)*, or *Listeria (23)* strains. Administration via bacteria may also contribute to the effectiveness of the vaccine by stimulating the innate immune response. Finally, despite a relatively short half-life in the circulation, studies of the intrasplenic administration of a DNA vaccine (24) demonstrated that strategies to promote uptake of DNA by splenocytes following intravenous administration might lead to induction of humoral and cellular immune responses.

The fact that all of these delivery routes results in antigen synthesis and induction of antigen-specific immune responses attests to the flexibility of PNI. It is important to note that these different routes of administration may lead to qualitatively different immune responses *(25,26)*, and the relative efficacy in humans remains to be determined.

Although typically composed of plasmid DNA encoding a defined tumor antigen, vaccine strategies using mRNA have also been developed. One potential disadvantage of RNA-based vaccines compared to DNA vaccines is the considerably shorter half-life of mRNA. Nevertheless, the use of mRNA in vivo may be advantageous for immunization against oncogenic antigens such as that encoded by the *HER-2/neu* gene because the theoretical risk of transgene integration into the genome is eliminated.

Qiu et al *(27)* used gene gun delivery of mRNA to demonstrate expression of the encoded genes in the mouse epidermis and induction of antigen-specific antibodies. Intramuscular delivery of mRNA encoding carcinoembryonic antigen (CEA) also led to detectable anti-CEA antibodies and partial protection against challenge with CEA-expressing tumor cells *(28)*.

The immune response elicited by mRNA-based vaccines is generally of lower magnitude than for DNA-based strategies, presumably because of the instability of the mRNA following delivery. To address this limitation, the use of self-replicating RNAs has emerged as a means to augment the efficacy of RNA-based immunization *(29–31)*. These vectors incorporate sequences into the RNA transcript that encode the RNA replicase polyprotein derived from alpha viruses (e.g., Sindbis or Semliki Forest virus). The replicase activity directs cytoplasmic replication of the entire transcript and also transcribes mRNA for the antigen from a subgenomic promoter, resulting in high levels of antigen expression. Further adaptation of the replicative RNA system has led to the development of plasmid DNA vectors encoding replicative RNA transcripts *(32)*, which combine the ease of plasmid DNA vaccine preparation with the advantages afforded by replicative RNAs.

3. MECHANISM OF IMMUNE RESPONSE INDUCTION FOLLOWING PNI

The ability of polynucleotide vaccines to elicit a cellular immune response paved the way for their development as a reagent for cancer immunotherapy. The mechanism for induction of the immune response following immunization is still not entirely clear, but appears to involve processing of the antigen through both endogenous and exogenous pathways, leading to presentation of the antigen in the context of both MHC class I and II. DNA may transfect both target cells (for example, myocytes after intramuscular delivery) as well as resident APCs. Although myocytes clearly synthesize the encoded protein, it is thought that only APCs are capable of delivering the costimulatory signals necessary to prime CTLs effectively.

A number of studies support the central role for bone marrow-derived APCs in induction of the immune response following DNA immunization *(33–36)*. The findings suggest a "cross-priming" scenario in which myocytes produce the antigenic protein and transfer it to APCs in such a way that the antigen is presented to T cells in the context of MHC class I, thereby allowing the APC to directly activate CTLs. Whereas proteins acquired exogenously by APCs are usually trafficked into the endolysosomal pathway for degradation and presentation by MHC class II molecules, in the case of PNI the processed antigen is available for both class I and II presentation, promoting both cellular and humoral immunity.

Alternatively, or more likely in addition, the APCs themselves may be transfected by the transferred nucleic acid *(37,38)*. The in vivo synthesis of the antigen in the cytoplasm promotes presentation of the peptide by MHC class I molecules. Proteins synthesized within the cell are endogenously processed into peptides by the proteasome. These peptides are loaded onto MHC class I molecules in the endoplasmic reticulum and transported to the cell surface. Presentation of the antigen in the context of both class I and II MHC and in the presence of the appropriate costimulatory molecules leads to the activation of both CD4$^+$ and CD8$^+$ T cells.

The importance of the CD8$^+$ CTLs in mediating tumor cell destruction by recognition of antigenic peptide presented in MHC class I on the tumor cell surface is well established. These cells are known to play an important role in tumor cell destruction and long-term protection against rechallenge. The importance of the CD4[+] cell in antitumor immunity has gained appreciation *(39,40)*. These CD4[+] T cells provide help for the induction of specific CD8[+] CTLs and secrete cytokines promoting the activation of CTL. In addition, they may activate nonspecific immune effector cells such as macrophages and eosinophils, which may further potentiate the destruction of tumor cells.

4. FACTORS INFLUENCING INDUCTION OF IMMUNE RESPONSE

A number of features of polynucleotide vaccines influence the nature and potency of the attendant immune response, from the composition of the nucleic acid itself, to the encoded antigen, to the microenvironment in which the vaccine is expressed. The composition of the DNA is an initial consideration for plasmid-based vaccines. The dinucleotide CpG is relatively underrepresented in the mammalian genome. Further, areas rich in CpG are frequently methylated as a mechanism of transcriptional regulation.

In contrast to this, preparation of DNA vaccines in bacterial hosts results in the presence of unmethylated CpG dinucleotides in the plasmid. These unmethylated sequences are recognized by the innate immune system as indicative of the presence of a pathogen and are immunostimulatory *(41)*. Specifically, the sequences are recognized by the toll-like receptor 9 and trigger activation of the innate immune system including DCs, macrophages, natural killer cells and natural killer T (NKT) cells *(42,43)*. The result is that CpGs, either present in the plasmid or delivered as purified oligodeoxynucleotides, are a potent adjuvant, biasing the immune system toward a Th1-type response *(44)*. The CpG-oligodeoxynucleotides also have an antiapoptotic effect on both CD4[+] and CD8[+] T cells, thereby expanding the pool of T cells and augmenting the immune response in an antigen-independent manner *(45)*. The presence of these CpG motifs contributes significantly to the overall immunogenicity of DNA vaccines.

Polynucleotide vaccines based on the RNA alpha viruses also are inherently immunostimulatory. These vaccines promote apoptosis in transfected cells, which may enhance immunogenicity *(46)*. The presence of a double-stranded RNA intermediate, which is generated during replication in the cytoplasm, activates the double-stranded protein kinase R *(47)* and NF-kappa B *(48)*, stimulating an innate antiviral pathway and thereby augmenting the immune response. An advantage of polynucleotide vaccines compared to viral vaccines is that the immunostimulatory pathways stimulated are nonspecific in nature and do not interfere with readministration of the vector.

In addition to the composition of the nucleic acids, an important determinant of immune response is level of transgene expression. In general, increased immunogene expression augments the immune response. Hence, a strong promoter is required to direct efficient transcription of the encoded protein, and optimized polyadenylation signals and untranslated regions may contribute to enhanced transgene expression *(49)*. The cytomegalovirus early promoter/enhancer has been widely used to drive expression of the encoded sequences and may be enhanced by the insertion of additional sequences, for example, those derived from the adeno-associated virus *(50)*.

Once an optimized vector has been developed, the route of administration may also influence the resulting immune response. As discussed in Section 3., a number of routes of PNI have led to induction of cellular and humoral immune responses, but the nature of the immune response elicited by different routes of administration may be qualitatively different *(51–53)*. In general, gene gun administration of DNA leads to a more T helper 2(Th2)-like immune response, with a strong humoral component that may be less effective for cancer therapy. However, this effect can be modified by coadministration of Th1-promoting cytokines *(54)*. The nature of the immune response can be further influenced by the vaccination dose and the schedule of administration *(55)*.

The antigenicity of the encoded protein is of considerable importance in generating an effective response. The fact that most tumor antigens are self-antigens represents a formidable challenge for all forms of active immunotherapy that rely on breaking immunological tolerance. Modifying the antigenicity of the protein or promoting its uptake by professional APCs (e.g., DCs) are key areas of

Table 1
Strategies to Enhance the Efficacy of Polynucleotide Vaccines for Cancer Therapy

Aspect of vaccine	Intervention	Reference
Improve nucleic acid delivery	Liposomes	*56*
	PLG microparticles	*57*
	Electroporation	*58,59*
Modify the antigen to target APCs	Fuse antigen with CD40L, FLT3L, CTLA4	*61–63*
Modify the antigen to increase immunogencity	Alter antigen processing	*64–66*
	Incorporate immunogenic eptiopes	*67*
	Use antigen from a different species	*78–81*
	Codon optimization	*68*
Modify the microenviroment	Add cytokines	*70,71*
	Add chemokines	*72,73*
	Decrease apoptosis in APCs	*74*
Incorporate alternative vectors into	Viral vectors (adenoviruses, vaccinia)	*84,86–88*
immunization schedule (prime–boost)	Protein	*89*

consideration in this respect. The local cytokine milieu also plays an important role in the immune response ultimately elicited. Optimizing all of these factors to maximize the effectiveness of the immune response following PNI has become a major focus for investigators in this area of research.

5. STRATEGIES TO ENHANCE THE IMMUNE RESPONSE

DNA vaccines have shown promise in eliciting effective CTL responses to neoantigens, but the weakly immunogenic antigens characteristic of most tumors will require polynucleotide vaccines to be more potent if they are to be clinically useful. Thus, many studies have focused on enhancing the immune response elicited by PNI. Approaches have focused on every aspect of the vaccine, from delivery of the nucleic acid, to modification of the encoded antigen, to the perturbation of the micro-environment to maximize and tailor the immune response to a Th1-type response (Table 1). The versatility of polynucleotide vaccines is a strength in this respect as both the nucleic acid and the encoded antigen of interest can be readily manipulated and evaluated.

Because the process of delivery of the nucleic acid to target cells is inefficient, approaches to increase the efficacy of delivery and/or increase the stability of the nucleic acid in vivo can result in higher and extended expression of the encoded antigen, increasing the magnitude of the immune response. To this end, incorporation of the nucleic acid into liposomes may protect it from endogenous nucleases and promote uptake into cells *(56)*. Adsorption of DNA onto the cationic microparticles composed of poly(DL-lactide-*co*-glycolide) (PLG) allows the slow release of the DNA and results in a more potent immune response compared to naked DNA *(57)*. To enhance the transport of nucleic acids into the target cells physically, electroporation into skin *(58)* or muscle *(59)* has proven an effective means of increasing gene transfer efficiency. Application of this technology in the clinical setting will require careful optimization in human subjects.

The ease of manipulation of recombinant complementary DNAs allows the encoded antigen to be readily altered in ways that may enhance immunogenicity; and possible manipulations in this respect are numerous and varied. Because uptake and appropriate presentation of the antigen are critical to induction of an effective immune response, several groups have modified encoded antigens to target them to for more efficient uptake by professional APCs *(60)*. Antigens fused to CD40 ligand *(61)*, the extracellular domain of the Fms-like tyrosine kinase-3 (FLT3) ligand *(62)*, or cytotoxic T-lymphocyte antigen 4 (CTLA4) *(63)* are examples in which the receptor for each ligand is found on surface of DCs, targeting the antigen to these cells for an enhanced immune response. Within the cell, the encoded antigen can be modified to promote degradation via the endosomal/lysosomal pathway *(64, 65)* as a means to enhance antigen presentation in MHC class II and increase CD4+ T-cell responses. In a similar approach targeting a different pathway, the proteolytic processing of the encoded antigen can be promoted by fusing it with sequences directing its ubiquitination *(66)*. Incorporation of heterologous immunogenic sequences, such as a tetanus toxin CTL epitope into a tumor antigen, resulted in rapid CTL induction against the tumor antigen with protection against tumor challenge *(67)*. For human papilloma virus (HPV)-based cancers such as cervical cancer, codon optimization of the antigen has proven an effective means of increasing protein expression and enhancing immune response *(68)*.

One common approach to enhance immunogenicity of nucleic acid vaccines is the codelivery of DNA-encoding cytokines, based on the rationale that a more potent immune response will be elicited if the antigen is presented in a favorable cytokine milieu. To this end, cytokines promoting a Th1-type response, including granulocyte-macrophage colony-stimulating factor, interferon-γ, interleukin 2, and interleukin 12 have been extensively evaluated in preclinical models of infectious disease *(69)* and cancer *(70,71)*, demonstrating the ability of this approach to influence favorably the nature and magnitude of the immune response.

Based on the rationale that more efficient delivery of the antigen to APCs will enhance immune responsiveness, chemokines have been used to draw APCs to the site of antigen synthesis. This has been accomplished either by fusion of the antigen to inflammatory chemokines *(72)* or by codelivery of the antigen with chemokines *(73)*. Additional alterations to the local environment that receives the polynucleotide vaccine include codelivery of antiapoptotic genes to enhance the survival of DNA-transfected DCs *(74)* and coadministration of the antigen-encoding DNA with the soluble lympho-cyte-activating gene-3 protein as a means to promote cross-presentation of the antigen *(75)*. In vivo expansion of the DCs to enhance immune responsiveness has been directed by delivery of a plasmid encoding the FLT3 ligand *(76)*. This approach can be used in combination with conventional peptide vaccines to enhance cellular immune response *(77)*.

Given that self-antigens are weakly immunogenic and that epitope spreading is known to occur on induction of an immune response, the concept of cross-species homologous immunization, also called xenogenic or orthologous immunization, has proven to be an effective method of breaking tolerance. For PNI, this strategy uses a tumor antigen gene derived from a different species than the vaccine recipient to induce a crossreactive immune response to the host autologous protein. For multiple proteins studied to date, the foreign species ortholog displays enhanced immunogenicity compared to the autologous or self-antigen. This approach leads to immunity that crossreacts with, and breaks tolerance to, the self-antigen. Orthologous immunization has been used successfully in animal models to induce antitumor immune responses against either endogenous tumor antigens *(78–80)* or tumor-promoting factors *(81)*. Initial clinical studies in prostate cancer using a protein/DC vaccine demonstrated induction of immune response to the self-antigen, suggesting the potential utility of this approach in the clinical setting *(82)*.

The ease of preparation and lack of vector-directed immune response associated with DNA vaccines have led to its incorporation into a variety of heterologous prime and boost strategies. These have proven more efficacious than DNA immunization alone in several preclinical models and with a variety of different strategies. Particularly effective among these prime and boost regimens is plasmid DNA priming, followed by boosting with a live viral vector. This approach leads to a more potent and expanded immune response compared to either vector alone. The strategy of priming the immune response with plasmid DNA-encoded antigen circumvents the ability of vector-specific immune responses to abrogate immunogen expression, which occurs on repeated delivery of live viral vectors. In turn, the potency of the viral vectors enhances the comparatively modest magnitude of the immune response elicited by plasmid DNA alone. The persistent expression afforded by DNA vaccines may generate T cells of high affinity, which can subsequently be expanded on boosting with viral vectors *(83–85)*.

Adenovirus is one replication-defective viral vector that has been successfully combined with DNA in a mouse model of hepatocellular carcinoma *(86)*. Vaccinia viral vectors are also promising in this regard *(87,88)*. Plasmid DNA can also be combined with protein boosts, for example, adsorbed to PLG microparticles *(89)*, with beneficial effects. Although such approaches will be somewhat more complicated to bring to the clinic, the increased potency of combination vaccines may override this consideration.

6. PRECLINICAL STUDIES

The use of appropriate preclinical models is a critical matter for all areas of cancer therapeutics development, and polynucleotide vaccines are no exception. Numerous preclinical models exist, with the majority of work performed in mouse models of cancer. The models have increased in stringency as the field has progressed, reflecting maturation of the technology to approximate more closely the clinical situation.

Initially, polynucleotide vaccine strategies for cancer were targeted to artificial tumor antigens such as ovalbumin or β-galactosidase. Demonstration of tumor protective effects in these model systems led to the development of tumor models in which human tumor antigens, such as *CEA (90)* and *MUC1 (91)*, were transfected into syngeneic mouse tumor cell lines. These studies were useful for proof of principle to demonstrate that CTLs generated to these tumor antigens could protect against a lethal challenge of tumor cells. However, the cross-species differences in amino acid composition between the human and mouse rendered these vaccines more immunogenic than what naturally occurs in the clinical setting. The development of transgenic mouse models expressing human tumor antigens provides more stringent conditions that better recapitulate the clinical scenario under which to optimize polynucleotide vaccines. These models allow investigation into the particular requirements for mounting an effective immune response in the face of existing tolerance to tumor antigens.

Another potentially fruitful area of investigation is in the treatment of companion pets, as recently reported in a study of dogs with spontaneously arising malignant melanoma *(92)*. The genetic diversity of this population better reflects the scenario that will be encountered with humans.

With respect to establishing the safety and feasibility of PNI, experience in large animals and non-human primates *(93,94)* has been useful to demonstrate the general safety of the approach prior to human clinical trials.

Preclinical models have also proven invaluable in understanding the molecular mechanisms involved in generating an effective antitumor immune response subsequent to PNI. The development of a number of mouse models with particular aspects of the immune system selectively disrupted (i.e., genetic knockouts) has allowed more clear delineation of the factors critical for the induction of an effective immune response *(95)*. Investigation of the mechanism of tumor rejection mediated by a therapeutic DNA vaccine in a transgenic mouse model of breast cancer demonstrated the coordinated role of CD4[+] and CD8[+] cells, antibodies, Fc receptors, perforin, interferon-γ, CD1d-restricted NKT, and macrophages, with an important role for activated neutrophils, which may directly lyse cancer cells and affect tumor vasculature *(96,97)*.

7. CLINICAL EXPERIENCE WITH POLYNUCLEOTIDE VACCINES

Although induction of both T- and B-cell responses to foreign antigens has been convincingly demonstrated in humans with respect to foreign antigens relevant to infectious disease *(98–102)*, tumor antigens are comparatively weak with respect to antigenicity. Induction of an effective antitumor immune response to such antigens represents a considerable challenge, and to date the clinical experience with polynucleotide vaccines has met with mixed results. The clinical studies have supported the general safety and low toxicity of the vectors, but the potency of the immune response has been disappointing, and antitumor efficacy has proven elusive.

Several human clinical trials have been completed. Direct intramuscular delivery of DNA encoding a cloned tumor antigen (CEA) has been reported for advanced-stage colon cancer *(103)*. Patients were immunized with a plasmid expressing both CEA and, as a control, hepatitis B surface antigen. Although protective levels of antibodies recognizing the hepatitis protein were detected in some patients, there was little evidence of immune response directed against CEA. Rosenberg and colleagues reported similar findings using a plasmid DNA encoding the melanoma antigen gp100 in a phase I clinical trial for patients with metastatic melanoma *(104)*. In this trial of 22 patients immunized either intramuscularly or intradermally, no evidence of gp100-specific immune responses was detected, although 1 patient exhibited a partial response. The authors concluded that no significant clinical or immunological response was generated. This contrasts with previous clinical trials involving the gp100 antigen delivered as a transgene in a fowlpox-based vaccine or as peptides and emphasizes the need for strategies to enhance immune response to plasmid DNA vaccines.

The immunogenicity of a plasmid DNA vaccine for patients with B-cell lymphoma was evaluated *(105)*. Previous clinical studies using proteins representing tumor-specific immunoglobulin idiotype for active immunization demonstrated clinical benefit for immunized patients *(106,107)*; however, preparation of patient-specific protein vaccines is laborious and not feasible for widespread application. DNA vaccination offers the advantage of comparatively rapid and inexpensive preparation. Immunization of patients with a DNA vaccine encoding a chimeric molecule consisting of the patient-specific idiotype fused to the immunoglobulin G2a and k mouse immunoglobulin constant region chains. Cohorts of patients were immunized with DNA encoding the chimeric vaccine intramuscularly and intradermally using the Biojector needle-free delivery device, with or without the addition of plasmid DNA encoding granulocyte-macrophage colony-stimulating factor. In all groups of patients, most patients generated an immune response to the murine immunoglobulin carrier protein, demonstrating that the encoded protein was produced and was capable of eliciting an immune response. Induction of an immune response to the Id portion of the encoded gene was infrequent, but was detected in some patients.

It should be noted that these clinical trials were performed in the setting of advanced disease, for which induction of an immune response may not be optimal. Nevertheless, collectively the experience with naked DNA transfer in humans for cancer immunotherapy suggests that first-generation plasmid DNA vaccines will not be sufficient to elicit a clinically effective immune response against nonmutated self-antigens. Translation of the most promising strategies outlined in Table 1 to the clinic may address the limitations of current methods.

Two phase I trials of DNA vaccines directed against HPV-related malignancies have been reported. Treatment of HPV-related malignancies may offer the advantage of expression of a foreign HPV antigen in the malignant cells. Plasmid DNA encoding HLA-A2 epitopes from HPV16 E7 protein was encapsulated in biodegradable polymer microparticles, PLG, and delivered intramuscularly *(108)*. This therapeutic trial for individuals with anal dysplasia led to increased T-cell responses as detected by enzyme-linked immunospot (ELISPOT) in 10 of 12 patients and partial histological responses in some subjects in the higher dose groups. Use of the same reagent delivered subcutaneously or intramuscularly to women with cervical intraepithelial neoplasia resulted in detectable immune response to HPV E7 in most patients (73%) and complete histological response in 33% of women *(109)*. No vaccine-related serious adverse events were reported. These studies suggest that DNA vaccines directed at HPV antigens may have a role in management of HPV-related malignancies.

8. CONCLUSIONS/FUTURE DIRECTIONS

The pace of tumor antigen identification has accelerated rapidly in the past few years *(110)* and will likely increase with new techniques, such as expression profiling *(111,112)*, SEREX *(113)*, and proteomic analysis *(114)* leading to the identification of new potential targets for active immunotherapy. The use of DNA vaccines in preclinical models may provide a relatively rapid means of evaluating the potential utility of these candidate antigens in mediating tumor rejection. In addition to traditional tumor-associated antigens, polynucleotide vaccines may also find a role in vaccines strategies directed against tumor vasculature *(115)*.

Studies of polynucleotide vaccines for the treatment of chronic infectious disease will continue to be valuable in developing novel strategies that can be incorporated into cancer vaccines. For example, building on encouraging preclinical studies, a clinical study targeting infectious disease suggested that DNA prime and viral boost also potentiate the immune response in humans *(116)*.

Although definitive clinical evidence of the efficacy of polynucleotide vaccines in cancer therapy remains to be demonstrated, there is reason to be optimistic about their potential in the management of a wide variety of malignancies. As a relatively nontoxic therapy, PNI may ultimately find its clinical application as an adjuvant in the setting of minimal residual disease, for which it may be useful in preventing disease recurrence. Eventually, use of polynucleotide vaccines may extend to the cancer prevention arena. The notable advantages of PNI and its proven safety thus far in clinical studies provides a sound basis for continued development and eventual incorporation into the management of malignant disease.

ACKNOWLEDGMENT

The U.S. Army Medical Research and Materiel Command under DAMD17-00-1-0122 and NIH 1 P50 CA89019 supported this work.

REFERENCES

1. Rosenberg, S. A., Zhai, Y., Yang, J. C., et al. (1998) Immunizing patients with metastatic melanoma using recombinant adenoviruses encoding MART-1 or gp100 melanoma antigens. *J. Natl. Cancer Inst.* **90,** 1894–1900.
2. Conry, R. M., Khazaeli, M. B., Saleh, M. N., et al. (1999) Phase I trial of a recombinant vaccinia virus encoding carcinoembryonic antigen in metastatic adenocarcinoma: comparison of intradermal vs subcutaneous administration. *Clin. Cancer Res.* **5,** 2330–2337.
3. Dunn, G. P., Bruce, A. T., Ikeda, H., Old, L. J., and Schreiber, R. D. (2002) Cancer immunoediting: from immunosurveillance to tumor escape. *Nat. Immunol.* **3,** 991–998.
4. Wolff, J. A, Malone, R. W., Williams, P., et al. (1990) Direct gene transfer into mouse muscle in vivo. *Science* **247,** 1465–1468.
5. Hansen, E., Fernandes, K., Goldspink, G., Butterworth, P., Umeda, P. K., and Chang, K. C. (1991) Strong expression of foreign genes following direct injection into fish muscle. *FEBS Lett.* **290,** 73–76.
6. Jiao, S., Williams, P., Berg, R. K., et al. (1992) Direct gene transfer into nonhuman primate myofibers in vivo. *Hum. Gene Ther.* **3,** 21–33.
7. Danko, I. and Wolff, J. A. (1994) Direct gene transfer into muscle. *Vaccine* **12,** 1499–1502.
8. Wolff, J. A., Dowty, M. E., Jiao, S., et al. (1992) Expression of naked plasmids by cultured myotubes and entry of plasmids into T tubules and caveolae of mammalian skeletal muscle. *J. Cell Sci.* **103,** 1249–1259.
9. Wolff, J. A., Ludtke, J. J., Acsadi, G., Williams, P., and Jani, A. (1992) Long-term persistence of plasmid DNA and foreign gene expression in mouse muscle. *Hum. Mol. Genet.* **1,** 363–369.
10. Ulmer, J. B., Donnelly, J. J., Parker, S. E., et al. (1993) Heterologous protection against influenza by injection of DNA encoding a viral protein. *Science* **259,** 1745–1749.
11. Tang, D. C., DeVit, M., and Johnston, S. A. (1992) Genetic immunization is a simple method for eliciting an immune response. *Nature* **356,** 152–154.
12. Williams, R. S., Johnston, S. A., Riedy, M., DeVit, M. J., McElligott, S. G., and Sanford, J. C. (1991) Introduction of foreign genes into tissues of living mice by DNA-coated microprojectiles. *Proc. Natl. Acad. Sci. USA* **88,** 2726–2730.
13. Barry, M. A. and Johnston, S. A. (1997) Biological features of genetic immunization. *Vaccine* **15,** 788–1791.
14. Fynan, E. F., Webster, R. G., Fuller, D. H., Haynes, J. R., Santoro, J. C., and Robinson, H. L. (1993) DNA vaccines: protective immunizations by parenteral, mucosal, and gene-gun inoculations. *Proc. Natl. Acad. Sci. USA* **90,** 11,478–11,482.
15. Ross, H. M., Weber, L. W., Wang, S., et al. (1997) Priming for T-cell-mediated rejection of established tumors by cutaneous DNA immunization. *Clin. Cancer Res.* **3,** 2191–2196.
16. Cui, Z., Baizer, L., and Mumper, R. J. (2003) Intradermal immunization with novel plasmid DNA-coated nanoparticles via a needle-free injection device. *J. Biotechnol.* **102,** 105–115.
17. Eriksson, K. and Holmgren, J. (2002) Recent advances in mucosal vaccines and adjuvants. *Curr. Opin. Immunol.* **14,** 666–672.

18. Rocha-Zavaleta, L., Alejandre, J. E., and Garcia-Carranca, A. (2002) Parenteral and oral immunization with a plasmid DNA expressing the human papillomavirus 16-L1 gene induces systemic and mucosal antibodies and cytotoxic T lymphocyte responses. *J. Med. Virol.* **66,** 86–95.

19. Darji, A., Guzman, C. A., Gerstel, B., et al. (1997) Oral somatic transgene vaccination using attenuated *S. typhimurium. Cell.* **91,** 765–775.

20. Niethammer, A. G., Primus, F. J., Xiang, R., et al. (2001) An oral DNA vaccine against human carcinoembryonic antigen (CEA) prevents growth and dissemination of Lewis lung carcinoma in CEA transgenic mice. *Vaccine* **20,** 421–429.

21. Pertl, U., Wodrich, H., Ruehlmann, J. M., Gillies, S. D., Lode, H. N., and Reisfeld, R. A. (2003) Immunotherapy with a posttranscriptionally modified DNA vaccine induces complete protection against metastatic neuroblastoma. *Blood* **101,** 649–654.

22. Sizemore, D. R., Branstrom, A. A., and Sadoff, J. C. (1995) Attenuated *Shigella* as a DNA delivery vehicle for DNA-mediated immunization. *Science* **270,** 299–302.

23. Pan, Z. K., Weiskirch, L. M., and Paterson, Y. (1999) Regression of established B16 F10 melanoma with a recombinant *Listeria monocytogenes* vaccine. *Cancer Res.* **59,** 5264–5269.

24. White, S. A., LoBuglio, A. F., Arani, R. B., et al. (2000) Induction of anti-tumor immunity by intrasplenic administration of a carcinoembryonic antigen DNA vaccine. *J. Gene Med.* **2,** 135–140.

25. Pertmer, T. M., Roberts, T. R., and Haynes, J. R. (1996) Influenza virus nucleoprotein-specific immunoglobulin G subclass and cytokine responses elicited by DNA vaccination are dependent on the route of vector DNA delivery. *J. Virol.* **70,** 6119–6125.

26. Feltquate, D. M., Heaney, S., Webster, R. G., and Robinson, H. L. (1997) Different T helper cell types and antibody isotypes generated by saline and gene gun DNA immunization. *J. Immunol.* **158,** 2278–2284.

27. Qiu, P., Ziegelhoffer, P., Sun, J., and Yang, N. S. (1996) Gene gun delivery of mRNA *in situ* results in efficient transgene expression and genetic immunization. *Gene Ther.* **3,** 262–268.

28. Conry, R. M., LoBuglio, A. F., Wright, M., et al. (1995) Characterization of a messenger RNA polynucleotide vaccine vector. *Cancer Res.* **55,** 1397–1400.

29. Lietner, W. W., Ying, H., and Restifo, N. P. (2000) DNA and RNA-based vaccines: principles, progress and prospects. *Vaccine* **18,** 765–777.

30. Lundstrom, K. (2002) Alphavirus vectors as tools in cancer gene therapy. *Technol. Cancer Res. Treat.* **1,** 83–88.

31. Rayner, J. O., Dryga, S. A., and Kamrud, K. I. (2002) Alphavirus vectors and vaccination. *Rev. Med. Virol.* **12,** 279–296.

32. Herweijer, H., Latendresse, J. S., Williams, P., et al. (1995) A plasmid-based self-amplifying Sindbis virus vector. *Hum. Gene Ther.* **6,** 1161–1167.

33. Doe, B., Selby, M., Barnett, S., Baenziger, J., and Walker, C. M. (1996) Induction of cytotoxic T lymphocytes by intramuscular immunization with plasmid DNA is facilitated by bone marrow-derived cells. *Proc. Natl. Acad. Sci. USA* **93,** 8578–8583.

34. Iwasaki, A., Torres, C. A., Ohashi, P. S., Robinson, H. L., and Barber, B. H. (1997) The dominant role of bone marrow-derived cells in CTL induction following plasmid DNA immunization at different sites. *J. Immunol.* **159,** 11–14.

35. Fu, T. M., Ulmer, J. B., Caulfield, M. J., et al. (1997) Priming of cytotoxic T lymphocytes by DNA vaccines: requirement for professional antigen presenting cells and evidence for antigen transfer from myocytes. *Mol. Med.* **3,** 362–371.

36. Corr, M., von Damm, A., Lee, D. J., and Tighe, H. (1999) In vivo priming by DNA injection occurs predominantly by antigen transfer. *J. Immunol.* **163,** 4721–4727.

37. Condon, C., Watkins, S. C., Celluzzi, C. M., Thompson, K., and Falo, L. D. Jr. (1996) DNA-based immunization by in vivo transfection of dendritic cells. *Nat. Med.* **2,** 1122–1128.

38. Casares, S., Inaba, K., Brumeanu, T. D., Steinman, R. M., and Bona, C. A. (1997) Antigen presentation by dendritic cells after immunization with DNA encoding a major histocompatibility complex class II-restricted viral epitope. *J. Exp. Med.* **186,** 1481–1486.

39. Ossendorp, F., Mengede, E., Camps, M., Filius, R., and Melief, C. J. (1998) Specific T helper cell requirement for optimal induction of cytotoxic T lymphocytes against major histocompatibility complex class II negative tumors. *J. Exp. Med.* **187,** 693–702.

40. Hung, K., Hayashi, R., Lafond-Walker, A., Lowenstein, C., Pardoll, D., and Levitsky, H. (1998) The central role of CD4(+) T cells in the antitumor immune response. *J. Exp. Med.* **188,** 2357–2368.

41. Klinman, D. M., Yi, A. K., Beaucage, S. L., Conover, J., and Krieg, A. M. (1996) CpG motifs present in bacteria DNA rapidly induce lymphocytes to secrete interleukin 6, interleukin 12, and interferon gamma. *Proc. Natl. Acad. Sci. USA* **93,** 2879–2883.

42. Ashkar, A. A. and Rosenthal, K. L. (2002) Toll-like receptor 9, CpG DNA and innate immunity. *Curr. Mol. Med.* **2,** 545–556.

43. Agrawal, S. and Kandimalla, E. R. (2002) Medicinal chemistry and therapeutic potential of CpG DNA. *Trends Mol. Med.* **8,** 114–121.

44. Dalpke, A., Zimmermann, S., and Heeg, K. (2002) Immunopharmacology of CpG DNA. *Biol. Chem.* **383,** 1491–1500.
45. Davila, E., Velez, M. G., Heppelmann, C. J., and Celis, E. (2002) Creating space: an antigen-independent, CpG-induced peripheral expansion of naïve and memory T lymphocytes in a full T-cell compartment. *Blood* **100,** 2537–2545.
46. Ying, H., Zaks, T. Z., Wang, R. F., et al. (1999) Cancer therapy using a self-replicating RNA vaccine. *Nat. Med.* **5,** 823–827.
47. Leitner, W. W., Hwang, L. N., deVeer, M. J., et al. (2003) Alphavirus-based DNA vaccine breaks immunological tolerance by activating innate antiviral pathways. *Nat. Med.* **9,** 33–39.
48. Alexopoulou, L., Holt, A. C., Medizhitov, R., and Flavell, R. A. (2001) Recognition of double-stranded RNA and activation of NF-kappa B by Toll like receptor 3. *Nature* **413,** 732–738.
49. Zinckgraf, J. W. and Silbart, L. K. (2003) Modulating gene expression using DNA vaccines with different 3'-UTRs influences antibody titer, seroconversion and cytokine profiles. *Vaccine* **21,** 1640–1649.
50. Xin, K. Q., Ooki, T., Jounai, N., et al. (2003) A DNA vaccine containing inverted terminal repeats from adeno-associated virus increases immunity to HIV. *J. Gene Med.* **5,** 438–445.
51. Hanke, T., Neumann, V. C., Blanchard, T. J., et al. (1999) Effective induction of HIV-specific CTL by multi-epitope using gene gun in a combined vaccination regime. *Vaccine* **17,** 589–596.
52. Smith, B. F., Baker, H. J., Curiel, D. T., Jiang, W., and Conry, R. M. (1998) Humoral and cellular immune responses of dogs immunized with a nucleic acid vaccine encoding human carcinoembryonic antigen. *Gene Ther.* **5,** 865–868.
53. Ito, K., Ito, K., Shinohara, N., and Kato, S. (2003) DNA immunization via intramuscular and intradermal routes using a gene gun provides different magnitudes and durations on immune response. *Mol. Immunol.* **39,** 847–854.
54. Tuting, T., Gambotto, A., Robbins, P. D., Storkus, W. J., and DeLeo, A. B. (1999) Co-delivery of T helper 1-biasing cytokine genes enhances the efficacy of gene gun immunization of mice: studies with the model tumor antigen beta-galactosidase and the BALB/c Meth A p53 tumor-specific antigen. *Gene Ther.* **6,** 629–636.
55. Leitner, W. W., Seguin, M. C., Ballou, W. R., et al. (1997) Immune responses induced by intramuscular or gene gun injection of protective deoxyribonucleic acid vaccines that express the circumsporozoite protein from *Plasmodium berghei* malaria parasites. *J. Immunol.* **159,** 6112–6119.
56. Gregoriadis, G., Bacon, A., Caparros-Wanderley, W., and McCormack, B. (2002) A role for liposomes in genetic vaccination. *Vaccine* **20(Suppl. 5),** B1–B9.
57. Singh, M., Briones, M., Ott, G., and O'Hagan, D. (2000) Cationic microparticles: a potent delivery system for DNA vaccines. *Proc. Natl. Acad. Sci. USA* **97,** 811–816.
58. Drabick, J. J., Glasspool-Malone, J., King, A., and Malone, R. W. (2001) Cutaneous transfection and immune responses to intradermal nucleic acid vaccination are significantly enhanced by in vivo electropermeabilization. *Mol. Ther.* **3,** 249–255.
59. Paster, W., Zehetner, M., Kalat, M., Schuller, S., and Schweighoffer, T. (2003) In vivo plasmid DNA electroporation generates exceptionally high levels of epitope-specific CD8⁺ T-cell responses. *Gene Ther.* **10,** 717–724.
60. Hung, C. F. and Wu, T. C. (2003) Improving DNA vaccine potency via modification of professional antigen presenting cells. *Curr. Opin. Mol. Ther.* **5,** 20–24.
61. Xiang, R., Primus, F. J., Ruehlmann, J. M., et al. (2001) A dual-function DNA vaccine encoding carcinoembryonic antigen and CD40 ligand trimer induces T cell-mediated protective immunity against colon cancer in carcinoembryonic antigen-transgenic mice. *J. Immunol.* **167,** 4560–4565.
62. Hung, C. F., Hsu, K. F., Cheng, W. F., et al. (2001) Enhancement of DNA vaccine potency by linkage of antigen gene to a gene encoding the extracellular domain of Fms-like tyrosine kinase 3-ligand. *Cancer Res.* **61,** 1080–1088.
63. Boyle, J. S., Brady, J. L., and Lew, A. M. (1998) Enhanced responses to a DNA vaccine encoding a fusion antigen that is directed to sites of immune induction. *Nature* **392,** 408–411.
64. Su, Z., Vieweg, J., Weizer, A. Z., et al. (2002) Enhanced induction of telomerase-specific CD4(+) T cells using dendritic cells transfected with RNA encoding a chimeric gene product. *Cancer Res.* **62,** 5041–5048.
65. Ji, H., Wang, T. L., Chen, C. H., et al. (1999) Targeting human papillomavirus type 16 E7 to the endosomal/lysosomal compartment enhances the antitumor immunity of DNA vaccines against murine human papillomavirus type 16 E7-expressing tumors. *Hum. Gene Ther.* **10,** 2727–2740.
66. Xiang, R., Lode, H. N., Chao, T. H., et al. (2000) An autologous oral DNA vaccine protects against murine melanoma. *Proc. Natl. Acad. Sci USA* **97,** 5492–5497.
67. Rice, J., Buchan, S., and Stevenson, F. K. (2002) Critical components of a DNA fusion vaccine able to induce protective cytotoxic T cells against a single epitope of a tumor antigen. *J. Immunol.* **169,** 3908–3918.
68. Cid-Arregui, A., Juarez, V., and zur Hausen, H. (2003) A synthetic E7 gene of human papillomavirus type 16 that yields enhanced expression of the protein in mammalian cells and is useful for DNA immunization studies. *J. Virol.* **77,** 4928–4937.
69. Scheerlinck, J. P., Casey, G., McWaters, P., et al. (2001) The immune response to a DNA vaccine can be modulated by co-delivery of cytokine genes using a DNA prime-protein boost strategy. *Vaccine* **19,** 4053–4060.
70. Conry, R. M., Widera, G., LoBuglio, A. F., et al. (1996) Selected strategies to augment polynucleotide immunization. *Gene Ther.* **3,** 67–74.

71. Irvine, K. R., Rao, J. B., Rosenberg, S. A., and Restifo, N. P. (1996) Cytokine enhancement of DNA immunization leads to effective treatment of established pulmonary metastases. *J. Immunol.* **156,** 238–245.
72. Biragyn, A., Surenhu, M., Yang, D., et al. (2001) Mediators of innate immunity that target immature, but not mature, dendritic cells induce antitumor immunity when genetically fused with nonimmunogenic tumor antigens. *J. Immunol.* **167,** 6644–6653.
73. Kim, J. J., Yang, J. S., Dentchev, T., Dang, K., and Weiner, D. B. (2000) Chemokine gene adjuvants can modulate immune responses induced by DNA vaccines. *J. Interferon Cytokine Res.* **20,** 487–498.
74. Kim, T. W. Hung, C. F., Ling, M., et al. (2003) Enhancing DNA vaccine potency by coadministration of DNA encoding antiapoptotic proteins. *J. Clin. Invest.* **112,** 109–117.
75. Cappello, P., Triebel, F., Iezzi, M., et al. (2003) LAG-3 Enables DNA vaccination to persistently prevent mammary carcinogenesis in HER-2/neu transgenic BALB/c mice. *Cancer Res.* **63,** 2518–2525.
76. He, Y., Pimenov, A. A., Nayak, J. V., Plowey, J., Falo, L. D. Jr., and Huang, L. (2002) Intravenous injection of naked DNA encoding secreted FLT3 ligand dramatically increases the number of dendritic cells and natural killer cells in vivo. *Hum. Gene Ther.* **11,** 547–554.
77. Fong, C. L. and Hui, K. M. (2002) Generation of potent and specific cellular immune responses via in vivo stimulation of dendritic cells by pNGVL3-hFLex plasmid DNA and immunogenic peptides. *Gene Ther.* **9,** 1127–1138.
78. Weber, L. W., Bowne, W. B., Wolchok, J. D., et al. (1998) Tumor immunity and autoimmunity induced by immunization with homologous DNA. *J. Clin. Invest.* **102,** 1258–1264.
79. Su, J. M., Wei, Y. Q., Tian, L., et al. (2003) Active immunogene therapy of cancer with vaccine on the basis of chicken homologous matrix metalloproteinase-2. *Cancer Res.* **63,** 600–607.
80. Hawkins, W. G., Gold, J. S., Blachere, N. E., et al. (2002) Xenogeneic DNA immunization in melanoma models for minimal residual disease. *J. Surg. Res.* **102,** 137–143.
81. Wei, Y. Q., Huang, M. J., Yang, L., et al. (2001) Immunogene therapy of tumors with vaccine based upon *Xenopus* homologous vascular endothelial growth factor as a model antigen. *Proc. Natl. Acad. Sci. USA* **98,** 11,545–11,550.
82. Fong, L., Brockstedt, D., Benike, C., et al. (2001) Dendritic cell-based xenoantigen vaccination for prostate cancer immunotherapy. *J. Immunol.* **167,** 7150–7156.
83. Ramshaw, I. A. and Ramsay, A. J. (2000) The prime-boost strategy: exciting prospects for improved vaccination. *Immunol. Today* **21,** 163–165.
84. Irvine, K. R., Chamberlain, R. S., Shulman, E. P., et al. (1997) Enhancing efficacy of recombinant anticancer vaccines with prime/boost regimens that use two different vectors. *J. Natl. Cancer Inst.* **89,** 1595–1601.
85. Woodberry, T., Gardner, J., Elliott, S. L., et al. (2003) Prime boost vaccination strategies: CD8 T cell numbers, protection, and Th1 bias. *J. Immunol.* **170,** 2599–2604.
86. Meng, W. S., Butterfield, L. H., Ribas, A., et al. (2001) Alpha-Fetoprotein specific tumor immunity induce by plasmid prime-adenovirus boost genetic vaccination. *Cancer Res.* **61,** 8782–8786.
87. Pasquini, S., Peralta, S., Missiaglia, E., Carta, L., and Lemoine, N. R. (2002) Prime-boost vaccines encoding an intracellular idiotype/GM-CSF fusion protein induce protective cell-mediated immunity in murine pre-B cell leukemia. *Gene Ther.* **9,** 503–510.
88. Chen, C. H., Wang, T. L., Hung, C. F., Pardoll, D. M., and Wu, T. C. (2000) Boosting with recombinant vaccinia increases HPE-16 E7-specific T cell precursor frequencies of HPV-16 E7-expressing DNA vaccines. *Vaccine* **18,** 2015–2022.
89. Otten, G., Schaefer, M., Greer, C., et al. (2003) Induction of broad and potent anti-human immunodeficiency virus immune responses in rhesus macaques by priming with a DNA vaccine and boosting with protein-adsorbed polylactide coglycolide microparticles. *J. Virol.* **77,** 6087–6092.
90. Conry, R. M., LoBuglio, A. F., Loechel, F., et al. (1995) A carcinoembryonic antigen polynucleotide vaccine has in vivo antitumor activity. *Gene Ther.* **2,** 59–65.
91. Graham, R. A., Burchell, J. M., Beverley, P., and Taylor-Papadimitriou, J. (1996) Intramuscular immunisation with MUC1 cDNA can protect C57 mice challenged with MUC1-expressing syngeneic mouse tumour cells. *Int. J. Cancer* **65,** 664–670.
92. Bergman, P. J., McKnight, J., Novosad, A., et al. (2003) Long-term survival of dogs with advanced malignant melanoma after DNA vaccination with xenogeneic human tyrosinase: a phase I trial. *Clin. Cancer Res.* **9,** 1284–1290.
93. Kim, J. J., Yang, J. S., Dang, K., Manson, K. H., and Weiner, D. B. (2001) Engineering enhancement of immune responses to DNA-based vaccines in a prostate cancer model in rhesus macaques through the use of cytokine gene adjuvants. *Clin. Cancer Res.* **7,** 882s–889s.
94. Conry, R. M., White, S. A., Fultz, P. N., et al. (1998) Polynucleotide immunization of nonhuman primates against carcinoembryonic antigen. *Clin. Cancer Res.* **4,** 2903–2912.
95. Song, K., Chang, Y., and Prud'homme, G. J. (2000) IL-12 plasmid-enhanced DNA vaccination against carcinoembryonic antigen (CEA) studied in immune-gene knockout mice. *Gene Ther.* **7,** 1527–1535.
96. Dranoff, G. (2003) Coordinated tumor immunity. *J. Clin. Invest.* **111,** 1116–1118.

97. Curcio, C., Di Carlo, E., Clynes, R., et al. (2003) Nonredundant roles of antibody, cytokines, and perforin in the eradication of established Her-2/neu carcinomas. *J. Clin. Invest.* **111,** 1161–1170.
98. Wang, R., Doolan, D. L., Le, T. P., et al. (1998) Induction of antigen-specific cytotoxic T lymphocytes in humans by a malaria DNA vaccine. *Science* **28,** 476–480.
99. Wang, R., Epstein, J., Baraceros, F. M., et al. (2001) Induction of CD4(+) T cell-dependent CD8(+) type 1 responses in humans by a malaria DNA vaccine. *Proc. Natl. Acad. Sci. USA* **98,** 10,817–10,822.
100. Roy, M. J., Wu, M. S., Barr, L. J., et al. (2000) Induction of antigen-specific CD8$^+$ T cells, T helper cells, and protective levels of antibody in humans by particle-mediated administration of a hepatitis B virus DNA vaccine. *Vaccine* **19,** 764–778.
101. MacGregor, R. R., Ginsberg, R., Ugen, K. E., et al. (2002) T-cell responses induced in normal volunteers immunized with a DNA-based vaccine containing HIV-1 env and rev. *AIDS* **16,** 2137–2143.
102. Calarota, S., Bratt, G., Nordlund, S., et al. (1998) Cellular cytotoxic response induced by DNA vaccination in HIV-1-infected patients. *Lancet* **351,** 1320–1325.
103. Conry, R. M., Curiel, D. T., Strong, T. V., et al. (2002) Safety and immunogenicity of a DNA vaccine encoding carcinoembryonic antigen and hepatitis B surface antigen in colorectal carcinoma patients. *Clin. Cancer Res.* **8,** 2782–2787.
104. Rosenberg, S. A., Yang, J. C., Sherry, R. M., et al. (2003) Inability to immunize patients with metastatic melanoma using plasmid DNA encoding the gp100 melanoma-melanocyte antigen. *Hum. Gene Ther.* **14,** 709–714.
105. Timmerman, J. M., Singh, G., Hermanson, G., et al. (2002) Immunogenicity of a plasmid DNA vaccine encoding chimeric idiotype in patients with B-cell lymphoma. *Cancer Res.* **62,** 5845–5852.
106. Timmerman, J. M. and Levy, R. (2000) The history of the development of vaccines for the treatment of lymphoma. *Clin. Lymphoma* **1,** 129–139.
107. Bendandi, M., Gocke, C. D., Kobrin, C. B., et al. (1999) Complete molecular remissions induced by patient-specific vaccination plus granulocyte-monocyte colony-stimulating factor against lymphoma. *Nat. Med.* **5,** 1171–1177.
108. Klencke, B., Matijevic, M., Urban, R. G., et al. (2002) Encapsulated plasmid DNA treatment for human papillomavirus 16-associated anal dysplasia: a phase I study of ZYC101. *Clin. Cancer Res.* **8,** 1028–1037.
109. Sheets, E. E., Urban, R. G., Crum, C. P., et al. (2003) Immunotherapy of human cervical high-grade cervical intraepithelial neoplasia with microparticle-delivered human papillomavirus 16 E7 plasmid DNA. *Am. J. Obstet. Gynecol.* **188,** 916–926.
110. Stevanovic, S. (2002) Identification of tumour-associated T-cell epitopes for vaccine development. *Nat. Rev. Cancer* **2,** 514–520.
111. Nelson, P. S. (2002) Identifying immunotherapeutic targets for prostate carcinoma through the analysis of gene expression profiles. *Ann. NY Acad. Sci.* **975,** 232–246.
112. Schultze, J. L. and Vonderheide, R. H. (2001) From cancer genomics to cancer immunotherapy: toward second-generation tumor antigens. *Trends Immunol.* **22,** 516–523.
113. Chen, Y. T. (2000) Cancer vaccine: identification of human tumor antigens by SEREX. *Cancer J.* **6(Suppl. 3),** S208–S217.
114. Naour, F. L., Brichory, F., Beretta, L., and Hanash, S. M. (2002) Identification of tumor-associated antigens using proteomics. *Technol. Cancer Res. Treat.* **1,** 257–262.
115. Niethammer, A. G., Xiang, R., Becker, J. C., et al. (2002) A DNA vaccine against VEGF receptor 2 prevents effective angiogenesis and inhibits tumor growth. *Nat. Med.* **8,** 1369–1375.
116. McConkey, S. J., Reece, W. H., Moorthy, V. S., et al. (2003) Enhanced T-cell immunogenicity of plasmid DNA vaccines boosted by recombinant modified vaccinia virus Ankara in humans. *Nat. Med.* **9,** 729–735.

13

Development of Oncolytic Replication-Competent Herpes Simplex Virus Vectors

Herpes Simplex Virus Vectors

The G207 Paradigm

Tomoki Todo and Samuel D. Rabkin

1. INTRODUCTION

Oncolytic virus therapy is a promising new strategy for treating cancer that involves replication-competent virus vectors that can replicate *in situ* in tumor cells, exhibit oncolytic activity by direct cytocidal effects, and then spread throughout the tumor. In addition, replication-competent virus vectors are capable of transferring and expressing foreign genes in host cells. These virus vectors are either genetically engineered (e.g., herpes simplex virus type 1 [HSV-1], adenovirus, vaccinia virus), naturally attenuated (e.g., Newcastle disease virus), or nonpathogenic in humans (e.g., reovirus), so they replicate selectively in tumor cells, but do not harm normal tissues *(1)*.

HSV-1 in particular has many features that make it attractive for cancer therapy *(2)*: (1) HSV-1 infects most tumor cell types; (2) its life cycle is well studied *(3)*; (3) the HSV-1 genome has been sequenced; (4) the functions of the majority of genes have been identified *(4)*; (5) genes can be manipulated; and (6) the large size of the genome (153 kb) provides space for insertion of large amounts of deoxyribonucleic acid (DNA) *(4)*. Furthermore, HSV-1 has the following features that are well suited for clinical application: (1) total tumor cell killing in vitro can be achieved at a relatively low multiplicity of infection (MOI); (2) antiviral drugs are available that enable optional termination of the therapy *(5)*; (3) animal models are available for preclinical evaluation of safety and efficacy; (4) the viral genome does not integrate into the host cell genome; and (5) it can exist in a latent state without causing detectable damage to the infected cell *(6)*. HSV-1 is a neurotropic virus, and many of the genes necessary for neuropathogenicity are nonessential and can be mutated *(7)*. Therefore, the use of HSV-1 is especially advantageous for brain tumor therapy.

Research on oncolytic HSV-1 therapy has advanced rapidly from a basic concept to clinical studies. In the early days, replication-competent HSV-1 vectors were genetically engineered to have mutations in one nonessential gene associated with either virulence or viral DNA synthesis to restrict viral replication to transformed cells *(2,8)*. These so-called first-generation vectors demonstrated that HSV-1 vectors could in fact efficiently inhibit the growth of tumors without lethally harming the host animal. They also showed that oncolytic HSV-1 therapy could be applied not only to brain tumors, but also to a broad range of solid tumors *(9)*. There were concerns, however, regarding the use of these first-generation vectors in humans because their pathogenicity may not have been sufficiently attenuated, and a single mutation could potentially revert to wild type. To address these concerns, so-called second-generation vectors were developed that had genetically engineered mutations in two different genes.

From: *Contemporary Cancer Research*
Cancer Gene Therapy
Edited by: D. T. Curiel and J. T. Douglas © Humana Press Inc., Totowa, NJ

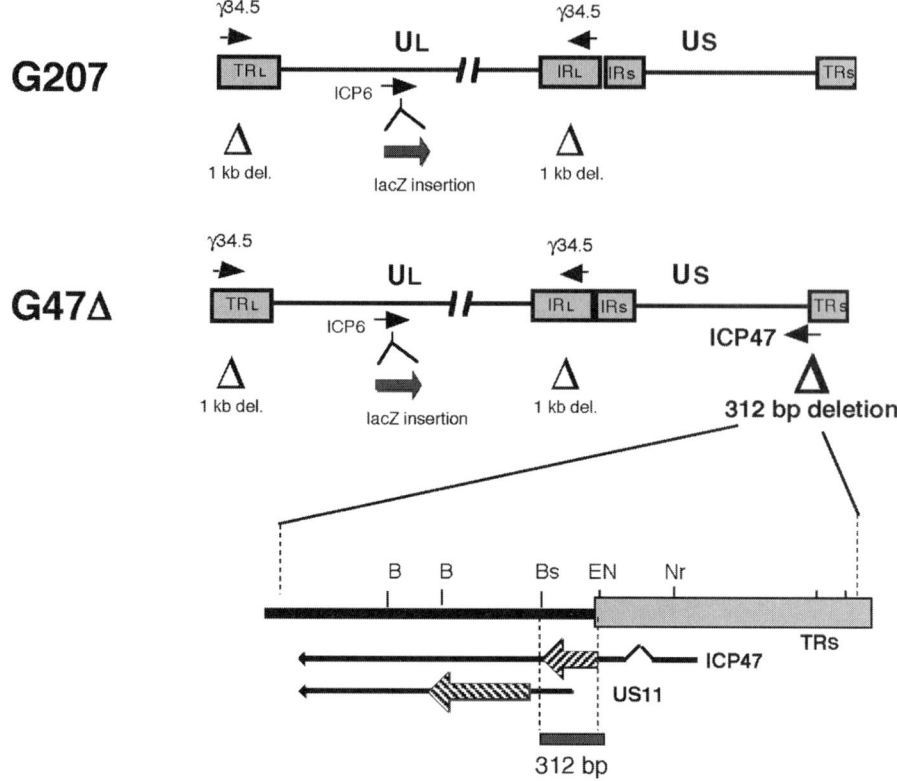

Fig. 1. Structures of G207 and G47Δ. The HSV-1 genome consists of long and short unique regions U$_L$ and U$_S$, respectively, each bounded by terminal (T) and internal (I) repeat regions R$_L$ and R$_S$, respectively. G207 was engineered from wild-type HSV-1 strain F by deleting 1 kb within both copies of the *γ34.5* gene and inserting the *E. coli lacZ* gene into the ICP6 coding region. G47Δ was derived from G207 by deleting 312 bp from the ICP47 locus. Because of the overlapping 3' coterminal transcripts of US11 and ICP47, the deletion also places the late gene US11 under control of the ICP47 immediate-early promoter. The ICP47 transcript contains an intron (indicated by Λ). Restriction site abbreviations: B, BamHI; Bs, BstEII; E, EcoRI, EN, EcoNI, Nr, NruI. (Modified from ref. *80*.)

2. G207

G207 was the first of the second-generation HSV-1 vectors *(10)*. It was originally designed for clinical application in patients with brain tumors, with an emphasis on employing ample safeguards. G207 has deletions in both copies of the γ34.5 gene (Fig. 1), the major determinant of HSV-1 neurovirulence *(11)*. The γ34.5-deficient HSV-1 vectors are considerably attenuated in normal cells, but retain their ability to replicate in neoplastic cells *(9)*.

In normal cells, HSV-1 infection induces activation of double-stranded RNA-dependent protein kinase R (PKR), which in turn leads to phosphorylation of the α-subunit of eukaryotic initiation factor 2α (eIF-2α) and a subsequent shutdown of host and viral protein synthesis *(12)*. The product of the γ34.5 gene antagonizes this PKR activity. However, in tumor cells with an activated Ras signaling pathway, it has been suggested that PKR activity is already inhibited, thereby allowing *γ34.5*-deficient HSV-1 vectors to replicate *(13,14)*. Many of the oncolytic HSV-1 vectors currently used have deletions in the *γ34.5* gene *(8)*, including R3616 *(11)*, the parent of G207, and 1716 *(15)*.

G207 also has an insertion of the *Escherichia coli lacZ* gene in the infected-cell protein 6 (ICP6) coding region (UL39), inactivating ribonucleotide reductase, a key enzyme for viral DNA synthesis in nondividing cells, but not in dividing cells *(16)*. This double mutation greatly minimizes the chances of G207 reverting to wild type or a pathogenic phenotype. It also confers favorable properties on the virus for treating human cancers; G207 replicates preferentially in tumor cells and is harmless in normal tissue because of attenuated virulence, G207 is about 10-fold more sensitive to ganciclovir/acyclovir than its parent virus R3616, and the reporter gene *lacZ* allows easy histochemical detection of G207-infected cells *(10)*. 3616UB is a similar, second-generation vector except uracil DNA glycosylase was inactivated instead of ICP6 *(17)*.

2.1. Antitumor Efficacy

G207 has been tested in more than 60 different cell lines, which revealed that the vast majority, although not all, of human tumor cell lines are susceptible to G207 infection and replication *(18)*. In human glioma and malignant meningioma cell lines, for example, G207 can achieve destruction of the entire cell population in culture within 2 to 6 days at an MOI of 0.1 *(10,19)*. In contrast, at the same MOI, G207 manifests no effect on primary cultures of rat cortical astrocytes or cerebellar neurons *(10)*.

This difference in G207 cytopathic effect observed in vitro between tumor cells and normal cells is directly reflected in the results of in vivo studies. In athymic mice harboring U87MG glioma or F5 malignant meningioma tumors intracranially or subcutaneously, a single intraneoplastic inoculation of G207 significantly inhibited tumor growth and prolonged animal survival *(10,19)*. Prominent *lacZ* expression from G207 replication within tumors could still be observed 24 days postinoculation *(19)*.

Besides brain tumors, G207 has proven efficacious in a variety of other animal tumor models in which human, mouse, rat, or hamster tumors have been generated subcutaneously or in various organs, including the liver, peritoneum, sciatic nerve, urinary bladder, and cheek pouch *(18)*.

In addition to direct intratumoral inoculation, G207 has been successfully administered intravenously *(20–22)*, via portal vein *(23)*, intraarterially *(24)*, and intraperitoneally *(25,26)*.

2.2. Safety

Because HSV-1 is the most common viral cause of fatal encephalitis *(27)* and G207 was the first replication-competent HSV-1 vector, along with 1716 *(28)*, to be used in human brains, it was extensively evaluated for its toxicity in the brain. In BALB/c mice, the highest dose of G207 (10^7 plaque forming units [pfu]) caused no symptoms for over 20 weeks when inoculated intracerebrally or intraventricularly *(29)*. In A/J mice, one of the most susceptible mouse strains to HSV-1 infection *(30)*, intracerebral inoculation of clinical-grade G207 at 2×10^6 pfu caused only a temporary and slight hunching in 2/8 mice *(31)*. Furthermore, in BALB/c mice that survived an intracerebral inoculation of wild-type HSV-1 (strain KOS) at an LD_{50} dose (~10^3 pfu), a subsequent challenge with an intracerebral inoculation of G207 (10^7 pfu) at the same stereotactic coordinates did not result in reactivation of latent HSV-1 *(29)*.

Aotus nancymae (New World owl monkeys) are among the most sensitive nonhuman primates to HSV-1 infection *(32,33)*. A total of 22 *Aotus* primates have been used for safety evaluation of G207 (intracerebral and/or intraprostatic inoculation) *(34–36)*. In *Aotus*, a single intracerebral inoculation of G207, up to 10^9 pfu or repeat inoculations of 10^7 pfu, caused neither virus-related disease nor detectable changes in the brain as assessed by magnetic resonance imaging (MRI) and pathological studies *(34)*.

In contrast, an intracerebral inoculation of 10^3 pfu of wild-type HSV-1 (strain F) caused acute viral encephalitis, with the animal becoming moribund within 5 days of inoculation. Four *Aotus* were used to evaluate the shedding and biodistribution of G207 after intracerebral inoculation of clinical-grade, column-purified G207 (3×10^7 pfu) *(35)*. Using polymerase chain reaction analyses and viral culture, neither infectious virus nor viral DNA was detected from tear, saliva, vaginal secretion, blood, or urine samples at any time-point up to 1 month postinoculation. Analyses of tissues obtained at necropsy at 1 month showed G207 DNA distribution restricted to the brain, with no infectious virus isolated. Histopathology revealed normal brain tissues, including the sites of inoculation *(35)*. All *Aotus* receiving an intracerebral G207 inoculation showed an increase in serum anti-HSV-1 antibody titers as early as 21 days postinoculation *(34,35)*.

2.3. Clinical Trial

A phase I clinical trial of G207 for recurrent malignant glioma was performed in 21 patients at two institutions in the United States *(37)*. This dose escalation study started at 10^6 pfu and increased to 3×10^9 pfu, with three patients at each dose. G207 was inoculated stereotactically into an enhancing region of the tumor, visualized by computerized tomographic scan with contrast enhancement. No acute, moderate-to-severe, adverse events attributable to G207 were observed *(37)*. Minor adverse events included seizure (2 cases) and brain edema (1 case). Among 7 biopsied or resected tumors analyzed, specimens from 2 patients were positive for G207 DNA by polymerase chain reaction analysis (56 and 157 days postinoculation). Of 19 patients, 5 were negative for serum anti-HSV-1 antibody prior to G207 treatment, and despite corticosteroid treatment of these patients, 1 patient seroconverted after G207 inoculation *(37)*.

The tools to evaluate efficacy included Karnofsky performance score and serial MRI *(37)*. An improvement in Karnofsky score was observed in 6 of 21 patients (29%) at some time after G207 inoculation. Of 20 patients that had serial MRI evaluations, 8 had a decrease in tumor volume (enhancing area) between 4 days and 1 month postinoculation. All patients, except 1 who died from cerebral infarction 10 months after G207 treatment, eventually showed tumor progression. Interestingly, this glioblastoma patient had no evidence of residual tumor at autopsy. Autopsy was performed in 5 cases, and histology of the brains showed no evidence of encephalitis, white matter degeneration, or inflammatory changes, and all were negative for HSV-1 immunoreactivity. In 3 cases, the tumor was localized to one region of the brain without significant tumor cell invasion into the surrounding brain tissue as usually observed with typical glioblastoma cases.

Overall, the phase I clinical trial confirmed the safety of G207 inoculated into the brain at doses up to 3×10^9 pfu. Currently, a phase Ib clinical trial for recurrent malignant glioma was performed [NIH 481 (2001-07)], and a phase II trial is planned. Similar results were obtained in phase I trials for glioma with 1716 in the United Kingdom *(28,38)*; 1716, which only contains deletions of $\gamma 34.5$ *(15)*, was tested at a lower dose range (up to 10^5 pfu) *(28,38)*.

3. USE OF ONCOLYTIC HSV VECTORS FOR IMMUNE THERAPY

Although G207 proved safe in glioma patients and efficacious in animal tumor models, G207 is considerably attenuated, not only for pathogenicity, but also in its tumor cell-killing capability compared to wild-type HSV-1. One way to improve the efficacy of oncolytic HSV therapy would be to harness antitumor immune responses induced in the course of the oncolytic activity of HSV vectors.

3.1. Antitumor Immune Responses

A difficulty in investigating the immune effects of oncolytic HSV therapy has been the lack of suitable animal tumor models susceptible to HSV-1 infection. Many mouse strains and a majority of murine cell lines are relatively resistant to HSV-1 *(18,30)*. It was not recognized until development of immunocompetent mouse tumor models suitable for HSV-1 evaluation that the host immune response plays an important role in the antitumor activity of oncolytic HSV-1 vectors both in the brain and in the periphery *(39,40)*. Initially, murine N18 neuroblastoma cells, one of the more susceptible murine cell lines tested for G207 susceptibility, were used in syngeneic A/J mice. In A/J mice harboring established N18 tumors subcutaneously or in the brain, intraneoplastic inoculation with G207 caused a significant reduction in tumor growth or prolongation of survival *(39)*. Moreover, in A/J mice bearing bilateral subcutaneous N18 tumors, intraneoplastic G207 inoculation into one tumor alone caused growth reduction and/or regression of both the inoculated and the noninoculated contralateral tumor, indicating induction of systemic antitumor immunity *(39)*. This inhibition of noninoculated tumor growth was also seen in animals bearing intracerebral brain tumors after subcutaneous tumor inoculation. Animals that were cured of their subcutaneous tumors by G207 were protected against tumor rechallenge, in either the periphery or the brain. Antitumor immunity was associated with cyto-toxic T lymphocyte (CTL) activity that was specific to N18 tumor cells and persisted for at least 13 months.

G207-induced, systemic antitumor immunity was also observed in BALB/c mice bearing subcuta-neous CT26 (colon carcinoma) tumors and DBA/2 mice bearing subcutaneous M3 (melanoma) tumors *(40)*. In the CT26 model, intraneoplastic inoculation of G207 induced CTL activity that recognized a dominant, tumor-specific, major histocompatibility complex (MHC) class I-restricted epitope (AH1) from CT26 cells. Similar systemic antitumor immunity induction by G207 was observed in Syrian hamsters bearing subcutaneous KIGB-5 (gallbladder carcinoma) tumors *(41)* and BALB/c mice bear-ing CT26 liver metastases *(42)*. Thus, in an immunocompetent condition, the oncolytic activity of G207 can be augmented by induction of specific and systemic antitumor immunity effective both in the periphery and in the brain.

When high-dose dexamethasone was given to A/J mice bearing subcutaneous N18 tumors for an extensive period (16 days), G207 retained antitumor activity and caused a significant suppression of tumor growth when inoculated into the tumors *(43)*. However, all immunosuppressed (dexamethasone-treated) mice treated with G207 displayed tumor regrowth despite initial shrinkage, whereas 50% of the G207-treated mice not immunosuppressed were cured. Dexamethasone administration signifi-cantly reduced neutralizing serum antibodies against G207 after intraneoplastic G207 inoculation, but this did not affect the amount of infectious G207 isolated from tumors. The most striking effect of dexamethasone administration was the abolition of G207-induced CTL activity against N18 cells *(43)*. These results further support the importance of tumor-specific CTL induction in the course of oncolytic HSV-1 antitumor activity.

The effect of circulating anti-HSV-1 antibodies on the efficacy of oncolytic HSV-1 therapy has been investigated because the majority of the population is HSV-1 seropositive *(44,45)*. A/J and BALB/c mice were immunized by repeated intraperitoneal inoculations of wild-type HSV-1 (strain KOS) and then the antitumor efficacy of G207 on established subcutaneous N18 and CT26 tumors was deter-mined *(46)*. In both tumor models, the antitumor efficacy of G207 was the same whether the mice were immunized or not for HSV-1.

In a study using intraocular immunization, treatment of M3 melanoma tumors in DBA/2 mice with HSV-1 1716 was actually more effective than in nonimmunized mice *(47)*. Because HSV-1 predomi-nantly spreads cell to cell, circulating antibodies known to neutralize free virus may have little effect on HSV-1 directly inoculated into tumors. When NV1020, at a low dose (10^6 pfu), was administered intra-venously to immunized BALB/c mice with CT26 tumors in the liver, there was a detectable decrease in efficacy *(48)*. This efficacy attenuation with intravenous delivery was overcome by administering a higher dose (10^7 pfu) of NV1020.

3.2. Third-Generation Oncolytic HSV-1 Vector

The therapeutic benefits of oncolytic HSV-1 vectors depend on the extent of both intratumoral viral replication and induction of host antitumor immune responses. We are developing new genera-tions of HSV-1 vectors by enhancing these properties and retaining the safety features of G207. G47Δ is one such vector created from G207 by introducing another genetic alteration, deletion of the α47 gene and the overlapping *US11* promoter region *(31)* (Fig. 1). Because the α47 gene product (ICP47) inhibits transporter associated with antigen presentation, which translocates peptides across the endoplasmic reticulum, the downregulation of MHC class I that normally occurs in human cells after infection with HSV-1 does not occur *(49)*. G47Δ-infected human cells in fact presented higher levels of MHC class I than cells infected with other HSV-1 vectors *(31)*. Further, human melanoma cells infected with G47Δ were better at stimulating their matched tumor-infiltrating lymphocytes in vitro than those infected with G207. Unfortunately, the interaction of ICP47 with transporter associated with antigen presentation is species specific and is exceedingly inefficient in rodent cells *(50)*. Therefore, it is not possible to test the immune effects in vivo in mouse tumor models.

The deletion also places the late *US11* gene under control of the immediate-early *α47* promoter, which results in suppression of the reduced growth phenotype of *γ34.5*-deficient HSV-1 mutants *(51)*, including G207. In the majority of cell lines tested in vitro, G47Δ replicated better than G207, resulting in the generation of higher virus titers, and exhibited greater cytopathic effect *(31)*. In athymic mice bearing subcutaneous U87MG human glioma tumors and A/J mice bearing subcutaneous Neuro2a neuroblastoma tumors, G47Δ was significantly more efficacious than G207 at inhibiting tumor growth when inoculated intraneoplastically *(31)*.

Improved antitumor efficacy of G47Δ has also been shown in other immunocompetent mouse tumor models, including prostate and breast cancer *(65)*. Nevertheless, this deletion does not suppress the attenuated pathogenicity of *γ34.5* deletion mutants *(52)*, and the safety of G47Δ remained unchanged from G207 following injection into the brains of HSV-1-sensitive A/J mice *(31)*.

Thus, compared with the parental virus G207, G47Δ demonstrated (1) better induction of human antitumor immune cells; (2) better growth properties, leading to higher virus yields and increased cytopathic effect in vitro; (3) better antitumor efficacy in both immunocompetent and immunoincompetent animals; and (4) preserved safety. These features make G47Δ highly attractive for clinical application.

3.3. Combination With Immune Gene Therapy

Our experience using various HSV-1 vectors to treat tumors, including wild-type HSV-1, indicates that there is a limit to improving the antitumor efficacy of oncolytic vectors by simply bringing the replication capability closer to that of wild-type viruses, putting aside the difficulty of doing so without increasing pathogenicity. In developing new vectors, therefore, more emphasis is currently placed on enhancing the ability to induce antitumor immunity. The combination of oncolytic HSV-1 vectors with defective vectors expressing immunostimulatory molecules can improve therapeutic efficacy significantly (Fig. 2) *(53–55)*. In this approach, the oncolytic HSV-1 vector acts as a helper virus for the propagation of plasmid-based defective vectors *(56)*. An advantage of this approach is that different defective vectors can be generated with different oncolytic helper viruses for a multiplicity of combinations without creating new vectors.

We have developed an immune gene therapy strategy that would work for brain tumors as well as other cancers. The brain is considered an immune-privileged site, and patients with brain tumors are often under an immune-suppressed condition because of immunosuppressive factors secreted by the brain tumor and/or corticosteroid administration. On the other hand, a robust, nonspecific inflammatory response in the brain can cause undesirable brain edema.

To meet these requirements, we created a defective HSV vector (dvB7Ig) expressing a soluble form of B7-1, one of the most potent costimulatory molecules, and used it in combination with G207 *(54)*. Soluble B7-1 was designed as a fusion protein of the extracellular domain of B7-1 and the Fc portion of immunoglobulin G, so that it is secreted by tumor cells rather than expressed on the cell surface. Secreted soluble B7-1 should provide antigen-presenting cells increased T-cell stimulatory activity, activate T cells in an anergic state, and because it is in a dimeric form, provide a strong stimulation to T cells by crosslinking neighboring CD28.

The in vivo efficacy was tested in the poorly immunogenic murine neuroblastoma Neuro2a in A/J mice. Intraneoplastic inoculation of dvB7Ig/G207 at a low titer successfully inhibited the growth of established subcutaneous tumors, despite the expression of B7-1-immunoglobulin detected in only 1% or fewer tumor cells at the inoculation site, and prolonged the survival of mice bearing intracerebral tumors *(54)*. Inoculation of dvB7Ig/G207 induced a significant influx of CD4$^+$ and CD8$^+$ T cells in the tumor. In vivo depletion of immune cell subsets further revealed that the antitumor effect

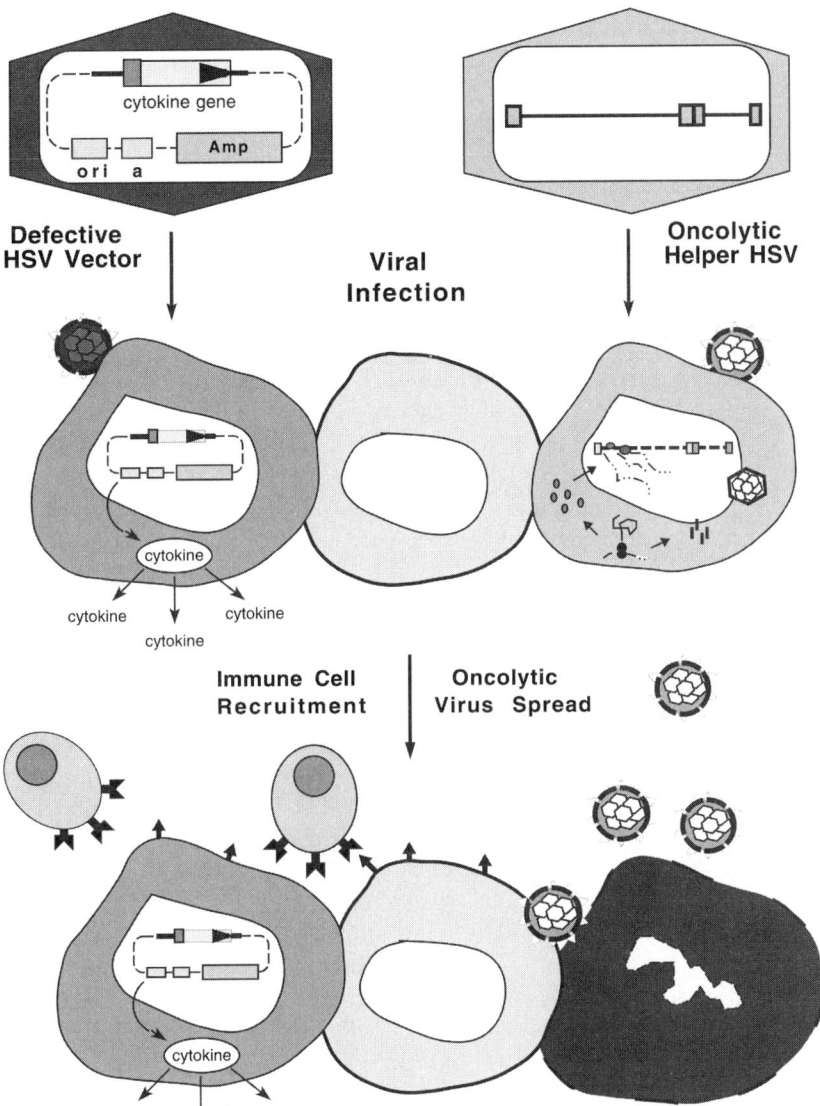

Fig. 2. Schematic diagram of immunomodulatory gene therapy using oncolytic HSV-1 vectors (like G207) as helper virus in combination with a defective HSV-1 vector expressing an immunomodulatory molecule. Defective HSV vector stocks are a mixture of defective particles (upper left) containing tandem repeats of an amplicon plasmid and HSV helper viruses (upper right) *(81)*. The amplicon plasmid consists of the cytokine/immunomodulatory gene, an HSV origin of replication (ori), and an HSV cleavage/packaging signal (a), but no viral coding sequences, and is packaged as a full viral genome length (~150 kb). Any conditional-lethal or replication-competent HSV mutant can be used as helper virus. When a mixture of helper and cytokine-expressing defective vector is inoculated into a tumor, the helper virus replicates, kills the infected cell, and spreads to other tumor cells (right side). On the other hand, tumor cells infected with the defective vector produce the cytokine and recruit immune cells (left side) that augment the antitumor immune response elicited by the oncolytic helper virus.

required CD8[+] T cells, but not CD4[+] T cells *(54)*. DvB7Ig/G207 treatment conferred tumor-specific protective immunity on cured animals. Thus, this approach proved to be a potent and clinically applicable means of treating brain tumors and other cancers.

A defective HSV vector expressing murine interleukin 12 (IL-12) in combination with G207 was very effective in treating subcutaneous CT26 tumors in BALB/c mice and inducing a tumor cell-specific CD8[+] CTL response *(53)*. An IL-2-expressing defective vector in combination with G207 had enhanced efficacy in murine squamous cell carcinoma and rat hepatocellular carcinoma models compared to G207 alone *(55,57)*. However, granulocyte-macrophage colony-stimulating factor (GM-CSF) expression from a defective vector did not have any increased efficacy over G207 alone in treating CT26 tumors (M. Toda and S. D. Rabkin, unpublished results, 1998). Whereas GM-CSF expression from replication-deficient HSV vectors did significantly enhance antitumor activity *(58, 59)*, as a tumor vaccine, GM-CSF-transduced cells have been found to be among the most effective *(60)*. This suggests that HSV infection may be inducing an immune response similar to that of GM-CSF expression, and that the spectrum of cytokines that will be effective in combination with oncolytic HSV vectors will be different from those used in tumor vaccines.

Replication-competent HSV-1 vectors that contain immunostimulatory molecule transgenes (i.e., IL-4, IL-10, IL-12, GM-CSF) have been created *(61–63)*. In particular, replication-competent HSV-1 vectors that express IL-12 have been shown in several animal tumor models to manifest direct oncolytic activity and express sufficient amounts of IL-12, which significantly augments antitumor activity without increasing toxicity, compared with the parental HSV-1 vectors *(62–65)*.

4. FUTURE DIRECTIONS

Now that it has been demonstrated in several clinical trials that oncolytic HSV-1 vectors can be administered safely in humans *(28,37,38,66)*, further development of oncolytic HSV-1 vectors will be directed toward improving antitumor efficacy. Doing so without compromising the safety of the vectors is the key to prevailing in this type of therapy. G47Δ is a good example of providing such an improvement in efficacy yet retaining safety features. A syncytial mutant (Fu-10) generated from G207, which forms tumor cell syncytium, was more efficacious in a lung metastases model than the parent, G207 *(22)*.

Expression of foreign transgenes, for example, "suicide" or immunostimulatory molecules, is another promising method to augment the activity of oncolytic HSV-1 vectors. A number of suicide genes, cytochrome P450 (CYP2B1) and cytosine deaminase (CD), have been incorporated into oncolytic HSV-1 vectors, and treatment with prodrugs significantly improved efficacy *(67,68)*. With the addition of foreign transgenes, it is important to be aware that they may increase the toxicity of the vector, decrease safety, and/or interfere with viral replication and decrease efficacy.

A practical method for improving the efficacy of oncolytic HSV-1 vectors is to combine them with conventional therapies. For example, a combination with cisplatin was shown to enhance the antitumor effect of G207 against human head and neck cancer *(69)*, and mitomycin C with 1716 was more effective than either treatment alone against human non-small cell lung cancer *(70)*.

Others have shown that ionizing radiation amplifies the replication of HSV-1 R3616 *(71)*, leading to improved survival of athymic mice bearing intracerebral U87MG tumors *(72)* and NV1020 (R7020) in some hepatoma tumor cell lines *(73)*. Although we did not observe such an enhancing effect of ionizing radiation with G207 in prostate cancer *(74)*, others have shown such an effect with G207 and cervical cancer *(75)*. Systemic delivery to brain tumors after intracarotid artery infusion can be enhanced by disruption of the blood–brain barrier using mannitol, bradykinin, or RMP-7 *(76–78)*. The replication and spread of oncolytic HSV-1 vector hrR3 in brain tumors after RMP-7 can be further enhanced by intraperitoneal administration of cyclophosphamide *(79)*. The combination of oncolytic HSV-1 vectors with established therapies should be rapidly translatable to the clinic.

5. CONCLUSION

Oncolytic virus therapy is an attractive treatment strategy because it is based on a new concept that the antitumor agent can amplify specifically at the tumor site after administration. This strategy also has features that make it attractive for clinical application: (1) tumor cells are targeted irrespective of their genetic makeup; (2) it can be combined with conventional therapies such as surgery, radiation therapy, and chemotherapy; (3) combination with immunotherapy has potential synergistic effects; and (4) it can act as a vehicle for gene delivery in vivo. An increasing number of clinical trials using oncolytic viruses have been initiated or planned in recent years. We anticipate that oncolytic virus therapy will be established as an important modality of cancer treatment in the near future.

ACKNOWLEDGMENTS

We thank the past and current members of the Molecular Neurosurgery Laboratory at Massachusetts General Hospital in Charlestown, especially Dr. Robert L. Martuza, who first developed the strategy of oncolytic virus therapy using replication-competent HSV-1 vectors and has been instrumental in all aspects of this research. S. D. Rabkin is a member of the Scientific Advisory Board of MediGene, which has an exclusive license from Georgetown University for G207. This research has been supported in part by grants from the National Institutes of Health, the Department of Defense, CaPCURE Foundation, NeuroVir Inc., the James S. McDonnell Foundation, and the Massachusetts General Hospital/Giovanni Armenise Neuro-Oncology and Related Disorders Grants Program.

REFERENCES

1. Kirn, D., Martuza, R. L., and Zwiebel, J. (2001) Replication-selective virotherapy for cancer: biological principles, risk management and future directions. *Nat. Med.* **7,** 781–787.
2. Martuza, R. L. (2000) Conditionally replicating herpes vectors for cancer therapy. *J. Clin. Invest.* **105,** 841–846.
3. Roizman, B. and Sears, A. E. (1996) Herpes simplex viruses and their replication. In *Fields Virology*, 3rd ed. (Fields, B. N., Knipe, D. M., and Howley, P. M., eds.), Lippincott-Raven, Philadelphia, pp. 2231–2296.
4. Roizman, B. (1996) The function of herpes simplex virus genes: a primer for genetic engineering of novel vectors. *Proc. Natl. Acad. Sci. USA* **93,** 11,307–11,312.
5. Balfour, H. H. Jr. (1999) Antiviral drugs. *N. Engl. J. Med.* **340,** 1255–1268.
6. Wagner, E. K. and Bloom, D. C. (1997) Experimental investigation of herpes simplex virus latency. *Clin. Microbiol. Rev.* **10,** 419–443.
7. Nishiyama, Y. (1996) Herpesvirus genes: molecular basis of viral replication and pathogenicity. *Nagoya J. Med. Sci.* **59,** 107–119.
8. Varghese, S. and Rabkin, S. D. (2002) Oncolytic herpes simplex virus vectors for cancer virotherapy. *Cancer Gene Ther.* **9,** 967–978.
9. Rabkin, S. D. and Hernaiz Driever, P. (2001) Replication-competent herpes simplex virus vectors for cancer therapy. In *Replication-Competent Viruses for Cancer Therapy* (Rabkin, S. D. and Hernaiz Driever, P., eds.), Karger, Basel, Switzerland, pp. 1–45.
10. Mineta, T., Rabkin, S. D., Yazaki, T., Hunter, W. D., and Martuza, R. L. (1995) Attenuated multi-mutated herpes simplex virus-1 for the treatment of malignant gliomas. *Nat. Med.* **1,** 938–943.
11. Chou, J., Kern, E. R., Whitley, R. J., and Roizman, B. (1990) Mapping of herpes simplex virus-1 neurovirulence to gamma 34.5, a gene nonessential for growth in culture. *Science* **250,** 1262–1266.
12. He, B., Gross, M., and Roizman, B. (1997) The gamma(1)34.5 protein of herpes simplex virus 1 complexes with protein phosphatase 1alpha to dephosphorylate the alpha subunit of the eukaryotic translation initiation factor 2 and preclude the shutoff of protein synthesis by double-stranded RNA-activated protein kinase. *Proc. Natl. Acad. Sci. USA* **94,** 843–848.
13. Farassati, F., Yang, A. D., and Lee, P. W. (2001) Oncogenes in Ras signalling pathway dictate host-cell permissiveness to herpes simplex virus 1. *Nat. Cell Biol.* **3,** 745–750.
14. Leib, D. A., Machalek, M. A., Williams, B. R., Silverman, R. H., and Virgin, H. W. (2000) Specific phenotypic restoration of an attenuated virus by knockout of a host resistance gene. *Proc. Natl. Acad. Sci. USA* **97,** 6097–6101.
15. MacLean, A. R., ul-Fareed, M., Robertson, L., Harland, J., and Brown, S. M. (1991) Herpes simplex virus type 1 deletion variants 1714 and 1716 pinpoint neurovirulence-related sequences in Glasgow strain 17⁺ between immediate early gene 1 and the "a" sequence. *J. Gen. Virol.* **72,** 631–639.
16. Goldstein, D. J. and Weller, S. K. (1988) Factor(s) present in herpes simplex virus type 1-infected cells can compensate for the loss of the large subunit of the viral ribonucleotide reductase: characterization of an ICP6 deletion mutant. *Virology* **166,** 41–51.
17. Pyles, R. B., Warnick, R. E., Chalk, C. L., Szanti, B. E., and Parysek, L. M. (1997) A novel multiply-mutated HSV-1 strain for the treatment of human brain tumors. *Hum. Gene Ther.* **8,** 533–544.

18. Todo, T., Ebright, M. I., Fong, Y., and Rabkin, S. D. (2001) Oncolytic herpes simplex virus (G207) therapy for cancer: from basic to clinical. In *Tumor Suppressing Viruses, Genes, and Drugs—Innovative Cancer Therapy Approaches* (Maruta, H., ed.), Academic Press, San Diego, CA, pp. 45–75.

19. Yazaki, T., Manz, H. J., Rabkin, S. D., and Martuza, R. L. (1995) Treatment of human malignant meningiomas by G207, a replication-competent multimutated herpes simplex virus 1. *Cancer Res.* **55,** 4752–4756.

20. Walker, J. R., McGeagh, K. G., Sundaresan, P., Jorgensen, T. J., Rabkin, S. D., and Martuza, R. L. (1999) Local and systemic therapy of human prostate adenocarcinoma with the conditionally replicating herpes simplex virus vector G207. *Hum. Gene Ther.* **10,** 2237–2243.

21. Oyama, M., Ohigashi, T., Hoshi, M., et al. (2000) Intravesical and intravenous therapy of human bladder cancer by the herpes vector G207. *Hum. Gene Ther.* **11,** 1683–1693.

22. Fu, X. and Zhang, X. (2002) Potent systemic antitumor activity from an oncolytic herpes simplex virus of syncytial phenotype. *Cancer Res.* **62,** 2306–2312.

23. Kooby, D. A., Carew, J. F., Halterman, M. W., et al. (1999) Oncolytic viral therapy for human colorectal cancer and liver metastases using a multi-mutated herpes simplex virus type-1 (G207) *FASEB J.* **13,** 1325–1334.

24. Carew, J. F., Kooby, D. A., Halterman, M. W., Federoff, H. J., and Fong, Y. (1999) Selective infection and cytolysis of human head and neck squamous cell carcinoma with sparing of normal mucosa by a cytotoxic herpes simplex virus type 1 (G207). *Hum. Gene Ther.* **10,** 1599–1606.

25. Bennett, J. J., Kooby, D. A., Delman, K., et al. (2000) Antitumor efficacy of regional oncolytic viral therapy for peritoneally disseminated cancer. *J. Mol. Med.* **78,** 166–174.

26. Coukos, G., Makrigiannakis, A., Montas, S., et al. (2000) Multi-attenuated herpes simplex virus-1 mutant G207 exerts cytotoxicity against epithelial ovarian cancer but not normal mesothelium and is suitable for intraperitoneal oncolytic therapy. *Cancer Gene Ther.* **7,** 275–283.

27. Whitley, R. J. and Gnann, J. W. (2002) Viral encephalitis: familiar infections and emerging pathogens. *Lancet* **359,** 507–513.

28. Rampling, R., Cruickshank, G., Papanastassiou, V., et al. (2000) Toxicity evaluation of replication-competent herpes simplex virus (ICP 34.5 null mutant 1716) in patients with recurrent malignant glioma. *Gene Ther.* **7,** 859–866.

29. Sundaresan, P., Hunter, W. D., Martuza, R. L., and Rabkin, S. D. (2000) Attenuated, replication-competent herpes simplex virus type 1 mutant G207: safety evaluation in mice. *J. Virol.* **74,** 3832–3841.

30. Lopez, C. (1975) Genetics of natural resistance to herpesvirus infections in mice. *Nature* **258,** 152–155.

31. Todo, T., Martuza, R. L., Rabkin, S. D., and Johnson, P. A. (2001) Oncolytic herpes simplex virus vector with enhanced MHC class I presentation and tumor cell killing. *Proc. Natl. Acad. Sci. USA* **98,** 6396–6401.

32. Katzin, D. S., Connor, J. D., Wilson, L. A., and Sexton, R. S. (1967) Experimental herpes simplex infection in the owl monkey. *Proc. Soc. Exp. Biol. Med.* **125,** 391–398.

33. Meignier, B., Martin, B., Whitley, R. J., and Roizman, B. (1990) In vivo behavior of genetically engineered herpes simplex viruses R7017 and R7020. II. Studies in immunocompetent and immunosuppressed owl monkeys (*Aotus trivirgatus*). *J. Infect. Dis.* **162,** 313–321.

34. Hunter, W. D., Martuza, R. L., Feigenbaum, F., et al. (1999) Attenuated, replication-competent herpes simplex virus type 1 mutant G207: safety evaluation of intracerebral injection in nonhuman primates. *J. Virol.* **73,** 6319–6326.

35. Todo, T., Feigenbaum, F., Rabkin, S. D., et al. (2000) Viral shedding and biodistribution of G207, a multimutated, conditionally-replicating herpes simplex virus type 1, after intracerebral inoculation in Aotus. *Mol. Ther.* **2,** 588–595.

36. Varghese, S., Newsome, J. T., Rabkin, S. D., et al. (2001) Preclinical safety evaluation of G207, a replication-competent herpes simplex virus type 1, inoculated intraprostatically in mice and nonhuman primates. *Hum. Gene Ther.* **12,** 999–1010.

37. Markert, J. M., Medlock, M. D., Rabkin, S. D., et al. (2000) Conditionally replicating herpes simplex virus mutant, G207 for the treatment of malignant glioma: results of a phase I trial. *Gene Ther.* **7,** 867–874.

38. Papanastassiou, V., Rampling, R., Fraser, M., et al. (2002) The potential for efficacy of the modified (ICP 34.5(−) herpes simplex virus HSV1716 following intratumoural injection into human malignant glioma: a proof of principle study. *Gene Ther.* **9,** 398–406.

39. Todo, T., Rabkin, S. D., Sundaresan, P., et al. (1999) Systemic antitumor immunity in experimental brain tumor therapy using a multimutated, replication-competent herpes simplex virus. *Hum. Gene Ther.* **10,** 2741–2755.

40. Toda, M., Rabkin, S. D., Kojima, H., and Martuza, R. L. (1999) Herpes simplex virus as an "*in situ* cancer vaccine" for the induction of specific anti-tumor immunity. *Hum. Gene Ther.* **10,** 385–393.

41. Nakano, K., Todo, T., Chijiiwa, K., and Tanaka, M. (2001) Therapeutic efficacy of G207, a conditionally replicating herpes simplex virus type 1 mutant, for gallbladder carcinoma in immunocompetent hamsters. *Mol. Ther.* **3,** 431–437.

42. Endo, T., Toda, M., Watanabe, M., et al. (2002) In situ cancer vaccination with a replication-conditional HSV for the treatment of liver metastasis of colon cancer. *Cancer Gene Ther.* **9,** 142–148.

43. Todo, T., Rabkin, S. D., Chahlavi, A., and Martuza, R. L. (1999) Corticosteroid administration does not affect viral oncolytic activity, but inhibits antitumor immunity in replication-competent herpes simplex virus tumor therapy. *Hum. Gene Ther.* **10,** 2869–2878.

44. Langenberg, A. G., Corey, L., Ashley, R. L., Leong, W. P., and Straus, S. E. (1999) A prospective study of new infections with herpes simplex virus type 1 and type 2. Chiron HSV Vaccine Study Group. *N. Engl. J. Med.* **341,** 1432–1438.

45. Xu, F., Schillinger, J. A., Sternberg, M. R., et al. (2002) Seroprevalence and coinfection with herpes simplex virus type 1 and type 2 in the United States, 1988–1994. *J. Infect. Dis.* **185,** 1019–1024.

46. Chahlavi, A., Rabkin, S., Todo, T., Sundaresan, P., and Martuza, R. (1999) Effect of prior exposure to herpes simplex virus 1 on viral vector-mediated tumor therapy in immunocompetent mice. *Gene Ther.* **6,** 1751–1758.

47. Miller, C. G. and Fraser, N. W. (2000) Role of the immune response during neuro-attenuated herpes simplex virus-mediated tumor destruction in a murine intracranial melanoma model. *Cancer Res.* **60,** 5714–5722.

48. Delman, K. A., Bennett, J. J., Zager, J. S., et al. (2000) Effects of preexisting immunity on the response to herpes simplex-based oncolytic viral therapy. *Hum. Gene Ther.* **11,** 2465–2472.

49. York, I. A., Roop, C., Andrews, D. W., Riddell, S. R., Graham, F. L., and Johnson, D. C. (1994) A cytosolic herpes simplex virus protein inhibits antigen presentation to CD8⁺ T lymphocytes. *Cell* **77,** 525–535.

50. Ahn, K., Meyer, T. H., Uebel, S., et al. (1996) Molecular mechanism and species specificity of TAP inhibition by herpes simplex virus ICP47. *EMBO J.* **15,** 3247–3255.

51. Mohr, I. and Gluzman, Y. (1996) A herpesvirus genetic element which affects translation in the absence of the viral GADD34 function. *EMBO J.* **15,** 4759–4766.

52. Mohr, I., Sternberg, D., Ward, S., Leib, D., Mulvey, M., and Gluzman, Y. (2001) A herpes simplex virus type 1 gamma34.5 second-site suppressor mutant that exhibits enhanced growth in cultured glioblastoma cells is severely attenuated in animals. *J. Virol.* **75,** 5189–5196.

53. Toda, M., Martuza, R. L., Kojima, H., and Rabkin, S. D. (1998) *In situ* cancer vaccination: an IL-12 defective vector/replication-competent herpes simplex virus combination induces local and systemic antitumor activity. *J. Immunol.* **160,** 4457–4464.

54. Todo, T., Martuza, R. L., Dallman, M. J., and Rabkin, S. D. (2001) *In situ* expression of soluble B7-1 in the context of oncolytic herpes simplex virus induces potent antitumor immunity. *Cancer Res.* **61,** 153–161.

55. Carew, J. F., Kooby, D. A., Halterman, M. W., Kim, S. H., Federoff, H. J., and Fong, Y. (2001) A novel approach to cancer therapy using an oncolytic herpes virus to package amplicons containing cytokine genes. *Mol. Ther.* **4,** 250–256.

56. Miyatake, S., Martuza, R. L., and Rabkin, S. D. (1997) Defective herpes simplex virus vectors expressing thymidine kinase for the treatment of malignant glioma. *Cancer Gene Ther.* **4,** 222–228.

57. Zager, J. S., Delman, K. A., Malhotra, S., et al. (2001) Combination vascular delivery of herpes simplex oncolytic viruses and amplicon mediated cytokine gene transfer is effective therapy for experimental liver cancer. *Mol. Med.* **7,** 561–568.

58. Toda, M., Martuza, R. L., and Rabkin, S. D. (2000) Tumor growth inhibition by intratumoral inoculation of defective herpes simplex virus vectors expressing granulocyte-macrophage colony-stimulating factor. *Mol. Ther.* **2,** 324–329.

59. Ali, S. A., Lynam, J., McLean, C. S., et al. (2002) Tumor regression induced by intratumor therapy with a disabled infectious single cycle (DISC) herpes simplex virus (HSV) vector, DISC/HSV/murine granulocyte-macrophage colony-stimulating factor, correlates with antigen-specific adaptive immunity. *J. Immunol.* **168,** 3512–3519.

60. Dranoff, G., Jaffee, E., Lazenby, A., et al. (1993) Vaccination with irradiated tumor cells engineered to secrete murine granulocye-macrophage colony-stimulating factor stimulates potent, specific, and long-lasting anti-tumor immunity. *Proc. Natl. Acad. Sci. USA* **90,** 3539–3543.

61. Andreansky, S., He, B., van Cott, J., et al. (1998) Treatment of intracranial gliomas in immunocompetent mice using herpes simplex viruses that express murine interleukins. *Gene Ther.* **5,** 121–130.

62. Parker, J. N., Gillespie, G. Y., Love, C. E., Randall, S., Whitley, R. J., and Markert, J. M. (2000) Engineered herpes simplex virus expressing IL-12 in the treatment of experimental murine brain tumors. *Proc. Natl. Acad. Sci. USA* **97,** 2208–2213.

63. Wong, R. J., Patel, S. G., Kim, S., et al. (2001) Cytokine gene transfer enhances herpes oncolytic therapy in murine squamous cell carcinoma. *Hum. Gene Ther.* **12,** 253–265.

64. Bennett, J. J., Malhotra, S., Wong, R. J., et al. (2001) Interleukin 12 secretion enhances antitumor efficacy of oncolytic herpes simplex viral therapy for colorectal cancer. *Ann. Surg.* **233,** 819–826.

65. Liu, R., Varghese, S., Martuza, R. L., and Rabkin, S. D. (2002) Oncolytic herpes simplex virus (HSV) therapy of breast and prostate cancer in C3(1)/SV40-TAg transgenic mice. *Mol. Ther.* **5,** S302.

66. Fong, Y., Kemeny, N., Jarnagin, W., et al. (2002) Phase 1 study of a replication-competent herpes simplex oncolytic virus for treatment of hepatic colorectal metastases. *Proc. Am. Soc. Clin. Oncol.* **21,** 8a.

67. Chase, M., Chung, R. Y., and Chiocca, E. A. (1998) An oncolytic viral mutant that delivers the CYP2B1 transgene and augments cyclophosphamide chemotherapy. *Nat. Biotechnol.* **16,** 444–448.

68. Nakamura, H., Mullen, J. T., Chandrasekhar, S., Pawlik, T. M., Yoon, S. S., and Tanabe, K. K. (2001) Multimodality therapy with a replication-conditional herpes simplex virus 1 mutant that expresses yeast cytosine deaminase for intra-tumoral conversion of 5-fluorocytosine to 5-fluorouracil. *Cancer Res.* **61,** 5447–5452.

69. Chahlavi, A., Todo, T., Martuza, R. L., and Rabkin, S. D. (1999) Replication-competent herpes simplex virus vector G207 and cisplatin combination therapy for head and neck squamous cell carcinoma. *Neoplasia* **1,** 162–169.

70. Toyoizumi, T., Mick, R., Abbas, A. E., Kang, E. H., Kaiser, L. R., and Molnar-Kimber, K. L. (1999) Combined therapy with chemotherapeutic agents and herpes simplex virus type 1 ICP34.5 mutant (HSV-1716) in human non-small cell lung cancer. *Hum. Gene Ther.* **10**, 3013–3029.

71. Advani, S. J., Sibley, G. S., Song, P. Y., et al. (1998) Enhancement of replication of genetically engineered herpes simplex viruses by ionizing radiation: a new paradigm for destruction of therapeutically intractable tumors. *Gene Ther.* **5**, 160–165.

72. Bradley, J. D., Kataoka, Y., Advani, S., et al. (1999) Ionizing radiation improves survival in mice bearing intracranial high-grade gliomas injected with genetically modified herpes simplex virus. *Clin. Cancer Res.* **5**, 1517–1522.

73. Chung, S. M., Advani, S. J., Bradley, J. D., et al. (2002) The use of a genetically engineered herpes simplex virus (R7020) with ionizing radiation for experimental hepatoma. *Gene Ther.* **9**, 75–80.

74. Jorgensen, T. J., Katz, S., Wittmack, E. K., et al. (2001) Ionizing radiation does not alter the antitumor activity of herpes simplex virus vector G207 in subcutaneous tumor models of human and murine prostate cancer. *Neoplasia* **3**, 451–456.

75. Blank, S. V., Rubin, S. C., Coukos, G., Amin, K. M., Albelda, S. M., and Molnar-Kimber, K. L. (2002) Replication-selective herpes simplex virus type 1 mutant therapy of cervical cancer is enhanced by low-dose radiation. *Hum. Gene Ther.* **13**, 627–639.

76. Muldoon, L. L., Nilaver, G., Kroll, R. A., et al. (1995) Comparison of intracerebral inoculation and osmotic blood-brain barrier disruption for delivery of adenovirus, herpesvirus, and iron oxide particles to normal rat brain. *Am. J. Pathol.* **147**, 1840–1851.

77. Rainov, N. G., Zimmer, C., Chase, M., et al. (1995) Selective uptake of viral and monocrystalline particles delivered intra-arterially to experimental brain neoplasms. *Hum. Gene Ther.* **6**, 1543–1552.

78. Barnett, F. H., Rainov, N. G., Ikeda, K., et al. (1999) Selective delivery of herpes virus vectors to experimental brain tumors using RMP-7. *Cancer Gene Ther.* **6**, 14–20.

79. Ikeda, K., Ichikawa, T., Wakimoto, H., et al. (1999) Oncolytic virus therapy of multiple tumors in the brain requires suppression of innate and elicited antiviral responses. *Nat. Med.* **5**, 881–887.

80. Todo, T. (2002) Oncolytic virus therapy using genetically engineered herpes simplex viruses. *Hum. Cell* **15**, 151–159.

81. Spaete, R. R. and Frenkel, N. (1982) The herpes simplex virus amplicon: a new eukaryotic defective-virus cloning-amplifying vector. *Cell* **30**, 295–304.

14

Development of Oncolytic Adenoviruses

From the Lab Bench to the Bedside

John A. Howe, Robert Ralston, and Murali Ramachandra

1. INTRODUCTION

Understanding of the molecular basis of oncogenesis has increased dramatically over the past 30 years, partly because of key discoveries about the biology of ribonucleic acid (RNA) and deoxyribonucleic acid (DNA) tumor viruses, enabled in turn by development of modern molecular biology. Despite great advances in basic research, progress in treatment has been limited, and cancer remains the second leading cause of death in the United States. Current drug therapy continues to be dominated by highly toxic drugs that increase susceptibility to severe infections and to long-term genetic damage that can result in secondary malignancies. These toxicities are primarily attributable to lack of specificity for tumor cells and consequent destruction of rapidly dividing normal cells in the bone marrow and GI tract. New agents with novel mechanisms of action and improved therapeutic indexes are therefore required.

Knowledge of the underlying mechanisms involved in neoplastic transformation has raised the prospect of developing molecularly targeted drugs with improved therapeutic indexes. Perhaps paradoxically, it has offered the possibility that human adenovirus, a "DNA tumor virus" that has provided many important insights into the molecular biology of neoplastic transformation, also could be developed as a targeted agent to fight cancer. Importantly, recombinant oncolytic adenoviruses have been designed using the understanding of neoplastic transformation combined with knowledge of virus biology, resulting in a new class of drugs that can kill tumor cells but cause minimal damage to normal cells.

Initial work with adenovirus as a targeted therapeutic agent focused on using replication-defective vectors carrying a therapeutic gene in place of the E1 region. Therapeutic genes used in these studies included the tumor suppressors such as p53, cytokines such as interleukin-2 (IL-2) and granulocyte-macrophage colony-stimulating factor, and prodrug activators such as herpes simplex virus thymidine kinase (HSV-TK) (for a review, *see* ref. *1*). Several replication-defective adenovirus vectors for cancer therapy are in late-stage clinical trials, including Advexin® (Introgen Therapeutics, Austin, TX), which expresses wild-type p53; and GVAX® (Cell Genesys, South San Francisco, CA), which expresses granulocyte-macrophage colony-stimulating factor and is used for ex vivo generation of autologous cancer vaccines. Other adenovirus-based gene therapies in early-stage trials include TNFerade® (GenVec, Gaithersburg, MD), which expresses tumor necrosis factor-α (TNF-α), and EG009 (Ark Therapeutics, London, UK), which expresses HSV-TK.

With the exception of Advexin, most of the adenovirus-based gene therapies rely on generation of cytokines or activated prodrugs as diffusible agents to compensate for inefficient distribution of the vector within tumor tissue. The poor distribution of adenovirus vectors relative to small molecule drugs or monoclonal antibodies is mainly because of its size and surface complexity. This inefficiency

From: *Contemporary Cancer Research*
Cancer Gene Therapy
Edited by: D. T. Curiel and J. T. Douglas © Humana Press Inc., Totowa, NJ

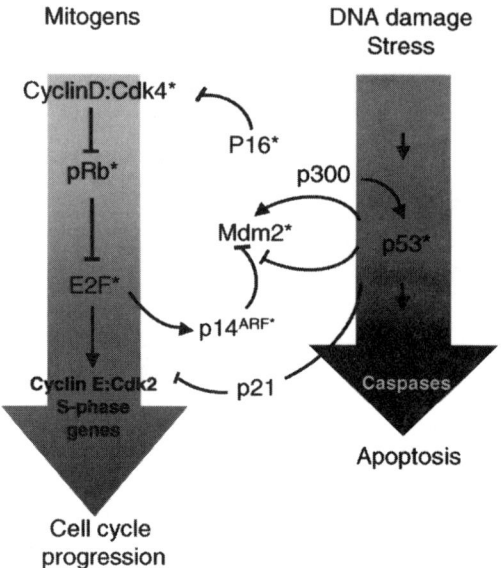

Fig. 1. p53 and pRb are the key pathways disrupted in tumor cells. Because of the inactivation of these two pathways (*see* Section 2.) in cancer cells, the balance between cell proliferation and death is disrupted, resulting in uncontrolled growth of cells. Proteins that exhibit altered functions in cancer cells are indicated with an asterisk.

could be overcome, however, if the virus were allowed to spread by replication. Indeed, the potential therapeutic use of adenoviruses as oncolytic agents was recognized soon after their discovery in the early 1950s, when it was noted that these newly discovered agents replicated particularly efficiently in HeLa cells. Although methods of virus preparation and characterization were primitive, the observation of robust replication and lysis of HeLa cells led to clinical trials using intratumoral, intraarterial, and intravenous administration of wild-type human and simian adenoviruses in patients with cervical carcinoma *(2)*. Such therapies were not pursued aggressively, possibly because of limitations inherent in virus preparation technology in the 1950s, which led to variable responses. However, there has been a renewed interest in the use of replicating viruses, with the realization that adenoviruses could be engineered for use as targeted oncolytic agents by taking advantage of the defects prevalent in cancer cells *(3,4)*.

2. EXPLOITING TUMOR-SPECIFIC DEFECTS IN REGULATORY PATHWAYS IN DEVELOPING ADENOVIRUS-BASED ANTICANCER AGENTS

Cancer cells possess multiple genetic defects that lead to abnormal growth because of increased cell proliferation and/or decreased apoptosis. Interestingly, consequences of most of these defects converge and result in aberrant function of the p53 and retinoblastoma protein (pRb) pathways (Fig. 1), which play key roles in control of cellular proliferation and survival. Depending on the state of the cell, p53 triggers either cell cycle arrest or apoptosis on damage to cellular DNA or in response to cellular stress. These crucial functions of p53 and pRb are lost in cancers.

The significance of p53 is exemplified by the findings that nearly all human cancers display a defect in p53 function, either through mutation in p53 itself (as in more than 50% of human cancers) or because of alterations in the pathway that regulates p53 activity. These alterations include overexpression of MDM2, an E3 ubiquitin ligase that targets p53 for degradation, hypermethylation, mutation, and deletion in p14[ARF], an inhibitor of MDM2, and expression of viral oncoproteins that affect p53 function in tumors, such as human papilloma virus E6 *(5)*.

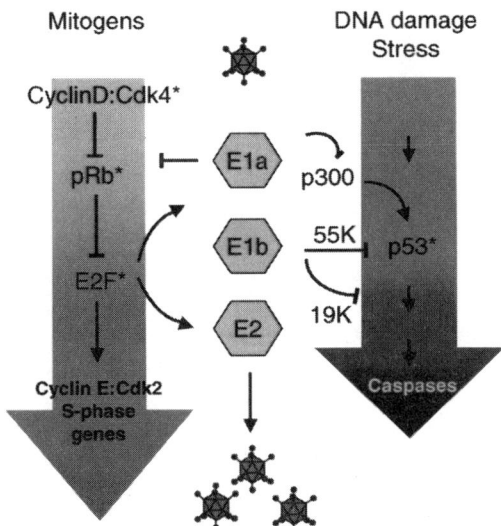

Fig. 2. The p53 and pRb pathways are also disrupted in cells infected with adenoviruses. For efficient replication of the virus, virus expresses proteins that interact with components of p53 and pRb pathways (*see* Section 2.), which leads to induction of cell cycle progression and inhibits apoptosis prior to viral replication. In addition to viral proteins shown, E4-orf6/7 and E4-orf6 bind and inhibit pRb and p53, respectively.

The transcription factor E2F, the functional target of pRb, promotes cell proliferation. Abnormal growth because of E2F is prevented by pRb, which under quiescent conditions binds to E2F and forms a potent transcriptional repressor complex, resulting in the repression of proliferation-associated genes. As cells progress into the cell cycle, cyclin-dependent kinases phosphorylate pRb, freeing E2F and allowing it to transactivate genes required for S-phase entry. Deregulation of E2F occurs in virtually all cancers as a result of alterations in various components of the pRb pathway, including mutations in pRb itself (approx 25% of tumors), overexpression of D-type cyclins, or activation of cyclin-dependent kinase 4 (CDK4), and inhibition of pRb function by direct-binding human papilloma virus E7 protein (*6*). Disruption of the pRb pathway also contributes to apoptosis through activation of E2F in both p53-dependent and p53-independent mechanisms by transcriptionally activating p14[ARF] and multiple caspases, which are essential components of the apoptotic machinery (*7*).

Interestingly, DNA tumor viruses such as adenovirus have evolved to seize and utilize the very same cellular regulatory machinery that is ultimately dysregulated in cancer cells. Following infection, adenovirus reprograms the cell in two major ways to accomplish its own replication (Fig. 2). First, the virus activates the cell cycle machinery that synthesizes new copies of cellular DNA and redirects it to produce viral DNA. This is accomplished by expression of proteins that lead to activation of E2F. Binding of viral E1a and E4-orf6/7 to pRb results in the dissociation of Rb/E2F complexes and stimulation of a number of cellular genes by E2F that are required for DNA synthesis and cell cycle progression (for a review, *see* ref. *8*).

Second, to complete its replication cycle without killing cells prematurely, the adenovirus takes control of the apoptotic machinery, which is triggered by induction of p53 because of increased levels of p14[ARF] a transcriptional target of E2F (*9*). Inhibition of premature apoptosis is accomplished by E1b-19K, a functional analogue of Bcl-2, and abrogation of p53 function by direct binding of p53 by E1b-55K and E4orf6 and sequestration by E1a of p300/CBP transcription coactivators (*10,11*). p300/CBP enhances the transcriptional activity of p53 by acetylation, and interaction of E1A with p300/CBP prevents acetylation of p53 (*12*). The net result of the ability of the virus to interfere in cellular p53 and pRb regulatory pathways is that the infected cell briefly resembles a tumor cell with one very important exception: the fate of the infected cell is to die following the generation of viral progeny.

2.1. Deletion of Viral Genes With Functions Dispensable for Virus Replication in Tumor Cells

If the primary roles of the E1a and E1b gene products in the viral replicative cycle are to inactivate cellular pRb and p53 pathways, respectively, then it is conceivable that, if these functions were deleted from the virus, replication would be restricted to cells with defects in these two regulatory pathways. However, as described in this section, for such as strategy to succeed, the alterations E1a or E1b need to abolish specifically their ability to inactivate pRb and p53 pathways without affecting other functions critical for the virus life cycle.

2.1.1. Deletion of E1b-55K

The major role of the E1b-55K protein in the early phase of the adenovirus life cycle is believed to inactivate the transcriptional activation capability of p53 to prevent p53-induced cell cycle arrest and apoptosis *(13,14)*. These observations led to the hypothesis that an E1b-55K mutated virus might replicate efficiently in p53-defective tumor cells, but not in normal cells, in which wild-type p53 function could block viral replication *(3)*.

To test this hypothesis, the replicative properties of an E1b-55K-deleted virus *dl*1520 *(13)*, also called ONYX-015 (Fig. 3), were analyzed in cell lines with wild-type or mutant p53 gene status. In initial reports, ONYX-015 was shown to replicate efficiently in p53-pathway-deficient tumor cells, but was attenuated in normal cells or tumor cells that expressed functional p53 *(3,15)*. Subsequently, in studies in which a wide range of cell types and assay conditions were used, a number of groups showed that replication of *dl*1520 in vitro was attenuated in tumor cells independent of p53 gene status (reviewed in ref. *16*). Viral DNA synthesis is not affected by the E1b-55K deletion in *dl*1520 *(17)*, but viral late protein synthesis is attenuated in most cell types regardless of p53 status *(18,19)*. These results suggested that the attenuation of *dl*1520 results primarily from the function of E1b-55K in the late phase of the infection cycle to facilitate the preferential transport and translation of viral messenger RNAs (mRNAs) at the expense of host macromolecule synthesis.

In an effort to design an adenovirus E1b-55K mutant that was defective for binding p53 but not affected for the late functions of E1b-55K, a series of point mutations in the overlapping region of the E1b-55K gene known to be required for p53 binding, viral mRNA transport, and host cell shutoff was created *(20)*. Among the mutant viruses, R240A (ONYX-051) was shown to interact poorly with p53, but to retain the late functions of wild-type E1b-55K, including expression of viral late proteins and host cell shut off. ONYX-051 showed higher cytolytic activity in tumor cells than ONYX-015, and efforts are under way to study the replication capacity of ONYX-051 in the presence or absence of normal p53 activity *(20)*. Although the ONYX-015 virus did not target p53 pathway defects as efficiently as new-generation vectors like ONYX-051 may, ONYX-015 has been used in a variety of phase I and II clinical trials and is reported to show an acceptable safety profile (*see* Section 6.).

2.1.2. Specific Deletions in E1a

The E1a gene encodes for two highly related proteins, 243R and 289R, which function to prepare the infected cell as an optimal environment for viral DNA replication. One of the roles of E1a, carried out primarily by the 289R protein, is to activate the transcription of the other viral early regions E1b, E2, E3, and E4 to provide factors required for viral DNA replication and to ensure timely progression of the virus lytic cycle. Another important function of E1a is to stimulate S phase in the normally quiescent cells that adenoviruses infect. As described earlier, this function is accomplished by the ability of the E1a proteins to bind to and deregulate the cellular factors, such as pRb, that function to regulate E2F. The rationale for specific deletions in E1a to restrict viral replication in tumor cell is

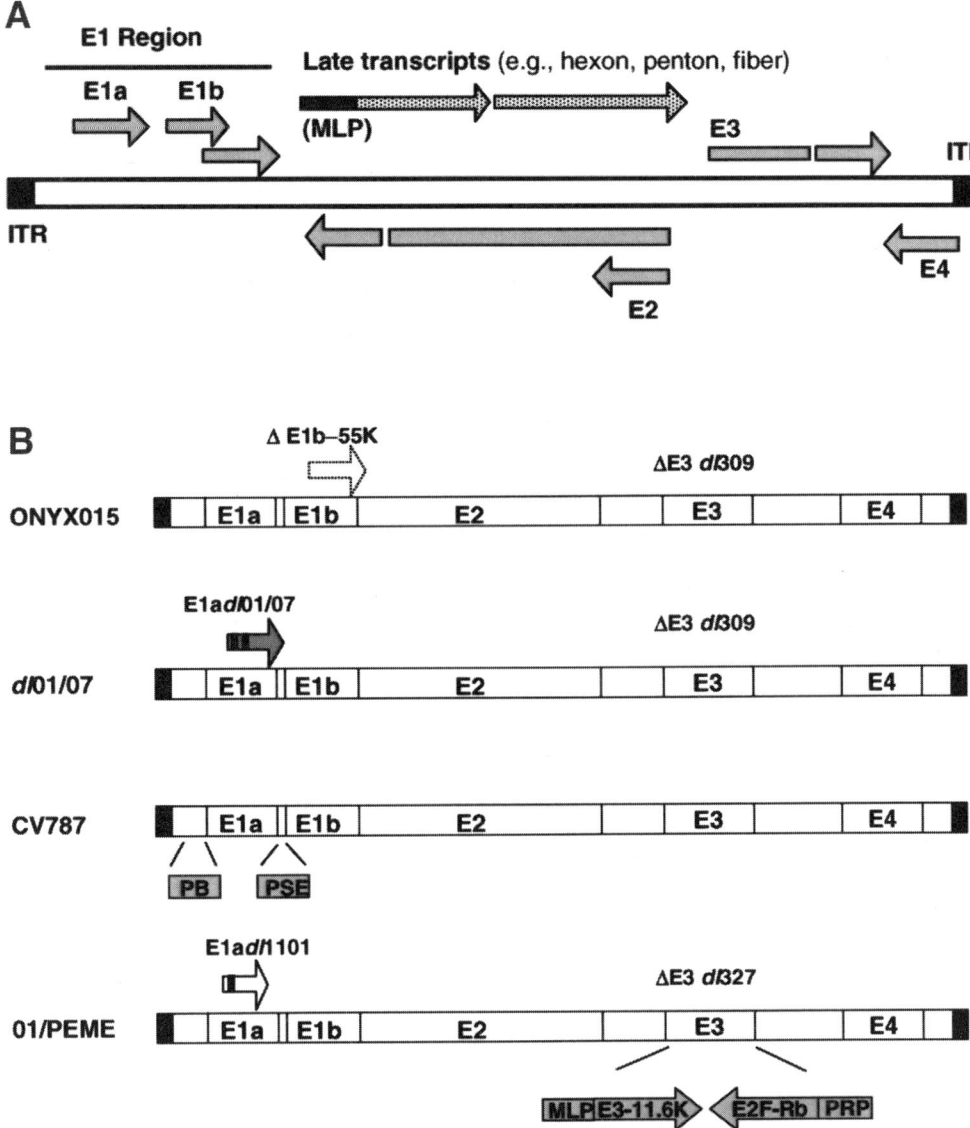

Fig. 3. Adenovirus genome structure and schematic of representative viruses. **(A)** The open bar represents the 36-kb adenoviral genome with inverted terminal repeats (black boxes). Shaded arrows indicate the gene transcription units, including the immediate early E1a; the early E1b, E2, E3, and E4 transcription units; and the late transcription region controlled by the MLP. **(B)** Major features of representative oncolytic adenoviruses are shown. **ONYX-015** contains a large deletion and insertion of a stop codon in the E1b-55K gene that together inhibit expression of the E1b-55K protein, but do not affect the E1b-19K gene. This virus was constructed in the *dl*309 backbone, which contains a deletion of the entire E3 region except for the genes encoding the 12.5K and E3-11.6K proteins. ***dl*01/07**, which was also constructed in the *dl*309 backbone, contains two small deletions, *dl*1101 and *dl*1107, in the E1a transcription unit (indicated by black boxes) that delete binding sites in the E1a proteins for the cellular proteins p300/CBP and pRb, respectively. The prostate-specific virus **CV787** contains the rat probasin promoter (PB) inserted upstream of the E1a transcription unit and the human prostate-specific enhancer/promoter (PSE) inserted in front of the E1b gene region. **01/PEME** contains the *dl*1101 mutation (see above) and insertion of two expression cassettes in the E3 region of the *dl*327 backbone (entire E3 deletion except the 12.5K gene), one of which contains the MLP promoter controlling production of the E3-11.6K, and the other is a p53-responsive promoter (PRP) to regulate expression of an E2F-Rb fusion protein.

that most tumor cells possess abnormalities in the control of E2F activity. Therefore, the role of E1a to deregulate E2F and stimulate the G1/S-phase transition, which is necessary for successful infection of quiescent cells, may not be required in tumor cells. The E1a proteins have been extensively studied, and separable functional domains have been delineated. Therefore, specific mutants that retain the trans-activation domain of E1a but are defective for the cell cycle effects of E1a were available for study.

Efforts to construct oncolytic adenovirus with specific E1a mutations initially focused on viruses with deletions in the CR2 region of E1a *(21,22)* as this region contains the major E1a binding site for pRb and the pRb family members p107 and p130. Ad-Δ24 (deletion of amino acids 121 to 128 of E1a) was found to be defective for induction of cytopathic effects (CPEs) in quiescent lung fibro-blasts or in cancer cells with restored pRb activity, but did induce CPEs in a number of glioma tumor lines known to contain mutations in *RB1* or *CDKN2A (21)*. A virus Ad*dl*922–947, with a slightly different mutation (deletion of amino acids 122 to 129 of E1a), was independently examined and found to be defective for viral growth in nonproliferating epithelial and endothelial cells, but replicated at wild-type or higher levels in tumor cells. Although both Ad-Δ24 and Ad*dl*922–947 were defective for viral growth in nonproliferating cells, *dl*922–947 was shown to replicate more efficiently than wild-type virus in proliferating normal cells *(22)*. In addition, Ad-Δ24 was found to have no selective replicative activity, as compared to wild-type virus, in organotypic cultures (graft cultures) of primary human keratinocytes *(23)*.

It is likely the limited selective replicative properties of E1a-CR2 mutants result from the ability of adenoviruses to deregulate pRb and induce S phase by two additional mechanisms, either through p300/CBP binding to E1a *(24)* or as a result of E4-orf6/7 protein binding to pRb directly *(25)*. These observations led to the study of Ad*dl*01/07, which produces an E1a protein defective for binding both pRb and p300/CBP *(26,27)* (Fig. 3). Ad*dl*01/07 has been shown to have attenuated CPEs in various proliferating or quiescent normal cells, including fibroblasts and epithelial and endothelial cells, but is almost as effective as wild-type virus in killing tumor cells. Ad*dl*01/07 has an antitumor effect that is comparable to wild-type virus in mouse models of human cancer and is more efficient for tumor-specific cell killing and antitumor effects than an E1b-55K mutant *(26)*. Another E1a double-mutant, CB016, which is also defective for binding both pRb and p300/CBP, has been shown to be severely attenuated for replication in organotypic keratinocyte cultures as compared to wild-type virus and Ad-Δ24, but to replicate and efficiently destroy organotypic keratinocyte cultures transformed with human papilloma virus E6/E7 genes *(23)*. Adenoviruses encoding E1a proteins that are defective for cell cycle stimulation, but retain the transactivation ability of E1a, display the desired characteristics of an anticancer agent: attenuation for destruction of normal cells and potent antitumor effects in mouse models. In addition, mutation of the E4-orf6/7 protein could potentially further enhance the tumor cell selective replicative properties of such mutant viruses.

2.2. Expression of E1a and Other Viral Early Proteins Using Transcription Factors Upregulated in Tumor Cells

Another strategy used to develop adenoviruses for cancer treatment involves modification of the viral genome to bring key regulatory genes such as E1a, E1b, E2, or E4 under the control of tumor-, or tissue-, selective promoters to target replication to specific cells. Pioneering efforts using this approach by Henderson's group were focused on targeting prostate cancer. The first virus generated CV706, which contains the minimal promoter/enhancer from the prostate-specific antigen (PSA) to regulate E1a expression, was shown to replicate preferentially in PSA-positive *(4)* cells and in clinical trials was well tolerated and safe and showed some antitumor activity *(28)*. A series of improved vectors was also developed, including CV739 and CV787, which contain the rat probasin prostate-specific promoter to drive E1a and the PSA promoter to regulate the E1b gene *(29)* (Fig. 3). CV739 and CV787 are identical except that CV787 contains a fully restored E3 region; CV739 is E3 deleted, and interestingly, although both viruses are highly cytopathic for PSA-positive cells in vitro, CV787 is capable of eliminating prostate tumor xenografts in mice following a single intravenous dose, but CV739 is not. The enhanced efficacy of CV787 is likely because of the inclusion of the E3-11.6K protein, also known as the adenovirus death protein, which promotes cell lysis in the late phase of the adenovirus replicative cycle. Clinical trials with CV787, which are under way, will determine if enhanced efficacy in preclinical studies will translate into increased clinical activity.

Efforts to generate adenoviruses with tumor type-specific replication for treatment for other cancer indications, including liver, lung, brain, breast, ovarian, and colon (*see* Table 1 for a summary), have also been undertaken. To target hepatocellular carcinoma (HCC) the α-fetoprotein (AFP) gene promoter, which is active in about 70% of patients with HCC but not in normal adults, was used to drive expression of E1a in a vector called AvE1a04i *(30)*. AvE1a04i was extensively tested in vitro and replicated well in human AFP-producing HCC cell lines, but was attenuated in non-AFP-producing human cell lines as well as primary cultures of normal human lung epithelial and endothelial cells. In an effort to enhance the selectivity of an oncolytic adenovirus vector for treatment of HCC, the AFP promoter has also been used to drive E1a expression in combination with deletion of the E1b-55K protein *(31,32)*.

Oncolytic vectors to target breast cancer have been constructed using either tumor-specific or tissue-specific promoter elements. The DF3/MUC1 promoter has been used to drive expression of E1a in an oncolytic vector, called Ad.DF3-E1, based on the observation that aberrant transcription control is responsible for overexpression of the DF3/MUC1 antigen in nearly 80% of primary human breast cancer cells *(34)*. Ad.DF3-E1 was reported to replicate selectively in MUC1-positive breast cancer cells and was efficacious for the treatment of human breast MCF-7 tumor xenografts in nude mice *(34)*. In an effort to target malignant breast cancer cells that retain expression of estrogen receptors (up to 70% of breast cancer cells), Ad5ERE2 was constructed by inserting promoters containing two estrogen response elements to control expression of E1a and E4 gene regions *(34)*. Ad5ERE2 was reported to be preferentially cytotoxic in estrogen receptor-positive tumor cells in the presence of 17β-estradiol; furthermore, replication of Ad5ERE2 could be inhibited by the antiestrogen tamoxifen, which is a desirable safety feature of this vector.

To design an oncolytic adenovirus for colon carcinomas, strategies that take advantage of the wnt signaling pathway, which is almost ubiquitously activated in colon cancer cells but not in normal colon cells, were evaluated *(35)*. A number of oncolytic adenoviruses in which the viral E2 and/or E1b promoters were under control of Tcf (a transcription factor activated by the wnt signaling) were first engineered and tested. Viruses with Tcf regulation were attenuated 50- to 100-fold in two cell lines without wnt activation, but replicated at wild-type levels in permissive SW480 colon cancer cells.

In an effort to improve the selectivity of the Tcf-regulated vectors, further modifications were made, including replacement of E1a promoter/enhancer elements and half of the left ITR with Tcf binding sites, relocation of the viral packaging signal from the left ITR to the right ITR, and addition of Tcf sites to the right ITR downstream of the E4 promoter to maintain symmetry of the terminal repeats *(36)*. Viruses with E1a, E1b, E2, and E4 promoters containing Tcf sites were greatly attenuated in cell lines such as HeLa and smooth airway epithelial cells in which the wnt pathway is not activated, but were also attenuated 100-fold in SW480 cells. Overall, the highly modified Tcf vectors were shown to have selectivity of up to 10^5-fold for wnt-activated cells in vitro; however, their activity in xenograft tumor models has not been evaluated.

In an effort to target adenoviral replication to a wide range of different tumor types, based on pRb-pathway defects, the E2F-1 promoter has been used to regulate viral early region function. To test the tumor-specific replication of a virus in which E1a gene expression was under E2F-1 control, Ad*E2F-1^{RC}* was constructed by inserting a fragment of the E2F-1 promoter downstream of the E1A promoter *(37)*. Ad*E2F-1^{RC}* was shown to replicate preferentially in tumor cells, but not a panel of normal cells, and to have antitumor efficacy in xenograft tumor models in mice. A series of viruses in which the E1a and/or E4 promoters of Ad*dl*922/947, an adenovirus with deletion in E1a that abolishes binding

Table 1
Tumor-/Tissue-Specific Promoter Regulation of Early Region Genes

Vector name (reference)	Target	Regulatory element	Adenovirus gene regulated	Reference
CN706	Prostate	PSA promoter	E1a	4
CN763	Prostate	Kallikrein 2 promoter	E1a	93
CN764	Prostate	PSA promoter	E1a	93
		Kallikrein 2 promoter	E1b	
CV739	Prostate	Rat probasin	E1a	29
		Human PSA	E1b	
CV787	Prostate	Rat probasin	E1a	29
		Human PSA	E1b (E3 region intact)	
Ad-OC-E1a	Prostate and bone metastasis	Osteocalcin C	E1a	94
AvE1A041	Liver	AFP	E1a	30
GT5610 +AdH$_B$	Liver	AFP	E1a, requires helper virus infection	95
CV890	Liver	AFP	E1a-IRES-E1b expression cassette	53
YKL-1001	Liver	AFP	E1a in a E1b 55K-deleted backbone	31
AdAFPep/Rep	Liver	AFP	E1a (13S cDNA), E1b 55K-deleted backbone	32
AdMKE1	Neuroblastoma	Midkine	E1a	96
Ad5ERE2	Breast	PS2/2-ERE	E1a and E4	34
Ad.DF3-E1	Breast	MUC 1promoter/enhancer	E1a	91
AdEHE2F	Breast	3-HRE/5-ERE	E1a	97
		E2F-1	E4	
Ad-Lp-E1A	Breast, ovary	L-Plastin truncated promoter	E1a	98
Ad-Tyr-E1A	Skin	Tyrosinase promoter/enhancer	E1a	98
AdTyrΔ24	Skin	Tyrosinase promoter/enhancer	E1a	99
			E1A Δ24 mutation	
AdTyrΔ2Δ24	Skin	Tyrosinase promoter/enhancer	E1a	99
			E1a Δ2Δ24 mutation	
KD-1-SPB	Lung	Surfactant protein B promoter	E4, E1A01/07 backbone, E3-deletion except ADP	27
CG8840	Bladder	Uroplakin II promoter	E1a-IRES-E1b, E1b-19K deletion	100
vMB19	Colon	Tcf4-binding sites (multiple copies)	E2, E1b	35
vCF62	Colon	Tcf4-binding sites (multiple copies)	E1a, E1b, E2, and E4	36
ONYX-411	Various	E2F1 promoter	E1a, E4	38
		E1a dl922/947 mutation		
AdE2F-1^{RC}	Various	E2F1 promoter	E1a	37
Ad.Flk-1	Angiogenic endothelial cells	Flk 1 promoter/enhancer	E1a	39
Ad.Flk-1-Endo	Angiogenic endothelial cells	Flk 1 promoter/enhancer, endoglin promoter	E1b	39

to pRb, were replaced with the human E2F-1 promoter has also been evaluated *(38)*. This work demonstrated that E2F-1 promoter control of the mutant E1a (ONYX-150) or E4 gene region (ONYX-410) was sufficient to attenuate virus DNA replication, and viral late gene expression, in normal small airway epithelial cells as compared to *dl*309 or Ad*dl*922/947, but not in a number of tumor cell lines. However, replacement of both the E1a and E4 promoters with the E2F-1 promoter in ONYX-411 resulted in further attenuation of virus growth in normal cells and, importantly, reduced liver toxicity in mice to levels comparable to a virus with a complete deletion of E1a. Finally, the demonstrated ability of ONYX-411 to exhibit antitumor efficacy in mice bearing C33A cervical carcinoma cells suggests that this virus may have great potential as a broad-based cancer therapeutic agent.

An attempt to design an oncolytic adenovirus to target lysis of dividing endothelial cells, and thus inhibit angiogenesis in tumor tissue, has been reported *(39)*. This approach also has the advantage that it could be used to treat a wide range of tumor types. The virus constructs (Ad.Flk-1 and Ad.Flk-Endo) use promoter elements from the *Flk-1* and endoglin genes because these genes are overexpressed in angiogenic endothelial cells, but not in normal endothelial cells. Both viruses use the Flk-1 promoter/enhancer to regulate E1a expression; Ad.Flk-Endo also contains the endoglin promoter inserted upstream of the E1b region. Evaluation of the replicative properties of the viruses showed that Ad-Flk-1 and Ad-Flk-Endo replicated as efficiently as wild-type virus in human umbilical vein endothelial cells, but were attenuated up to 30- and 600-fold, respectively, in human tumor control cell lines control. In addition, both Ad.Flk-1 and Ad.Flk-Endo efficiently inhibited the differentiation of human umbilical vein endothelial cells into capillarylike structures in an in vitro assay. One potential drawback of Ad.Flk and Ad.Flk-Endo, as noted by the authors, is that the relatively low level of infectivity of the endothelial cells may limit the use of these viruses to local or regional therapy until enhanced endothelial cell targeting can be engineered into the viruses.

2.3. Strategies That Take Advantage of Both p53 and pRb Pathway Defects in Tumor Cells

As described above, specific alterations in E1a and E1b were evaluated with the idea of exploiting either pRb or p53 pathway defects. Because adenovirus has evolved to commandeer both pRb and p53 pathways for its replication, it should be possible to abort or reverse conditionally the virus regulatory circuit that interferes in these two key pathways. Functional p53 and pRb pathways can be exploited to attenuate the viral growth in normal cells instead of depending on tumor cell defects to complement viral gene inactivation or to drive viral gene expression (Fig. 4) *(40)*. Because of the heterogeneity in tumors compared to normal cells, such strategies that take advantage of normal cell functions to inhibit virus replication may be useful for the treatment of a broad range of tumors.

To exploit defects in both p53 and pRb pathways to confer selectivity to oncolytic viruses, a dominant-negative inhibitor of viral replication was expressed using a p53-responsive promoter (PRP) *(40)*. An E2F antagonist composed of a fusion protein with the DNA-binding domain of E2F and the transrepression domain of pRb (E2F-Rb) was used as the dominant-negative inhibitor in the construct 01/PEME. Such E2F-Rb fusion proteins are potent repressors of E2F-dependent promoters *(41)*. Viral E2 and E1a promoters and many of the cellular S-phase genes are regulated by E2F; therefore, repression of E2F-dependent promoters leads to inhibition of critical events required for viral replication, such as viral gene expression and S-phase induction.

Following infection of normal cells with 01/PEME, cellular p53 drives expression of E2F-Rb and inhibits viral replication (Fig. 4). In contrast, tumor cells with p53-inactivating mutations do not permit expression of E2F-Rb from 01/PEME and thus allow replication of 01/PEME to proceed unhindered. Tumor cells with functional p53 also allow replication of 01/PEME because higher E2F activity as the result of prevalent disruption of the pRb pathway in tumor cells promotes transcription from E2F-dependent viral E1a and E2a promoters immediately after the virus enters the cells and prior to expression of sufficient quantities of E2F-Rb. In addition, because inhibition by E2F-Rb depends on

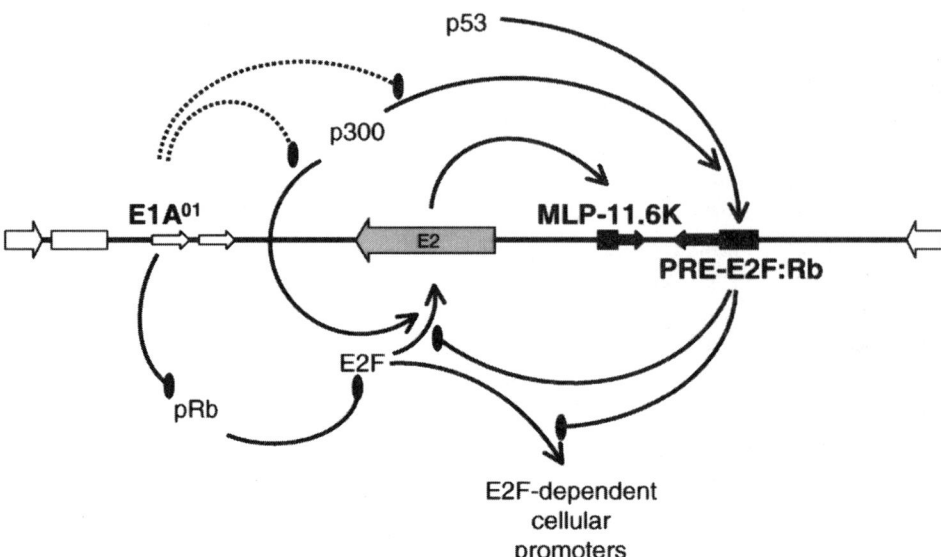

Fig. 4. The p53-dependent expression of an E2F antagonist in 01/PEME selectively attenuates viral replication in normal cells. In a strategy that exploits both p53 and pRb pathway defects, expression of an E2F antagonist constructed with the DNA-binding domain of E2F and transcriptional repression domain of pRb is regulated by the functional p53 pathway prevalent in normal cells (PRE-E2F-Rb), but not in tumor cells with defective p53 pathway. Unlike wild-type E1a, E1a[01] (*dl*1101 deletion in E1a; *101*) does not sequester the transcriptional coactivator p300/CBP *(11,102)* (shown as dotted line) and allows for the optimum activity of cellular p53 in driving E2F antagonist expression. Repression of E2F-dependent promoters, including viral E2 promoter, leads to inhibition of critical events required for viral replication, such as early viral gene expression and S-phase induction, resulting in attenuation of virus growth (*see* Section 2.3.). Because E3-11.6K is under the control of an extra copy of the MLP, which is strictly dependent on viral DNA replication for its activity, enhanced expression and cell killing occur in tumor cells *(40)*.

competition with endogenous E2F activity, E2F-Rb would be less effective in inhibiting adenoviral early promoters when E2F activity is upregulated in tumor cells. In contrast, p53-dependent E2F-Rb expression would be effective in attenuating the virus in normal cells because of both functional p53 and tightly regulated E2F pathways.

3. MANIPULATION OF THE VIRAL GENOME TO ENHANCE ONCOLYTIC ACTIVITY

Efficient killing of tumor cells and rapid spread of the virus within a tumor are essential for maximum efficacy. Strategies evaluated to achieve this include specific alterations in the viral genome and incorporation of transgenes (*see* below). Because of the limitations in the size and type of transgene that can be inserted without compromising the replication potential of the virus, engineering the viral regulatory pathways may be more desirable. Alterations evaluated within the viral genome include functional inactivation of antiapoptotic viral protein such as E1b-19K and overexpression of viral proteins involved in induction of cell death. In infected cells, E1b-19K prevents premature killing of infected cells *(42)*, whereas E3-11.6K *(43,44)* and E4orf4 *(45–47)* promote cell death following replication and assembly of the virus. Consistent with the antiapoptotic function of E1b-19K, E1b-19K-deleted viruses were found to induce apoptosis very efficiently, resulting in faster spread of the virus than for the wild type. AdH5 dL118, a virus that lacks expression of both E1b-19K and E1b-55K proteins, and Ad337, a virus that lacks E1b-19K, showed enhanced cytolytic activity on tumor cell lines in vitro and in vivo *(48,49)*. Furthermore, increased chemosensitization to DNA-damaging agents in vitro and in vivo was observed with the use of E1b-19K-deleted viruses *(50)*.

Overexpression of E3-11.6K late in the infection as a means to enhance the cytolytic activity without interfering in virus replication has also been investigated *(27,40)*. E3-11.6K is expressed at low levels at early times, but synthesized in large amounts from mRNAs derived from the major late promoter (MLP) *(51)*. E3-11.6K overexpression, as opposed to functional inactivation of E1b-19K, may be desirable in light of the findings that E1b-19K mutations also affect viral replication in some tumor cells *(18)*. E3-11.6K overexpression and enhanced oncolytic activity in xenograft tumor models were achieved on removal of all other open reading frames in the E3 region except that of E3-11.6K in the virus KD1, with *dl*01/07 deletion in the E1a gene *(27)*. Overexpression of E3-11.6K and increased in vitro and in vivo oncolytic activity were also achieved using an extra copy of the viral MLP inserted in the E3 region upstream of the E3-11.6K coding sequence *(40)*. The use of the major late promoter, which becomes active after the onset of DNA replication, couples E3-11.6K overexpression and cell killing to viral DNA replication and thus provides another level of control in oncolytic viruses *(40)*.

4. COMBINATION WITH CHEMO- AND RADIATION THERAPIES TO ENHANCE ONCOLYTIC ACTIVITY AND POSSIBLY INCREASE SELECTIVITY

It is likely that any new treatments will be used in combination with chemotherapeutic drugs widely accepted for therapy. In the clinical studies with ONYX-015, significant antitumor activity was reported only when viral therapy was combined with chemotherapeutic agents 5-fluorouracil (5-FU) or cisplatin *(33)*. Enhanced antitumor activity has also been reported in preclinical studies for oncolytic viruses with deletions in E1b-55K and E1b-19K and with conditional expression of E1a or E4 regulated by tumor-specific promoters *(52–54)* when combined with chemotherapeutic agents such as 5-FU, cisplatin, doxorubicin, paclitaxel, or docetaxel. Of potential significance, in preclinical studies with the prostate-specific CV787, healthier animals were observed when treated in combination with docetaxel than treatment with either agent alone, and toxicology studies in Balb/C mice did not show synergistic or additive toxicity because of combined treatment of docetaxel and CV787 *(54)*.

It is likely that the demonstrated antitumor synergistic or additive activities of viral oncolysis and chemotherapeutic agents are the result of multiple mechanisms. Among viral proteins, E1a is known to sensitize infected cells for killing by various chemotherapeutic agents in both a p53-dependent and a p53-independent manner *(55–59)*. The p53-dependent sensitization could occur through stabilization of p53 through increased transcriptional upregulation p14^{ARF} as a result of E2F activation *(60)* (Fig. 1). The p53-independant sensitization by E1a might be the result of E2F activation and subsequent transcriptional activation of multiple caspases *(7)*. Based on the finding that E1b-19K-deleted viruses are much more efficient in inducing apoptosis of infected cells, it is believed that virus-generated proapoptotic signals might contribute to sensitized killing of infected cells by chemotherapeutic agents.

Increased expression of inflammatory cytokines such TNF-α, which is a known chemosensitizer *(61–63)*, following adenovirus infection might also contribute to the enhanced oncolytic activities *(64)*. With a secreted mediator of chemosensitization such as TNF-α, it is possible that even the uninfected cells in the tumor are killed because of increased sensitization.

Enhanced oncolytic activity with combination treatment may also be the result of enhanced viral activity in tumor cells. Greater antitumor activity has been shown to be the result of increased transduction rate for combination of paclitaxel with a replication-defective recombinant adenovirus vector *(65)*. A number of chemotherapeutic agents that induce cells to arrest in the G2 phase of the cell cycle have been shown to increase virus replication *(66)*. In addition, increased cell killing by chemotherapeutic agents might contribute to greater spread of the virus in the tumor.

It is likely that, depending on the modification introduced into oncolytic viruses, the antitumor synergy with chemotherapeutic agents may vary *(66)*. Therefore, it will be important to choose the optimized combination of drug and virus for use in the clinic.

Additive or synergistic oncolytic activities have also been observed in combination with radiation for oncolytic viruses, including E1b-55K-deleted ONYX-015 *(67)*, the PSA promoter-driven CV706 *(68)* and Ad5-d24RGD, a virus with deletion in the pRb-binding domain of E1a and an Arg-Gly-Asp motif inserted in the fiber knob *(69)*. It is likely that many of the same mechanisms, such as activation of E2F because of expression of E1a, expression of pro-death viral proteins, and cytokines that sensitize to killing by chemotherapeutic agents, may also be involved in radiosensitization. Studies with ONYX-015 in combination with radiation have indicated that the radiation does not alter virus replication *(67)*.

It is possible that, similar to chemotherapeutic agents *(66)*, radiation may enhance replication at subtoxic doses by arresting cells in the G2 phase of the cell cycle. This idea is supported by the findings that radiation at synergistic dose significantly increased virus replication *(68)*. Increased sensitivity to killing and rapid spread of the virus, together with enhanced replication within the tumor prior to generation of immune response toward the virus, will be clinically valuable. Radiation may also complement the oncolytic utility of viruses by effectively targeting tumor cell populations resistant to virus-mediated killing *(67)*. Furthermore, because of synergistic interactions, it might be possible to use considerably lower doses of virus as well as chemotherapeutic agents or radiation to achieve antitumor efficacy with lower toxicity in the clinic.

In oncolytic viruses such as 01/PEME, in which selectivity is conferred by expression of an E2F antagonist with a PRP *(40)* (Fig. 4), the use of radiation and chemotherapies has the potential to enhance the therapeutic index by attenuating the virus in p53 functional normal cells and increase the potency in p53-defective tumor cells. Induction of p53 as a result of DNA damage by radiation and chemotherapeutic agents leads to increased expression of E2F antagonist encoded in the virus and further attenuation of the virus in those cells (M. Ramachandra, 2003, unpublished observations). In contrast, in tumor cells with defective p53, E2F antagonist is not upregulated because of radiation and chemotherapy. As a result, viral replication proceeds unhindered in those tumor cells, resulting in high-level expression of viral proteins, including E1a, that are known to sensitize to killing by radiation and chemotherapeutic agents.

5. THERAPEUTIC GENES IN REPLICATING ADENOVIRUSES

Although pathway-targeted oncolytic viruses offer great potential as anticancer agents, in practice, issues of delivery and tumor cell heterogeneity may still prevent lysis of the majority of cells within the tumor tissue. One approach to enhance the efficacy of replication-selective vectors is to take advantage of the replicative properties of adenovirus to deliver therapeutic proteins efficiently at levels higher than with replication-defective adenovirus vectors. The choice of transgene in such an approach is important so as not to inhibit the replicative properties of the virus. Potential inhibitory activities of the transgene product may be overcome by timing the expression of the transgene to the late phase of the replicative cycle *(27,40,70–73)*. The various strategies in which oncolytic vectors have been used to deliver therapeutic genes, including cytokines, prodrug-converting enzymes, and proapoptotic genes, are summarized in Table 2.

In an early study, Ad/IFN, a replicating adenovirus not targeted to tumor cells, was used to deliver the cytokine interferon (IFN) and was found to be efficacious in a number of tumor models *(74)*. The breast tumor-targeted Ad.DF3-E1 (described above) was used to express the antitumor cytokine TNF-α. At a low-level infection in vitro, Ad.DF3-E1/CMV–TNF produced TNF-α at levels as much as 10^6-fold higher than a replication-defective vector for TNF-α delivery, a clear demonstration of the potential ability of replicating vectors to produce high local concentrations of antitumor molecules. Potential efficacy was also demonstrated as tumors treated with Ad.DF3-E1/CMV-TNF were significantly smaller than tumors treated with a control vector or the replication-defective Ad.CMV-TNF.

Table 2
Oncolytic Adenovirus to Express Therapeutic Genes

Vector name (reference)	Backbone	Transgene	Reference
Ad 5/IFN	E3 deletion	Human consensus IFN inserted in the E3 region under MLP control	74
Ad5-CD/TKrep	E1b-55K/E3 deletion	CD/HSV-tk fusion	75
Ad.TK^{RC} (II)	E1b-55K/E3 deletion	CMV promoter drives HSV-*tk*/IRES E1a	90
Ad.DF3-E1/CMV-TNF	DF3 promoter insertion regulates E1a	CMV promoter drives TNF expression in E1 region	91
Ad.E1A(+)HS-CDTK	E1b^{ve}/E3 deletion	Hsp70 promoter regulates CD/TK fusion expression	92
Adp53rc	E3 deletion	p53 gene inserted into fiber transcription unit with IRES	72
AdΔ24-p53	E1aΔ24 (deletion of pRb binding site in E1a)/E3 deletion	Insertion of SVE promoter to regulate p53 in E3 region	73
Ad.IR-SG	E1/E3 deleted	Secreted B-glucuronidase (expression dependent on homologous recombination)	66
Ad.IR-CodAupp	E1/E3 deleted	CD/uracil phosphoribosyltransferase (expression dependent on homologous recombination)	66

E1b-55K⁻ adenoviruses have been used to enhance the delivery of prodrug-activating enzymes, which are used to convert prodrugs to DNA synthesis inhibitors. In one set of studies, the ONYX-015 backbone was used to deliver a cytosine deaminase (CD)/HSV*tk* fusion gene expressed from the CMV promoter *(75)*. The CD/HSV*tk* fusion has also been shown to sensitize cells to radiation, potentially allowing a three-prong treatment approach combining double-suicide gene therapy, oncolysis, and radiation therapy. In vitro studies showed that Ad5-CD/TKrep exhibited the same tumor cell specificity and replication kinetics as the E1b-55K-deleted virus, but incorporation of the CD/HSV-TK fusion gene enhanced the CPE of the virus and sensitized tumors to radiation following 5-fluorocytosine and ganciclovir (GCV) treatment.

Wildner and coworkers evaluated an E1b-55K-deleted adenovirus vector, Ad.TK^{RC}, engineered to express HSV*tk* transcriptional linked to E1a and E1b-19K from a CMV promoter. In tumor xenograft models, AdTK^{RC}(II) showed increased efficacy in combination with the GCV treatment compared to an E1b-55K⁻-deleted control virus or a replication-defective HSV*tk* encoding adenovirus vector *(76,77)*. In contrast, the efficacy of E1b-55K⁺ virus encoding HSV-TK, called AdOW34, was not improved, and in fact was significantly reduced in one tumor treatment model, with GCV treatment *(73)*. Similar lack of improved efficacy with a TK-encoding virus in combination with GCV was noted in an independent study *(78)*.

It would be interesting to determine if expression of HSV*tk* from the MLP rather than the CMV promoter or optimization of the timing of prodrug treatment would allow for effective prodrug treatment with E1b-55K⁺ vectors designed to deliver suicide enzymes. A potential advantage of suppression of viral replication with prodrug treatment is that it provides a fail-safe mechanism to control viral spread.

One way to improve the oncolytic effect of adenovirus vectors might be to deliver proapoptotic transgenes that accelerate oncolysis and improve lateral spread of the virus in tumor tissue. Coinfection of the replication-competent breast tumor-targeted Ad5ERE2 (*see* above) with a replication-defective adenovirus to deliver the proapoptotic Bcl-xs led to a dramatic increase in cell death and efficacy for tumor xenografts as compared to treatment with Ad5ERE2 alone *(34)*. The tumor suppressor p53 has also been expressed in replicating adenovirus, in a virus called Adp53rc, as part of the fiber transcription unit using an internal ribosomal entry site. In vitro characterization of this vector showed that p53 expression occurred in the late phase of the replication cycle, was dependant on viral replication, and improved virus release and spread. In addition, inclusion of a p53 expression cassette in the E3 region increased the oncolytic potency of AdΔ24 *(73)*.

6. CLINICAL STUDIES

E1b-55K-deleted virus ONYX-015, viruses with E1a under the control of tumor-specific promoters, and a virus with prodrug-activating enzyme have been studied in the clinic (Table 3). More than 230 patients have been treated with ONYX-015 via intratumoral and intracavity such as intraperitoneal, intraarterial, and intravenous routes. ONYX-015 was reported to be well tolerated even at the highest feasible doses (2×10^{12} to 2×10^{13} particles) by all routes of administration. Common toxicities observed were fever, nausea, chills, and flulike symptoms, which were more severe following intravascular treatment.

Following repeated intraarterial and intravenous delivery, circulating levels of inflammatory cytokines, including IL-1, IL-6, TNF-α, and IFN-γ, increased. Increase in neutralizing antibodies against the virus was observed in almost all patients. The half-life of the virus in the plasma by intravenous administration *(79)* was approx 20 minutes. Demonstration of viral replication was reported in head and neck and colorectal tumors following intratumoral or intraarterial administration, respectively. Viral replication was not observed in pancreatic and ovarian tumors following intratumoral and intraperitoneal administration, respectively. However, antitumor efficacy with ONYX-015 as a single agent has been limited in patients with head and neck, pancreatic, colorectal, or ovarian carcinomas.

After establishing the safety of ONYX-015 alone, chemotherapy combinations with 5-FU and cisplatin were also studied in the clinic *(33)*. The combination treatment also was well tolerated, with no apparent change in chemotherapy toxicity because of viral therapy. Potentially synergistic interactions with chemotherapy have been reported in trials with patients with head and neck tumors following intratumoral administration and colorectal liver metastases following hepatic arterial administration. Responses observed in these studies were independent of the p53 status. Partial or complete response of 63%, including 27% complete response in the head-and-neck trial, was higher than the expected 30–40% partial or complete response rate in similar patients receiving the same chemotherapy regimen *(33)*. Based on these results, a phase III clinical trial of ONYX-015 for the treatment of recurrent head and neck cancer has been initiated. This phase III trial will be a randomized, two-arm study comparing intratumoral injection of ONYX-015 plus standard chemotherapy (5-FU and cisplatin) against chemotherapy alone.

Viruses with E1a under the control of tumor-specific promoters CG7060 (previously known as CV706) *(28)* and CG7870 (previously CV787) *(28)* have been reported to show acceptable safety profiles and suggestions of antitumor activity based on decrease in PSA levels in phase I/II studies following direct intratumoral administration in patients with prostate cancer *(28)*. The virus was detected in the plasma with a half-life of 23 minutes. A phase I clinical study has also been performed using a replication-competent adenovirus with E1b-55K deletion, but encoding CD/HSV-1-TK fusion protein (Ad5-CD/TK*rep*) for the treatment of locally recurrent prostate cancer *(80)*. Administration of the virus by intraprostatic injection under transrectal ultrasound guidance was followed by treatment with prodrugs 5-fluorocytosine and GCV (Table 3). Similar to other viruses, observed toxicities were mild to moderate, with no dose-limiting toxicity. Antitumor activity was suggested by a decrease in serum PSA levels *(80)*.

7. FUTURE DIRECTIONS

Oncolytic adenoviruses provide a unique therapeutic approach that could supply a new weapon for the clinician's armamentarium of anticancer drugs. The initial hurdles of moving oncolytic adenoviruses from basic to clinical research have largely been overcome. Complete development of these agents as successful drugs will require filling in a number of gaps in the knowledge of their basic pharmacology and toxicology, learning how to deliver them systemically as well as locally, and understanding how to use them in combination with other anticancer agents.

7.1. Mechanisms of Action: Unanswered Questions

Numerous studies have demonstrated that lytic replication of adenovirus is the primary mechanism of cell killing in vitro, and that adenoviral transcription and replication functions can be modified to provide relative selectivity for killing of tumor cells vs normal cells. However, it has been difficult to demonstrate that tumor-selective replication is the primary in vivo mechanism of oncolytic activity of these agents both in clinical studies, in which the use of biopsy-based analytical methods is limited, and in preclinical studies, in which the restricted host range of adenovirus requires use of human xenograft tumors in immunodeficient mice. Further improvements in bioanalytical methods to measure viral replication, selectivity for tumor cells, and pharmacodynamic effects would be very useful in support of early-phase clinical development.

Other factors that may play a role in oncolytic activity in vivo include direct CPEs at high doses of virus and development of inflammatory responses as well as adaptive immunity. Among these factors, induction of inflammatory responses may be particularly significant because inflammatory cytokines such as TNF-α and IFN-γ and inflammatory cells, including macrophages, natural killer cells, granulocytes, and NKT cells have well-characterized antitumor activity. Increases in serum levels of TNF-α and IFN-γ are a consistent observation in clinical *(79)* and preclinical studies using systemic administration of oncolytic adenoviruses and adenovirus vectors; these cytokines presumably are expressed

Table 3
Published Clinical Trials of Replicating Adenoviruses

Study type/virus	Tumor type	Route, dose, and treatment schedule	Toxicity	Response	Evidence of virus presence and replication
Phase I/ ONYX-015 (83)	Recurrent head and neck cancer	Intratumoral; 10^7 to 10^{11} pfu; single injection	No DLT; flulike symptoms and injection site pain	No objective response; 22% response at the tumor site; no correlation between response and p53 status or preexisting adenovirus antibodies	No evidence of virus in plasma on days 3, 8, 15, 22, and 29 posttreatment PCR
Phase II/ ONYX-015 (84)	Recurrent head and neck cancer	Intratumoral; 2×10^{11} particles; days 1–5, every 21 days; additional arm with twice daily for 5 days and repeated the following week	Mild-to-moderate fever and injection site pain	Complete or partial response in 14% of patients; 7 of 12 p53-altered tumors responded, whereas 0 of 7 wild-type p53 tumors responded; no correlation between preexisting adenovirus antibodies and response	Assessed for viral replication by in situ hybridization, IHC for E1a and EM; virus detected between days 1 and 10 in 7 of 11 samples only in tumor not in surrounding normal tissue; virus detected by PCR in 41% of patients 24 hours after last injection and in 9% of patients 10 days after treatment, suggesting virus replication
Phase II/ ONYX-015 (33)	Recurrent head and neck cancer	Intratumoral; 10^{10} pfu; days 1–5, every 21 days; in combination with cisplatin and 5-FU; some patients with two tumors, only the large one was injected	Flulike symptoms and injection site pain	33% Partial response, 27% complete response; no correlation between response and adenovirus antibodies, p53 status, tumor size, or prior treatment; among patients with two tumors in 6 of 11 only injected tumor, 3 of 11 both and 2 of 11 none responded	Analysis by in situ hybridization revealed viral replication in 4 of 7 biopsies taken between days 5 and 15; no viral DNA in normal tissue
Phase I/ ONYX-015 (85)	Pancreatic carcinoma	Intratumoral; 2×10^9 to 2×10^{12} particles in a volume of 20% tumor size; every 4 weeks until tumor regression	Flulike symptoms resolved in 2 days	No objective tumor response; stable disease in 10 of 23 patients	Virus detected in the blood at 15 minutes after dosing, but not the following day or 2 weeks later; no demonstration of virus replication

226

Phase I/dl1520 (not supplied by ONYX) (86)	HCC	Percutaneous injection; 5 patients with 3×10^{11} pfu intravenous then it on days 2, 25, 16, 29, and 30	Flulike symptoms; liver function tests not elevated 2 weeks after treatment	1 of 5 patients partial response, progressive disease in other 4 patients	Virus detected in the blood 30 minutes after treatment; blood samples negative 4 hours after dosing
Phase I/ONYX-015 (87)	Ovarian cancer	Intraperitoneal; 1×10^9 to 1×10^{11} pfu infused in a volume of 500 mL over 15 minutes; daily for five days, every 21 days	Flulike symptoms, abdominal pain, and diarrhea	No tumor response	Peritoneal washes from days 5 and 15 positive for virus by PCR; of 10 cytology specimens (only 10 of 26 evaluable) positive by *in situ* hybridization; plasma cells negative
Phase I/ONYX-015 (88)	Colorectal cancer liver metastases	Intrahepatic artery infusion; 2×10^8 to 2×10^{12} particles; days 1 and 8; every 28 days; 5-FU and leucovorin combination in the later cycle (day 28)	No DLT; low-grade transaminitis; flulike symptoms; treatment with virus and chemotherapy did not worsen toxicity associated with chemotherapy	Partial response in 9% of patients; dose-dependent tumor responses noted in combination with chemotherapy	Input virus was cleared in the blood within 6 hours after infusion; on day 4, viral genomes detected by PCR at doses of $\geq 2 \times 10^{11}$ particles, suggesting replication
Phase II/ONYX-015 (89)	Gastrointestinal cancer liver metastases	Intrahepatic artery infusion; 2×10^{12} particles; days 1 and 8 as single agent; starting on day 22, in combination with intravenous; 5-FU and leucovorin every 28 days	Generally well tolerated alone or in combination with chemotherapy; adverse events with ONYX-015 alone were flulike symptoms, including fever, myalgias, asthenia, and/or chills; chemotherapy-related toxicities were similar to those expected for those agents when treated without the virus	11% partial response; increase in neutralizing antibody titers did not prevent efficacy or replication; increase in the levels of TNF-α, IFN-γ, and IL-6 within 3 hours, followed by an increase in IL-10 level at 18 hours	Virus cleared to undetectable levels within 6 hours, but concentration increased to 1.7×10^5 to 4×10^6 genomes/mL, suggesting viral replication

(continued)

Table 3 (Continued)

Study type/virus	Tumor type	Route, dose, and treatment schedule	Toxicity	Response	Evidence of virus presence and replication
Phase I/ ONYX-015 (79)	Various metastatic solid tumors	Intravenous; 2×10^{10} to 2×10^{13} particles; days 1, 8, 15, every 21 days	No DLT; fever and rigor; transient elevation in serum transaminase with $>2 \times 10^{12}$ particles; no changes in toxicity in combination with taxol and carboplatin	No objective tumor response when most patients had stable disease; elevated IL-6, IL-10, TNF-α, and IFN-γ in serum with $>2 \times 10^{12}$ particles; no increase in IL-1α, IL-1β, or IL-2; serum cytokine returned to baseline within 7 days; transient elevation in circulating lymphocytes noted; neutralizing antibody titers increased within 2–3 weeks	Virus detected in the plasma 6 hours after infusion; half-life was ~20 minutes; 3 of 4 patients with $>2 \times 10^{12}$ particles showed increased virus concentration for 6–48 hours after infusion, suggesting virus replication; positive staining for capsid antigen
Phase I/ CV706 (28)	Recurrent prostate cancer	Intratumoral (ultrasound guided); 1×10^{11} to 1×10^{13} particles	Local pain at the injection site; no DLT; frequent fever and prostatitis; no irreversible grade 3 or any grade 4 toxicity	Partial response of >50% reduction in PSA for at least 4 weeks in 5 of 11 patients at two highest doses; increase in neutralizing antibody titer in all patients; no correlation between baseline antibody titer and PSA response	Late gene expression and nuclear inclusion bodies in biopsy samples, suggesting replication; virus detected in the plasma at 30 minutes that dropped to baseline by 12–24 hours with a half-life of 23 minutes; virus detected in the circulation between 1 and 8 days; secondary peak returned to baseline by day 15; patients with greatest secondary peaks had lower antiadenovirus titers
Phase I/Ad5-CD/TK*rep* (80)	Recurrent prostate cancer	Intratumoral (ultrasound guided); maximum dose of 1×10^{12} particles; 2 days after virus dosing, treatment with prodrugs 5-FU and GCV for a week	Frequent pain at the injection site; no DLT; 95% of the adverse events observed were mild or moderate (grade 1/2)	44% of patients demonstrated a ≥25% decrease in serum PSA, and 19% of patients demonstrated ≥50% decrease in serum PSA; 2 patients negative for adenocarcinoma at 1 year after treatment	Transgene expression and tumor destruction at the injection site confirmed at 2 weeks; viral DNA detected in blood even at day 76, but no infectious virus detected in serum or urine

CD, cytosine deaminase; DLT, dose-limiting toxicity; 5-FU, 5-fluorouracil; GCV, ganciclovir; PCR, polymerase chain reaction; pfu, plaque-forming unit (particle-to-pfu ratio is 20:1 for ONYX-015; *81*); TK, thymidine kinase.

locally following intratumoral injection. Because TNF-α and IFN-γ also have significant toxicity to normal tissues and organs, understanding the role of these responses in overall antitumor activity of oncolytic adenoviruses will be important for safe and effective use of these agents and for determining whether inflammation is a mechanism-based toxicity.

7.2. Challenges for Delivery of Effective Doses and Clinical Development

Although oncolytic adenoviruses have been reported to be well tolerated in clinical studies using various routes of administration at doses up to 2×10^{12} viral particles for multiple cycles or single doses up to 2×10^{13} viral particles, evidence of single-agent efficacy has been limited *(81)*. Intratumoral administration of ONYX-015 in combination with systemic administration of 5-FU and cisplatin for treatment of recurrent/refractory head and neck cancer showed a significant response in the injected tumors compared to noninjected control tumors *(81)*. Based on these results, phase III trials have been initiated with end-points including tumor response, progression-free survival, durable tumor response, patient quality-of-life measurements, and overall survival.

Consideration of the challenges for clinical development of oncolytic adenoviruses illustrates the interrelationship between dose and route and mechanisms of efficacy and toxicity. ONYX-015, as well as other oncolytic adenoviruses in clinical trials, has shown the best evidence of local antitumor response when administered intralesionally. Volume limitations for intratumoral injection are typically 1–2 mL, effectively limiting the total dose to approx 2×10^{12} viral particles at the maximum obtainable virus concentration. Although doses of up to 2×10^{13} viral particles have been administered intravascularly, there appears to be a consensus that this is probably very near or at the upper limit for safety *(81)*. With intravascular administration of ONYX-015, toxicities such as fever, chills, and asthenia were more common and more severe than with intratumoral administration, and AST/ALT levels were elevated to three to five times normal at the highest doses (6×10^{12} to 2×10^{13} viral particles) *(81)*.

Because cancer generally presents as or progresses to a disseminated disease, the goal for development is to identify a disease type and stage at which safe delivery at a sufficient dose can be achieved and meaningful clinical benefit can be demonstrated, possibly as increased time to progression (for accelerated approval) and ultimately as improved overall survival *(82)*. Demonstrating improved overall survival using intratumoral administration generally presents a significant challenge, although some settings, such as head and neck cancer or glioblastoma, may provide an opportunity *(81)*. For the latter tumor type, however, the potential role of inflammatory response in antitumor efficacy could present a problem because efforts to control inflammation also might reduce efficacy. Alternatively, treatment of disseminated tumors by intravenous administration would potentially provide a survival benefit, provided that therapeutic levels in the tumor can be achieved without unacceptable toxicity.

8. CONCLUSIONS

Overall, significant advances have been made in development of engineered oncolytic adenoviruses as cancer drugs. Clinical testing of the current generation of viruses may yield commercially successful products and certainly will provide important information for development of safer and more potent agents. The use of specific transgenes to "arm" viruses to increase potency and modification of the virus coat to improve intravenous delivery can address many of the general limitations of current-generation oncolytic viruses. Defining the mechanisms of activity and toxicity, including the role of the host immune response, will provide the specific information helpful for selecting the most effective transgenes and coat modifications.

ACKNOWLEDGMENT

We thank Stephen Chang, Paul Shabram, Bill Demers, and Chuck Baum for helpful discussions.

REFERENCES

1. Swisher, S. G., Roth, J. A., and Carbone, D. P. (2002) Genetic and immunologic therapies for lung cancer. *Semin. Oncol.* **29,** 95–101.
2. Smith, R. R., Huebner, R. J., Rowe, W. P., Schatten, W. F., and Thomas, L. B. (1956) Studies on the use of viruses in the treatment of carcinoma of the cervix. *Cancer* **9,** 1211–1218.
3. Bischoff, J. R., Kirn, D. H., Williams, A., et al. (1996) An adenovirus mutant that replicates selectively in p53-deficient human tumor cells. *Science* **274,** 373–376.
4. Rodriguez, R., Schuur, E. R., Lim, H. Y., Henderson, G. A., Simons, J. W., and Henderson, D. R. (1997) Prostate attenuated replication competent adenovirus (ARCA) CN706: a selective cytotoxic for prostate-specific antigen-positive prostate cancer cells. *Cancer Res.* **57,** 2559–2563.
5. Prives, C. and Hall, P. A. (1999) The p53 pathway. *J. Pathol.* **187,** 112–126.
6. Sherr, C. J. and Weber, J. D. (2000) The ARF/p53 pathway. *Curr. Opin. Genet. Dev.* **10,** 94–99.
7. Nahle, Z., Polakoff, J., Davuluri, R. V., et al. (2002) Direct coupling of the cell cycle and cell death machinery by E2F. *Nat. Cell Biol.* **4,** 859–864.
8. Dyson, N. (1998) The regulation of E2F by pRB-family proteins. *Genes Dev.* **12,** 2245–2262.
9. de Stanchina, E., McCurrach, M. E., Zindy, F., et al. (1998) E1A signaling to p53 involves the p19(ARF) tumor suppressor. *Genes Dev.* **12,** 2434–2442.
10. Yew, P. R. and Berk, A. J. (1992) Inhibition of p53 transactivation required for transformation by adenovirus early 1B protein. *Nature* **357,** 82–85.
11. Somasundaram, K. and El-Deiry, W. S. (1997) Inhibition of p53-mediated transactivation and cell cycle arrest by E1A through its p300/CBP-interacting region. *Oncogene* **14,** 1047–1057.
12. Chakravarti, D., Ogryzko, V., Kao, H. Y., et al. (1999) A viral mechanism for inhibition of p300 and PCAF acetyltransferase activity. *Cell* **96,** 393–403.
13. Barker, D. D. and Berk, A. J. (1987) Adenovirus proteins from both E1B reading frames are required for transformation of rodent cells by viral infection and DNA transfection. *Virology* **156,** 107–121.
14. Babiss, L. E. and Ginsberg, H. S. (1984) Adenovirus type 5 early region 1b gene product is required for efficient shutoff of host protein synthesis. *J. Virol.* **50,** 202–212.
15. Heise, C., Sampson-Johannes, A., Williams, A., McCormick, F., Von Hoff, D. D., and Kirn, D. H. (1997) ONYX-015, an E1B gene-attenuated adenovirus, causes tumor-specific cytolysis and antitumoral efficacy that can be augmented by standard chemotherapeutic agents. *Nat. Med.* **3,** 639–645.
16. Alemany, R., Balague, C., and Curiel, D. T. (2000) Replicative adenoviruses for cancer therapy. *Nat. Biotechnol.* **18,** 723–727.
17. Goodrum, F. D. and Ornelles, D. A. (1998) p53 status does not determine outcome of E1B 55-kilodalton mutant adenovirus lytic infection. *J. Virol.* **72,** 9479–9490.
18. Pilder, S., Moore, M., Logan, J., and Shenk, T. (1986) The adenovirus E1B-55K transforming polypeptide modulates transport or cytoplasmic stabilization of viral and host cell mRNAs. *Mol. Cell. Biol.* **6,** 470–476.
19. Harada, J. N. and Berk, A. J. (1999) p53-Independent and -dependent requirements for E1B-55K in adenovirus type 5 replication. *J. Virol.* **73,** 5333–5344.
20. Shen, Y., Kitzes, G., Nye, J. A., Fattaey, A., and Hermiston, T. (2001) Analyses of single-amino-acid substitution mutants of adenovirus type 5 E1B-55K protein. *J. Virol.* **75,** 4297–4307.
21. Fueyo, J., Gomez-Manzano, C., Alemany, R., et al. (2000) A mutant oncolytic adenovirus targeting the Rb pathway produces anti-glioma effect in vivo. *Oncogene* **19,** 2–12.
22. Heise, C., Hermiston, T., Johnson, L., et al. (2000) An adenovirus E1A mutant that demonstrates potent and selective systemic anti-tumoral efficacy. *Nat. Med.* **6,** 1134–1139.
23. Balague, C., Noya, F., Alemany, R., Chow, L. T., and Curiel, D. T. (2001) Human papillomavirus E6E7-mediated adenovirus cell killing: selectivity of mutant adenovirus replication in organotypic cultures of human keratinocytes. *J. Virol.* **75,** 7602–7611.
24. Wang, H. G., Draetta, G., and Moran, E. (1991) E1A induces phosphorylation of the retinoblastoma protein independently of direct physical association between the E1A and retinoblastoma products. *Mol. Cell Biol.* **11,** 4253–4265.
25. O'Connor, R. J. and Hearing, P. (2000) The E4-6/7 protein functionally compensates for the loss of E1A expression in adenovirus infection. *J. Virol.* **74,** 5819–5824.
26. Howe, J., Demers, G. W., Johnson, D. E., et al. (2000) Evaluation of E1-mutant adenoviruses as conditionally replicating agents for cancer therapy. *Mol. Ther.* **2,** 485–495.
27. Doronin, K., Toth, K., Kuppuswamy, M., Ward, P., Tollefson, A. E., and Wold, W. S. (2000) Tumor-specific, replication-competent adenovirus vectors overexpressing the adenovirus death protein. *J. Virol.* **74,** 6147–6155.
28. DeWeese, T. L., van der Poel, H., Li, S., et al. (2001) A phase I trial of CV706, a replication-competent, PSA selective oncolytic adenovirus, for the treatment of locally recurrent prostate cancer following radiation therapy. *Cancer Res.* **61,** 7464–7472.

29. Yu, D. C., Chen, Y., Seng, M., Dilley, J., and Henderson, D. R. (1999) The addition of adenovirus type 5 region E3 enables calydon virus 787 to eliminate distant prostate tumor xenografts. *Cancer Res.* **59,** 4200–4203.

30. Hallenbeck, P. L., Chang, Y. N., Hay, C., et al. (1999) A novel tumor-specific replication-restricted adenoviral vector for gene therapy of hepatocellular carcinoma. *Hum. Gene Ther.* **10,** 1721–1733.

31. Kim, J., Lee, B., Kim, J. S., et al. (2002) Antitumoral effects of recombinant adenovirus YKL-1001, conditionally replicating in alpha-fetoprotein-producing human liver cancer cells. *Cancer Lett.* **180,** 23–32.

32. Takahashi, M., Sato, T., Sagawa, T., et al. (2002) E1B-55K-deleted adenovirus expressing E1A-13S by AFP-enhancer/promoter is capable of highly specific replication in AFP-producing hepatocellular carcinoma and eradication of established tumor. *Mol. Ther.* **5,** 627–634.

33. Khuri, F. R., Nemunaitis, J., Ganly, I., et al. (2000) A controlled trial of intratumoral ONYX-015, a selectively-replicating adenovirus, in combination with cisplatin and 5-fluorouracil in patients with recurrent head and neck cancer. *Nat. Med.* **6,** 879–885.

34. Hernandez-Alcoceba, R., Pihalja, M., Wicha, M. S., and Clarke, M. F. (2000) A novel, conditionally replicative adenovirus for the treatment of breast cancer that allows controlled replication of E1a-deleted adenoviral vectors. *Hum. Gene Ther.* **11,** 2009–2024.

35. Brunori, M., Malerba, M., Kashiwazaki, H., and Iggo, R. (2001) Replicating adenoviruses that target tumors with constitutive activation of the wnt signaling pathway. *J. Virol.* **75,** 2857–2865.

36. Fuerer, C. and Iggo, R. (2002) Adenoviruses with Tcf binding sites in multiple early promoters show enhanced selectivity for tumour cells with constitutive activation of the wnt signalling pathway. *Gene Ther.* **9,** 270–281.

37. Tsukuda, K., Wiewrodt, R., Molnar-Kimber, K., Jovanovic, V. P., and Amin, K. M. (2002) An E2F-responsive replication-selective adenovirus targeted to the defective cell cycle in cancer cells: potent antitumoral efficacy but no toxicity to normal cell. *Cancer Res.* **62,** 3438–3447.

38. Johnson, L., Shen, A., Boyle, L., et al. (2002) Selectively replicating adenoviruses targeting deregulated E2F activity are potent, systemic antitumor agents. *Cancer Cell* **1,** 325–337.

39. Savontaus, M. J., Sauter, B. V., Huang, T. G., and Woo, S. L. (2002) Transcriptional targeting of conditionally replicating adenovirus to dividing endothelial cells. *Gene Ther.* **9,** 972–979.

40. Ramachandra, M., Rahman, A., Zou, A., et al. (2001) Re-engineering adenovirus regulatory pathways to enhance oncolytic specificity and efficacy. *Nat. Biotechnol.* **19,** 1035–1041.

41. Antelman, D., Gregory, R. J., and Wills, K. N. (2000) Retinoblastoma fusion polypeptides. In *US Patent and Trademark Office*. Canji, San Diego, CA, patent number 6,074,850.

42. White, E., Faha, B., and Stillman, B. (1986) Regulation of adenovirus gene expression in human WI38 cells by an E1B-encoded tumor antigen. *Mol. Cell. Biol.* **6,** 3763–3773.

43. Tollefson, A. E., Ryerse, J. S., Scaria, A., Hermiston, T. W., and Wold, W. S. (1996) The E3-11.6-kDa adenovirus death protein (ADP) is required for efficient cell death: characterization of cells infected with adp mutants. *Virology* **220,** 152–162.

44. Tollefson, A. E., Scaria, A., Hermiston, T. W., Ryerse, J. S., Wold, L. J., and Wold, W. S. (1996) The adenovirus death protein (E3-11.6K) is required at very late stages of infection for efficient cell lysis and release of adenovirus from infected cells. *J. Virol.* **70,** 2296–2306.

45. Lavoie, J. N., Nguyen, M., Marcellus, R. C., Branton, P. E., and Shore, G. C. (1998) E4orf4, a novel adenovirus death factor that induces p53-independent apoptosis by a pathway that is not inhibited by zVAD-fmk. *J. Cell Biol.* **140,** 637–645.

46. Marcellus, R. C., Chan, H., Paquette, D., Thirlwell, S., Boivin, D., and Branton, P. E. (2000) Induction of p53-independent apoptosis by the adenovirus E4orf4 protein requires binding to the Balpha subunit of protein phosphatase 2A. *J. Virol.* **74,** 7869–7877.

47. Marcellus, R. C., Lavoie, J. N., Boivin, D., Shore, G. C., Ketner, G., and Branton, P. E. (1998) The early region 4 orf4 protein of human adenovirus type 5 induces p53-independent cell death by apoptosis. *J. Virol.* **72,** 7144–7153.

48. Duque, P. M., Alonoso, C., Sanchez-Prieto, R., et al. (1999) Adenovirus lacking the 19-kDa and 55-kDa E1B genes exerts a marked cytotoxic effect in human malignant cells. *Cancer Gene Ther.* **6,** 554–563.

49. Harrison, D., Sauthoff, H., Heitner, S., Jagirdar, J., Rom, W. N., and Hay, J. G. (2001) Wild-type adenovirus decreases tumor xenograft growth, but despite viral persistence complete tumor responses are rarely achieved—deletion of the viral E1b-19-kD gene increases the viral oncolytic effect. *Hum. Gene Ther.* **12,** 1323–1332.

50. Sauthoff, H., Heitner, S., Rom, W. N., and Hay, J. G. (2000) Deletion of the adenoviral E1b-19kD gene enhances tumor cell killing of a replicating adenoviral vector. *Hum. Gene Ther.* **11,** 379–388.

51. Tollefson, A. E., Scaria, A., Saha, S. K., and Wold, W. S. (1992) The 11,600-MW protein encoded by region E3 of adenovirus is expressed early but is greatly amplified at late stages of infection. *J. Virol.* **66,** 3633–3642.

52. You, L., Yang, C. T., and Jablons, D. M. (2000) ONYX-015 works synergistically with chemotherapy in lung cancer cell lines and primary cultures freshly made from lung cancer patients. *Cancer Res.* **60,** 1009–1013.

53. Li, Y., Yu, D. C., Chen, Y., et al. (2001) A hepatocellular carcinoma-specific adenovirus variant, CV890, eliminates distant human liver tumors in combination with doxorubicin. *Cancer Res.* **61,** 6428–6436.

54. Yu, D. C., Chen, Y., Dilley, J., et al. (2001) Antitumor synergy of CV787, a prostate cancer-specific adenovirus, and paclitaxel and docetaxel. *Cancer Res.* **61,** 517–525.
55. Zhou, Z., Jia, S. F., Hung, M. C., and Kleinerman, E. S. (2001) E1A sensitizes HER2/neu-overexpressing Ewing's sarcoma cells to topoisomerase II-targeting anticancer drugs. *Cancer Res.* **61,** 3394–3398.
56. Ueno, N. T., Yu, D., and Hung, M. C. (1997) Chemosensitization of HER-2/neu-overexpressing human breast cancer cells to paclitaxel (Taxol) by adenovirus type 5 E1A. *Oncogene* **15,** 953–960.
57. Sanchez-Prieto, R., Quintanilla, M., Cano, A., et al. (1996) Carcinoma cell lines become sensitive to DNA-damaging agents by the expression of the adenovirus E1A gene. *Oncogene* **13,** 1083–1092.
58. Samuelson, A. V. and Lowe, S. W. (1997) Selective induction of p53 and chemosensitivity in RB-deficient cells by E1A mutants unable to bind the RB-related proteins. *Proc. Natl. Acad. Sci. USA* **94,** 12,094–12,099.
59. Lowe, S. W., Ruley, H. E., Jacks, T., and Housman, D. E. (1993) p53-dependent apoptosis modulates the cytotoxicity of anticancer agents. *Cell* **74,** 957–967.
60. James, M. C. and Peters, G. (2000) Alternative product of the p16/CKDN2A locus connects the Rb and p53 tumor suppressors. *Prog. Cell Cycle Res.* **4,** 71–81.
61. Krosnick, J. A., Mule, J. J., McIntosh, J. K., and Rosenberg, S. A. (1989) Augmentation of antitumor efficacy by the combination of recombinant tumor necrosis factor and chemotherapeutic agents in vivo. *Cancer Res.* **49,** 3729–3233.
62. Metcalf, J. P. (1996) Adenovirus E1A 13S gene product upregulates tumor necrosis factor gene. *Am. J. Physiol.* **270,** L535–L540.
63. Rhoades, K. L., Golub, S. H., and Economou, J. S. (1996) The adenoviral transcription factor, E1A 13S, transactivates the human tumor necrosis factor-alpha promoter. *Virus Res.* **40,** 65–74.
64. Lieber, A., He, C. Y., Meuse, L., et al. (1997) The role of Kupffer cell activation and viral gene expression in early liver toxicity after infusion of recombinant adenovirus vectors. *J. Virol.* **71,** 8798–8807.
65. Nielsen, L. L., Lipari, P., Dell, J., Gurnani, M., and Hajian, G. (1998) Adenovirus-mediated p53 gene therapy and paclitaxel have synergistic efficacy in models of human head and neck, ovarian, prostate, and breast cancer. *Clin. Cancer Res.* **4,** 835–846.
66. Bernt, K. M., Steinwaerder, D. S., Ni, S., Li, Z. Y., Roffler, S. R., and Lieber, A. (2002) Enzyme-activated prodrug therapy enhances tumor-specific replication of adenovirus vectors. *Cancer Res.* **62,** 6089–6098.
67. Rogulski, K. R., Freytag, S. O., Zhang, K., et al. (2000) In vivo antitumor activity of ONYX-015 is influenced by p53 status and is augmented by radiotherapy. *Cancer Res.* **60,** 1193–1196.
68. Chen, Y., DeWeese, T., Dilley, J., et al. (2001) CV706, a prostate cancer-specific adenovirus variant, in combination with radiotherapy produces synergistic antitumor efficacy without increasing toxicity. *Cancer Res.* **61,** 5453–5460.
69. Lamfers, M. L., Grill, J., Dirven, C. M., et al. (2002) Potential of the conditionally replicative adenovirus Ad5-Delta24RGD in the treatment of malignant gliomas and its enhanced effect with radiotherapy. *Cancer Res.* **62,** 5736–5742.
70. Hawkins, L. K. and Hermiston, T. (2001) Gene delivery from the E3 region of replicating human adenovirus: evaluation of the E3B region. *Gene Ther.* **8,** 1142–1148.
71. Hawkins, L. K. and Hermiston, T. W. (2001) Gene delivery from the E3 region of replicating human adenovirus: evaluation of the ADP region. *Gene Ther.* **8,** 1132–1141.
72. Sauthoff, H., Pipiya, T., Heitner, S., et al. (2002) Late expression of p53 from a replicating adenovirus improves tumor cell killing and is more tumor cell specific than expression of the adenoviral death protein. *Hum. Gene Ther.* **13,** 1859–1871.
73. van Beusechem, V. W., van den Doel, P. B., Grill, J., Pinedo, H. M., and Gerritsen, W. R. (2002) Conditionally replicative adenovirus expressing p53 exhibits enhanced oncolytic potency. *Cancer Res.* **62,** 6165–6171.
74. Zhang, J. F., Hu, C., Geng, Y., et al. (1996) Treatment of a human breast cancer xenograft with an adenovirus vector containing an interferon gene results in rapid regression due to viral oncolysis and gene therapy. *Proc. Natl. Acad. Sci. USA* **93,** 4513–4518.
75. Freytag, S. O., Rogulski, K. R., Paielli, D. L., Gilbert, J. D., and Kim, J. H. (1998) A novel three-pronged approach to kill cancer cells selectively: concomitant viral, double suicide gene, and radiotherapy. *Hum. Gene Ther.* **9,** 1323–1333.
76. Wildner, O., Blaese, R. M., and Morris, J. C. (1999) Therapy of colon cancer with oncolytic adenovirus is enhanced by the addition of herpes simplex virus-thymidine kinase. *Cancer Res.* **59,** 410–413.
77. Wildner, O., Morris, J. C., Vahanian, N. N., Ford, H. Jr., Ramsey, W. J., and Blaese, R. M. (1999) Adenoviral vectors capable of replication improve the efficacy of HSVtk/GCV suicide gene therapy of cancer. *Gene Ther.* **6,** 57–62.
78. Lambright, E. S., Amin, K., Wiewrodt, R., et al. (2001) Inclusion of the herpes simplex thymidine kinase gene in a replicating adenovirus does not augment antitumor efficacy. *Gene Ther.* **8,** 946–953.
79. Nemunaitis, J., Cunningham, C., Buchanan, A., et al. (2001) Intravenous infusion of a replication-selective adenovirus (ONYX-015) in cancer patients: safety, feasibility and biological activity. *Gene Ther.* **8,** 746–759.
80. Freytag, S. O., Khil, M., Stricker, H., et al. (2002) Phase I study of replication-competent adenovirus-mediated double suicide gene therapy for the treatment of locally recurrent prostate cancer. *Cancer Res.* **62,** 4968–4976.

81. Kirn, D. (2001) Clinical research results with dl1520 (ONYX-015), a replication-selective adenovirus for the treatment of cancer: what have we learned? *Gene Ther.* **8**, 89–98.

82. Pazdur, R. (2000) Response rates, survival, and chemotherapy trials. *J. Natl. Cancer Inst.* **92**, 1552–1553.

83. Ganly, I., Kirn, D., Eckhardt, S. G., et al. (2000) A phase I study of ONYX-015, an E1B attenuated adenovirus, administered intratumorally to patients with recurrent head and neck cancer. *Clin. Cancer Res.* **6**, 798–806.

84. Nemunaitis, J., Ganly, I., Khuri, F., et al. (2000) Selective replication and oncolysis in p53 mutant tumors with ONYX-015, an E1B-55kD gene-deleted adenovirus, in patients with advanced head and neck cancer: a phase II trial. *Cancer Res.* **60**, 6359–6366.

85. Mulvihill, S., Warren, R., Venook, A., et al. (2001) Safety and feasibility of injection with an E1B-55 kDa gene-deleted, replication-selective adenovirus (ONYX-015) into primary carcinomas of the pancreas: a phase I trial. *Gene Ther.* **8**, 308–315.

86. Habib, N., Salama, H., Abd El Latif Abu Median, A., et al. (2002) Clinical trial of E1B-deleted adenovirus (dl1520) gene therapy for hepatocellular carcinoma. *Cancer Gene Ther.* **9**, 254–259.

87. Vasey, P. A., Shulman, L. N., Campos, S., et al. (2002) Phase I trial of intraperitoneal injection of the E1B-55-kd-gene-deleted adenovirus ONYX-015 (dl1520) given on days 1 through 5 every 3 weeks in patients with recurrent/refractory epithelial ovarian cancer. *J. Clin. Oncol.* **20**, 1562–1569.

88. Reid, T., Galanis, E., Abbruzzese, J., et al. (2001) Intra-arterial administration of a replication-selective adenovirus (dl1520) in patients with colorectal carcinoma metastatic to the liver: a phase I trial. *Gene Ther.* **8**, 1618–1626.

89. Reid, T., Galanis, E., Abbruzzese, J., et al. (2002) Hepatic arterial infusion of a replication-selective oncolytic adenovirus (dl1520): phase II viral, immunologic, and clinical endpoints. *Cancer Res.* **62**, 6070–6079.

90. Wildner, O. and Morris, J. C. (2000) Therapy of peritoneal carcinomatosis from colon cancer with oncolytic adenoviruses. *J. Gene Med.* **2**, 353–360.

91. Kurihara, T., Brough, D. E., Kovesdi, I., and Kufe, D. W. (2000) Selectivity of a replication-competent adenovirus for human breast carcinoma cells expressing the MUC1 antigen. *J. Clin. Invest.* **106**, 763–771.

92. Lee, Y. J., Galoforo, S. S., Battle, P., Lee, H., Corry, P. M., and Jessup, J. M. (2001) Replicating adenoviral vector-mediated transfer of a heat-inducible double suicide gene for gene therapy. *Cancer Gene Ther.* **8**, 397–404.

93. Yu, D. C., Sakamoto, G. T., and Henderson, D. R. (1999) Identification of the transcriptional regulatory sequences of human kallikrein 2 and their use in the construction of calydon virus 764, an attenuated replication competent adenovirus for prostate cancer therapy. *Cancer Res.* **59**, 1498–1504.

94. Matsubara, S., Wada, Y., Gardner, T. A., et al. (2001) A conditional replication-competent adenoviral vector, Ad-OC-E1a, to cotarget prostate cancer and bone stroma in an experimental model of androgen-independent prostate cancer bone metastasis. *Cancer Res.* **61**, 6012–6019.

95. Alemany, R., Lai, S., Lou, Y. C., Jan, H. Y., Fang, X., and Zhang, W. W. (1999) Complementary adenoviral vectors for oncolysis. *Cancer Gene Ther.* **6**, 21–25.

96. Adachi, Y., Reynolds, P. N., Yamamoto, M., et al. (2001) A midkine promoter-based conditionally replicative adenovirus for treatment of pediatric solid tumors and bone marrow tumor purging. *Cancer Res.* **61**, 7882–7888.

97. Hernandez-Alcoceba, R., Pihalja, M., Qian, D., and Clarke, M. F. (2002) New oncolytic adenoviruses with hypoxia- and estrogen receptor-regulated replication. *Hum. Gene Ther.* **13**, 1737–1750.

98. Zhang, L., Akbulut, H., Tang, Y., et al. (2002) Adenoviral vectors with E1A regulated by tumor-specific promoters are selectively cytolytic for breast cancer and melanoma. *Mol. Ther.* **6**, 386–393.

99. Nettelbeck, D. M., Rivera, A. A., Balague, C., Alemany, R., and Curiel, D. T. (2002) Novel oncolytic adenoviruses targeted to melanoma: specific viral replication and cytolysis by expression of E1A mutants from the tyrosinase enhancer/promoter. *Cancer Res.* **62**, 4663–4670.

100. Zhang, J., Ramesh, N., Chen, Y., et al. (2002) Identification of human uroplakin II promoter and its use in the construction of CG8840, a urothelium-specific adenovirus variant that eliminates established bladder tumors in combination with docetaxel. *Cancer Res.* **62**, 3743–3750.

101. Howe, J. A., Mymryk, J. S., Egan, C., Branton, P. E., and Bayley, S. T. (1990) Retinoblastoma growth suppressor and a 300-kDa protein appear to regulate cellular DNA synthesis. *Proc. Natl. Acad. Sci. USA* **87**, 5883–5887.

102. Lill, N. L., Grossman, S. R., Ginsberg, D., DeCaprio, J., and Livingston, D. M. (1997) Binding and modulation of p53 by p300/CBP coactivators. *Nature* **387**, 823–827.

15

Conditionally Replicating
Adenoviruses for Cancer Treatment

Ramon Alemany

1. INTRODUCTION

Adenovirus is characterized by an icosahedral protein capsid 80 nm in diameter; it packages a 36-kb linear double-stranded deoxyribonucleic acid (DNA). A fiber protein projects from the 12 vertices of the capsid to interact with the cellular receptor. Among the more than 50 different types of human adenoviruses, type 5 has been mainly used to study the molecular biology of adenoviruses. This virus infects mainly epithelial cells (origin of most tumors) and causes a mild pathology with flulike symptoms. On infection, the DNA reaches the nucleus and is efficiently transcribed without insertion in the host genome.

These traits placed adenovirus at the front line of different gene vehicles used since the inception of cancer gene therapy. After more than a decade, efficient gene expression has not been enough to offer a new cancer therapy. Cancer gene therapy requires every tumor cell to be affected directly or indirectly by the therapeutic effect of the transduced gene. However, the poor penetration of adenovirus-size particles throughout a solid tumor mass has hampered this requisite.

A different and much older therapeutic approach against cancer that uses adenovirus is virotherapy. Replication-competent viruses with preferential replication in cancer cells represent antitumoral agents that can multiply and disseminate through the tumor mass and thus compensate the main limitation found with nonreplicative adenoviral vectors.

Some viruses, such as Newcastle disease virus, vesicular stomatitis virus, parvovirus, or reovirus, show a natural tropism for transformed cells compared to normal cells because of their sensitivity to interferons (IFNs) or their dependence on an active cell cycle or signal transduction pathway. Others, such herpes simplex virus or adenovirus, can be genetically modified to acquire conditional replication. The transcriptional control of key viral genes using promoters active in tumor cells or the deletion of viral functions that are dispensable in tumor cells are two strategies in this direction.

The combination of gene therapy and virotherapy using replicating adenoviruses that carry exogenous genes to enhance their antitumoral activity is emerging as a potent strategy to attack tumors selectively. Furthermore, to treat disseminated tumors, adenovirus should be injected systemically, targeted to the tumor, and untargeted from hepatocytes and Kupffer cells. This chapter reviews the work done with conditionally replicating adenoviruses (CRAds) and their use as vectors in the emerging field of cancer gene virotherapy.

2. TRANSCRIPTIONAL CONTROL OF EARLY VIRAL GENES

E1a is the first viral gene to be transcribed when the viral genome reaches the cell nucleus. Although viral proteins can regulate this transcription, it relies initially only in cellular factors present in most

From: *Contemporary Cancer Research*
Cancer Gene Therapy
Edited by: D. T. Curiel and J. T. Douglas © Humana Press Inc., Totowa, NJ

cells. Transcriptions of the rest of early viral genes mostly depend on *E1a*; here, the importance is to regulate *E1a* to achieve conditional replication. However, the regions that stimulate E1a transcription cannot be easily removed to construct a CRAd.

Several regulatory regions that control *E1a* transcription can be distinguished: the proximal promoter, enhancers, and elements in the coding region *(1)*. The proximal promoter contains a TATA box at nucleotide 468 of Ad5, 31 nucleotides upstream of the *E1a* cap site (nucleotide 499, numbering from GenBank M73260), that binds to TFIID (transcription complex formed by the TATA-binding protein (TBP) and several associated proteins). A TGACGT sequence at nucleotide 456 binds to ATF (activating transcription factor). Then, further upstream, at nucleotide 296, an enhancer (element I) that regulates *E1a* transcription is found, and it is repeated at nucleotide 229 and 199. Between this repeated enhancer I are found inverted repeats of enhancer element II, from nucleotides 248 to 282, that stimulate transcription of all early viral genes. Removal of these enhancer elements I and II reduces E1A expression 20-fold. Transcription factors that bind to the core sequence of the enhancer element I were named EF1-A and E1A-F. An OCT-1-binding site at nucleotide 300 and an ATF-binding 24-bp enhancer element at nucleotide 153 can also activate E1a expression in infected cells.

In the E1a enhancer region, there are also two binding sites for E2F (nucleotides 215 and 279). Although their deletion does not seem to affect E1a expression, they may be useful in CRAd strategies targeted to E2 repression via E2F binding. In addition, the inverted terminal repeat (ITR) also has ATF-binding sites (TGACGT) and SP1-binding sites (GC-rich GGGTGG), both with E1a transcriptional activity. Thus, the ITR can initiate transcription when placed next to the E1a TATA box or even linked to a gene without promoter *(2)*.

To control E1a expression, the tumor-selective promoter is usually inserted between the E1a cap site (nucleotide 499) and the first E1a codon (nucleotide 559) (using either a convenient Age I at the nucleotide 522 site or polymerase chain reaction). Because Enhancer I and II overlap with the A repeats that form the packaging signal of adenovirus and the ATF- and the Sp1-binding sites of the ITR overlap with the origin of viral DNA replication, these cannot be removed and remain upstream of the inserted promoter. Another transcriptional stimulation supplied in *cis* to E1a that is difficult to avoid is found in the E1a-coding sequence itself at nucleotide 900 *(3)*.

How these elements affect the tumor- or tissue-selective promoter is a case-by-case issue. It is expected that promoters regulated by transcriptional repression in normal cells (presence of silencers on the inserted promoter) would behave better than promoters with selectivity conferred solely by enhancers because they can inhibit enhancer activity.

Several promoters have been used to control E1A expression. Comparison of these studies could help elucidate the traits that maintain proper regulation in the viral genome. Since the studies of Hitt and Graham *(4)*, it is accepted that the levels of E1A do not correlate with virus production, and that low E1A levels are enough to engage other viral early promoters. If this were the case, it would be expected that different promoters do not result as much in different viral yields in permissive cells as in different defectiveness in nonpermissive cells. This also means that, in contrast to other strategies that use adenoviral vectors with tumor-selective promoters to drive therapeutic genes, promoter strength is not as critical for CRAds.

Most studies use tumor cell lines that do not express the selective promoter as nonpermissive cells. Less often, normal cells such as bronchial human epithelial cells or hepatocytes are used. Although it is true that the normal cell that would receive the virus differs when the virus is injected local-regionally, in any case, and especially for intravascular delivery, the hepatocyte is a critical common target that could be used for standardization. The level of basal or leaky activity of the endogenous promoter in the nonpermissive cell has been studied using different techniques (e.g., Northern blotting, reverse transcriptase polymerase chain reaction) and that of the plasmid-isolated promoter using CAT or luciferase reporter assays.

Cells in which the activity of the cloned promoter is as low as the basic plasmid without promoter are useful to discover interference from the viral genome. Some information of selectivity, however, can be inferred as a comparison to the production of wild-type adenovirus. CN706 with prostate-specific antigen promoter/enhancer driving E1A (PSE-E1A) and CV763 with kallikrein enhancer/promoter driving E1A (hK2-E1A) are restricted 2 to 3 logs. E1A under the α-fetoprotein promoter restricted replication by 4 logs in α-fetoprotein-negative cells *(5)* and under the MUC1 promoter by 5 to 6 logs in Muc1 negative cells *(6)*. The presence of silencers in these promoters may be one reason for such differences.

The E2F promoter has also been used to restrict E1A expression *(7)*. An advantage of this promoter is that the CRAd should replicate in all tumor cells because the disregulation of the pRB pathway is the most common trait of cancer. In normal quiescent cells, the complex formed between RB and E2F1 represses E2F1promoter, and E2F1 levels become undetectable *(8)*. The replication of a virus with E1A under the control of E2F1 promoter, however, is not completely abrogated in normal resting cells (from 2 to 4 logs of attenuation) *(7)*. In infected normal lung fibroblasts, E1A can be detected even in the absence of endogenous E2F-1, which indicates that the E2F1 promoter is not tightly regulated in the viral context.

Loose promoter control in the viral context has also been detected in a CRAd with E1A under the midkine promoter *(9)*. In this study, an E1A under a stronger promoter (cytomegalovirus) gave viral yields higher than under the midkine or even the natural E1A promoters, challenging the concept that high E1A levels do not increase virus production.

To increase the specificity of replication, other early genes can also be considered targets for regulation with tumor-selective promoters. In fact, several CRAds have been designed to control E1a and E1B, E2, or E4 expression *(10,11)*. E1-deleted vectors express low levels of early proteins that are recognized by the immune system, revealing that early transcription units have E1A-independent expression. The E1B promoter is a simple promoter formed by a GC box (SP1-binding site) at nucleotide 1654 and TATA box at nucleotide 1670. Four enhancers near the E1A stop codon have been described. There is a basal activity in the absence of E1A expression that, added to the fact that E1B-19K can activate E1A, E2, E3, and E4 promoters and E1B-55K can activate the E2 late promoter, it could diminish CRAd selectivity. E4 expression is not as E1A independent as E1B because it needs to be activated by E1A-13S through ATF-2 and p50E4F factors. P50E4F is the proteolytic product of p120E4F, which in turn is a repressor of E4 and is inactivated by E1a by phosphorylation *(12)*. However, the E2-transcriptional activity of E4-ORF6/7 is more important than that of E1B19K, and if expressed at high levels, it can produce E1A-independent replication *(13)*.

E4 promoter has been replaced with surfactant protein B promoter to confer further selectivity to a CRAd (named KD1-SPB) that contains a first level of selectivity by means of E1A deletions *(see* Section 3.) *(14)*. The E4 promoter replacement in KD1-SPB attenuated viral production by 4 logs compared to KD1 in tumor cells that do not express SPB. Such a high level of attenuation could be related to the fact that, placed between the E4 and the right ITR, the inserted promoter is not affected by the enhancer element I of E1A promoter, although interference from the ITR still remains. Leaky replication occurred, as revealed by a single-step growth curve assay showing that the titer of virus in the supernatant of infected cells increased with time. With this in mind, it would be interesting to quantify the attenuation of this virus in normal cells in which the 4 logs of attenuation gained with E4 control are combined with the 3 logs of attenuation gained with E1A deletions *(see* Section 3.).

E2 has also been target of transcriptional control. It has two promoters, one that controls early transcription formed mainly by E2F- and ATF-binding sites and highly dependent on E1A transactivation and another one that controls late transcription formed by Sp1-binding sites and CCAAT boxes and repressed by E1A but activated by E1B-55K *(15)*. E2 is an attractive candidate for regulation because E2 products are components of the viral DNA replication system, not proteins that regulate other early genes or the cell status, and hence cannot be bypassed by other early viral genes or cellular functions.

E2F- and ATF-binding sites in E2 early promoter have been replaced with Tcf sites that drive transcription when the wnt signaling pathway is active, such as in colon cancer *(16)*. E2 control by Tcf reduced replication 2 logs in nonpermissive cells. Interestingly, to achieve this selectivity, the adjacent E3 enhancer had to be mutated.

A different strategy did not rely on changing E2 early and E3 promoters, but on the production of an E2F-binding domain fused to an Rb-repressor domain *(10)*. This repressor was placed under a p53-responsive promoter in E3 to achieve p53-dependent repression in normal cells. In tumor cells, even in those with wild-type p53 activity, the virus replicated efficiently, probably to the high level of free E2F competing with the repressor for the E2F-binding sites. This strategy resulted also in an attenuation of 2 logs in normal cells.

So far the regulation of E2 has allowed normal levels of replication in permissive cells, but the attenuation achieved has been lower than with E1A or E4 control. The control of E2 late promoter may be necessary; in that case, the combination of E1B and E2 early regulation could increase attenuation.

Several factors need to be taken into consideration to study the benefit of multiple regulation. Different cell lines or cell types allow different levels of E1A-independent expression of early viral genes. For example, HeLa cells allow E1A-independent expression at high multiplicity of infection (MOI). The status of differentiation of the cell is also a key factor that affects early gene expression. For example, the F9 teratocarcinoma cells allow E1A-independent expression when undifferentiated.

Selectivity should be compared at low and high MOI as E1A-deleted mutants can express viral genes and replicate when used at high MOI. The concerted regulation of early units along the viral life cycle will be also more affected in multiple-unit regulated CRAds, and it could affect viral production and oncolytic potency.

Finally, the use of the same promoter elements to control several units is very prone to cause viral DNA rearrangements, and viral DNA stability should be monitored *(17)*. Attenuation of multiple-unit regulated CRAds in nonpermissive cells is very pronounced, although the benefit of multiple regulation is sometimes not known because comparisons to their single-unit counterparts is missing. CV787 with probasin-E1A and PSE-E1B is restricted 5 logs *(18)*. CV876 and CG8840, both with uroplakin II promoter driving E1a and E1b connected through an internal ribosome entry site, are restricted 4 logs *(19)*.

Some studies have tried to quantify the benefit of multiple-unit regulation. Compared to a virus with E1A promoter, CV764 with PSE-E1A and hK2-E1B was restricted 5 logs, but viruses with either of these promoters just regulating E1A were restricted 3 logs *(20)*. Therefore, E1A-E1B double regulation added 100 times the selectivity in this case. In contrast, E1B placed under Tcf sites did not add any selectivity beyond the simple regulation of E2 by these sites, despite the fact that E1B expression was reduced *(16)*. The effects of promoter control could be evident only with particular combinations of early regions.

Despite the high levels of selectivity achieved in some cases (4–5 logs), an emerging problem recognized for several promoters inserted in the viral genome is the loss of proper regulation. This problem was noted when tyrosine kinase was placed under the ErbB2 promoter in an E1-deleted adenoviral vector *(21)*. Flanking the expression cassette with bovine growth hormone transcription stop signals restored promoter selectivity. Another promoter that loses selectivity in the adenoviral genome is the myosin promoter *(22)*. As in previous reports, a transcriptional start site was identified within the E1A enhancer. In this case, however, a transcriptional terminator could not restore promoter specificity.

A different approach that restored promoter fidelity in E1-deleted vectors has been the use of insulators to flank the expression cassette. Insulators are DNA sequences that flank genomic domains transcribed independently from their surroundings. Among different functions, these elements dock enhancer-blocking proteins such as CTCF that, in contrast to transcription terminators, can block *cis*-activation by distant enhancers. The HS4 insulator that flanks the chicken β-globin locus is active in a heterologous context, and it has been used to produce transgenic animals. HS4 can shield a metal-inducible promoter from the effects of adenoviral enhancers present in E1-deleted vectors *(23)*. Optimal shielding reduced noninduced expression 200-fold in vitro and 15-fold in vivo and required one copy of the 1.2-kb insulator in 5' to 3' orientation at each side of the expression cassette. Because of size constraints, their application to CRAds will require an artificial insulator formed by two repeats of the 250-bp active core of HS4.

Finally, it is probable that the combination of insulators to avoid the effects of enhancers and terminators to avoid "read-through" transcription from the ITR-packaging signal will be needed. Long insulators or long promoters could solve the fidelity problem, but the capacity for exogenous DNA of CRAds is limited to a few kilobases. Splitting the genome of the CRAd in two mutually dependent viruses has been used as an approach to insert large promoters and exogenous DNA, but these dual systems have lower virus yield and spread slowly as they depend on coinfection *(24)*.

Other transcriptional or translational regulatory elements with tissue- or tumor-selective properties can be attached to viral genes to construct a CRAd. Splicing signals or messenger ribonucleic acid (mRNA) stabilization elements are good examples. For example, a CRAd with E1A linked to the 3' untranslated region of COX-2 is highly attenuated in non-Ras transformed cell lines because this region is selectively stabilized by Ras (R. Vile, personal communication).

3. EXPLOITING THE FUNCTIONAL SIMILARITIES OF ADENOVIRUS AND CANCER

Several adenoviral proteins have functions that interfere with cell signaling pathways, activate cell proliferation, and inhibit apoptosis in a similar way as occurs in tumor cells. Therefore, a normal cell, when infected with adenovirus, resembles a tumor cell in various aspects. The viral functions that bring the cell to this tumorlike phenotype are recognized as oncogenic traits of adenoviruses. The overlap is not complete, however, because adenovirus also has functions that induce an epithelial-like phenotype to the infected cell, and these are recognized as antitumoral traits *(25,26)*. These functions combined lie behind the preference of adenovirus for activated epithelial cells.

The overlap between adenoviral functions and oncogenesis can be used to achieve selective replication of adenoviruses in tumors. In fact, the first selective adenovirus proposed and tested relies on the analogy of p53 inactivation produced by the adenovirus E1B-55K protein and by the tumor cell *(27)*.

When adenovirus genome reaches the nucleus of the infected cell, its DNA remains anchored to centers of active transcription in which the expression of the first viral genes starts (Fig. 1). E1A 243R (12S) and 289R (13S) are the first proteins synthesized. E1a contains three domains, CR1 to CR3, conserved among serotypes. CR3 is present only in the 289R protein, and it is a transcriptional activator domain that binds to the TBP and ATF. Also, p53 binds to TBP, acting as a transcriptional repressor, and it is displaced by CR3.

For CRAd design, CR1, CR2, and the nonconserved amino-terminal domain of E1A are more attractive because they are involved in the activation of the cell cycle and are the domains that confer transformation properties to E1A of certain serotypes in rodent cells. CR1 and CR2 are essential for E1A to bind pRB, p130, and p107 family protein members. Binding of pRB dissociates the E2F-pRB complex that functions as a transcriptional repressor recruiting histone deacetylase. At the same time, free E2F is a transcriptional activator of viral genes and cellular genes involved in the control of the cell cycle (e.g., cdk2; cdk4; cyclins a, D, and E) or DNA synthesis (e.g., PCNA, DNA polymerase, ribocucleotide reductase). E1A binds to p300 by its amino-terminal domain and the C-terminal half of CR1. This binding increases the ability of p300 to stimulate EF2 transcriptional activity. E1A thus removes the E2F inhibitor (pRB) and stimulates the E2F activator (p300) with the same final outcome. Either p300 or Rb binding is enough to induce cellular DNA synthesis, but binding to both is necessary to pass G2/M.

Several CRAds have been constructed based on deletions of E1A. A single CR2 deletion (residues 122–129: LTCHEAGF) that affects binding to pRB and the pRB-related proteins p130 and p107 has been shown to confer selectivity for tumor cells *(28)*. This CR2 deletion was able to attenuate viral

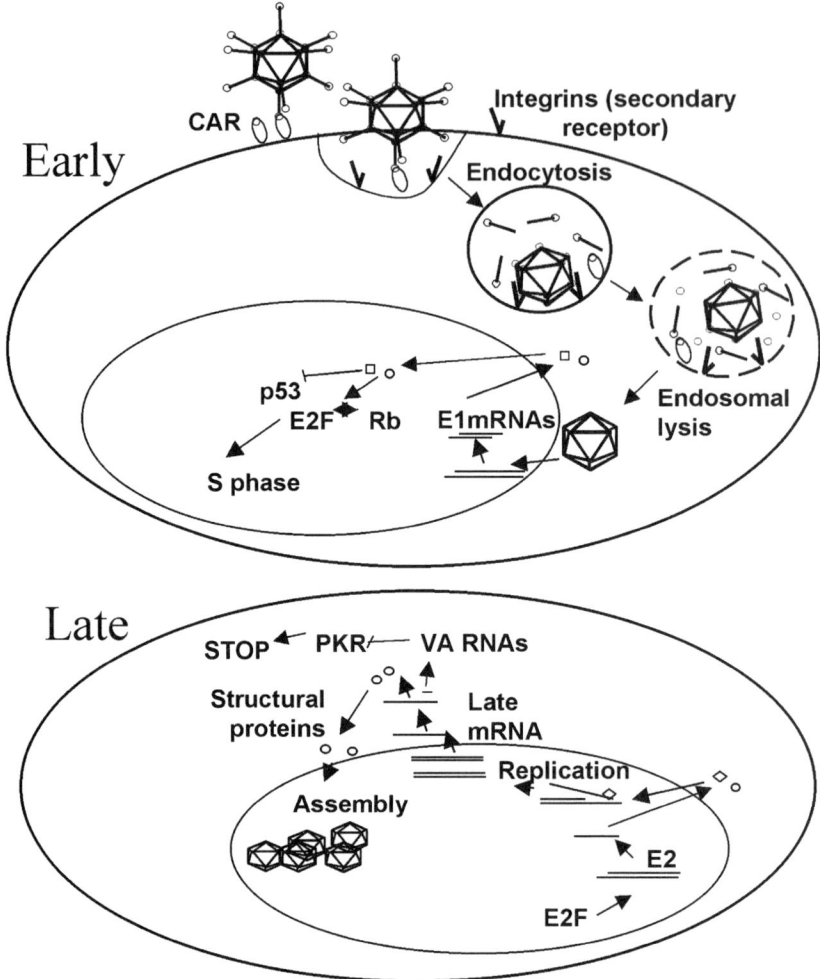

Fig. 1. Adenovirus infection cycle and its similarity to cancer. The functional analogy of E1A with pRB, E1B-55K with p53, and VA-RNAs with Ras has been used to achieve conditional replication.

production in normal fibroblasts grown at low serum concentration to arrest them in G1. When a similar G1 arrest was induced in tumor cells by Rb gene transfer, the CR2 mutant (AdΔ24) was also unable to replicate. Further studies with an adenovirus with the same CR2 mutation (dl922–947) have confirmed that this mutant cannot induce S phase and demonstrated its selectivity in terms of viral yields.

Comparing the mutant adenovirus yield in several tumor cell lines vs airway epithelial and microvascular endothelial normal cells (defined as the therapeutic index), a reduction of 2 logs is observed when the normal cells are proliferating and 4 logs when they are arrested. Compared to that of wild type, dl922–947 yield is attenuated 3 logs in the arrested normal cells *(29)*. Thus, 3 of the 4 logs of the therapeutic index (difference between tumor and normal) are because of selectivity conferred by the mutation. Some cytopathic effects, however, could be observed in normal arrested cells. The p300-binding ablation could be a possibility to reduce toxicity in normal cells. However, dl1101, a mutant with a deletion in the p300-binding CR1 region (amino acids 4–25) showed similar toxicity in normal cells and an undesired attenuation in tumor cells *(29)*. Independent studies with dl1101 also suggested some attenuation in tumor and normal cells. Nevertheless, this CR1 mutation may have value to increase the selectivity of certain CR2 mutants *(30)*. For example, dl01/07, a CRAd with this CR1 deletion combined with a CR2 deletion that only affects pRB binding (residues 111–123), is selective for tumor cells, as opposed to viruses that contain either mutation. Most interestingly, this double-ablated E1A is attenuated 1 log in proliferating normal lung fibroblasts. Other efforts using dl01/07 as the basis for further CRAd development showed the same 1-log attenuation compared to wild type in proliferating lung fibroblasts and an additional 2 logs on arrest *(31)*. Based on comparisons with wild type, pRb-binding deletion combined with p300-binding deletion therefore renders the same attenuation levels as the pRB plus p130–p107 deletions. However, the p300-pRb combination is more restricting in proliferating normal cells. This is in accord with the observation that the double p300-pRb-binding deletion mutant E1a has more limited effects on the cell cycle compared to single mutants *(32)*. Furthermore, in organotypic cultures of primary human keratinocytes representing a good model of normal human epithelial cells permissive to adenovirus, the combined CR1 and CR2 deletion that abrogates p300, p107, and pRB binding is necessary to restrict replication *(33)*.

E1B is also an important target for CRAd design. In the early viral phase, E1B-55K forms a complex with E4orf6 and p53 that leads to the ubiquitin-mediated proteolysis of p53. This would favor viral replication, allowing the infected cell to remain in S phase, but the dependence of viral replication on p53 status is not clear. During the late phase, E1B-55K forms a different complex with E4orf6 that shuts off host mRNA nuclear export and host protein synthesis. It also facilitates the nuclear localization of transcription factor YB1 to activate the E2 late promoter *(15)*. Tumor cells often have inactivated p53, counteract protein shutoff and contain nuclear YB1. Defects of 55K are then complemented accordingly. In general, however, the replication efficiency of 55K mutant seldom reaches the level of E1A mutants *(29,30)*. The use of 55K mutants that separate these multiple functions is under way, and it will help to obtain mutants not attenuated in tumor cells and to clarify correlation of viral selectivity and specific cellular traits such as p53 inactivation *(34)*.

E1B 19K is a homologue of Bcl-2 that inhibits the p53-independent apoptosis induced by E1A via the interaction of Bak and Bax *(35)*. In normal cells and in many tumor cell lines (e.g., HeLa), 19K mutants do not replicate because of the premature apoptotic death of the infected cell. In other tumor cells particularly resistant to apoptosis, the 19K function can be complemented. A virus with a complete E1B deletion could then replicate in certain cell lines or tumors (B-cell lymphoma caused by the overexpression of Bcl-2, melanoma caused by deficiency of caspase 9 coactivator Apaf-1, etc.). However, the replication of such viruses will be impaired at various degrees in most tumors *(35)*. On the other hand, it seems that the release of viral particles from the infected cell is not efficient, and apoptosis at this late stage could help viral spread (*see* Section 4.).

E4 is also a region with cell cycle regulatory functions and thus of CRAd design interest. It remains, however, quite unexplored regarding the role of mutations in cancer selectivity. E4orf6 is able to accelerate tumor growth in rat cells already transformed with E1A and E1B, and this correlates with a reduction in p53 levels *(36)*. E4orf6 binds to p53, but its effects on blocking p53-mediated transcriptional activation and repression are controversial *(12)*. E4orf6/7 binds to free E2F to promote its binding to the inverted repeats of E2F-binding sites present in the early E2 promoter and the cellular E2F-1 promoter. Most important, this binding has some capability to displace pRb and p107 from E2F complexes and thus to release free E2F that would activate the E2 promoter without the aid of E1A. Thus, if orf6/7 is produced at high levels (such as under a cytomegalovirus promoter in a viral vector), it can complement E1A. The deletion of orf6/7 is a potentially attractive trait of CRAds. E4 orf1 may also be a target for selective replication as it binds to proteins with signal transudation functions.

Besides these deletions that affect early viral genes, there are other possible areas of intervention based on the similarities between adenovirus infection and cancer. One common trait is the inactivation of the cellular RNA-dependent protein kinase (PKR). PKR is a serine-threonine kinase activated by double-stranded RNAs produced during cellular stress or viral infections. PKR bound to double-

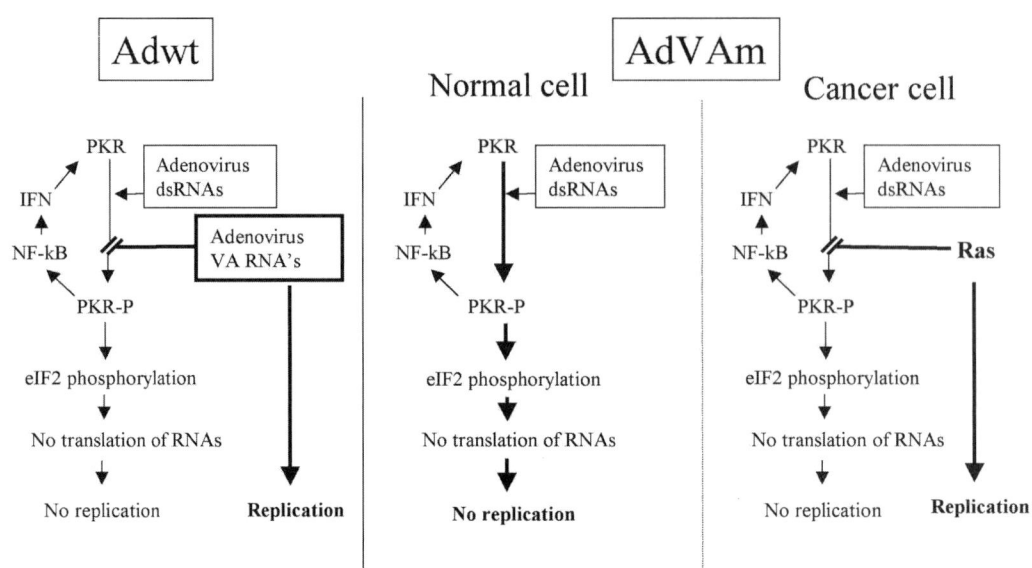

Fig. 2. The deletion of VA-RNA genes represents a strategy to achieve replication conditional to an active Ras pathway. *See* Section 3. for details.

stranded RNA is activated by autophosphorylation and in turn phosphorylates eukaryotic initiation factor eIF2 to stop protein translation. In tumor cells, this stress-response pathway can be blocked by downstream effectors of Ras *(37)*. Adenovirus also blocks PKR activity by synthesizing two small PKR-binding virus-associated RNAs (VA-RNAs) *(38)*. Regarding PKR activation, the oncogenic Ras pathway is analogous to the function of VA-RNAs, making the genomic deletion of these RNA genes a way to achieve Ras-dependent replication (Fig. 2). We have found that a VAI mutant (dl331) replicates 40 times better in cells with an active Ras pathway than in cells in which this pathway is not active (unpublished observations at June 2003). This mechanism of selectivity is inherent to viruses that cannot inactivate PKR, such as reovirus *(39)*, or it has been introduced in other viruses, deleting their respective PKR-inactivating proteins, such as NS1 of influenza A virus *(40)* or ICP34.5 of herpes simplex virus *(41)*.

In general, it is considered that the Ras pathway is activated in 80% of all tumors either by mutations of ras (90% of pancreatic tumors, 50% of colon tumors, 30% of lung tumors, etc.), or by overexpression of EGFR or c-erbB2. Furthermore, this selectivity could have even a broader application because PKR needs to be induced by IFN to be present in a significant amount in the cytoplasm. Often, tumor cells are refractory to IFN effects, and the amount of PKR in the cytoplasm is kept at very low levels. It is well established that tumor cells present defects in the IFN response pathway *(42)*. In general, viruses that are very sensitive to the inhibition mediated by IFN have been used to treat tumors selectively, and VA-deleted adenoviruses could be used accordingly.

An important point to keep in mind when using all of the above deletions to confer selectivity is that at least E1A, mutated or not, is going to be expressed in normal cells with toxic consequences. This E1A-induced toxicity is manifested in vivo, especially in liver. Thus, when systemic administration is considered, it is important to combine the promoter regulation approach with these genetic mutations. The combination of strategies not only reduces the toxicity of the CRAds, but also multiplies the selectivity of the replication. For example, if an E1A mutation restricts replication 2 logs in normal proliferating cells, the addition of a promoter such as the tyrosinase promoter results in another 2 logs of selectivity toward cells that express tyrosinase such as melanoma cells *(43)*.

4. MAXIMIZING THE RELEASE OF VIRIONS FROM THE CELL

The mechanism of adenovirus release from the infected cell is not clearly understood. It is a rather inefficient process because, in vitro, when the cytopathic effects are completed, only 10% of virions are released, and the rest remain arrayed in the nucleus of the infected cell. Nevertheless, certain viral genes seem to play an active role in this process. Among them, the best characterized is the E3-encoded adenovirus death protein (ADP). ADP is expressed at the late phase of the viral life cycle and accelerates cell death and release of virions. Although E3 is usually removed from adenovirus vectors, CRAds retain a better oncolytic potency when ADP is preserved, and this potency can be further enhanced over the levels of Adwt by overexpression of ADP *(10,31)*. This role of ADP can be substituted by the expression of p53 in the late phase, suggesting that apoptosis induction at this phase could be beneficial for virus propagation, in contrast to what happens at the early phase *(44)*. E4orf1 could have a late lytic function similar to ADP, and in the same way, it could be considered to enhance oncolysis *(12)*. Another adenovirus protein implicated in cell death and virion release that could be used for oncolysis enhancement is the L3 protease that cleaves cytokeratin 8.

E1B19K is the main adenovirus-encoded apoptosis inhibitor, and it has been considered a target to enhance cell lysis and virion release *(45)*. As mentioned, E1B-19K mutants can grow more efficiently than wild type. This has been observed under apoptotic blockage *(46)* or in specific cell types *(47)*, for example, in WI38, A549 but not in H411, H446, Calu1, and 293 *(45)*. Results seem to indicate that the 19K deletion could result in enhanced oncolysis in tumor cells, in which its early apoptotic inhibitory function is complemented.

Early apoptosis inhibition and late apoptosis induction may be optimal for virus release, but this hypothesis does not match with the regulation of 19K during the viral cycle in normal cells. The E1B region transcribes a 22S and a 13S mRNA. Both 55K and 19K are produced from the larger messenger, but 19K can also be produced from the shorter one. Curiously, the abundance of 13S mRNA increases at late times of infection and so does the ratio 19K to 55K. It is possible that the function of 19K in normal cells needs to be studied in more detail to understand which tumor cell will produce 19K mutants more efficiently.

5. ARMED AND TARGETED CRADS

If the poor transduction of injected tumors has been the main reason behind the deceiving results of the first decade of cancer gene therapy, a replicating vector now offers the possibility to multiply the transduction efficiency. Conversely, genes with antitumoral activity can complement oncolysis to enhance the attack against the tumor. It is natural, then, to combine gene therapy and virotherapy in a conditionally replicative vector. As adenovirus has been the main player in these two fields, the gene–virotherapy combination appears straightforward.

The rationale to include a transgene in a CRAd is not as much to produce the death of the transduced cell (eventually induced by virus replication) as it is to affect untransduced surrounding cells (bystander effects) or to favor the oncolytic process. Suicide gene therapy was the first kind of gene therapy tested in the context of a conditionally replicating adenovirus *(48)*. Antitumor activity of an E1b-55K-deleted CRAd expressing thymidine kinase increased only when the prodrug ganciclovir was administered several days after the CRAd, indicating that replication is necessary to enhance the suicide gene therapy. In a double suicide gene therapy strategy with a CRAd armed with thymidine kinase and cytosine deaminase, only the combined application of ganciclovir and 5-fluorouracil (5-FU) prodrugs increased the antitumoral activity of the CRAd, and inhibition of viral replication was noted *(49)*.

As expected, if not timed appropriately, cytotoxic gene therapy can counteract viral replication. To avoid this problem, expression can be rendered dependent on replication. Driving the expression of the transgene by the major late promoter or substituting the transgene for late-phase viral genes are strategies to achieve this replication-dependent expression and avoid the interference of the two therapeutic approaches. Besides distributing the transgene throughout the tumor, an armed CRAd can also increase the levels of expression of the transgene up to 2000-fold because of the high copy number of the replicated genome *(50)*. However, eventual cell lysis will halt gene expression, and transgene expression levels in vivo may be more erratic.

Tumor suppressor gene therapy has also been combined with virotherapy. As mentioned in Section 4., p53 has been expressed in a CRAd, producing an increase of virus release. It is expected that a p53-expressing CRAd can combine the gene therapy effect of p53, such as angiogenic inhibition with the oncolytic effect. Fusogenic therapy is another type of cytotoxic gene therapy that has been combined with virotherapy *(51)*. In a concept model using the human immunodeficiency virus env and CD4$^+$ cells, the formation of small syncytia did not seem to interfere with adenovirus production, and the combination showed improved cytotoxicity compared to fusogenesis or oncolysis separately. It remains to be seen whether fusogenesis and replication get along when other fusogenic proteins that can target tumors of epithelial origin are used.

Another example of gene virotherapy used a CRAd-expressing tumor necrosis factor *(6)*. In this case, the expression level of tumor necrosis factor from a replicative vector was 10^6-fold higher than with a nonreplicative vector and was sufficient to induce tumor regression. Immunogene therapy could also benefit from a replication-competent vector if the vector-induced cell lysis favors the presentation of tumor antigens. On the other hand, the presence of immune-dominant viral antigens could mask responses to tumor antigens. These hypotheses are difficult to test because of the lack of immuno-competent animal models that allow human adenovirus replication.

Approaches applied to cancer gene therapy to improve the delivery of the adenoviral vector to the tumor can be used as well in cancer virotherapy. Genetic and nongenetic capsid modifications used to increase the infectivity of adenoviral vectors have already been applied to CRAds, with the expected enhancement of oncolytic potency *(52,53)*. Although means to modify the capsid genetically beyond the addition of small peptides are explored, a nongenetic approach based on adaptor molecules of high specificity such as antibodies and natural ligands can be used. Adaptors need to be expressed by the CRAd to target its progeny. In this case, the length of exogenous DNA in a CRAd is limited because few viral sequences are deleted, and the total capacity of packaged DNA cannot exceed 105% of its genome length. Splitting the genome of the CRAd in several complementary vectors could solve this problem *(24)*.

6. COMBINATION WITH OTHER ANTICANCER THERAPIES AND THE EFFECTS OF THE IMMUNE SYSTEM

For a rational use of CRAds in combination with chemotherapy and radiotherapy, a distinction should be made between the effect of the virus on susceptibility to these therapies and the effect of these therapies on virus replication. Adenovirus E1A can induce S phase and hence the susceptibility to S-phase-specific antineoplastic agents like cisplatin or topotecan. Accordingly, initial in vitro and preclinical studies with ONYX-015 showed synergistic efficacy in combination with cisplatin and 5-FU without decreasing replication *(27,54)*, and these results have been corroborated in clinical trials *(55)*.

The hypothesis of virus-mediated sensitization to chemotherapy is supported by the fact that best results are observed when the virus is given prior to administration of the drug. However, a negative effect on viral replication is suggested by the facts that cisplatin reduces the flulike symptoms associated with CRAd injection *(55)*, and on the other hand, topotecan does not increase the antitumoral effect of CRAds *(48)*. E1A can also induce topoisomerase levels and thus the toxicity of topoisomerase inhibitors such as camptothecin (TopoI inhibitor) and etoposide and daunorubicin (TopoII inhibitors). These drugs enhance viral replication more than cisplatin or 5-FU, a favorable interaction that seems to be related to G2 cell arrest *(56)*. Nocodazole also arrests cells in G2 and enhances virus production, but it has an additional effect via upregulation of CAR and integrins *(57,58)*. CRAds enhance the susceptibility to doxorubicin; conversely, doxorubicin enhances CRAd replication *(59)*. The synergistic antitumoral effect of taxanes (paclitaxel and docetaxel) has been demonstrated in vitro and in vivo *(19,60)*, but the M-phase block they produce is not beneficial to virus replication. A G1-phase block, such as the one produced by actinomycin D, is also detrimental for replication *(56)*. Mitomycin C, thiotepa, mitoxantrone, and vinblastine are also synergic with CRAds when cell death is measured *(19)*, but the impact of these agents on virus production remains to be determined.

A negative effect on replication is particularly important in an in vivo situation, for which, because of diffusion constraints, the therapeutic effect depends on more virus replication cycles. Therefore, a small negative effect could represent a noticeable decrease in efficacy. Besides the effect of chemotherapeutic drugs, CRAds also enhance the effects of radiation therapy *(61)*.

The patient immune response against the CRAd is expected to have a negative impact on the therapy outcome. Activated cytotoxic T cells can destroy infected tumor cells and thereby block the virus spread before it has reached all tumor cells. Antiadenovirus antibodies can directly neutralize infectivity or cause the opsonization of the virus by macrophages. The clinical experience via intratumoral injection, however, indicates that antiadenovirus antibodies do not diminish efficacy because they do not penetrate into the tumor *(55)*. Certainly, control of the immune response will be more relevant for systemic delivery of CRAds. Preexisting neutralizing antibodies, as well as those raised after a first CRAd administration, block antitumor efficacy in murine models in a dose-dependent manner *(62)*. Immunosuppression, either with chemotherapeutic drugs or with drugs specifically administered for this purpose, could avoid the formation of antiadenovirus antibodies, but preexisting antibodies would remain. It will then be important to correlate dose responses with preexisting antibody levels to find threshold doses that overcome the neutralization of the inoculated CRAd. Transient removal of antiadenovirus antibodies through immunoapheresis is also an attractive solution under investigation.

7. CONCLUSION AND FUTURE DIRECTIONS

During the early 1990s, cancer gene therapy drew in much enthusiasm among basic and clinical researchers. A bright decade of molecular biology had revealed the genetic defects that cause cancer and offered the opportunity for rational treatments. At the preclinical level, each strategy of cancer gene therapy tested showed an unprecedented specificity and efficacy. Investment and expectations increased. Clinical trials fell like a cold shower that tempered the hypes and put things in their place. Multiple combinations with radio- and chemotherapy looked for hints of efficacy without clear results. Lack of toxicity prevailed as the most-praised achievement.

Through a different and much longer path, cancer virotherapy has progressed over a century of hopes and failures. However, a continuous trend toward strains or mutants with preferential replication in cancer cells endured. Genetic engineering techniques and better understanding of how viruses use cell metabolism allowed viruses designed with these preferential replication traits. Pioneering efforts explored mutations in nucleotide metabolism genes using herpes simplex virus *(63)*.

The design of mutations targeting the genetic defects that cause cancer represented a conceptual leap toward a truly tumor-specific virotherapy *(27)*. Targeting the genetic defects central to cancer genesis is synonymous with selectivity and efficacy. Loss of tumor suppressors is the main trait of cancer, and it is very difficult for conventional drugs to detect their absence. Even more difficult is making a drug that it amplifies itself until it reaches the entire tumor. This therapeutic chain reaction is the appeal of the immune system, but tumors evolve in the presence of the immune system, and they are selected until they evade it.

The design of viruses that target the genetic origin of cancer shares objectives and tools with cancer gene therapy. Both fields rely on viruses and on the expression of genes central to cancer development. At the time when cancer gene therapy was losing stamina and cancer gene therapists recognized the importance of reaching all tumor cells to succeed in the clinic, this new kind of virotherapy lighted an explosion of interest.

Replication-competent viruses can also be used to deliver therapeutic genes to cancer cells to have a further impact on the destruction of tumors or to help the virus replication. Viral and gene therapy mingle in a new approach against cancer, and adenovirus plays a major role in this new field. The reasons for this popularity are multiple: proven safety, epithelial tropism, amenability to capsid modifications, high levels of episomal gene expression, interactions of viral proteins and cellular proteins involved in cancer, high titers, easy manipulation of the genome, and more. High expectations will face the clinical test, and only after stepwise improvements on systemic delivery, intratumoral dissemination, and control of the neutralizing responses may these expectations be fulfilled.

ACKNOWLEDGMENTS

I am grateful to Cristina Balague for reviewing the manuscript and to Joanne T. Douglas for her invitation to write it.

REFERENCES

1. Yoshida, K., Higashino, F., and Fujinaga, K. (1995) Transcriptional regulation of the adenovirus E1A gene. *Curr. Top. Microbiol. Immunol.* **199**, 113–130.
2. Hatfield, L. and Hearing, P. (1991) Redundant elements in the adenovirus type 5 inverted terminal repeat promote bidirectional transcription in vitro and are important for virus growth in vivo. *Virology* **184**, 265–276.
3. Osborne, T. F., Arvidson, D. N., Tyau, E. S., Dunsworth-Browne, M., and Berk, A. J. (1984) Transcription control region within the protein-coding portion of adenovirus E1A genes. *Mol. Cell Biol.* **4**, 1293–1305.
4. Hitt, M. M. and Graham, F. L. (1990) Adenovirus E1A under the control of heterologous promoters: wide variation in E1A expression levels has little effect on virus replication. *Virology* **179**, 667–678.
5. Hallenbeck, P. L., Chang, Y. N., Hay, C., et al. (1999) A novel tumor-specific replication-restricted adenoviral vector for gene therapy of hepatocellular carcinoma. *Hum. Gene Ther.* **10**, 1721–1733.
6. Kurihara, T., Brough, D. E., Kovesdi, I., and Kufe, D. W. (2000) Selectivity of a replication-competent adenovirus for human breast carcinoma cells expressing the MUC1 antigen. *J. Clin. Invest.* **106**, 763–771.
7. Tsukuda, K., Wiewrodt, R., Molnar-Kimber, K., Jovanovic, V. P., and Amin, K. M. (2002) An E2F-responsive replication-selective adenovirus targeted to the defective cell cycle in cancer cells: potent antitumoral efficacy but no toxicity to normal cell. *Cancer Res.* **62**, 3438–3447.
8. Black, A. R. and Azizkhan-Clifford, J. (1999) Regulation of E2F: a family of transcription factors involved in proliferation control. *Gene* **237**, 281–302.
9. Adachi, Y., Reynolds, P. N., Yamamoto, M., et al. (2001) A midkine promoter-based conditionally replicative adenovirus for treatment of pediatric solid tumors and bone marrow tumor purging. *Cancer Res.* **61**, 7882–7888.
10. Ramachandra, M., Rahman, A., Zou, A., et al. (2001) Re-engineering adenovirus regulatory pathways to enhance oncolytic specificity and efficacy. *Nat. Biotechnol.* **19**, 1035–1041.
11. Hernandez-Alcoceba, R., Pihalja, M., Wicha, M. S., and Clarke, M. F. (2000) A novel, conditionally replicative adenovirus for the treatment of breast cancer that allows controlled replication of E1a-deleted adenoviral vectors. *Hum. Gene Ther.* **11**, 2009–2024.
12. Tauber, B. and Dobner, T. (2001) Molecular regulation and biological function of adenovirus early genes: the E4 ORFs. *Gene* **278**, 1–23.
13. O'Connor, R. J. and Hearing, P. (2000) The E4-6/7 protein functionally compensates for the loss of E1A expression in adenovirus infection. *J. Virol.* **74**, 5819–5824.
14. Doronin, K., Kuppuswamy, M., Toth, K., et al. (2001) Tissue-specific, tumor-selective, replication-competent adenovirus vector for cancer gene therapy. *J. Virol.* **75**, 3314–3324.
15. Holm, P. S., Bergmann, S., Jurchott, K., et al. (2002) YB-1 relocates to the nucleus in adenovirus-infected cells and facilitates viral replication by inducing E2 gene expression through the E2 late promoter. *J. Biol. Chem.* **277**, 10,427–10,434.
16. Brunori, M., Malerba, M., Kashiwazaki, H., and Iggo, R. (2001) Replicating adenoviruses that target tumors with constitutive activation of the wnt signaling pathway. *J. Virol.* **75**, 2857–2865.
17. Carlson, C. A., Steinwaerder, D. S., Stecher, H., Shayakhmetov, D. M., and Lieber, A. (2002) Rearrangements in adenoviral genomes mediated by inverted repeats. *Methods Enzymol.* **346**, 277–292.
18. Yu, D. C., Chen, Y., Seng, M., Dilley, J., and Henderson, D. R. (1999) The addition of adenovirus type 5 region E3 enables calydon virus 787 to eliminate distant prostate tumor xenografts. *Cancer Res.* 59, 4200–4203; published erratum appears in *Cancer Res.* 2000, **60**, 1150.
19. Zhang, J., Ramesh, N., Chen, Y., et al. (2002) Identification of human uroplakin II promoter and its use in the construction of CG8840, a urothelium-specific adenovirus variant that eliminates established bladder tumors in combination with docetaxel. *Cancer Res.* **62**, 3743–3750.

20. Yu, D. C., Sakamoto, G. T., and Henderson, D. R. (1999) Identification of the transcriptional regulatory sequences of human kallikrein 2 and their use in the construction of calydon virus 764, an attenuated replication competent adenovirus for prostate cancer therapy. *Cancer Res.* **59,** 1498–1504.
21. Vassaux, G., Hurst, H. C., and Lemoine, N. R. (1999) Insulation of a conditionally expressed transgene in an adenoviral vector. *Gene Ther.* **6,** 1192–1197.
22. Buvoli, M., Langer, S. J., Bialik, S., and Leinwand, L. A. (2002) Potential limitations of transcription terminators used as transgene insulators in adenoviral vectors. *Gene Ther.* **9,** 227–231.
23. Steinwaerder, D. S. and Lieber, A. (2000) Insulation from viral transcriptional regulatory elements improves inducible transgene expression from adenovirus vectors in vitro and in vivo. *Gene Ther.* **7,** 556–567.
24. Alemany, R., Lai, S., Lou, Y. C., Jan, H. Y., Fang, X., and Zhang, W. W. (1999) Complementary adenoviral vectors for oncolysis. *Cancer Gene Ther.* **6,** 21–25.
25. Frisch, S. M. (1996) Reversal of malignancy by the adenovirus E1a gene. *Mutat. Res.* **350,** 261–266.
26. Frisch, S. M. and Mymryk, J. S. (2002) Adenovirus-5 E1A: paradox and paradigm. *Nat. Rev. Mol. Cell Biol.* **3,** 441–452.
27. Bischoff, J. R., Kirn, D. H., Williams, A., et al. (1996) An adenovirus mutant that replicates selectively in p53-deficient human tumor cells. *Science* **274,** 373–376.
28. Fueyo, J., Gomez-Manzano, C., Alemany, R., et al. (2000) A mutant oncolytic adenovirus targeting the Rb pathway produces anti-glioma effect in vivo. *Oncogene* **19,** 2–12.
29. Heise, C., Hermiston, T., Johnson, L., et al. (2000) An adenovirus E1A mutant that demonstrates potent and selective systemic anti-tumoral efficacy. *Nat. Med.* **6,** 1134–1139.
30. Howe, J. A., Demers, G. W., Johnson, D. E., et al. (2000) Evaluation of E1-mutant adenoviruses as conditionally replicating agents for cancer therapy. *Mol. Ther.* **2,** 485–495.
31. Doronin, K., Toth, K., Kuppuswamy, M., Ward, P., Tollefson, A. E., and Wold, W. S. (2000) Tumor-specific, replication-competent adenovirus vectors overexpressing the adenovirus death protein. *J. Virol.* **74,** 6147–6155.
32. Moran, E. (1994) Mammalian cell growth controls reflected through protein interactions with the adenovirus E1A gene products. *Semin. Virol.* **5,** 327–340.
33. Balague, C., Noya, F., Alemany, R., Chow, L. T., and Curiel, D. T. (2001) Human papillomavirus E6E7-mediated adenovirus cell killing: selectivity of mutant adenovirus replication in organotypic cultures of human keratinocytes. *J. Virol.* **75,** 7602–7611.
34. Shen, Y., Kitzes, G., Nye, J. A., Fattaey, A., and Hermiston, T. (2001) Analyses of single-amino-acid substitution mutants of adenovirus type 5 E1B-55K protein. *J. Virol.* **75,** 4297–4307.
35. Cuconati, A., Degenhardt, K., Sundararajan, R., Anschel, A., and White, E. (2002) Bak and Bax function to limit adenovirus replication through apoptosis induction. *J. Virol.* **76,** 4547–4558.
36. Nevels, M., Spruss, T., Wolf, H., and Dobner, T. (1999) The adenovirus E4orf6 protein contributes to malignant transformation by antagonizing E1A-induced accumulation of the tumor suppressor protein p53. *Oncogene* **18,** 9–17.
37. Mundschau, L. J. and Faller, D. V. (1992) Oncogenic ras induces an inhibitor of double-stranded RNA-dependent eukaryotic initiation factor 2 alpha-kinase activation. *J. Biol. Chem.* **267,** 23,092–23,098.
38. Thimmappaya, B., Weinberger, C., Schneider, R. J., and Shenk, T. (1982) Adenovirus VAI RNA is required for efficient translation of viral mRNAs at late times after infection. *Cell* **31,** 543–551.
39. Strong, J. E., Coffey, M. C., Tang, D., Sabinin, P., and Lee, P. W. (1998) The molecular basis of viral oncolysis: usurpation of the Ras signaling pathway by reovirus. *EMBO J.* **17,** 3351–3362.
40. Bergmann, M., Romirer, I., Sachet, M., et al. (2001) A genetically engineered influenza A virus with ras-dependent oncolytic properties. *Cancer Res.* **61,** 8188–8193.
41. Bolovan, C. A., Sawtell, N. M., and Thompson, R. L. (1994) ICP34.5 mutants of herpes simplex virus type 1 strain 17syn+ are attenuated for neurovirulence in mice and for replication in confluent primary mouse embryo cell cultures. *J. Virol.* **68,** 48–55.
42. Stojdl, D. F., Lichty, B., Knowles, S., et al. (2000) Exploiting tumor-specific defects in the interferon pathway with a previously unknown oncolytic virus. *Nat. Med.* **6,** 821–825.
43. Nettelbeck, D. M., Rivera, A. A., Balague, C., Alemany, R., and Curiel, D. T. (2002) Novel oncolytic adenoviruses targeted to melanoma: specific viral replication and cytolysis by expression of E1A mutants from the tyrosinase enhancer/promoter. *Cancer Res.* **62,** 4663–4670.
44. Sauthoff, H., Pipiya, T., Heitner, S., et al. (2002) Late expression of p53 from a replicating adenovirus improves tumor cell killing and is more tumor cell specific than expression of the adenoviral death protein. *Hum. Gene Ther.* **13,** 1859–1871.
45. Sauthoff, H., Heitner, S., Rom, W. N., and Hay, J. G. (2000) Deletion of the adenoviral E1b-19kD gene enhances tumor cell killing of a replicating adenoviral vector. *Hum. Gene Ther.* **11,** 379–388.
46. Chiou, S. K. and White, E. (1998) Inhibition of ICE-like proteases inhibits apoptosis and increases virus production during adenovirus infection. *Virology* **244,** 108–118.
47. White, E., Faha, B., and Stillman, B. (1986) Regulation of adenovirus gene expression in human WI38 cells by an E1B-encoded tumor antigen. *Mol. Cell Biol.* **6,** 3763–3773.

48. Wildner, O., Blaese, R. M., and Morris, J. C. (1999) Therapy of colon cancer with oncolytic adenovirus is enhanced by the addition of herpes simplex virus-thymidine kinase. *Cancer Res.* **59,** 410–413.

49. Rogulski, K. R., Wing, M. S., Paielli, D. L., Gilbert, J. D., Kim, J. H., and Freytag, S. O. (2000) Double suicide gene therapy augments the antitumor activity of a replication-competent lytic adenovirus through enhanced cytotoxicity and radiosensitization. *Hum. Gene Ther.* **11,** 67–76.

50. Freytag, S. O., Rogulski, K. R., Paielli, D. L., Gilbert, J. D., and Kim, J. H. (1998) A novel three-pronged approach to kill cancer cells selectively: concomitant viral, double suicide gene, and radiotherapy. *Hum. Gene Ther.* **9,** 1323–1333.

51. Li, H., Haviv, Y. S., Derdeyn, C. A., et al. (2001) Human immunodeficiency virus type 1-mediated syncytium formation is compatible with adenovirus replication and facilitates efficient dispersion of viral gene products and de novo-synthesized virus particles. *Hum. Gene Ther.* **12,** 2155–2165.

52. Suzuki, K., Fueyo, J., Krasnykh, V., Reynolds, P. N., Curiel, D. T., and Alemany, R. (2001) A conditionally replicative adenovirus with enhanced infectivity shows improved oncolytic potency. *Clin. Cancer Res.* **7,** 120–126.

53. Hemminki, A., Dmitriev, I., Liu, B., Desmond, R. A., Alemany, R., and Curiel, D. T. (2001) Targeting oncolytic adenoviral agents to the epidermal growth factor pathway with a secretory fusion molecule. *Cancer Res.* **61,** 6377–6381.

54. Heise, C., Lemmon, M., and Kirn, D. (2000) Efficacy with a replication-selective adenovirus plus cisplatin-based chemotherapy: dependence on sequencing but not p53 functional status or route of administration. *Clin. Cancer Res.* **6,** 4908–4914.

55. Khuri, F. R., Nemunaitis, J., Ganly, I., et al. (2000) A controlled trial of intratumoral ONYX-015, a selectively-replicating adenovirus, in combination with cisplatin and 5-fluorouracil in patients with recurrent head and neck cancer. *Nat. Med.* **6,** 879–885.

56. Bernt, K. M., Steinwaerder, D. S., Ni, S., Li, Z. Y., Roffler, S. R., and Lieber, A. (2002) Enzyme-activated prodrug therapy enhances tumor-specific replication of adenovirus vectors. *Cancer Res.* **62,** 6089–6098.

57. Seidman, M. A., Hogan, S. M., Wendland, R. L., Worgall, S., Crystal, R. G., and Leopold, P. L. (2001) Variation in adenovirus receptor expression and adenovirus vector-mediated transgene expression at defined stages of the cell cycle. *Mol. Ther.* **4,** 13–21.

58. Steinwaerder, D. S., Carlson, C. A., and Lieber, A. (2000) DNA replication of first-generation adenovirus vectors in tumor cells. *Hum. Gene Ther.* **11,** 1933–1948.

59. Li, Y., Yu, D. C., Chen, Y., et al. (2001) A hepatocellular carcinoma-specific adenovirus variant, CV890, eliminates distant human liver tumors in combination with doxorubicin. *Cancer Res.* **61,** 6428–6436.

60. Yu, D. C., Chen, Y., Dilley, J., et al. (2001) Antitumor synergy of CV787, a prostate cancer-specific adenovirus, and paclitaxel and docetaxel. *Cancer Res.* **61,** 517–525.

61. Rogulski, K. R., Freytag, S. O., Zhang, K., et al. (2000) In vivo antitumor activity of ONYX-015 is influenced by p53 status and is augmented by radiotherapy. *Cancer Res.* **60,** 1193–1196.

62. Chen, Y., Yu, D. C., Charlton, D., and Henderson, D. R. (2000) Pre-existent adenovirus antibody inhibits systemic toxicity and antitumor activity of CN706 in the nude mouse LNCaP xenograft model: implications and proposals for human therapy. *Hum. Gene Ther.* **11,** 1553–1567.

63. Martuza, R. L., Malick, A., Markert, J. M., Ruffner, K. L., and Coen, D. M. (1991) Experimental therapy of human glioma by means of a genetically engineered virus mutant. *Science* **252,** 854–856.

16

Reovirus as an Oncolytic Agent

Megan K. Patrick, Kara L. Norman, and Patrick W. K. Lee

1. INTRODUCTION

As the incidence of cancer continues to escalate, the demand for alternative anticancer therapeutics increases. The use of viruses in cancer treatment is well documented *(1)*; however, as knowledge in the fields of virology, cell biology, and oncology expands, refined techniques and novel viral-based therapeutics emerge. The oncolytic potential of a wide spectrum of viruses has been explored, such as adenovirus *(2,3)*, herpes simplex virus (HSV) *(4,5)*, vesicular stomatitis virus *(6)*, vaccinia virus *(7)*, poliovirus *(8)*, and mammalian reovirus *(9)*.

To date, numerous engineered adenovirus mutants have been described *(10–13)*. For example, ONYX-015 lacks E1B55Kd adenoviral protein expression *(14)*, known to block p53 tumor suppressor activity *(15)*. This variant selectively replicates in cells with aberrant p53 function *(14,16,17)*, a feature common to 50% of all cancers *(18,19)*, through a mechanism not yet fully understood *(20–22)*. Clinical trials suggested that treatment with ONYX-015 is nontoxic and demonstrates increased efficacy when administered in combination with conventional chemotherapeutics *(23)*.

In humans, HSV infections are highly pathogenic *(24)*; however, manipulation of the viral genome has led to the development of several oncolytic HSV mutants with attenuated pathogenicity *(5)*. For example, G207 harbors defects in UL39 and ICP34.5 function *(25–29)*, promoting replication in tumor cells with increased ribonucleotide reductase activity and Ras activity, respectively *(26,27)*. G207 treatment of human tumor xenografts in mice inhibits tumor growth in vivo *(29–35)*, with enhanced effects when delivered in conjunction with traditional chemotherapeutic drugs or radiotherapy *(34, 36,37)*. Moreover, phase I clinical trials indicated that G207 therapy of human malignant gliomas has no overtly toxic side effects *(38)*.

Finally, reoviral infections are nonpathogenic in humans *(39,40)* and historically have served as a model to study related, more clinically threatening viruses, such as rotavirus *(41)*. The recent emergence of reovirus as a potential oncolytic agent has sparked much interest in the field of reovirology. Along with its lack of pathogenicity, mammalian reovirus offers several other therapeutic advantages. Reovirus does not require genetic alteration because it selectively replicates within cells bearing an activated Ras pathway *(42)*, a feature common to 30% of all human cancers *(43,44)*. Thus, this virus may represent a safe and effective oncolytic agent that can be exploited to combat a wide variety of human cancers. Phase I and II clinical trials testing reovirus are currently under way.

2. BACKGROUND

Mammalian reovirus is a member of the orthoreovirus genus in the family Reoviridae. Based on hemaglutination assays, reoviruses can be categorized into three different serotypes: type 1 (prototype T1 Lang), type 2 (prototype T2 Jones), and type 3 (prototype T3 Dearing [T3D]). Notably, T3D is the primary strain exploited in oncolysis studies. Reovirus is ubiquitous in nature, found predominantly

From: *Contemporary Cancer Research*
Cancer Gene Therapy
Edited by: D. T. Curiel and J. T. Douglas © Humana Press Inc., Totowa, NJ

in stagnant and fresh water and sewage *(45,46)*. The virus can be isolated from several natural hosts, such as mice, cats, sheep, pigs, cattle, monkeys, chimpanzees, and humans *(47)*. Similarly, reovirus infects cells from a variety of species in vitro *(41)*. These characteristics permit evaluation of reovirus-induced oncolysis in both allograft and human tumor xenograft mouse models prior to use in a clinical setting.

Reovirus is commonly isolated from human respiratory and enteric tracts; however, infections are typically subclinical. In 1959, Sabin introduced the name reovirus (for respiratory enteric orphan) to reflect this lack of pathogenicity *(48)*. In contrast, reovirus infection of immune-deficient mice induces significant morbidity and mortality. Human reoviral infections are extremely common, with the reported prevalence of antireovirus antibodies varying from 50% of the adults in some studies *(41,47,49)* to 70–100% in others *(50,51)*.

In 1963, Rosen et al. *(39)* published the most convincing evidence supporting the nonpathogenic nature of reovirus. In this study, inmates in an American federal correctional institution were enlisted and intranasally challenged with mammalian reovirus serotype 1, 2, or 3. Of 27 volunteers, 9 developed mild coldlike symptoms that were not definitively attributed to the infection itself. Serologic and virologic testing identified that not all symptomatic patients were productively infected; moreover, some asymptomatic patients were seropositive. The absence of reovirus-induced human disease has led to its development as a model to study related, more pathogenic viruses and more recently as an oncolytic agent.

Mammalian reovirus is a nonenveloped icosahedral particle composed of eight structural proteins arranged in two concentric capsid layers. The virion encases 10 linear double-stranded ribonucleic acid (dsRNA) gene segments that encode 11 proteins. The viral genome and protein complement are classified into three size classes based on electrophoretic migration profiles and are designated as large, medium, and small or λ, μ, and σ, respectively *(52–54)*.

To initiate infection, the cell attachment protein σ1 *(55)* binds the host cellular receptors sialic acid, junction adhesion molecule, and potentially several others *(56–59)*. Virus entry occurs via the receptor-mediated endocytic pathway *(60–62)*, in which the endolysosomal low pH and proteases aid in viral uncoating *(63,64)*. Proteolytic processing results in the loss of σ3 and cleavage of μ1 to μ1c, producing an intermediate subviral particle (ISVP). The ISVP is further uncoated with the loss of σ1 and μ1 *(65)*, which permits the release of the transcriptionally active core particle into the cytoplasm. The core initiates primary transcription of 5' capped, nonpolyadenylated messenger RNA (mRNA) from each of the 10 genomic strands *(66,67)*, which are translated by the host translational machinery. These reoviral proteins associate with each of the 10 primary transcripts in RNA assortment complexes. Core-like replicase intermediate particles are subsequently assembled *(68,69)*, and synthesis of the genomic RNA-minus strand ensues. This provides the template for transcription of secondary uncapped mRNAs *(70)*, which are later translated by host cellular ribosomes and represent the predominant source of reoviral proteins during infection *(71)*. In the final stage of the reoviral lifecycle, viral proteins and genome are assembled and released by host cell lysis.

3. THE REOVIRUS–CANCER LINK

Early investigations implicated an association between reoviral infection and cellular transformation; however, these initial clues were not understood until recently. In 1977, Hashiro et al. reported transformed cell lines were susceptible to reovirus infection, whereas untransformed cells from various species were resistant *(72)*. Similarly, in 1978 Duncan et al. stated normal WI-38 cells failed to support reoviral infection, in contrast to reovirus-permissive SV-40 large T-antigen-transformed WI-38 cell lines *(73)*.

Reovirus receptor and attachment studies unexpectedly uncovered the molecular basis of this specificity for cancer cells. Reovirus binds to sialic acid moieties that are ubiquitously expressed on host cells; however, not all cells support the reoviral lifecycle. In 1993, Strong et al. reported that epidermal growth factor receptor (EGFR)-deficient 3T3 murine fibroblasts (designated NR6) were resistant to T3D, whereas cells expressing EGFR (designated HER5) were not *(74)*. Furthermore, reovirus was capable of binding to the EGFR directly *(75)*. This suggested that EGFR functions directly in viral attachment and entry; alternatively, it creates a reovirus-compatible intracellular environment. Further investigation revealed the latter scenario was in fact the case.

Transformation of reovirus-resistant NIH 3T3 cells with the constitutively active v-*erbB* oncogene derived from retroviral transduction of an EGFR homologue that lacks the extracellular binding domain and confers reovirus susceptibility *(76)*. This evidence confirmed that EGFR is not required for viral entry; rather, the virus exploits the environment created on overactivation of EGFR signaling cascades. A more detailed understanding of these intracellular signaling pathways is essential to employ reovirus effectively and conscientiously as a therapeutic human anticancer agent.

4. EGF SIGNALING AND THE RAS PATHWAY

Activation of the EGFR signal transduction cascade stimulates numerous effector molecules that facilitate several cellular responses. The Ras pathway represents a major regulatory pathway downstream of EGFR. Activating mutations in *ras* are associated with 30% of all human cancers *(43,44)*; moreover, mutations in many Ras pathway effector molecules are also associated with several other human cancers *(77–87)*. Thus, activation of the Ras pathway may be responsible for the cellular modifications that favor the reoviral life cycle in transformed cells.

Ras pathway activation can occur in several different ways (Fig. 1). Extracellular ligand binding to EGFR induces receptor dimerization and cytoplasmic tail autophosphorylation *(88–90)*. An EGFR cytoplasmic phosophotyrosine residue provides a docking site for several signaling molecules, such as adapter proteins Shc and Grb2 *(91,92)*. However, Grb2 may be indirectly recruited to EGFR through association with Shc phosphotyrosine residues *(93,94)*. The GTP exchange factor SOS interacts with Grb2 at the cytoplasmic membrane and catalyzes GDP–GTP exchange and thus activates the small G protein Ras *(95)*. Alternatively, Ras activation can occur in a receptor-independent fashion. This strategy involves activation of intracellular tyrosine kinases such as Src, which stimulate tyrosine phosphorylation of Shc, recruitment of Grb2 and Sos, and ultimately the production of Ras-GTP.

Accumulation of Ras-GTP can stimulate activation of many downstream signal transduction pathways *(89,96)*, such as those involving Raf-1, phosphatidylinositol 3 kinase (PI3K), and Ral guanine nucleotide exchange factors (Ral GEFs) (Fig. 1). Ras activation of Raf-1 kinase at the cytoplasmic membrane induces phosphorylation and activation of MEK, a dual-specificity serine/threonine and tyrosine kinase. Activated MEK phosphorylates extracellular signal regulated kinase (ERK) and induces ERK nuclear translocation and phosphorylation of other enzymes and transcription factors, such as Elk1 (reviewed in refs. *89* and *96*).

Alternatively, Ras-GTP interaction with PI3K induces phosphorylation of phosphatidylinositides. For example, phosphorylation of PIP_2 to PIP_3 facilitates its interaction with Rac GDP–GTP exchange factors (Rac GEFs) such as vav, leading to Rac activation and NF-κB translocation to the nucleus (reviewed in refs. *89* and *96*). Ras-GTP can interact with Ral GEFs, for example, Ral GDS or Rlf, which in turn activate the small GTPase Ral *(89,96,97)*. Activated Ral interacts with several downstream effectors, such as phospholipase D1, Ral-binding protein 1 (RalBP1), and filamin (reviewed in refs. *89* and *96*). In addition to the above-mentioned Ras-GTP effectors, several others have been reported, such as RIN1, p120GAP, MEKK, NF1GAP, and AF-6 (reviewed in ref. *89*).

5. THE REOVIRAL INFECTION MECHANISM

As mentioned in Section 3., untransformed 3T3 murine fibroblasts fail to support productive reovirus infection. These cells permit viral entry and early transcript synthesis; however, viral protein production is not detectable as measured by ^{35}S-methionine labeling *(42)*. This resistance may reflect induction of an innate cellular antiviral response (Fig. 2).

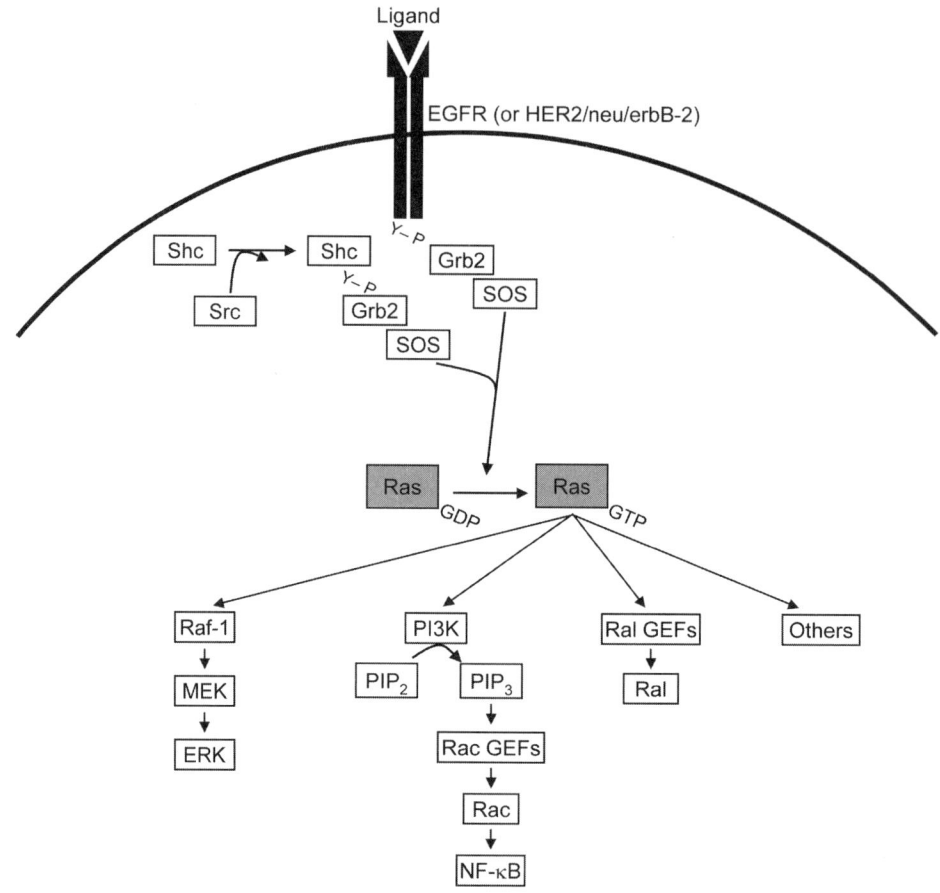

Fig. 1. EGFR activation of Ras pathway signaling. Ligand-induced EGFR dimerization and autophosphor-ylation activate Grb2 directly or indirectly through receptor-independent Shc activation. Grb2 interacts with the GTP exchange factor SOS, catalyzing GDP–GTP exchange and activation of Ras. Ras-GTP stimulates numerous effector molecules, such as Raf-1, PI3K, Ral GEFs, and several others.

Following viral infection, transcription ensues, generating viral mRNAs such as s1, which form extensive dsRNA secondary structures. These viral dsRNA replication intermediates induce host dsRNA-activated protein kinase (PKR) activity *(98)*. In this process, two PKR molecules interact with dsRNA structures, which activate PKR through intermolecular autophosphorylation *(99)*. Active PKR induces phosphorylation of eIF-2α, a component of the cellular translational initiation apparatus. Ultimately, another initiation factor, eIF-2B, is sequestered, preventing the eIF-2 GDP–GTP exchange required for translation initiation *(100,101)*. Viral translation is specifically inhibited, and the infection is aborted; the host cell continues to thrive. The role of PKR in reovirus resistance was confirmed because loss of PKR function conferred cellular susceptibility. In these studies, infection of PKR$^{-/-}$ mouse embryo fibroblasts or PKR inhibitor (2-aminopurine)-treated untransformed 3T3 cells was productive *(42)*.

In contrast to untransformed cells, 3T3 fibroblasts transformed with the v-*erbB* oncogene, a con-stitutively active truncated form of EGFR, support the reoviral life cycle *(76)*. Ras is a major down-stream effector of EGFR signaling; furthermore, mutations in Ras or members of the Ras pathway are commonly associated with several human cancer types. These characteristics implicate Ras signal-ing in reovirus susceptibility. Infection of cells transformed with an activated mutant of Ras results in

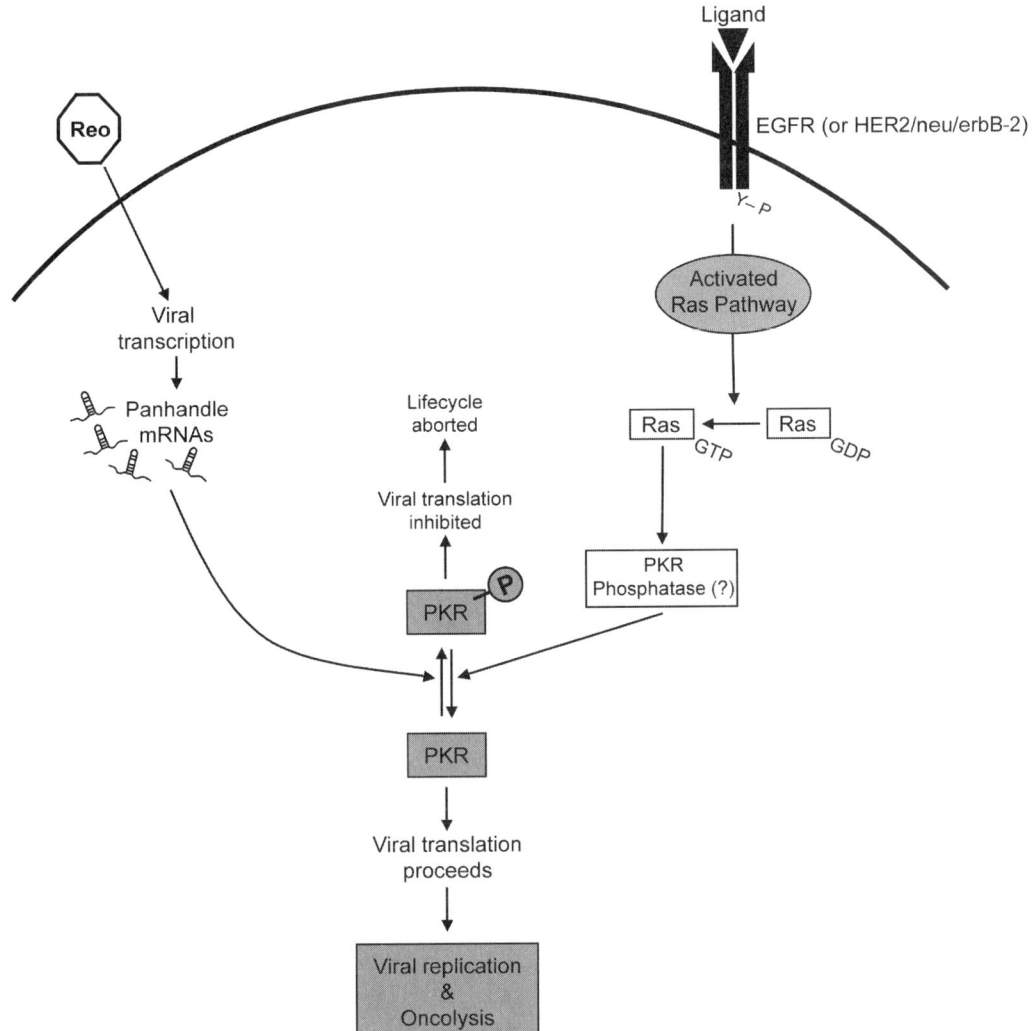

Fig. 2. The proposed mechanism of reovirus-induced oncolysis. In reovirus-infected untransformed cells, mRNA panhandle structures activate host PKR. Active, phosphorylated PKR halts viral protein synthesis, and the infection is terminated. In transformed cells with an activated Ras signaling pathway, the reoviral life cycle is completed. This productive infection is accompanied by a loss of phosphorylated PKR through an unknown mechanism.

transcription, translation, and host cell lysis *(42)* (Fig. 2). Moreover, infection coincides with a lack of PKR phosphorylation *(42)*, indicating the cellular antiviral response is impaired. Also, infection of cells expressing zinc-inducible active Ras was only productive in the presence of zinc *(42)*. This confirms the involvement of the Ras pathway in cellular susceptibility and that long-term transformation alone does not impart susceptibility. Similarly, transformation of 3T3 cells with SOS, a GTP exchange factor upstream of Ras in the EGFR signaling cascade, permits reoviral infection with an accompanying lack of PKR phosphorylation *(42)*.

Previous reports suggested a relationship between Ras transformation of BALB cells and PKR inhibition *(102)*. In these studies, a 100-kDa Ras-inducible kinase inhibitor prevented PKR autophosphorylation and thus its activity; however, the nature of the involvement of Ras-inducible kinase inhibitors in the Ras-PKR pathway is not completely understood.

The elements downstream of Ras that signal to PKR are currently under intense investigation. An association between ERK activity and reoviral susceptibility has been noted, but is inconsistent (103; unpublished, Norman and Lee, 2004). Moreover, elimination of ERK activity using an MEK inhibitor (PD98059) did not alter Ras regulation of PKR in Ras-transformed cells or negatively affect reovirus infection (42). This suggests the critical signal transduction that promotes reoviral infection does not involve the MEK/ERK pathway, but likely involves alternative Ras effector pathways. Several potential mediators are currently under examination in our laboratory. Notably, experiments involving Ras effector mutants impaired in specific downstream signaling events suggest that retention of Ras signaling to Ral GEF enhances reovirus susceptibility (unpublished, Norman and Lee, 2004).

Activation of the Ras pathway promotes inhibition of innate antiviral defense mechanisms, such as PKR; however, the mechanism of PKR inhibition is yet to be elucidated. Ras-related negative regulation of PKR may be a reflection of an initial block in PKR phosphorylation or a result of PKR dephosphorylation. In vitro experiments suggested Ras transformed cell lysates dephosphorylate phosphorylated PKR (unpublished data, Zhao and Lee, 2004), supporting the existence of a potential Ras-regulated PKR phosphatase. The nature of this phosphatase is currently under investigation in our laboratory.

Reovirus infection of transformed cell lines induces extensive cytopathic effects and cell death and is likely attributed to life cycle completion through host cell lysis. However, Clarke et al. reported reovirus-induced death of human cancer cells occurs via an apoptotic mechanism (104). In this study, infection was associated with increased caspase 8 activity and release of tumor necrosis factor-related apoptosis inducing ligand. In contrast, other reports have indicated host receptor interactions and ISVP formation, but not subsequent viral transcription or replication, are required for reovirus-induced apoptosis (105). To date, the precise mechanism of cell death in Ras-transformed, reovirus-susceptible cells has not been examined.

6. REOVIRUS AND ONCOLYSIS

Activation of the Ras pathway is commonly associated with cellular transformation and cancer. Approximately 30% of all human cancers have mutations in one of three Ras genes (K-, H-, N-Ras) at residues 12, 13, or 61. This genetic alteration restricts the ability of Ras-GTPase-activating proteins to induce Ras-GTPase activity (106,107), leading to accumulation of active Ras-GTP. Mutant K-Ras is expressed in 50% of colorectal cancers (107,108) and 95% of adenocarcinomas of the exocrine pancreas (109). The presence of Ras mutations found in ovarian cancer studies varied between 4 and 48% (110–112). Lung adenocarcinomas (113), thyroid neoplasms, seminomas, and acute myelogenous, chronic myelomonocytic, and acute lymphoblastic leukemias (114) have been found to harbor Ras mutations, suggesting reovirus may represent an effective anticancer therapeutic against a wide variety of human tumor types.

Moreover, activating mutations in other members of the Ras pathway are often associated with human cancers, expanding the number of potentially reovirus-treatable tumors. In human gliomas, EGFR and platelet-derived growth factor receptor, proto-oncogenes that activate Ras, are often overexpressed (77–81). Similarly, 30% of human breast cancers exhibit amplified expression of HER-2 (NEU/ErbB-2), an EGFR family member with a transforming ability that is dependent on Ras activity (82,83). Overexpression of EGFR itself (84,85) or increased activation Src family nonreceptor tyrosine kinases (86,87) is also often associated with human breast carcinomas.

Initially, the ability of reovirus to infect, replicate in, and kill human cancer cells was examined in vitro in several human cancer cell lines. Human breast tumor cell lines that possess increased Src family kinase activity and overexpress Her-2 and EGFR were susceptible to reovirus infection, replication, and host cell lysis, in contrast to normal breast epithelial cell lines (115). Similarly, all colon and ovarian cancer cell lines tested were susceptible to reoviral infection compared to reovirus-resistant normal cell lines, and this susceptibility correlated with elevated Ras activity (116). Diffuse, large, non-Hodgkin B-cell lymphoma cells lines *(117)*, some Burkitt lymphoma cell lines *(117)*, and 83% of malignant glioma cell lines tested supported the reovirus life cycle *(103)*. Furthermore, pancreatic and prostate human cancer cell lines tested also supported reovirus infection (unpublished, Coffey and Lee, 2004). These preliminary in vitro studies indicated that the virus may function as a tumor-specific oncolytic agent and led to more detailed in vivo investigations.

The oncolytic potential of mammalian reovirus can be directly analyzed in vivo as the virus naturally infects a wide variety of species *(47)*. Consequently, viral oncolysis can be evaluated in both human tumor cell line xenograft or in tumor allograft rodent models. This permits assessment of reovirus efficacy against human or murine tumor implants in immune-compromised hosts or in the face of an elicited immune response, respectively.

Intratumoral inoculation of orthotopic human breast cancer xenografts in SCID/nonobese diabetic (NOD) mice led to dramatic tumor regression compared to ultraviolet-inactivated virus or uninfected controls *(115)*. Similarly, intratumoral infection of human colon or ovarian xenografts in SCID or CD-1 nude mice, respectively, reduced the tumor size compared to controls *(116)*. Moreover, in a murine model of advanced-stage human ovarian cancer, repeated intraperitoneal reoviral injections facilitated a 90% survival rate *(116)*. Intraneoplastic infection of intracerebral human malignant gliomas in SCID/ NOD and in less-immune-compromised CD-1 nude mice also resulted in tumor regression *(103)*.

To further confirm reoviral infection of human cancerous tissues, surgical tumor biopsy specimens were studied ex vivo. Human breast cancer (*n* = 3) *(115)*, ovarian endometrioid adenocarcinoma and papillary serous adenocarcinoma (*n* = 3) *(116)*, chronic lymphocytic leukemia (*n* = 15) *(117)*, and glioma (*n* = 9) *(103)* biopsies all supported reovirus replication to varying degrees. Interestingly, only 6 of 12 primary non-Hodgkin lymphoma samples *(117)* and none of the meningioma biopsy specimens tested (*n* = 7) supported reovirus infection *(103)*.

Metastases represent a significant obstacle in traditional cancer treatments because they are often widespread and less responsive to chemotherapeutic treatment. Metastatic cancers are commonly associated with an activated Ras pathway and may be susceptible to reovirus-induced lysis. Reovirus is a replication-competent, infectious, oncolytic agent, characteristics that may facilitate replication at sites remote from the primary tumor. In a bilateral human breast cancer model, xenografts were implanted subcutaneously in both hind flanks of SCID/NOD mice *(115)*. Intratumoral reovirus injection in the left hind flank resulted in tumor regression in both the injected and contralateral tumor. Reoviral detection in the blood and delayed viral appearance in the contralateral flank suggest regression of the untreated tumor is attributed to systemic viral spread *(115)*.

In several experimental models of lung metastases, intravenous infection resulted in improved survival or inhibition of metastatic development *(118)*. Intravenous treatment of immune-competent C3H mice implanted with Ras-transformed allografts resulted in early tumor inhibition followed later by regrowth *(118)*. This inefficiency may reflect an elicited antiviral immune response as reovirus delivered in combination with immune-suppressing drugs enhanced tumor regression and prolonged survival in localized and metastatic models, respectively *(118)*.

The high incidence of previous reoviral exposure and presence of antireovirus antibodies in the population may reduce the efficacy of reovirus oncolytic therapy. Consequently, reovirus delivered in combination with immune suppressants may represent a realistic alternative in the clinical setting.

7. CURRENT ALTERNATIVE ANTI-RAS THERAPIES

The high incidence of Ras pathway activation in human cancers suggests that exploitation or inhibition of this pathway may provide an effective cancer therapeutic. Reovirus utilizes cells with an enhanced Ras pathway as a suitable environment to carry out its natural life cycle, which inevitably leads to host cell death. It is important to acknowledge that several other groups have explored alternate approaches by which molecular modulators that attenuate Ras activity (reviewed in ref. *119*) or its downstream effector molecules *(120,121)* are utilized.

For example, several studies focused on inhibition of Ras anchorage to the cell membrane. Farnesylation of Ras at the carboxy terminal CAAX motif by the cellular enzyme farnesyltransferase is a critical modification required for cell membrane association. Reports suggested farnesyltransferase inhibitors (FTIs) *(122,123)* induce tumor regression in experimental animals *(124,125)*; however, this may not directly reflect FTI-induced Ras inhibition, but rather its effects on other cellular targets *(126,127)*. Similarly, the drug *trans*-farnesylthiosalicylic acid, which specifically mimics the farnesylcysteine of Ras and directly competes for anchorage sites *(128,129)*, inhibits Ras transformation in vitro and tumor growth in vivo *(130)*. However, downregulation of Ras activity may affect normal Ras functions such as cell growth, differentiation, survival, and migration and thus may present human toxicity concerns. Nonetheless, the ability of FTI or *trans*-farnesylthiosalicylic acid to cause tumor regression in humans remains to be seen.

8. CONCLUDING REMARKS

To date, the ability of reovirus to function as a selective oncolytic agent is promising in vitro, in vivo, ex vivo, and in ongoing human clinical trials. However, the precise mechanism of Ras-related PKR inhibition and the potential involvement of other cellular processes in reovirus-induced oncolysis remains to be elucidated. In attempts to maximize the efficacy of reovirus treatment, reoviral infection in combination with traditional or alternative anticancer therapeutics must be more thoroughly investigated. Moreover, as most individuals carry antireovirus antibodies, the addition of immune-suppressive drugs to the treatment regime may be advantageous. Although many questions remain, reovirus serves as a promising oncolytic agent both in the laboratory and in ongoing clinical trials. Thus, future reovirus-based therapies may improve patient prognosis and minimize human suffering in the face of the cancer epidemic.

REFERENCES

1. Sinkovics, J. and Horvath, J. (1993) New developments in the virus therapy of cancer: a historical review. *Intervirology* **36**, 193–214.
2. McCormick, F. (1999) Cancer therapy based on p53. *Cancer J. Sci. Am.* **5**, 139–144.
3. McCormick, F. (2000) ONYX-015 selectivity and the p14ARF pathway. *Oncogene* **19**, 6670–6672.
4. Rampling, R., Cruickshank, G., Papanastassiou, V., et al. (2000) Toxicity evaluation of replication-competent herpes simplex virus (ICP 34.5 null mutant 1716) in patients with recurrent malignant glioma. *Gene Ther.* **7**, 859–866.
5. Martuza, R. L. (2000) Conditionally replicating herpes vectors for cancer therapy. *J. Clin. Invest.* **105**, 841–846.
6. Stojdl, D. F., Lichty, B., Knowles, S., et al. (2000) Exploiting tumor-specific defects in the interferon pathway with a previously unknown oncolytic virus. *Nat. Med.* **6**, 821–825.
7. McCart, J. A., Ward, J. M., Lee, J., et al. (2001) Systemic cancer therapy with a tumor-selective vaccinia virus mutant lacking thymidine kinase and vaccinia growth factor genes. *Cancer Res.* **61**, 8751–8757.
8. Gromeier, M., Lachmann, S., Rosenfeld, M. R., Gutin, P. H., and Wimmer, E. (2000) Intergeneric poliovirus recombinants for the treatment of malignant glioma. *Proc. Natl. Acad. Sci. USA* **97**, 6803–6808.
9. Coffey, M. C., Strong, J. E., Forsyth, P. A., and Lee, P. W. (1998) Reovirus therapy of tumors with activated Ras pathway. *Science* **282**, 1332–1334.
10. Hemminki, A., Dmitriev, I., Liu, B., Desmond, R. A., Alemany, R., and Curiel, D. T. (2001) Targeting oncolytic adenoviral agents to the epidermal growth factor pathway with a secretory fusion molecule. *Cancer Res.* **61**, 6377–6381.
11. Dmitriev, I., Krasnykh, V., Miller, C. R., et al. (1998) An adenovirus vector with genetically modified fibers demonstrates expanded tropism via utilization of a Coxsackievirus and adenovirus receptor-independent cell entry mechanism. *J. Virol.* **72**, 9706–9713.
12. van der Poel, H. G., Molenaar, B., van Beusechem, V. W., et al. (2002) Epidermal growth factor receptor targeting of replication competent adenovirus enhances cytotoxicity in bladder cancer. *J. Urol.* **168**, 266–272.
13. Shayakhmetov, D. M., Li, Z. Y., Ni, S., and Lieber, A. (2002) Targeting of adenovirus vectors to tumor cells does not enable efficient transduction of breast cancer metastases. *Cancer Res.* **62**, 1063–1068.
14. Bischoff, J. R., Kirn, D. H., Williams, A., et al. (1996) An adenovirus mutant that replicates selectively in p53-deficient human tumor cells. *Science* **274**, 373–376.
15. Yew, P. R. and Berk, A. J. (1992) Inhibition of p53 transactivation required for transformation by adenovirus early 1B protein. *Nature* **357**, 82–85.

16. Ries, S. J., Brandts, C. H., Chung, A. S., et al. (2000) Loss of p14ARF in tumor cells facilitates replication of the adenovirus mutant dl1520 (ONYX-015). *Nat. Med.* **6,** 1128–1133.
17. Yang, C. T., You, L., Uematsu, K., Yeh, C. C., McCormick, F., and Jablons, D. M. (2001) p14(ARF) modulates the cytolytic effect of ONYX-015 in mesothelioma cells with wild-type p53. *Cancer Res.* **61,** 5959–5963.
18. Levine, A. J., Momand, J., and Finlay, C.A. (1991) The p53 tumour suppressor gene. *Nature* **351,** 453–456.
19. Hollstein, M., Sidransky, D., Vogelstein, B., and Harris, C. C. (1991) p53 mutations in human cancers. *Science* **253,** 49–53.
20. Hall, A. R., Dix, B. R., O'Carroll, S. J., and Braithwaite, A. W. (1998) p53-dependent cell death/apoptosis is required for a productive adenovirus infection. *Nat. Med.* **4,** 1068–1072.
21. Dix, B. R., O'Carroll, S. J., Myers, C. J., Edwards, S. J., and Braithwaite, A. W. (2000) Efficient induction of cell death by adenoviruses requires binding of E1B55k and p53. *Cancer Res.* **60,** 2666–2672.
22. Goodrum, F. D. and Ornelles, D. A. (1998) p53 status does not determine outcome of E1B 55-kilodalton mutant adenovirus lytic infection. *J. Virol.* **72,** 9479–9490.
23. Khuri, F. R., Nemunaitis, J., Ganly, I., et al. (2000) A controlled trial of intratumoral ONYX-015, a selectively-replicating adenovirus, in combination with cisplatin and 5-fluorouracil in patients with recurrent head and neck cancer. *Nat. Med.* **6,** 879–885.
24. Whitley, R. J., Kimberlin, D. W., and Roizman, B. (1998) Herpes simplex viruses. *Clin. Infect. Dis.* **26,** 541–553; quiz 554–545.
25. Mineta, T., Rabkin, S. D., and Martuza, R. L. (1994) Treatment of malignant gliomas using ganciclovir-hypersensitive, ribonucleotide reductase-deficient herpes simplex viral mutant. *Cancer Res.* **54,** 3963–3966.
26. Boviatsis, E. J., Scharf, J. M., Chase, M., et al. (1994) Antitumor activity and reporter gene transfer into rat brain neoplasms inoculated with herpes simplex virus vectors defective in thymidine kinase or ribonucleotide reductase. *Gene Ther.* **1,** 323–331.
27. Mineta, T., Rabkin, S. D., Yazaki, T., Hunter, W. D., and Martuza, R. L. (1995) Attenuated multi-mutated herpes simplex virus-1 for the treatment of malignant gliomas. *Nat. Med.* **1,** 938–943.
28. Hunter, W. D., Martuza, R. L., Feigenbaum, F., et al. (1999) Attenuated, replication-competent herpes simplex virus type 1 mutant G207: safety evaluation of intracerebral injection in nonhuman primates. *J. Virol.* **73,** 6319–6326.
29. Oyama, M., Ohigashi, T., Hoshi, M., et al. (2000) Intravesical and intravenous therapy of human bladder cancer by the herpes vector G207. *Hum. Gene Ther.* **11,** 1683–1693.
30. Kooby, D. A., Carew, J. F., Halterman, M. W., et al. (1999) Oncolytic viral therapy for human colorectal cancer and liver metastases using a multi-mutated herpes simplex virus type-1 (G207). *FASEB J.* **13,** 1325–1334.
31. Coukos, G., Makrigiannakis, A., Montas, S., et al. (2000) Multi-attenuated herpes simplex virus-1 mutant G207 exerts cytotoxicity against epithelial ovarian cancer but not normal mesothelium and is suitable for intraperitoneal oncolytic therapy. *Cancer Gene Ther.* **7,** 275–283.
32. Toda, M., Rabkin, S. D., and Martuza, R. L. (1998) Treatment of human breast cancer in a brain metastatic model by G207, a replication-competent multimutated herpes simplex virus 1. *Hum. Gene Ther.* **9,** 2177–2185.
33. Walker, J. R., McGeagh, K. G., Sundaresan, P., Jorgensen, T. J., Rabkin, S. D., and Martuza, R. L. (1999) Local and systemic therapy of human prostate adenocarcinoma with the conditionally replicating herpes simplex virus vector G207. *Hum. Gene Ther.* **10,** 2237–2243.
34. Chahlavi, A., Todo, T., Martuza, R. L., and Rabkin, S. D. (1999) Replication-competent herpes simplex virus vector G207 and cisplatin combination therapy for head and neck squamous cell carcinoma. *Neoplasia* **1,** 162–169.
35. Randazzo, B. P., Bhat, M. G., Kesari, S., Fraser, N. W., and Brown, S. M. (1997) Treatment of experimental subcutaneous human melanoma with a replication-restricted herpes simplex virus mutant. *J. Invest. Dermatol.* **108,** 933–937.
36. Bradley, J. D., Kataoka, Y., Advani, S., et al. (1999) Ionizing radiation improves survival in mice bearing intracranial high-grade gliomas injected with genetically modified herpes simplex virus. *Clin. Cancer Res.* **5,** 1517–1522.
37. Coukos, G., Makrigiannakis, A., Kang, E. H., Rubin, S. C., Albelda, S. M., and Molnar-Kimber, K. L. (2000) Oncolytic herpes simplex virus-1 lacking ICP34.5 induces p53-independent death and is efficacious against chemotherapy-resistant ovarian cancer. *Clin. Cancer Res.* **6,** 3342–3353.
38. Markert, J. M., Medlock, M. D., Rabkin, S. D., et al. (2000) Conditionally replicating herpes simplex virus mutant, G207 for the treatment of malignant glioma: results of a phase I trial. *Gene Ther.* **7,** 867–874.
39. Rosen, L., Evans, H. E., and Sickard, A. (1963) Reovirus infections in human volunteers. *Am. J. Hyg.* **77,** 29–37.
40. Rosen, L., Hovis, J. F., Mastrota, F. M., Bell, J. A., and Huebner, R. J. (1960) Observations on a newly recognized virus (Abney) of the reovirus family. *Am. J. Hyg.* **71,** 258–265.
41. Tyler, K. L., Fields, B. N. (1996) Reoviruses. In *Fields Virology* (Fields, B. N., Knipe, D. M., and Howley, P. M., ed.), Lippincott-Raven, Philadelphia, PA, pp. 1597–1623.
42. Strong, J. E., Coffey, M. C., Tang, D., Sabinin, P., and Lee, P. W. (1998) The molecular basis of viral oncolysis: usurpation of the Ras signaling pathway by reovirus. *EMBO J.* **17,** 3351–3362.
43. Lowe, P. N. and Skinner, R. H. (1994) Regulation of Ras signal transduction in normal and transformed cells. *Cell Signal.* **6,** 109–123.

44. Levitzki, A. (1994) Signal-transduction therapy. A novel approach to disease management. *Eur. J. Biochem.* **226**, 1–13.
45. Ridinger, D. N., Spendlove, R. S., Barnett, B. B., George, D. B., and Roth, J. C. (1982) Evaluation of cell lines and immunofluorescence and plaque assay procedures for quantifying reoviruses in sewage. *Appl. Environ. Microbiol.* **43**, 740–746.
46. Stanley, N. F. (1967) Reoviruses. *Br. Med. Bull.* **23**, 150–154.
47. Jackson, G. G. and Muldoon, R. L. (1973) Viruses causing common respiratory infection in man. IV. Reoviruses and adenoviruses. *J. Infect. Dis.* **128**, 811–866.
48. Sabin, A. (1959) Reoviruses: a new group of respiratory and enteric viruses formerly classified as ECHO type 10 is described. *Science* **130**, 1387–1389.
49. Stanley, N. F. (1974) The reovirus murine models. *Prog. Med. Virol.* **18**, 257–272.
50. Minuk, G. Y., Rascanin, N., Paul, R. W., Lee, P. W., Buchan, K., and Kelly, J. K. (1987) Reovirus type 3 infection in patients with primary biliary cirrhosis and primary sclerosing cholangitis. *J. Hepatol.* **5**, 8–13.
51. Minuk, G. Y., Paul, R. W., and Lee, P. W. (1985) The prevalence of antibodies to reovirus type 3 in adults with idiopathic cholestatic liver disease. *J. Med. Virol.* **16**, 55–60.
52. Both, G. W., Lavi, S., and Shatkin, A. J. (1975) Synthesis of all the gene products of the reovirus genome in vivo and in vitro. *Cell* **4**, 173–180.
53. McCrae, M. A. and Joklik, W. K. (1978) The nature of the polypeptide encoded by each of the 10 double-stranded RNA segments of reovirus type 3. *Virology* **89**, 578–593.
54. Shatkin, A. J., Sipe, J. D., and Loh, P. (1968) Separation of ten reovirus genome segments by polyacrylamide gel electrophoresis. *J. Virol.* **2**, 986–991.
55. Lee, P. W., Hayes, E. C., and Joklik, W. K. (1981) Protein sigma 1 is the reovirus cell attachment protein. *Virology* **108**, 156–163.
56. Choi, A. H., Paul, R. W., and Lee, P. W. (1990) Reovirus binds to multiple plasma membrane proteins of mouse L fibroblasts. *Virology* **178**, 316–320.
57. Gentsch, J. R. and Hatfield, J. W. (1984) Saturable attachment sites for type 3 mammalian reovirus on murine L cells and human HeLa cells. *Virus Res.* **1**, 401–414.
58. Barton, E. S., Forrest, J. C., Connolly, J. L., et al. (2001) Junction adhesion molecule is a receptor for reovirus. *Cell* **104**, 441–451.
59. Paul, R. W., Choi, A. H., and Lee, P. W. (1989) The alpha-anomeric form of sialic acid is the minimal receptor determinant recognized by reovirus. *Virology* **172**, 382–385.
60. Borsa, J., Morash, B. D., Sargent, M. D., Copps, T. P., Lievaart, P. A., and Szekely, J. G. (1979) Two modes of entry of reovirus particles into L cells. *J. Gen. Virol.* **45**, 161–170.
61. Georgi, A., Mottola-Hartshorn, C., Warner, A., Fields, B., and Chen, L. B. (1990) Detection of individual fluorescently labeled reovirions in living cells. *Proc. Natl. Acad. Sci. USA* **87**, 6579–6583.
62. Rubin, D. H., Weiner, D. B., Dworkin, C., Greene, M. I., Maul, G. G., and Williams, W. V. (1992) Receptor utilization by reovirus type 3: distinct binding sites on thymoma and fibroblast cell lines result in differential compartmentalization of virions. *Microb. Pathog.* **12**, 351–365.
63. Sturzenbecker, L. J., Nibert, M., Furlong, D., and Fields, B. N. (1987) Intracellular digestion of reovirus particles requires a low pH and is an essential step in the viral infectious cycle. *J. Virol.* **61**, 2351–2361.
64. Canning, W. M. and Fields, B. N. (1983) Ammonium chloride prevents lytic growth of reovirus and helps to establish persistent infection in mouse L cells. *Science* **219**, 987–988.
65. Dryden, K. A., Wang, G., Yeager, M., et al. (1993) Early steps in reovirus infection are associated with dramatic changes in supramolecular structure and protein conformation: analysis of virions and subviral particles by cryoelectron microscopy and image reconstruction. *J. Cell Biol.* **122**, 1023–1041.
66. Faust, M., Hastings, K. E., and Millward, S. (1975) m7G5'ppp5'GmptcpUp at the 5' terminus of reovirus messenger RNA. *Nucleic Acids Res.* **2**, 1329–1343.
67. Furuichi, Y., Morgan, M., Muthukrishnan, S., and Shatkin, A. J. (1975) Reovirus messenger RNA contains a methylated, blocked 5'-terminal structure: m-7G(5()ppp(5()G-MpCp. *Proc. Natl. Acad. Sci. USA* **72**, 362–366.
68. Zou, S. and Brown, E. G. (1992) Identification of sequence elements containing signals for replication and encapsidation of the reovirus M1 genome segment. *Virology* **186**, 377–388.
69. Chapell, J. D., Goral, M. I., Rodgers, S. E., dePamphilis, C. W., and Dermody, T. S. (1994) Sequence diversity within the reovirus S2 gene: reovirus genes reassort in nature, and their termini are predicted to form a panhandle motif. *J. Virol.* **68**, 750–756.
70. Zarbl, H., Skup, D., and Millward, S. (1980) Reovirus progeny subviral particles synthesize uncapped mRNA. *J. Virol.* **34**, 497–505.
71. Ito, Y. and Joklik, W. K. (1972) Temperature-sensitive mutants of reovirus. I. Patterns of gene expression by mutants of groups C, D, and E. *Virology* **50**, 189–201.
72. Hashiro, G., Loh, P. C., and Yau, J. T. (1977) The preferential cytotoxicity of reovirus for certain transformed cell lines. *Arch. Virol.* **54**, 307–315

73. Duncan, M. R., Stanish, S. M., and Cox, D. C. (1978) Differential sensitivity of normal and transformed human cells to reovirus infection. *J. Virol.* **28,** 444–449.

74. Strong, J. E., Tang, D., and Lee, P. W. (1993) Evidence that the epidermal growth factor receptor on host cells confers reovirus infection efficiency. *Virology* **197,** 405–411.

75. Tang, D., Strong, J. E., and Lee, P. W. (1993) Recognition of the epidermal growth factor receptor by reovirus. *Virology* **197,** 412–414.

76. Strong, J. E. and Lee, P. W. (1996) The v-erbB oncogene confers enhanced cellular susceptibility to reovirus infection. *J. Virol.* **70,** 612–616.

77. Libermann, T. A., Nusbaum, H. R., Razon, N., et al. (1985) Amplification, enhanced expression and possible rearrangement of EGF receptor gene in primary human brain tumours of glial origin. *Nature* **313,** 144–147.

78. Guha, A., Dashner, K., Black, P. M., Wagner, J. A., and Stiles, C. D. (1995) Expression of PDGF and PDGF receptors in human astrocytoma operation specimens supports the existence of an autocrine loop. *Int. J. Cancer* **60,** 168–173.

79. Shamah, S. M., Stiles, C. D., and Guha, A. (1993) Dominant-negative mutants of platelet-derived growth factor revert the transformed phenotype of human astrocytoma cells. *Mol. Cell Biol.* **13,** 7203–7212.

80. Helseth, E., Unsgaard, G., Dalen, A., et al. (1988) Amplification of the epidermal growth factor receptor gene in biopsy specimens from human intracranial tumours. *Br. J. Neurosurg.* **2,** 217–225

81. Guha, A. (1998) Ras activation in astrocytomas and neurofibromas. *Can. J. Neurol. Sci.* **25,** 267–281.

82. Slamon, D. J., Godolphin, W., Jones, L. A., et al. (1989) Studies of the HER-2/neu proto-oncogene in human breast and ovarian cancer. *Science* **244,** 707–712.

83. Ross, J. S. and Fletcher, J. A. (1998) The HER-2/neu oncogene in breast cancer: prognostic factor, predictive factor, and target for therapy. *Oncologist* **3,** 237–252

84. Koenders, P. G., Beex, L. V., Geurts-Moespot, A., Heuvel, J. J., Kienhuis, C. B., and Benraad, T. J. (1991) Epidermal growth factor receptor-negative tumors are predominantly confined to the subgroup of estradiol receptor-positive human primary breast cancers. *Cancer Res.* **51,** 4544–4548.

85. Shackney, S. E., Pollice, A. A., Smith, C. A., et al. (1998) Intracellular coexpression of epidermal growth factor receptor, Her-2/neu, and p21ras in human breast cancers: evidence for the existence of distinctive patterns of genetic evolution that are common to tumors from different patients. *Clin. Cancer Res.* **4,** 913–928.

86. Jacobs, C. and Rubsamen, H. (1983) Expression of pp60c-src protein kinase in adult and fetal human tissue: high activities in some sarcomas and mammary carcinomas. *Cancer Res.* **43,** 1696–1702.

87. Verbeek, B. S., Vroom, T. M., Adriaansen-Slot, S. S., et al. (1996) c-Src protein expression is increased in human breast cancer. An immunohistochemical and biochemical analysis. *J. Pathol.* **180,** 383–388.

88. Schlessinger, J. (1993) How receptor tyrosine kinases activate Ras. *Trends Biochem. Sci.* **18,** 273–275.

89. Campbell, S. L., Khosravi-Far, R., Rossman, K. L., Clark, G. J., and Der, C. J. (1998) Increasing complexity of Ras signaling. *Oncogene* **17,** 1395–1413.

90. Vojtek, A. B. and Der, C. J. (1998) Increasing complexity of the Ras signaling pathway. *J. Biol. Chem.* **273,** 19,925–19,928.

91. Kavanaugh, W. M. and Williams, L. T. (1994) An alternative to SH2 domains for binding tyrosine-phosphorylated proteins. *Science* **266,** 1862–1865.

92. Batzer, A. G., Blaikie, P., Nelson, K., Schlessinger, J., and Margolis, B. (1995) The phosphotyrosine interaction domain of Shc binds an LXNPXY motif on the epidermal growth factor receptor. *Mol. Cell Biol.* **15,** 4403–4409.

93. Egan, S. E., Giddings, B. W., Brooks, M. W., Buday, L., Sizeland, A. M., and Weinberg, R. A. (1993) Association of Sos Ras exchange protein with Grb2 is implicated in tyrosine kinase signal transduction and transformation. *Nature* **363,** 45–51.

94. Pelicci, G., Lanfrancone, L., Grignani, F., et al. (1992) A novel transforming protein (SHC) with an SH2 domain is implicated in mitogenic signal transduction. *Cell* **70,** 93–104.

95. Buday, L. and Downward, J. (1993) Epidermal growth factor regulates p21ras through the formation of a complex of receptor, Grb2 adapter protein, and Sos nucleotide exchange factor. *Cell* **73,** 611–620.

96. Shields, J. M., Pruitt, K., McFall, A., Shaub, A., and Der, C. J. (2000) Understanding Ras: "it ain't over 'til it's over." *Trends Cell Biol.* **10,** 147–154.

97. Wolthuis, R. M., de Ruiter, N. D., Cool, R. H., and Bos, J. L. (1997) Stimulation of gene induction and cell growth by the Ras effector Rlf. *EMBO J.* **16,** 6748–6761.

98. Bischoff, J. R. and Samuel, C. E. (1989) Mechanism of interferon action. Activation of the human P1/eIF-2 alpha protein kinase by individual reovirus s-class mRNAs: s1 mRNA is a potent activator relative to s4 mRNA. *Virology* **172,** 106–115.

99. Thomis, D. C. and Samuel, C. E. (1993) Mechanism of interferon action: evidence for intermolecular autophosphorylation and autoactivation of the interferon-induced, RNA-dependent protein kinase PKR. *J. Virol.* **67,** 7695–7700.

100. Levin, D. H., Petryshyn, R., and London, I. M. (1980) Characterization of double-stranded-RNA-activated kinase that phosphorylates alpha subunit of eukaryotic initiation factor 2 (eIF-2 alpha) in reticulocyte lysates. *Proc. Natl. Acad. Sci. USA* **77,** 832–836.

101. Panniers, R. and Henshaw, E. C. (1983) A GDP/GTP exchange factor essential for eukaryotic initiation factor 2 cycling in Ehrlich ascites tumor cells and its regulation by eukaryotic initiation factor 2 phosphorylation. *J. Biol. Chem.* **258,** 7928–7934.

102. Mundschau, L. J. and Faller, D. V. (1992) Oncogenic ras induces an inhibitor of double-stranded RNA-dependent eukaryotic initiation factor 2 alpha-kinase activation. *J. Biol. Chem.* **267,** 23,092–23,098.

103. Wilcox, M. E., Yang, W., Senger, D., et al. (2001) Reovirus as an oncolytic agent against experimental human malignant gliomas. *J. Natl. Cancer Inst.* **93,** 903–912.

104. Clarke, P., Meintzer, S. M., Spalding, A. C., Johnson, G. L., and Tyler, K. L. (2001) Caspase 8-dependent sensitization of cancer cells to TRAIL-induced apoptosis following reovirus-infection. *Oncogene* **20,** 6910–6919.

105. Connolly, J. L. and Dermody, T. S. (2002) Virion disassembly is required for apoptosis induced by reovirus. *J. Virol.* **76,** 1632–1641.

106. Clark, G. J., Westwick, J. K., and Der, C. J. (1997) p120 GAP modulates Ras activation of Jun kinases and transformation. *J. Biol. Chem.* **272,** 1677–1681.

107. Bos, J. L. (1989) ras oncogenes in human cancer: a review. *Cancer Res.* **49,** 4682–4689.

108. Forrester, K., Almoguera, C., Han, K., Grizzle, W. E., and Perucho, M. (1987) Detection of high incidence of K-ras oncogenes during human colon tumorigenesis. *Nature* **327,** 298–303.

109. Almoguera, C., Shibata, D., Forrester, K., Martin, J., Arnheim, N., and Perucho, M. (1988) Most human carcinomas of the exocrine pancreas contain mutant c-K-ras genes. *Cell* **53,** 549–554.

110. Varras, M. N., Sourvinos, G., Diakomanolis, E., et al. (1999) Detection and clinical correlations of ras gene mutations in human ovarian tumors. *Oncology* **56,** 89–96.

111. Caduff, R. F., Svoboda-Newman, S. M., Ferguson, A. W., Johnston, C. M., and Frank, T. S. (1999) Comparison of mutations of Ki-RAS and p53 immunoreactivity in borderline and malignant epithelial ovarian tumors. *Am. J. Surg. Pathol.* **23,** 323–328.

112. Haas, C. J., Diebold, J., Hirschmann, A., Rohrbach, H., and Lohrs, U. (1999) In serous ovarian neoplasms the frequency of Ki-ras mutations correlates with their malignant potential. *Virchows Arch.* **434,** 117–120.

113. Slebos, R. J., Kibbelaar, R. E., Dalesio, O., et al. (1990) K-ras oncogene activation as a prognostic marker in adenocarcinoma of the lung. *N. Engl. J. Med.* **323,** 561–565.

114. Beaupre, D. M. and Kurzrock, R. (1999) RAS and leukemia: from basic mechanisms to gene-directed therapy. *J. Clin. Oncol.* **17,** 1071–1079.

115. Norman, K. L., Coffey, M. C., Hirasawa, K., et al. (2002) Reovirus oncolysis of human breast cancer. *Hum. Gene Ther.* **13,** 641–652.

116. Hirasawa, K., Nishikawa, S. G., Norman, K. L., Alain, T., Kossakowska, A., and Lee, P. W. (2002) Oncolytic reovirus against ovarian and colon cancer. *Cancer Res.* **62,** 1696–1701.

117. Alain, T., Hirasawa, K., Pon, K. J., et al. (2002) Reovirus therapy of lymphoid malignancies. *Blood* **100,** 4146–4153.

118. Hirasawa, K., Nishikawa, S. G., Norman, K. L., et al. (2003) Systemic reovirus therapy of metastatic cancer in immune-competent mice. *Cancer Res.* **63,** 348–353.

119. Kloog, Y. and Cox, A. D. (2000) RAS inhibitors: potential for cancer therapeutics. *Mol. Med. Today* **6,** 398–402.

120. Dudley, D. T., Pang, L., Decker, S. J., Bridges, A. J., and Saltiel, A. R. (1995) A synthetic inhibitor of the mitogen-activated protein kinase cascade. *Proc. Natl. Acad. Sci. USA* **92,** 7686–7689.

121. Herrmann, C., Block, C., Geisen, C., et al. (1998) Sulindac sulfide inhibits Ras signaling. *Oncogene* **17,** 1769–1776.

122. James, G. L., Goldstein, J. L., Brown, M. S., et al. (1993) Benzodiazepine peptidomimetics: potent inhibitors of Ras farnesylation in animal cells. *Science* **260,** 1937–1942.

123. Kohl, N. E., Mosser, S. D., deSolms, S. J., et al. (1993) Selective inhibition of ras-dependent transformation by a farnesyltransferase inhibitor. *Science* **260,** 1934–1937.

124. Kohl, N. E., Omer, C. A., Conner, M. W., et al. (1995) Inhibition of farnesyltransferase induces regression of mammary and salivary carcinomas in ras transgenic mice. *Nat. Med.* **1,** 792–797.

125. Liu, M., Bryant, M. S., Chen, J., et al. (1998) Antitumor activity of SCH 66336, an orally bioavailable tricyclic inhibitor of farnesyl protein transferase, in human tumor xenograft models and wap-ras transgenic mice. *Cancer Res.* **58,** 4947–4956.

126. Sepp-Lorenzino, L., Ma, Z., Rands, E., et al. (1995) A peptidomimetic inhibitor of farnesyl:protein transferase blocks the anchorage-dependent and -independent growth of human tumor cell lines. *Cancer Res.* **55,** 5302–5309.

127. Whyte, D. B., Kirschmeier, P., Hockenberry, T. N., et al. (1997) K- and N-Ras are geranylgeranylated in cells treated with farnesyl protein transferase inhibitors. *J. Biol. Chem.* **272,** 14,459–14,464.

128. Marom, M., Haklai, R., Ben-Baruch, G., Marciano, D., Egozi, Y., and Kloog, Y. (1995) Selective inhibition of Ras-dependent cell growth by farnesylthiosalisylic acid. *J. Biol. Chem.* **270,** 22,263–22,270.

129. Haklai, R., Weisz, M. G., Elad, G., et al. (1998) Dislodgment and accelerated degradation of Ras. *Biochemistry* **37,** 1306–1314.

130. Jansen, B., Schlagbauer-Wadl, H., Kahr, H., et al. (1999) Novel Ras antagonist blocks human melanoma growth. *Proc. Natl. Acad. Sci. USA* **96,** 14,019–14,024.

17

Antiangiogenic Gene Therapy of Cancer

Steve Gyorffy, Jack Gauldie, A. Keith Stewart, and Xiao-Yan Wen

1. ANTIANGIOGENIC GENE THERAPY OF CANCER

It has been well established that tumor growth depends on angiogenesis, the process of continued expansion of endothelial cells from preexisting blood vessels *(1,2)*. Tumors *in situ*, which are smaller than 3 mm in diameter, exist in a prevascular state and are limited in their ability to grow without perfusion from the blood supply. Without such a neovascularization process, these dormant tumors remain microscopic in size and quiescent for years *(1,3)*. The recruitment of new blood vessels increases the availability of oxygen and metabolites to the tumor and removes waste products. Moreover, this newly formed vasculature facilitates the escape of tumor cells to distant regions of the body, where they may form detectable metastases *(4,5)*. Evidence suggests that new vessel growth from bone marrow-derived endothelial precursor cells also contributes to tumor blood vessel development *(6,7)*.

The inhibition of tumor angiogenesis, therefore, is an important potential therapy for all types of malignancies, including both solid tumors and the bone marrow in hematological malignancies. The inhibition or regression of a single capillary can have an impact on the growth of a large number of tumor cells. Therapies designed to inhibit new blood vessel formation have the advantage that they target the genetically stable endothelial cells supporting the tumor growth, and it is potentially less likely that resistance to antiangiogenic therapy will develop. In contrast, current standard chemotherapies designed to attack genetically unstable tumor cells can result in rapid resistance to the chemotherapeutic agent *(8,9)*.

Angiogenesis is a complex, multistep process that in the adult also involves normal physiological processes, including the female reproductive system *(10,11)* and wound healing *(12)*. In addition to tumor growth, neovascularization plays an important role in many pathological processes, including arthritis *(13,14)*, endometriosis *(15)*, diabetic retinopathy, and macular degeneration *(16,17)*.

The angiogenic process has been well described in the literature by numerous groups *(1,18)*. Endothelial cells within a capillary or postcapillary venule receive proangiogenic stimuli from soluble growth factors, including vascular endothelial growth factor (VEGF) and basic fibroblast growth factor (bFGF), in a paracrine manner from surrounding tumor or stromal cells and from the extracellular matrix pool. Degradation of the basement membrane by serine proteases, such as plasmin and matrix metalloproteinases (MMPs), occurs following endothelial cell activation, enabling endothelial cells to migrate from the established vessel toward the angiogenic stimuli *(1,18,19)*. Normally quiescent endothelial cells trailing behind the migrating cells rapidly proliferate and replace cells that have moved toward the developing capillary sprouts. The sprouting endothelial cells form tubes and connect to other blood vessels, permitting blood to flow. These primordial capillaries do not yet have supporting pericytes, but begin to express the formation of basement membrane.

From: *Contemporary Cancer Research*
Cancer Gene Therapy
Edited by: D. T. Curiel and J. T. Douglas © Humana Press Inc., Totowa, NJ

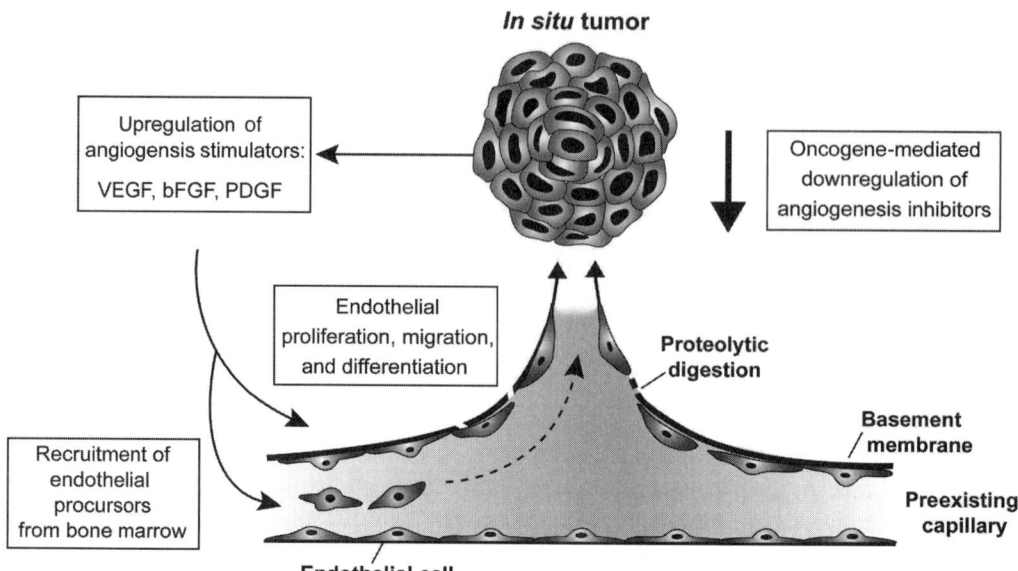

Fig. 1. The mechanism of tumor angiogenesis. Proangiogenic factors produced by tumor cells, including vascular endothelial growth factor (VEGF), stimulate quiescent endothelial cells in nearby preexisting capillaries. The activated endothelial cells proliferate and secrete proteolytic enzymes that degrade the extracellular matrix, allowing the cells to migrate toward the tumor. The migrating cells deposit new basement membrane along the newly sprouting blood vessel. In addition, endothelial precursor cells may be recruited from the bone marrow into the newly formed capillary. Vessel stabilization is achieved by the recruitment of pericytes, which are attracted by platelet-derived growth factor (PDGF) released by the endothelial cells.

Angiopoietin 1/Tie2 (tyrosine kinase 2)receptor activation initiates endothelial quiescence, vessel maturation with the completion of the basement membrane, and the recruitment of mesenchymal cells, which will eventually become pericytes *(20–22)*. Unlike physiological angiogenesis in normal tissue, tumor blood vessels do not undergo this maturation process. These vessels remain immature and leaky as a result of angiopoietin 2, the antagonist to angiopoietin 1, which provides a destabilization signal to blood vessels, promoting additional vascular remodeling in the presence of angiogenic growth factors *(23,24)* (Fig. 1).

Tumor neovascularization does not simply arise from the overexpression of proangiogenic growth factors. Folkman and Hanahan proposed the presence of an "angiogenic switch" to describe the shift in the balance between positive and negative regulatory factors controlling endothelial growth, proliferation and vascular formation within a tumor *(25)*. Genetic regulation via lowered expression of negative regulators of angiogenesis, under the normal control of tumor suppressor genes and the upregulation of angiogenic stimuli related to oncogene expression, contributes to the development of the angiogenic phenotype (Fig. 1).

In addition to angiogenic growth factors such as VEGF and bFGF, over 28 positive mediators of angiogenesis have been identified. Counteracting these factors are more than 50 known endogenous angiogenic inhibitors. A number of these inhibitors are proteolytic fragments of larger molecules identified as possessing antiangiogenic activity. They include angiostatin, endostatin, canstatin, vasostatin, and the two recently identified peptides tumstatin and endorepellin *(26–30)*.

Systemic administration of recombinant protein angiogenesis inhibitors has been effective in regressing tumors in preclinical mouse models *(31–33)*. Moreover, with exception of the antiangiogenic cytokines *(34)*, the inhibitors angiostatin and endostatin in particular have been safe on prolonged administration, with no apparent side effects reported. This is likely because of the specificity of these inhibitors for endothelial cells contributing to tumor angiogenesis *(12,31,32)*. Animal studies have indicated that recombinant antiangiogenic proteins will have to be administered to patients repeatedly, over extended periods, at high therapeutic doses to achieve successful tumor regressions *(9,35,36)*. These recombinant proteins are difficult to manufacture and purify in large quantities for practical clinical use. The recombinant proteins have also been reported to be unstable and may exhibit short plasma half-lives as a result of altered glycosylation *(32,37)*. Given the technical and inherent cost for manufacturing endogenous recombinant angiogenesis inhibitors for clinical use, gene therapy could deliver sustained levels of circulating proteins made directly from within the cells of a patient infused with the vector.

2. ANTIANGIOGENIC GENE THERAPY STRATEGIES

Two gene therapy strategies have been proposed for the delivery of antiangiogenic proteins. The first involves systemic gene therapy, by which vectors injected into the patient would produce high circulating levels of the angiogenic inhibitor *(38)*. The rationale is based on the lack of toxicity seen in preclinical mouse models and early phase I clinical trials using angiostatin or endostatin protein *(27,39)*. However, toxicity from systemic administration of the vector could be a potential side effect, especially when using viral vectors.

The second strategy, local, tumor-directed antiangiogenic gene therapy, aims to increase levels of antiangiogenic proteins in the tumor environment *(40)*. This approach would maintain high levels of protein in the tumor and could limit systemic toxicity because of the biological properties of the protein or the vector. However, potential limitations may occur with this approach, especially when treating tumors that are not accessible for vector delivery or in treating multiple metastases.

As with other antiangiogenic therapies, including recombinant proteins, monoclonal antibodies, or small molecular weight signal transduction inhibitors, potential transgenes can be categorized as "direct" or "indirect" inhibitors of angiogenesis *(2)*. Direct inhibitors specifically target the endothelial cells in the tumor, whereas the indirect approach targets the ability of the tumor or other bystander cells to produce angiogenic growth factors such as VEGF or bFGF *(38)*. These factors add a layer of complexity to how antiangiogenic gene therapy would be applied to different tumor types. Although inhibition of neovascularization conceptually may be a ubiquitous therapy to cancer treatment, in practice the success of antiangiogenic gene therapy will depend on the ability to optimize the vector system with a suitable transgene and may be specific for a tumor type.

Antiangiogenic gene therapy employing nonviral, such as plasmid or naked deoxyribonucleic acid (DNA) administration, and viral strategies, such as adenovirus, adeno-associated virus, retrooncovirus, and lentivirus has been employed in numerous rodent tumor models (Table 1). The majority of these approaches have used transgenes directly cytotoxic to tumor endothelium, such as angiostatin and endostatin. Other approaches have examined inhibiting the proangiogenic growth factors as well as the invasive process by targeting MMPs or serine protease pathways (Fig. 2).

3. PLASMID- AND CELL-BASED THERAPIES

Polymer-encapsulated DNA plasmid-based therapy expressing human endostatin was effective in delaying the growth of subcutaneous Renca and Lewis lung carcinoma (LLC) in mice. This study demonstrated that an intramuscular injection of a polymer–plasmid complex could maintain detectable levels of circulating endostatin in treated mice for 14 days *(41)*. In a lung metastases model, pretreatment of mice with a single intramuscular injection of the plasmid, followed by a second injection 1 week later could significantly reduce the number of lung tumor nodules *(41)*. The results of this study demonstrated the feasibility of using repeated intramuscular injections of plasmid complexes to induce modest inhibition of tumor growth without the development of an immune response to the vector. The lack of an immune response, safety, and the relative ease of preparation of the polymer–plasmid complex for delivery are attractive features of this system.

Table 1
Examples of Antiangiogenic Cancer Gene Therapy in Rodent Models

Vector	Gene	Reference
Plasmid	Endostatin	*41*
	Angiostatin	*42,43*
Plasmid-transfected cells	Endostatin, angiostatin	*44*
	Endostatin	*45,46*
	Thrombospondin	*49*
Endothelial precursor stem cell	Soluble VEGFR2 (Flk-1)	*47*
Adenovirus	Angiostatin	*53,54*
	IL-12	*54*
	Endostatin	*56–60*
	Soluble VEGFR1 (Flt-1)	*61*
	Soluble VEGFR2 (Flk-1)	*60,62*
	TIE-2	*60*
	TIMPs	*65,66*
Adeno associated virus	VEGF antisense	*70*
	Angiostatin	*71,72*
	Soluble VEGFR1 (Flt-1)	*73*
Lentivirus/stem cells	(Tie2/Tek) promoter/thymidine kinase	*48*
Moloney murine leukemia virus	Endostatin, angiostatin	*75*
	Platelet factor 4 (PF4)	*76*
	Dominant negative Flk-1	*77*

Local injection of liposome-plasmid vectors expressing angiostatin or endostatin reduced tumor growth by 36 and 49%, respectively, following three intratumor injections in a breast cancer model *(42)*. In a parallel study, the intravenous systemic administration of the liposome-plasmid complex expressing endostatin reduced tumor size by 40% compared to controls *(42)*.

In a transgenic mouse model of breast cancer in which the HER2/neu oncogene is driven by the murine mammary tumor virus (MMTV) promoter, a liposome-plasmid vector expressing angiostatin was injected into the mammary glands of mice before detectable tumors had formed. Mice receiving the angiostatin gene had a significant decrease in the number and size of breast tumors compared to controls. Lung metastases were absent in the treated animals, demonstrating a local and systemic effect of the antiangiogenic therapy *(43)*.

Implantation of cells transfected ex vivo with plasmids carrying angiostatin or endostatin complementary DNA have been reported to inhibit tumor growth locally and systemically. Transfection of the highly angiogenic murine T241 fibrosarcoma with angiostatin suppressed the primary tumor growth and could inhibit the development of micrometastases in the lungs of mice *(44)*. Microencapsulation of baby hamster kidney cells transfected with endostatin into alginate-poly-L-lysine beads was demonstrated to inhibit the growth of human glioblastoma in a subcutaneous nude mouse model *(45)*. A single subcutaneous injection of 2×10^5 engineered cells continuously secreted endostatin and inhibited tumor growth by 62% over a 3-week period *(45)*.

In an intracerebral model of brain cancer, encapsulated endostatin plasmid transfected 293 cells implanted into the brain reduced tumor blood vessel formation, increasing survival of animals by 85% *(46)*. The implanted cells were viable and secreted endostatin for 4 months. Long-term expression and minimal development of an immune response against the encapsulated cells is an attractive feature of this antiangiogenic gene therapy procedure.

Stem cells or endothelial precursor cells have been shown to be important in tumor neovascularization *(7)*. Potentially, these cells transduced with antiangiogenic genes may be important delivery

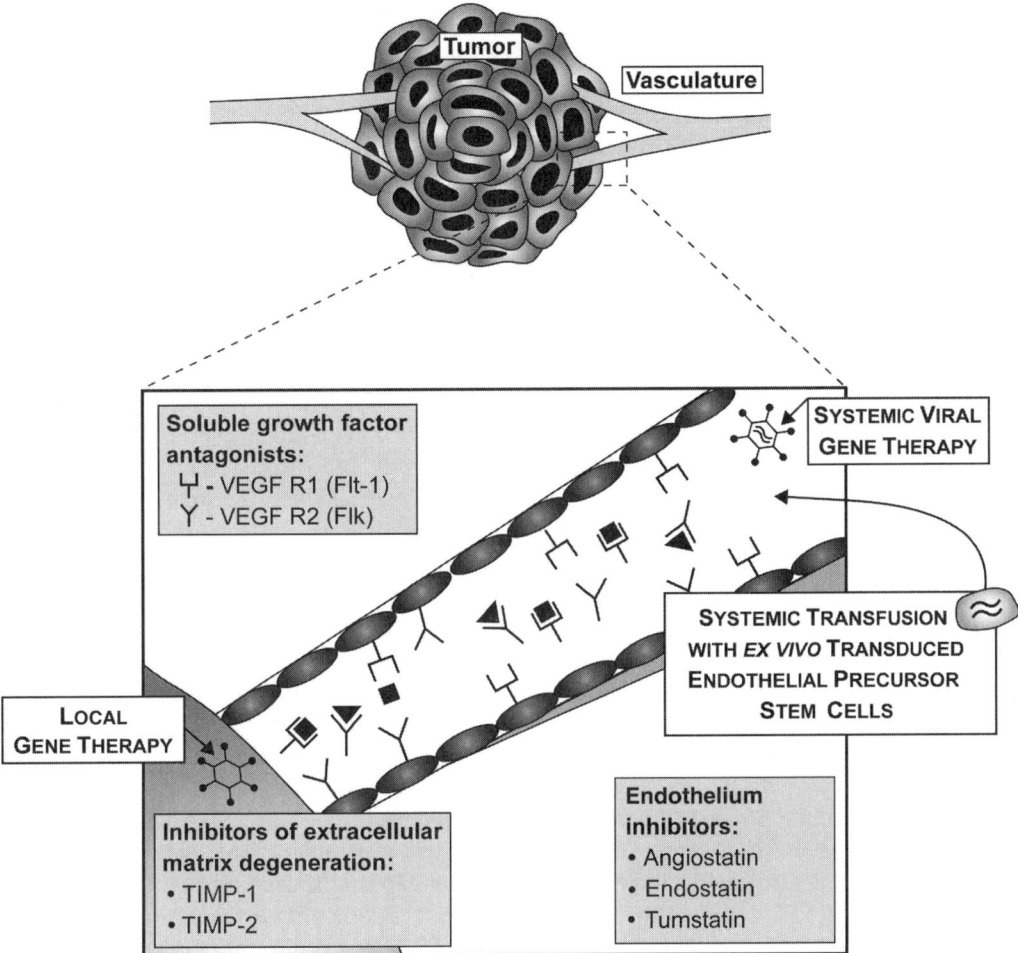

Fig. 2. Modes of inhibition by direct antiangiogenic gene therapy. Direct antiangiogenesis gene therapy targets the active tumor endothelial cells. Vectors may be injected directly into the tumor or delivered systemically via the circulation. Ex vivo-transduced endothelial precursor cells injected systemically, home to sites of angiogenesis, providing local production of angiogenic inhibitor. Inhibition of new vessel growth is accomplished with transgenes expressing endothelial cell inhibitors, blockage of proangiogenic endothelial growth factors, and impeding extracellular matrix degradation.

vehicles that could be injected systemically, yet home directly to regions of tumor growth *(47,48)*. This form of cell therapy could be practical given that autologous endothelial precursor cells could be isolated from the patient's bone marrow or directly from the blood *(49)*.

An alternative ex vivo approach has used cell factories grown on scaffold implants. Interperitoneal implants of biodegradable polyglycolic acid sheets seeded with NIH3T3 fibroblasts transfected with a retrovirus expressing thrombospondin-2 demonstrated inhibition of angiogenesis and tumor growth in squamous cell carcinoma, melanoma, and LLC tumor models *(50)*. The success of ex vivo-implanted transfected cells in human studies to inhibit tumor neovascularization may be dependent on finding suitable cells that can be safely implanted into the host.

A novel targeting strategy utilizing nanoparticles has been reported. Hood and colleagues developed a cationic nanoparticle coupled to a small organic ligand targeting the integrin $\alpha_v\beta_3$ of angiogenic endothelium *(51)*. Intravenous delivery of the $\alpha_v\beta_3$ ligand-NP conjugated to the signal transduction molecule Raf, which was mutated to be incapable of binding adenosine triphosphate, blocked endothelial signaling pathways and angiogenesis. This resulted in apoptosis of tumor-associated endothelium and induced regression of established primary and metastatic tumors (51). The use of nanoparticles may have significant advantages over viral vectors because they are not immunogenic and may be applied repeatedly for sustained treatment of tumor and metastases.

3.1. Adenoviral Delivery of Angiogenesis Inhibitors

Replication-deficient, first-generation adenoviral vectors have been used in the majority of antiangiogenic gene therapy studies in murine tumor models. These vectors have numerous advantages for gene therapy, including the ability to infect replicating and nonreplicating cells, high transient gene expression, no association with human malignancy, and the ability to manufacture high titers of virus. The application of these vectors is limited, however, by host cellular and humoral immune responses that develop after the initial vector administration (52,53).

A human type 5 adenoviral vector expressing murine angiostatin (Ad-angiostatin) has been described. This vector was shown to be effective in vitro, inhibiting the growth of cultured endothelial cells and neovascularization in a bFGF-driven matrigel model of angiogenesis. The addition of 10^9 plaque-forming units (pfu) of virus resulted in apoptosis of the migrating endothelial cells in a matrigel plug 1 week after subcutaneous implantation (54). In a pulmonary metastatic breast cancer model, intranasal delivery of the vector into the lungs significantly reduced the tumor burden and could delay the appearance of visible tumor nodules. Local 5- to 10-day overexpression by direct injection of Ad-angiostatin into transgenic mice bearing implanted transgenic breast tumors delayed tumor growth and increased the survival of treated mice by 3 weeks compared to controls. Microvessel density as measured by CD31 staining was significantly decreased, whereas tumor necrosis and apoptosis increased in the angiostatin-treated tumors (55).

Similar results were found when using the potent antiangiogenic cytokine interleukin 12 (IL-12) expressed locally from the tumor. Tumor growth kinetics during the initial 2 weeks was similar for both Ad-angiostatin- or Ad-IL-12-treated tumors. During this period, microvessel density of the tumors decreased to levels seen with angiostatin (55). Unlike the angiostatin-treated mice, a small percentage of mice treated with IL-12 continued to have total tumor regression. These regressions were a result of this cytokine's immune stimulatory ability to mount a T-cell-specific immune response (55,56). The results from both the primary and metastatic breast cancer models demonstrated that, although the expression of angiostatin could delay tumor growth, this was insufficient to induce total regression of established tumors. The combination of angiostatin and IL-12 was significantly more potent in decreasing microvessel density and inhibiting tumor growth. Mice treated with this combination therapy had a significant increase in life-span and an overall total tumor regression of 54% (55).

Mice treated with Ad-angiostatin by intratumoral, intranasal, or intraperitoneal administration had a 30% increase in weight gain (15). This side effect occurred within 2 weeks of the vector administration in both FVB and C57Bl/6 female mice. Examination of these mice revealed impaired ovarian function and decreased estradiol and progesterone levels consistent with the onset of menopause (15). The data strongly indicated that high circulating levels of angiostatin can affect normal physiological angiogenesis of the female reproductive system (15). These results indicated that careful monitoring of female patients of reproductive age might be required during antiangiogenic gene therapy treatment regimes.

Numerous groups have reported the efficacy of adenoviral gene transfer of endostatin in a variety of tumor models (57–61). The results of Wen and coworkers indicated that systemic intravenous administration of the vector resulted in high circulating endostatin protein levels for more than 2 months in 129/J mice. In contrast, Balb/c mice receiving an identical dose of vector had significantly lower endostatin levels that persisted for only a short time (62). These results may indicate a stain difference in how genes are regulated from the expression cassette of the vector. In a metastatic lung tumor model, systemic injection of the vector significantly reduced EOMA metastases compared to vector control-treated 129/J mice. However, no reduction in B16 metastatic melanoma growth was found using the identical viral dose in C57Bl/6 mice *(62)*.

In an orthotopic colon metastases model to the liver, systemic adenoviral endostatin gene therapy protected 25% of mice from developing metastatic lesions. This study took advantage of the tropism of the adenoviral vector for the liver and aimed at creating a poor angiogenic environment for the developing colon metastases *(58)*. Preadministration of adenoviral vectors expressing endostatin was also effective at inhibiting tumor development in a transgenic breast cancer mouse model. Angioprevention, via systemic administration of the vector, could delay the switch from per-invasive mammary lesions to invasion carcinomas *(60)*.

Adenoviral gene therapy using receptor antagonists targeting angiogenic growth factors has been reported to be effective. Vectors expressing soluble receptors to VEGF have demonstrated promising results in animal models. Intramuscular injection of a vector producing soluble VEGFR1 (Flt-1 [fms-like tyrosine kinase]) fused to the Fc portion of immunoglobulin G could inhibit the growth of a high-VEGF-secreting lung tumor *(63)*. Circulating levels of the VEGF antagonist could be detected for 21 days, and no toxicity to the animals was found. Soluble Flt-1 was also effective in reducing the growth of T241 fibrosarcoma and LLC when the vector was given intravenously *(61)*. This report also demonstrated the effectiveness of an adeno vector producing soluble VEGFR2 (Flk-Fc [fatal liver kinase-FC]) at inhibiting the growth of subcutaneous prostate and colon tumors in SCID mice. These results demonstrated the effectiveness of both VEGF receptors in inhibiting the growth of various tumor types. However, unexplained toxicity, the formation of ascites followed by mortality, was reported when the Flt-1 vector was used *(61)*.

Adenovirus expressing soluble Tie2 inhibited the growth of primary and metastatic tumors. Lin and coworkers *(64)* demonstrated that systemic delivery of this vector acted in a manner mimicking the actions of angiopoitein 2, inducing vascular disruption, resulting in regression of tumor vessels.

Delivery of tissue inhibitors of metalloproteinases (TIMPs), the natural antagonists of MMPs, has been studied for inhibition of tumor cell invasion and angiogenesis. Vectors expressing TIMP1 or TIMP2 inhibited the tumor invasiveness of intraperitoneal pancreatic cancer cells in mice when the adenovirus was administered early in tumor development *(65)*. Direct injection of a vector expressing Ad-TIMP2 was effective at inhibiting the growth of primary LLC as well as reducing the number of metastases to the lung *(66)*. Significant reduction in microvessel density was observed by vWF staining; however, the overall survival benefit was just 12 days as compared to control-treated animals.

The shortcomings of current adenoviral gene transfer aimed at the inhibition of angiogenesis may be alleviated by the third-generation, "helper-dependent" adenoviral systems. Parks and coworkers developed a helper-dependent adenovirus vector system with the removal of all viral coding sequences. These vectors can subsequently be used to carry up to 33.6 kb of exogenous DNA *(67,68)*. Moreover, because these vectors do not express viral proteins, they have much-reduced host immune responses, leading to prolonged expression of transgenes, ideal for antiangiogenic therapy. The advantages of this system have not yet been implemented in any in vitro or in vivo angiogenesis studies.

3.2. Adeno-Associated Virus Delivery of Antiangiogenic Genes

Recombinant adeno-associated viruses (rAAV) are replication-deficient, nonpathogenic vectors belonging to the group of human parvovirus. These vectors have great potential for cancer gene therapy because they can transduce both dividing and nondividing cells, are less immunogenic than other vectors, and can integrate into the host genome, allowing long-term transgene expression *(69)*. However, as with other integrating vector systems, a potential concern of insertional mutagenesis may limit applications.

Few reports have used these vectors to deliver antiangiogenic genes for cancer therapy. Nguyen and coworkers developed rAAV vectors containing the genes for angiostatin, endostatin, and antisense VEGF messenger ribonucleic acid *(70)*. The study demonstrated the production of active angiostatin and endo-statin protein and the ability to inhibit VEGF production from infected cultured tumor cells. How-ever, the study did not extend to animal models.

Ma and coworkers successfully treated rat models of brain tumors using intracranial or intramus-cular injection of rAAV-expressing angiostatin *(71,72)*. Stable transfection of C6 glioma cells with rAAV-angiostatin followed by intracranial implantation resulted in significant inhibition of tumor growth. Tumors reached a maximum volume 2 weeks after implantation, but shrank considerably by 5 weeks. In contrast, control transduced tumor cells achieved lethal tumor volumes within 3 weeks *(71)*. Similar regressions were observed by direct injection of the vector into preexisting brain tumors. Sur-vival increased significantly, with 40% of treated rats having small, poorly vascularized tumors at 6 months. This survival was further enhanced to 55% when an adenovirus expressing the suicide gene RSV*tk* was coinjected. Toxicity related to subsequent ganciclovir treatment limited higher survival rates *(71)*. In a follow-up study, a single injection of rAAV-angiostatin into the leg muscles of nude mice inhibited tumor vascularization and the intracranial growth of U87 cells. High circulating levels of angiostatin increased the long-term survival of the treatment group, with 40% of mice surviving more than 10 months *(71)*.

Long-term expression is a key benefit of rAAV vectors. Portal vein injection of a vector producing soluble Flk-1 demonstrated expression of the protein from the liver for up to 6 months *(73)*. This was shown to be effective in reducing tumor vessel density and the subsequent size of SK-NEP-1 tumors in subcutaneous and orthotopic mouse models *(73)*.

3.3. Retroviral Inhibition of Tumor Neovascularization

Retroviral-mediated gene therapy has been used by numerous groups to deliver long-term expression of angiogenic inhibitors in tumor models. The majority of these studies have used Moloney murine leu-kemia (MMuLv) retrooncoviruses. Replication-deficient, third-generation lentiviral vectors based on human immunodeficiency virus 1 have been developed for antiangiogenesis applications *(74)*. This is an effort to overcome the restriction of the ability of the MMuLv vectors to infect only dividing cells.

Combined retroviral delivery of angiostatin and endostatin was shown to act in a synergistic man-ner in treating models of melanoma and leukemia *(75)*. Mice implanted with MMuLv-transduced L1210 leukemia cells expressing both angiogenesis inhibitors had an overall tumor-free survival of 40%, whereas there was no survival advantage for the groups receiving cells transduced by angiostatin or endostatin alone *(75)*.

Retroviral vectors have also been used in rodent glioma models to deliver platelet factor 4 (PF4) and a dominant negative Flk1. Tanaka and coworkers demonstrated that, 14 days after implantation, RT2 glioma cells transduced with PF4 produced tumors that were small and with reduced vasculature *(76)*. In contrast, control tumors were hypervascularized and significantly larger. In a rat GS-9L glioma study, cells transduced with the dominant negative Flk1, lacking the intracellular signaling domain, could inhibit tumor growth when injected into the brain. No significant tumor reduction occurred when virus-containing supernatant was injected into preexisting tumors, highlighting the poor in vivo transduction efficiency of retroviral vectors *(77)*.

The major shortcomings of these studies are illustrated by the fact that tumor cells were stably trans-duced in vitro, followed by implantation of the cells into animals. This methodology runs counter to the previously described vector technologies, which were administered to preestablished tumors. Although these retroviral studies are important in demonstrating the beneficial effects of long-term angiogen-esis inhibitor expression, practical applications to the treatment of human tumors may be limited.

4. CONCLUSIONS

The study of angiogenesis is a field that has only been established in the last 30 years. During this period, it has been conclusively demonstrated that cancers require blood vessels to progress from premalignant, noninvasive growths into aggressive tumors that can metastasize to distant points in the body. The last decade has seen the emergence of numerous angiogenesis inhibitors, many of which are endogenous proteins or fragments of proteins found in the body. At present, clinical trials are evaluating the safety and efficacy of these inhibitors. These recombinant proteins have unique properties, and numerous hurdles have to be overcome to understand the mechanisms of action, the dosing schedule, and the biologic effectiveness in the clinic.

It has become evident that many of these protein inhibitors are structurally complex, and it is difficult to manufacture cost-effectively large quantities for use in cancer patients. The promise of gene therapy would alleviate this shortcoming as the patients could make the inhibitors directly in their own cells.

As with other cancer gene therapy applications, the major hurdle in the use of antiangiogenic approaches is the development of appropriate and safe vectors. The optimal gene therapy vector for antiangiogenesis therapy would deliver consistent, therapeutically efficacious amounts of the transgene for extended periods. In addition, the vector would have to be safe and poorly immunogenic to allow multiple applications because cancer patients may have to remain on these inhibitors for months to establish stabilization and ultimate regression of the disease. Ultimately, the appropriate vector used may depend on the type of cancer and the biological properties of the antiangiogenic transgene it carries. There is no doubt, however, that antiangiogenic gene therapy will be a significant treatment for cancer in the near future.

REFERENCES

1. Folkman, J. (1996) Clinical applications of research on angiogenesis. *N. Engl. J. Med.* **333,** 1757–1763.
2. Kerbel, R. and Folkman, J. (2002) Clinical translation of angiogenesis inhibitors. *Nat. Rev. Cancer* **2,** 727–739.
3. Udagawa, T., Fernandez, A., Achilles, E. G., Folkman, J., and D'Amato, R. J. (2002) Persistence of microscopic human cancers in mice: alterations in the angiogenic balance accompanies loss of tumor dormancy. *FASEB J.* **16,** 1361–1370.
4. Folkman, J. and Shing, Y. (1992) Angiogenesis. *J. Biol. Chem.* **267,** 10,931–10,934.
5. Fidler, I. J. and Ellis, L. M. (1994) The implications of angiogenesis for the biology and therapy of cancer metastasis. *Cell* **79,** 185–188.
6. Asahara, T., Takahashi, T., Masuda, H., et al. (1999) VEGF contributes to postnatal neovascularization by mobilizing bone marrow-derived endothelial progenitor cells. *EMBO J.* **18,** 3964–3972.
7. Lyden, D., Hattori, K., Dias, S., et al. (2001) Impaired recruitment of bone-marrow-derived endothelial and hematopoietic precursor cells blocks tumor angiogenesis and growth. *Nat. Med.* **7,** 1194–1201.
8. Kerbel, R. S. (1997) A cancer therapy resistant to resistance. *Nature* **390,** 335–336.
9. Boehm, T., Folkman, J., Browder, T., and O'Reilly, M. S. (1997) Anti-angiogenic therapy of experimental cancer does not induce drug resistance. *Nature* **390,** 404–407.
10. Klauber, N., Rohan, R. M., Flynn, E., and D'Amato, R. J. (1997) Critical components of the female reproductive pathway are suppressed by the angiogenesis inhibitor AGM-1470. *Nat. Med.* **3,** 443–446.
11. Torry, R. J. and Rongish, B. J. (1992) Angiogenesis in the uterus: potential regulation and relation to tumor angiogenesis. *Am. J. Reprod. Immunol.* **27,** 171–179.
12. Berger, A. C., Feldman, A. L., Gnant, M. F., et al. (2000) The angiogenesis inhibitor, endostatin, does not affect murine cutaneous wound healing. *J. Surg. Res.* **91,** 26–31.
13. Gouze, E., Pawliuk, R., Pilapil, C., et al. (2002) In vivo gene delivery to synovium by lentiviral vectors. *Mol. Ther.* **5,** 397–404.
14. Firestein, G. S. (1999) Starving the synovium: angiogenesis and inflammation in rheumatoid arthritis. *J. Clin. Invest.* **103,** 3–4.
15. Dabrosin, C., Gyorffy, S., Margetts, P., Ross, C., and Gauldie, J. (2002) Therapeutic effect of angiostatin gene transfer in a murine model of endometriosis. *Am. J. Pathol.* **161,** 909–918.
16. D'Amato, R. J. and Adamis, A. P. (1995) Angiogenesis inhibition in age-related macular degeneration. *Ophthalmology* **102,** 1261–1262.
17. Adamis, A. P. and D'Amato, R. J. (1995) Shedding light on diabetic retinopathy. *Ophthalmology* **120,** 1127–1128.
18. Klagsbrun, M. and Moses, M. A. (1999) Molecular angiogenesis. *Chem. Biol.* **6,** R217–R224.
19. Jain, R. K., Schlenger, K., Hockel, M., and Yuan, F. (1997) Quantitative angiogenesis assays: progress and problems. *Nat. Med.* **3,** 1203–1208.
20. Suri, C., Jones, P. F., Patan, S., et al. (1996) Requisite role of angiopoietin-1, a ligand for the TIE2 receptor during embryonic angiogenesis. *Cell* **87,** 1171–1180.

21. Davis, S., Aldrich, T. H., Jones, P. F., et al. (1996) Isolation of angiopoietin-1 a ligand for the TIE2 receptor, by secretion trap expression cloning. *Cell* **87,** 1161–1169.
22. Vikkula, M., Boon, L., Carraway, K., et al. (1996) Vascular dysmorphogenesis caused by an activating mutation in the receptor tyrosine kinase TIE2. *Cell* **87,** 1181–1190.
23. Holash, J., Maisonpierre, P. C., Compton, D., et al. (1999) Vessel cooption, regression and growth in tumors mediated by angiopoitins and VEGF. *Science* **284,** 1994–1998.
24. Maisonpierre, P. C., Suri, C., Jones, P. F., et al. (1997) Angiopoietin-2, a natural antagonist for Tie2 that disrupts in vivo angiogenesis. *Science* **277,** 55–60.
25. Hanahan, D. and Folkman, J. (1996) Patterns and emerging mechanisms of the angiogenic switch during tumorgenesis. *Cell* **86,** 353–364.
26. O'Reilly, M. S., Holmgren, L., Shing, Y., et al. (1994) Angiostatin: a novel angiogenesis inhibitor that mediates the suppression of metastases by a Lewis lung carcinoma. *Cell* **79,** 315–328.
27. O'Reilly, M. S., Boehm, T., Shing, Y., et al. (1997) Endostatin: an endogenous inhibitor of angiogenesis and tumor growth. *Cell* **88,** 277–285.
28. Mongiat, M., Sweeney, S. M., San Antonio, J. D., Fu, J., and Iozzo, R. V. (2003) Endorepellin, a novel inhibitor of angiogenesis derived from the C terminus of perlecan. *J. Biol. Chem.* **278,** 4238–4249.
29. Pike, S. E., Yao, L., Jones, K. D., et al. (1998) Vasostatin, a calreticulin fragment, inhibits angiogenesis and suppresses tumor growth. *J. Exp. Med.* **188,** 2349–2356.
30. Maeshima, Y., Sudhakar, A., Lively, J. C., et al. (2002) Tumstatin, an endothelial cell-specific inhibitor of protein synthesis. *Science* **295,** 140–143.
31. Wu, Z., O'Reilly, M. S., Folkman, J., and Shing, Y. (1997) Suppression of tumor growth with recombinant murine angiostatin. *Biochem. Biophys. Res. Commun.* **236,** 651–654.
32. Sim, B. K., O'Reilly, M. S., Liang, H., et al. (1997) A recombinant human angiostatin protein inhibits experimental primary and metastatic cancer. *Cancer Res.* **57,** 1329–1334.
33. O'Reilly, M. S., Pirie-Shepherd, S., Lane, W. S., and Folkman, J. (1999) Anti-angiogenic activity of the cleaved conformation of the serpin antithrombin. *Science* **285,** 1926–1928.
34. Hendrzak, J. A. and Brunda, M. J. (1995) Interleukin-12: biological activity, therapeutic utility and role in disease. *Lab. Invest.* **72,** 619–637.
35. Tanaka, T., Cao, Y., Folkman, J., and Fine, H. A. (1998) Viral vector-targeted antiangiogenic gene therapy utilizing an angiostatin complementary DNA. *Cancer Res.* **58,** 3362–3369.
36. Kisker, O., Becker, C. M., Prox, D., et al. (2001) Continuous administration of endostatin by intraperitoneally implanted osmotic pump improves the efficacy and potency of therapy in a mouse xenograft tumor model. *Cancer Res.* **61,** 7669–7674.
37. Barinaga, M. (1997) Designing therapies that target tumor blood vessels. *Science* **275,** 482–484.
38. Folkman, J. (1998) Anti-angiogenic gene therapy. *Proc. Natl. Acad. Sci. USA* **95,** 9064–9066.
39. Herbst, R. S., Hess, K. R., Tran, H. T., et al. (2002) Phase I study of recombinant human endostatin in patients with advanced solid tumors. *J. Clin. Oncol.* **20,** 3792–3803.
40. Kong, H. L. and Crystal, R. G. (1998) Gene therapy strategies for tumor anti-angiogenesis. *J. Natl. Cancer Inst.* **90,** 273–286.
41. Blezinger, P., Wang, J., Gondo, M., et al. (1999) Systemic inhibition of tumor growth and tumor metastases by intramuscular administration of the endostatin gene. *Nat. Med.* **17,** 343–348.
42. Chen, Q. R., Kumar, D., Stass, S. A., and Mixson, A. J. (1999) Liposomes complexed to plasmids encoding angiostatin and endostatin inhibit breast cancer in nude mice. *Cancer Res.* **59,** 3308–3312.
43. Sacco, M. G., Caniatti, M., Cato, E. M., et al. (2000) Liposome-delivered angiostatin strongly inhibits tumor growth and metastatization in a transgenic model of spontaneous breast cancer. *Cancer Res.* **60,** 2660–2665.
44. Cao, Y., O'Reilly, M. S., Marshall, B., Flynn, E., Ji, R. W., and Folkman, J. (1998) Expression of angiostatin cDNA in a murine fibrosarcoma suppresses primary tumor growth and produces long-term dormancy of metastases. *J. Clin. Invest.* **101,** 1055–1063.
45. Joki, T., Machluf, M., Atala, A., et al. (2001) Continuous release of endostatin from microencapsulated engineered cells for tumor therapy. *Nat. Biotechnol.* **19,** 35–39.
46. Read, T. A., Sorensen, D. R., Mahesparan, R., et al. (2001) Local endostatin treatment of gliomas administered by microencapsulated producer cells. *Nat. Biotechnol.* **19,** 29–34.
47. Davidoff, A. M., Ng, C. Y., Brown, P., et al. (2001) Bone marrow-derived cells contribute to tumor neovasculature and, when modified to express an angiogenesis inhibitor, can restrict tumor growth in mice. *Clin. Cancer Res.* **7,** 2870–2879.
48. De Palma, M., Venneri, M. A., Roca, C., and Naldini, L. (2003) Targeting exogenous genes to tumor angiogenesis by transplantation of genetically modified hematopoietic stem cells. *Nat. Med.* **9,** 789–795.
49. Hill, J. M., Zalos, G., Halcox, J. P., et al. (2003) Circulating endothelial progenitor cells, vascular function, and cardiovascular risk. *N. Engl. J. Med.* **348,** 593–600.
50. Streit, M., Stephen, A. E., Hawighorst, T., et al. (2002) Systemic inhibition of tumor growth and angiogenesis by thrombospondin-2 using cell-based anti-angiogenic gene therapy. *Cancer Res.* **62,** 2004–2014.

51. Hood, J. D., Bednarski, M., Frausto, R., et al. (2002) Tumor regression by targeted gene delivery to the neovasculature. *Science* **296,** 2404–2407.

52. Douglas, J. T. and Curiel, D. T. (1997) Adenoviruses as vectors for gene therapy. *Sci. Med.* **4,** 44–53.

53. Stewart, A. K., Lassam, N. J., Graham, F. L., et al. (1997) A phase I study of adenovirus mediated gene transfer of inter-leukin 2 cDNA into metastatic breast cancer or melanoma. *Hum. Gene Ther.* **8,** 1403–1414.

54. Gyorffy, S., Palmer, K., and Gauldie, J. (2001) Adenoviral vector expressing murine angiostatin inhibits a model of breast cancer metastatic growth in the lungs of mice. *Am. J. Pathol.* **159,** 1137–1147.

55. Gyorffy, S., Palmer, K., Podor, T. J., Hitt, M., and Gauldie, J. (2001) Combined treatment of a murine breast cancer model with type 5 adenovirus vectors expressing murine angiostatin and IL-12: a role for combined anti-angiogenesis and immunotherapy. *J. Immunol.* **166,** 6212–6217.

56. Tahara, H. and Lotze, M. T. (1995) Antitumor effects of interleukin-12 (IL-12): applications for the immunotherapy and gene therapy of cancer. *Gene Ther.* **2,** 96–106.

57. Feldman, A. L., Restifo, N. P., Alexander, H. R., et al. (2000) Anti-angiogenic gene therapy of cancer utilizing a recombinant adenovirus to elevate systemic endostatin levels in mice. *Cancer Res.* **60,** 1503–1506.

58. Chen, C. T., Lin, J., Li, Q., et al. (2000) Anti-angiogenic gene therapy for cancer via systemic administration of adenoviral vectors expressing secretable endostatin. *Hum. Gene Ther.* **11,** 1983–1996.

59. Regulier, E., Paul, S., Marigliano, M., et al. (2001) Adenovirus-mediated delivery of anti-angiogenic genes as an anti-tumor approach. *Cancer Gene Ther.* **8,** 45–54.

60. Calvo, A., Feldman, A. L., Libutti, S. K., and Green, J. E. (2002) Adenovirus-mediated endostatin delivery results in inhibition of mammary gland tumor growth in C3(1)/SV40 T-antigen transgenic mice. *Cancer Res.* **62,** 3934–3938.

61. Kuo, C. J., Farnebo, F., Yu, E. Y., et al. (2001) Comparative evaluation of the anti-tumor activity of anti-angiogenic proteins delivered by gene transfer. *Proc. Natl. Acad. Sci. USA* **98,** 4605–4610.

62. Wen, X. Y., Bai, Y., and Stewart, A. K. (2001) Adenovirus-mediated human endostatin gene delivery demonstrates strain- specific anti-tumor activity and acute dose-dependent toxicity in mice. *Hum. Gene Ther.* **12,** 347–358.

63. Takayama, K., Ueno, H., Nakanishi, Y., et al. (2000) Suppression of tumor angiogenesis and growth by gene transfer of a soluble form of vascular endothelial growth factor receptor into a remote organ. *Cancer Res.* **60,** 2169–2177.

64. Lin, P., Buxton, J. A., Acheson, A., et al. (1998) Anti-angiogenic gene therapy targeting the endothelium-specific receptor tyrosine kinase Tie2. *Proc. Natl. Acad. Sci. USA* **95,** 8829–8834.

65. Rigg, A. S. and Lemoine, N. R. (2001) Adenoviral delivery of TIMP1 or TIMP2 can modify the invasive behavior of pancreatic cancer and can have a significant anti-tumor effect in vivo. *Cancer Gene Ther.* **8,** 869–878.

66. Li, H., Lindenmeyer, F., Grenet, C., et al. (2001) AdTIMP-2 inhibits tumor growth, angiogenesis, and metastasis, and prolongs survival in mice. *Hum. Gene Ther.* **12,** 515–526.

67. Parks, R. J., Chen, L., Anton, M., Sankar, U., Rudnicki, M. A., and Graham, F. L. (1996) A helper-dependent adeno-virus vector system: removal of helper virus by Cre-mediated excision of the viral packaging signal. *Proc. Natl. Acad. Sci. USA* **93,** 13,565–13,570.

68. Parks, R. J. and Graham, F. L. (1997) A helper-dependent system for adenovirus vector production helps define a lower limit for efficient DNA packaging. *J. Virol.* **71,** 3293–3298.

69. Ponnazhagan, S., Curiel, D. T., Shaw, D. R., Alvarez, R. D., and Siegal, G. P. (2001) Adeno-associated virus for cancer gene therapy. *Cancer Res.* **61,** 6313–6321.

70. Nguyen, J. T., Wu, P., Clouse, M. E., Hlatky, L., and Terwilliger, E. F. (1998) Adeno-associated virus-mediated delivery of anti-angiogenic factors as an anti-tumor strategy. *Cancer Res.* **58,** 5673–5677.

71. Ma, H. I., Lin, S. Z., Chiang, Y. H., et al. (2002) Intratumoral gene therapy of malignant brain tumor in a rat model with angiostatin delivered by adeno-associated viral (AAV) vector. *Gene Ther.* **9,** 2–11.

72. Ma, H. I., Guo, P., Li, J., et al. (2002) Suppression of intracranial human glioma growth after intramuscular adminis-tration of an adeno-associated viral vector expressing angiostatin. *Cancer Res.* **62,** 756–763.

73. Davidoff, A. M., Nathwani, A. C., Spurbeck, W. W., Ng, C. Y., Zhou, J., and Vanin, E. F. (2002) rAAV-mediated long-term liver-generated expression of an angiogenesis inhibitor can restrict renal tumor growth in mice. *Cancer Res.* **62,** 3077–3083.

74. Shichinohe, T., Bochner, B. H., Mizutani, K., et al. (2001) Development of lentiviral vectors for anti-angiogenic gene delivery. *Cancer Gene Ther.* **8,** 879–889.

75. Scappaticci, F. A., Smith, R., Pathak, A., et al. (2001) Combination angiostatin and endostatin gene transfer induces synergistic anti-angiogenic activity in vitro and anti-tumor efficacy in leukemia and solid tumors in mice. *Mol. Ther.* **3,** 186–196.

76. Tanaka, T., Manome, Y., Wen, P., Kufe, D. W., and Fine, H. A. (1997) Viral vector-mediated transduction of a modi-fied platelet factor 4 cDNA inhibits angiogenesis and tumor growth. *Nat. Med.* **3,** 437–442.

77. Machein, M. R., Risau, W., and Plate, K. H. (1999) Anti-angiogenic gene therapy in a rat glioma model using a dominant-negative vascular endothelial growth factor receptor 2. *Hum. Gene Ther.* **10,** 1117–1128.

18

Proapoptotic Strategy in Cancer Gene Therapy

David H. Holman, Marc L. Hyer,
Ahmed El-Zawahry, Gina M. Keller, and James S. Norris

1. PROAPOPTOSIS STRATEGIES

With the recent availability of the human genome sequence and development of bioinformatic tools to analyze these results, the promise of gene therapy is broad. Further, our understanding of the causes of cancer are rapidly expanding with the developing tools of genomics, proteomics, and metabolomics, which when analyzed with continually developing bioinformatics tools will provide insight into the myriad cellular signaling pathways that become disturbed in cancer. Thus, there is now an abundance of genes available for introduction into cancer to correct better-understood growth aberrations.

The difficulty lies not in the choice of genes *per se*, but in the ability to deliver a corrective or lethal gene to every cell in the cancer, as required in many gene therapy applications. This is further compounded by the necessity of delivering the therapeutic gene to tumors at distant metastatic sites. Presently, state-of-art of gene therapy does not allow this practice. Orthotopic introduction of genes, via virus, naked deoxyribonucleic acid (DNA), or encapsulated in liposomes, at best is able to transduce 25 to 30% of cells in the tumor. Regarding viral delivery, many tumor cells have variable expression of the receptors that allow viral interaction and gene delivery, so in many cases the multiplicity of infection of virus needs to be relatively high to achieve even the 25–30% infectivity. Thus, it is hoped that improved viral vectors will be developed. A large group of individuals is working on this subject.

Another complementary approach might be to define and deliver genes that not only cause apoptotic cell death, but also transmit additional death signals to adjacent tumor cells, allowing the so-called bystander effect. This chapter discusses the use of molecules that induce apoptosis, some of which also exhibit the capacity to activate bystander activity. The chapter first discusses prodrug bystander therapies, *Bcl-2* family proteins, death receptor genes, death ligand systems, and functional replacement of tumor suppressor genes. We finish by discussing the current status of clinical trials using proapoptotic gene therapy along with combination therapies to elicit bystander activity.

2. PRODRUG THERAPIES

Prodrug therapy utilizes exogenously delivered genes to convert nontoxic prodrugs into toxic analogues capable of inducing apoptosis. These toxic analogues interfere with DNA synthesis by incorporation into growing DNA strands to terminate DNA replication *(1,2)*. Perhaps the two best examples of this strategy are thymidine kinase (TK) and cytosine deaminase (CD), which convert ganciclovir (GCV) and 5-fluorocytosine, respectively, into their toxic drug forms *(3)*. There have been a number

From: *Contemporary Cancer Research*
Cancer Gene Therapy
Edited by: D. T. Curiel and J. T. Douglas © Humana Press Inc., Totowa, NJ

of reports of preclinical and clinical trials using this type of approach, although overall the results are generally disappointing *(4)*. One approach using orthotopic delivery of an adenovirus-expressing TK under a tissue-specific promoter demonstrated modest efficacy in prostate cancer *(5)*.

Other studies have contributed to understanding the cell-signaling mechanisms that occur following TK-GCV treatment. For example, TK-GCV has been shown to induce cytochrome-*c* release from mitochondria in glioblastoma tumor cells; furthermore, this study demonstrated that effector caspase activation was mitochondrial dependent *(6)*. It has also been shown that TK-GCV-induced cell death is enhanced by death receptor agonists CD95L (Fas ligand) *(5–8)*.

Prodrug therapy has been combined with gene therapy using caspase 3 introduction in combination with TK to treat ovarian carcinoma cells. This article by the LeMoine group demonstrated that expression of TK from an adenoviral vector plus GCV led to cell death in ovarian carcinoma cells in vitro, which could be significantly amplified if the ovarian cancer cells were engineered to express caspase 3 *(9)*. This linked procaspase 3 activation to this prodrug pathway. The concern for this approach, however, is that a cancer cell would have to be infected by both a TK-expressing virus and a virus expressing procaspase 3 to achieve amplification under clinical conditions.

3. *BCL-2* FAMILY PROTEIN

There are more than 20 proteins in the *Bcl-2* family that exhibit either pro- or antiapoptotic function. Most of them contain a hydrophobic c-terminal transmembrane domain that serves to anchor them to membranes. However, there are a few members of the family that appear to be cytoplasmic *(10–12)*. *Bcl-2* family proteins are characterized by the *Bcl-2* homology (BH) domains.

There are four different BH domains, and some *Bcl-2* family proteins contain all four. Typically, BH1 and BH2 domains allow heterodimerization with Bax to repress programmed cell death (PCD). The BH3 domain appears to function by allowing heterodimerization between Bcl-x_L and *Bcl-2* and agonistic family members (Bax, Bak) to promote PCD *(13–17)*. The BH4 domain is conserved in antagonist members of the family (e.g., Bcl-x_L), but tends to be absent in the agonistic members, and functions to allow interaction with death regulatory proteins such as Apaf-1 and Bad.

Many *Bcl-2* family members can be regulated posttranslationally by phosphorylation of the variable-loop domain, which alters activity. Studies using Bcl-x_L and Bax are demonstrative of the ability of *Bcl-2* family members to form ion-selective pores in membranes. Some of these molecules, such as *Bcl-2*, inhibit the permeability transition phase and prevent apoptosis; others, such as Bax, counter this effect. Many cancers appear to upregulate antiapoptotic members of the *Bcl-2* family; therefore, a therapeutic strategy has been to overexpress proapoptotic members (e.g., Bax, as discussed in the next section).

One of the main functions of the proapoptotic members of this family is to alter and permeabilize the inner and outer membranes of the mitochondria to release cytochrome-*c*. Cytochrome-*c* interacts with Apaf-1 and caspase 9 to form the apoptosome, which transmits the apoptotic signal by activating caspase 9 *(18)*. When molecules like *Bcl-2* and Bcl-x_L are overexpressed in cancer, the release of cytochrome-*c* from mitochondria is reduced or blocked, preventing activation of the apoptosome-mediated death-signaling pathway *(19)*. To determine their therapeutic role in inducing apoptosis, a number of *Bcl-2* family members have been used in gene therapy experiments, including Bax, Bak, Bad, Bcl-x_S, Bcl-Rambo, Blk, Bik, Harakiri, and Bim.

3.1. Bax

Bax is perhaps the most well-studied member of this family in relationship to gene therapy. Bax is primarily a cytosolic 21-kDa protein mobilized in response to cell death signals; it translocates to the mitochondrial membrane, where it forms a membrane-bound structure through a c-terminal conformational change *(20)*. A number of studies have focused on the role of Bax, delivered by adenovirus to ovarian *(21,22)*, prostate *(23)*, or glial cell *(24)* models growing in syngenic or nude mice. In most of these studies, effective therapeutic results have been demonstrated, revealing that Bax is a relatively strong inducer of apoptosis.

Bax has also been successfully used in conjunction with proapoptotic Bad in a study by Marcelli et al. *(25)*, who demonstrated that androgen-regulated expression of Bad in the LNCaP human prostate cancer cell line was able to delay the growth of xenograft tumors in nude mice. However, it was determined that LNCaP tumors, following treatment with the Bad-expressing adenovirus, eventually regained the ability to grow. If they combined treatment using Bad- and Bax-expressing adenovirus, several of the tumors disappeared completely at the end of the treatment period and did not reoccur in the 8-week follow-up.

Why this approach succeeded is unclear because delivery of adenovirus to solid tumors in vivo is at best only 25–35% efficient. It can therefore be concluded that the Bad/Bax combination described in ref. *25* induces either a bystander activity in the tumor bed or an immune-mediated inflammatory response in the nude mouse model. This is likely mediated by either neutrophils or natural killer cell-targeted tumor killing. These systems are not well understood and are in need of more in-depth study, not only with the introduction of the *Bcl-2* family members, but also with many other forms of gene therapy.

3.2. Bik, Blk, Bcl-Rambo, Bak, Bid, Bim, and Harakiri

The proapoptotic Bik, which is found on chromosome 22Q, has been linked to the development of breast and colorectal cancers when downregulated. This protein has a molecular weight of 18,000 kDa and contains a single BH3 domain, which allows it to form heterodimers with *Bcl-2* and Bcl-x_L *(26)*. This association creates a proapoptotic phenotype through a p53-independent pathway *(14)*. In studies carried out at MD Anderson *(27)*, Bik was administered as a plasmid DNA/cationic lipid emulsion to treat human breast cancer cell lines and xenografts and was demonstrated to induce apoptosis in these models. When administered systemically to mice by intravenous injection, there was good induction of apoptosis in the tumor, as assayed by TUNEL, with little to no apoptosis present in the liver. This treatment greatly prolonged the survival of nude mice bearing MDA-MB-468 metastatic xenografts. The mechanisms that prolonged survival are not entirely clear because of the caveat mentioned in Section 3.1. concerning efficiency of Bik gene delivery to tumor cells.

Bik-related murine protein Blk, which has some identity to human Bik, including conservation of the BH3 domain, has been studied for its ability to induce PCD in mouse tissues *(28)*. It was present in the kidneys, lungs, and heart, but not in the skeletal muscles, spleen, and brain. Highest expression was observed in the liver and kidney, and this pattern of expression differed from Bik. Further, this protein was localized to the mitochondrial membrane and demonstrated a potent death effector with its activity related to inhibition of *Bcl-2* and Bcl-x_L antiapoptotic proteins. Blk appears to function through the mitochondria because it activates caspase 9 *(9)*. Blk has not as yet been delivered to xenograft tumors for functional studies.

There are a number of other potential proapoptotic molecules that could be applied to gene therapy approaches for treatment of cancer. The protein Bcl-Rambo, which is a novel *Bcl-2* homologue, induces apoptosis via a unique c-terminal extension *(28)*. This molecule appears to be localized to mitochondria and, when overexpressed, induces apoptosis that can be blocked by a downstream IAP family member by inhibition of effector caspases. Upstream caspase inhibitors such as FLIP and dominant-negative FADD had no effect, strongly suggesting Bcl-Rambo exerts its proapoptotic effects through the mitochondria.

Bak is another proapoptotic molecule efficient in the treatment of cancer cells both in vivo and in vitro. In vivo, Bak has successfully been delivered to cancer cells using an adenoviral system *(29)*. Bak functions in a fashion similar to Bax by suppressing *Bcl-2* function and inducing apoptosis by cytochrome-*c* release from the mitochondria *(30)*. Moreover, signaling through Bak appears to be via caspase 3 (MCF-7) because, in at least one study *(31)* in which the cell lacked a functional caspase 3,

Bak had little effect on inducing apoptosis. This differs slightly from Bax, in which both caspase-dependent and caspase-independent pathways of activation exist. Both Bax and Bak are ideal agents for treatment of cancers that have excessive expression of *Bcl-2* because adenovirus typically over-expresses the transgene, making it possible to overcome even high levels of the antiapoptotic *Bcl-2* member in the cell and induce PCD.

Another molecule deserving consideration for molecular therapy is Bid, a BH3-containing molecule. Bid becomes activated (t-Bid) following caspase 8 cleavage and translocates to the mitochondria, in which it facilitates Bax oligomerization, allowing cytochrome-*c* release and subsequent apoptosis *(32)*. We were unable to find any reference to use of this molecule in gene therapy to date.

A molecule named Harakiri (HRK) was cloned and determined to interact selectively with *Bcl-2* and Bcl-x$_L$ to promote apoptosis *(33)*. HRK lacks both BH1 and BH2 homology regions, but has a BH3 region of high homology to the *Bcl-2* family. This member of the *Bcl-2* family appears to act by direct interaction with *Bcl-2* and Bcl-x$_L$ to effect mitochondrial apoptotic signaling. To our knowledge, its use in a gene therapy approach has not yet been attempted.

Finally, a splice variant of Bcl-x$_L$, Bcl-x$_S$, is proapoptotic and has been demonstrated in a gene therapy approach to induce apoptosis of human mammary tumor xenografts *(34)*. This study was carried out with a first-generation adenovirus, perhaps limiting its efficacy; however, apoptosis was noted in the study.

In summary, much has been learned concerning the mechanism of action of *Bcl-2*, its many family members, and their collective role in tumor apoptosis inhibition or induction. Some surprisingly positive results on the efficacy of these molecules in the induction of apoptosis in vitro and in vivo were discussed and suggest that induction of apoptosis in the tumor setting is a valid and promising gene therapy approach.

4. DEATH RECEPTOR AND LIGAND SYSTEMS AND PATHWAYS

There are a number of death receptor/ligand systems that can function to regulate apoptosis in cells. These include tumor necrosis factor-α, tumor necrosis factor-related apoptosis inducing ligand (TRAIL), and Fas ligand (FasL). In general, these ligands function at the proximal end of the apoptotic induction pathway by causing conformational changes to their corresponding receptors. These changes generate the death-inducing signaling complex (DISC), which is able to recruit additional molecules, leading to activation of caspase 8 or 10 by autocatalytic cleavage mechanisms. Caspases 8 and 10 then directly activate the executioner caspases, for example, caspase 3 and 7. Alternatively, the initiator caspases can also cleave the full-length proapoptotic Bid molecule into its truncated version t-Bid, which interacts with Bax, Bak, and other molecules on the mitochondrial membrane ultimately to release cytochrome-*c*. Cytochrome-*c* then interacts with Apaf-1 and caspase 9 in a complex known as the apoptosome to activate caspase 9, which subsequently activates caspase 3, 7, and/or other caspases *(35)* and induces apoptosis.

Numerous studies have been carried out using TRAIL, FasL, and a dominant-negative FADD (integral component of FasL signaling in the DISC) to induce apoptosis in tumor cells *(24,36–45)*. There are several interesting aspects relative to these approaches. First, it has been widely observed that the administration of TRAIL and FasL as native or crosslinked molecules is frequently not effective on a number of different types of cancer cell lines *(36,42,46,47)*. The reason for this is typically not because of the lack of death receptors, but because of the presence of molecules that inhibit DISC formation and autocatalytic cleavage of caspase 8, such as cFLIP *(48–50)*. Of interest, when viral systems have been used to deliver FasL or TRAIL to these cells, the ineffective external death receptor signaling pathways are overcome by downregulation of cFLIP *(48)* and/or the IAPs or by other mechanisms, including *de novo* ceramide synthesis to initiate a stress response-mediated apoptosis.

In the case of both TRAIL and FasL, virally induced cell death results in apoptotic vesicles that form in the dying cells and are capable of presenting TRAIL or FasL to adjacent cells *(40,51)*. If the adjacent cells are responsive to FasL or TRAIL then bystander-mediated apoptosis occurs (i.e., an amplification of the death signal). However, if tumor cells belong to the subset of tumors resistant to exogenous signaling, little benefit would be predicted in relation to bystander-mediated cell death unless recruitment of the immune system occurs. Although the immune system is not covered in this chapter, it is likely highly relevant to tumor eradication.

There are many laboratories investigating ways to downregulate the cellular apoptotic inhibitory molecules such as cFLIP and the IAPs to sensitize cancer to apoptotic signals. Combination therapies with small molecule therapeutics, including anthracyclines, triterpenoids, nucleoside chemotherapeutic analogs, Taxol, ceramides, and ceramidase inhibitors, may amplify death ligand bystander activity by downregulating apoptotic inhibitory molecules *(45,48–50,52–54)*.

There have also been numerous studies demonstrating caspase overexpression induces apoptosis in tumor cells *(25,55–60)*. Although caspases have the potential for causing cell death in the transduced cell, they suffer from similar pitfalls as those of the *Bcl-2* family of proteins in that many of these proteins do not induce a bystander effect. Thus, there is little chance for complete tumor eradication because of the limited delivery of adenovirally expressed genes into all the cells of the tumor. In contrast, use of both TRAIL and the FasL viruses appears to have an advantage in gene therapy in that they generate apoptotic vesicles, which continue to express functional death ligand.

5. TUMOR SUPPRESSOR GENES THAT CAN FUNCTION TO INDUCE APOPTOSIS

Tumor suppressor genes function to regulate cellular division and apoptosis. As a result, malignant neoplasms often arise because of a functional defect or absence of one or more tumor suppressor genes. In fact, deregulation of the p53/MDM/p14^{ARF} and pRb/p16/CDK4/cycD pathways is thought to be a fundamental requirement for the genesis of most human cancers because it results in disruption of cell cycle regulation and deactivation of the apoptotic response *(61,62)*. Therefore, one of the strategies used in cancer gene therapy is tumor suppressor gene replacement. This can either restore the normal function of a defective tumor suppressor gene or eliminate the abnormal function of an oncogene *(63,64)*.

One of the most widely studied tumor suppressor genes is p53. The p53 gene encodes a transcription factor that acts on hundreds of different promoter elements, many belonging to genes involved in cell cycle regulation or apoptosis *(65)*. Over 50% of all human cancers contain mutations in p53. Many of these p53 mutant tumors are more resistant to conventional therapies, such as chemotherapy or ionizing radiation. Roth et al. *(66)* were the first group to demonstrate in a clinical trial that tumor suppressor gene replacement could induce tumor regression in human cancer. In this study, non-small cell lung cancer (NSCLC) patients were treated with a retroviral vector containing the wild-type p53 gene under control of the β-actin promoter. Three of the seven patients evaluated showed signs of tumor regression, and no vector-associated toxicity was evident. Limitations in the study arose from the low transduction efficiency of retroviral vectors as well as difficulties in producing high titers of the virus.

A similar clinical trial involving NSCLC was later carried out using replication-defective adenoviral vectors containing the wild-type p53 gene *(67)*. This approach yielded disease stabilization in 64% of the patients and partial response in 8% of the patients.

The p53 gene therapy has been studied in cancers of other tissues as well, and many of those studies have produced encouraging results. Cancer tissues such as breast *(68,69)*, brain *(70,71)*, prostate *(69, 72–74)*, colorectal *(75,76)*, pancreatic, *(77)*, thyroid *(78)*, uterine *(79)*, ovarian, and head and neck *(69)* have all shown potential benefit from p53 gene therapy.

Many studies using oncolytic viruses are also based on the characteristic p53 deficiency observed in many cancers. The first replication-competent adenovirus genetically engineered for tumor selectivity based on p53 mutation was ONYX-015. The efficacy of ONYX-015 was originally thought to be because of its selective replication in tumor cells harboring an inactive p53 *(80,81)*. However, recent data have shown ONYX-015 will replicate in tumor cells regardless of p53 status *(82–84)*. The role of p14^{ARF} status in the selective replication of ONYX-015 is also a source of controversy *(81,83)*.

Other tumor suppressor genes under study for gene therapy include the retinoblastoma susceptibility gene (Rb), pHyde, p16, p21, and MDA-7. Much like p53, a pRb mutation can result in deregulated growth and/or apoptosis *(85)*. pRb gene therapy has been shown to reduce transformation progression in a number of Rb$^{+/-}$ mouse tissues as well as to suppress lung metastasis *(86,87)*. Use of an adenovirus expressing a constitutively active form of pRb has also shown efficacy in treatment of human vascular proliferative disorders *(88)*.

The more recently cloned tumor suppressor gene known as pHyde has demonstrated its proapoptotic function in prostate cancer cell lines *(89,90)*. Infecting human PCa cell lines with a pHyde-expressing adenovirus resulted in inhibition of proliferation in vitro as well as suppression of xenograft tumor growth in vivo. This inhibition was because of induction of apoptosis and is apparently dependent on the activation of caspase 3.

The p16 gene (*INK4a, CDKN2, MTS*) maps to the 9*P21* chromosomal region *(91,92)*. p16, also known as the major tumor suppressor 1 gene, was isolated and characterized during studies of Adp53 *(93)*. It encodes a protein that specifically binds to and inhibits cyclin-dependent kinase 4 (CDK4) and CDK6. The CDKs are essential enzymes with activities that are tightly regulated by protein phosphorylation in association with other proteins called cyclins *(94)*. The activation of CDK–cyclin complexes is responsible for cell cycle progression via phosphorylation of pRb. In contrast, CDK inhibitors, which include p15, p16, p21, and p27, prevent the activation of CDK–cyclin complexes. Thus, hypophosphorylated pRb remains bound to the E2F transcription factor, resulting in an arrest in the G1 phase of cell cycle and inhibition of entry into S phase *(91,92)*. The abnormal activation of CDK or overexpression of cyclins may lead to the uncontrolled growth characteristic of cancer.

It also has been demonstrated that levels of p16 gradually increase as cells proceed toward senescence in response to Ras activation. This action likely constitutes the basis of its role as a tumor suppressor gene in many cancers *(95,96)*. p16 has also been implicated in other fundamental cellular processes, such as angiogenesis *(97)*, tumor invasion *(98)*, contact inhibition *(99)*, and apoptosis *(100,101)*.

The tumor suppressor gene p16 is an important negative regulator of the cell cycle; its functional loss may significantly contribute to malignant transformation. Overexpression of p16 arrests cell division in cell lines with an intact pRb protein *(102)*. Many tumors, including transitional cell carcinoma, melanoma, leukemia, and glioma, contain heterozygous or homozygous deletions of the 9*P21* region *(103–106)*.

Subtle mutations of the p16 gene have also been reported in a variety of tumor cell lines and in some primary tumors. Germline alterations of p16 have been found in a subset of patients with familial melanoma *(107)*. Moreover, deletion of p16 has been found in brain tumors *(108,109)*, adult T-cell leukemia *(110)*, childhood acute lymphoblastic leukemia *(111)*, NSCLC *(112)*, primary malignant mesothelioma *(113)*, prostate cancer *(114)*, and human pancreatic cell carcinoma lines *(115)*.

Taking into account the significance of p16 as a tumor suppressor gene, studies were carried out based on adenovirus-mediated transduction of p16. Adenovirus-mediated p16 gene transfer has been studied in lung cancer *(116,117)*, breast cancer *(118,119)*, ovarian cancer *(120,121)*, prostate cancer *(122–124)*, pancreatic cancer *(125)*, glioblastoma *(126)*, head and neck squamous cell carcinoma *(127)*, and melanoma *(128)* with variable degrees of success. It seems likely that delivery to all tumor cells will be required by this approach.

Another gene that is a negative regulator of Rb phosphorylation is p21 (also called *WAF1, CAP20, Cip 1,* and *Sdi1*) *(129,130)*. p21 is the founding member of the Cip/Kip family of CKIs, which includes p27 *(131,132)* and p57 *(133)*. As a CDK inhibitor, p21 functions by binding to and inactivating a number of the cyclin/CDK complexes involved in the G1-S transition in the cell cycle *(129,134)*. By preventing the CDKs from phosphorylating their targets, the cell cycle will arrest. p21 can mediate cell cycle arrest in both a p53-dependent *(130)* and p53-independent *(130,134,135)* manner.

Under normal circumstances, p21 is induced following DNA damage *(130)*, and this induction blocks cell cycle progression from G1 to S phase *(136)*. This pause in the cell cycle progression allows for DNA repair to occur before the replication of DNA in S phase. p21 is also shown to inhibit both PCNA-dependent DNA replication and phosphorylation.

A number of studies suggested that p21 displays proapoptotic characteristics under certain conditions in specific systems. The utility of p21 as an antitumor agent in a number of human cancer cell lines has been reported. Introduction of p21 into human prostate cancer *(137)*, brain tumor *(138)*, esophageal carcinoma *(139)*, and colon carcinoma cells *(140)* can significantly inhibit cell growth and tumorigenesis. p21 can also enhance the apoptotic response to the chemotherapeutic agent cisplatin in glioma *(141)* and ovarian carcinoma cell lines *(142)*. Overexpression of p21-promoted C6-ceramide-induced apoptosis in a p53-deficient human hepatoma cell line *(143)*. Transducing cervical cancer cell lines with a p21-expressing adenovirus resulted in growth inhibition and apoptosis *(144)*. p21 has also been shown to promote Fas/CD95-mediated apoptosis in T lymphocytes *(145)*.

In summary, it would appear that tumor suppressor gene replacement has promise as a therapeutic modality, and it would appear that p53 and p21 hold the most promise as gene therapies to date. Although there is evidence that p53 mediates bystander activity, diminishing the requirement for delivery to all cells in the tumor bed, the same cannot be said for p16- or p21-mediated therapies.

6. CLINICAL TRIALS USING p53 GENE THERAPY

There are a number of approaches for cancer gene therapy presently in clinical trials. Many of these approaches are based on replacement of a defective gene, such as p53, with the functional wild-type gene. Of all the tumor suppressor genes under study for cancer gene therapy, p53 has shown the most promise *(67)*. p53 gene therapy has great potential in that tumor cells expressing wild-type p53 are often more sensitive to chemotherapeutic agents and radiation than those lacking functional p53 *(24)*. The p53 approach has been applied with some efficacy in head and neck, ovarian, and lung cancer.

As discussed in Section 5., Roth et al. *(160)* were the first to use p53 gene therapy clinically. The group used a retroviral vector to deliver the wild-type p53 gene to nine patients with NSCLC who previously failed conventional therapy. In addition to being safe and feasible, results showed tumor regression in three patients and tumor growth stabilization in three others *(160)*.

Swisher et al. later carried out a similar study involving adenovirus-mediated p53 gene transfer. Investigators in this study treated 28 patients with NSCLC with Adp53, which resulted in disease stabilization in 64% of the patients and a partial response in 8% *(67)*.

Prostate cancer also has the potential to benefit from p53 gene therapy. One study involved treatment of 30 patients with prostate cancer with Adp53 delivered by intraprostatic injection. Results of this study demonstrated production of p53 proteins without significant side effects *(161)*.

Gene transfer of p53 has also been studied in combination with chemotherapeutic drugs. Clinically, this approach has been investigated in NSCLC, head and neck cancer, breast cancer, prostate cancer, and hepatic metastasis of colon cancer *(162,163)*. Adp53 gene therapy has also been studied in combination with radiotherapy. NSCLC has received a great deal of attention regarding this therapeutic approach.

An additional approach taking advantage of p53 gene therapy is cancer vaccine development. For example, a current phase I/II study is designed using an autologous dendritic cell-Adp53 vaccine following standard chemotherapy for treatment of extensive stage small cell lung cancer. This approach uses the patients' dendritic cells and a p53-expressing adenovirus to construct the vaccine. If in fact gene therapy approaches can be utilized to harness the immune system and eradicate cancer, we will likely be well ahead of most current chemotherapy modalities in use today in the oncology clinic setting.

7. COMBINATION THERAPIES

Combining proapoptotic gene therapy with another treatment can often result in a synergistic effect. Adp53 gene therapy has been linked to many different combination therapies, such as chemotherapy

(69), ionizing radiation *(74,75)*, histone deacetylase inhibitors *(78)*, and polygene therapy *(77,146–148)*. Enzyme prodrug therapies such as herpes simplex virus-TK or CD have also proven beneficial if combined with other gene therapies. For example, herpes simplex virus-TK suicide gene therapy has been used in a variety of polygene therapy studies, including genes that encode for antiangiogenesis factors *(149)*, connexins *(150)*, cytokines *(151–153)*, caspases *(9)*, and double-suicide gene therapy *(3)*.

Strategies using apoptotic genes like Bax can also be beneficial if combined with other agents. Lee et al. *(154)* showed that a Bax-expressing herpes virus enhanced the efficacy of BCNU treatment in a rat glioma model. Bax polygene therapy has also been studied in combination with Bad *(155)*, Bak, and p53 *(148)*. Additional apoptotic molecules such as FasL or TRAIL can also exhibit synergistic effects when combined with other treatment modalities, such as doxorubicin or p53 *(42,146,156–159)*.

REFERENCES

1. Moolten, F. L. (1986) Tumor chemosensitivity conferred by inserted herpes thymidine kinase genes: paradigm for a prospective cancer control strategy. *Cancer Res.* **46**, 5276–5281.
2. Reid, R., Mar, E. C., Huang, E. S., and Topal, M. D. (1988) Insertion and extension of acyclic, dideoxy, and ara nucleotides by herpesviridae, human alpha and human beta polymerases. A unique inhibition mechanism for 9-(1,3-dihydroxy-2-propoxymethyl)guanine triphosphate. *J. Biol. Chem.* **263**, 3898–3904.
3. Uckert, W., Kammertons, T., Haack, K., et al. (1998) Double suicide gene (cytosine deaminase and herpes simplex virus thymidine kinase) but not single gene transfer allows reliable elimination of tumor cells in vivo. *Hum. Gene Ther.* **9**, 855–865.
4. Shand, N., Weber, F., Mariani, L., et al. (1999) A phase 1–2 clinical trial of gene therapy for recurrent glioblastoma multiforme by tumor transduction with the herpes simplex thymidine kinase gene followed by ganciclovir. GLI328 European-Canadian Study Group. *Hum. Gene Ther.* **10**, 2325–2335.
5. Seino, K., Kayagaki, N., Okumura, K., and Yagita, H. (1997) Antitumor effect of locally produced CD95 ligand. *Nat. Med.* **3**, 165–170.
6. Klatzmann, D., Valery, C. A., Bensimon, G., et al. (1998) A phase I/II study of herpes simplex virus type 1 thymidine kinase "suicide" gene therapy for recurrent glioblastoma. Study Group on Gene Therapy for Glioblastoma. *Hum. Gene Ther.* **9**, 2595–2604.
7. Friesen, C., Herr, I., Krammer, P. H., and Debatin, K. M. (1996) Involvement of the CD95 (APO-1/FAS) receptor/ligand system in drug-induced apoptosis in leukemia cells. *Nat. Med.* **2**, 574–577.
8. Heise, C., Ganly, I., Kim, Y. T., et al. (2000) Efficacy of a replication-selective adenovirus against ovarian carcinomatosis is dependent on tumor burden, viral replication and p53 status. *Gene Ther.* **7**, 1925–1929.
9. McNeish, I. A., Tenev, T., Bell, S., Marani, M., Vassaux, G., and Lemoine, N. (2001) Herpes simplex virus thymidine kinase/ganciclovir-induced cell death is enhanced by co-expression of caspase-3 in ovarian carcinoma cells. *Cancer Gene Ther.* **8**, 308–319.
10. Antonsson, B. and Martinou, J. C. (2000) The Bcl-2 protein family. *Exp. Cell Res.* **256**, 50–57.
11. Guo, B., Godzik, A., and Reed, J. C. (2001) Bcl-G, a novel pro-apoptotic member of the Bcl-2 family. *J. Biol. Chem.* **276**, 2780–2785.
12. Ke, N., Godzik, A., and Reed, J. C. (2001) Bcl-B, a novel Bcl-2 family member that differentially binds and regulates Bax and Bak. *J. Biol. Chem.* **276**, 12,481–12,484.
13. Chittenden, T., Harrington, E. A., O'Connor, R., et al. (1995) Induction of apoptosis by the Bcl-2 homologue Bak. *Nature* **374**, 733–736.
14. Han, J., Sabbatini, P., and White, E. (1996) Induction of apoptosis by human Nbk/Bik, a BH3-containing protein that interacts with E1B 19K. *Mol. Cell. Biol.* **16**, 5857–5864.
15. Simonian, P. L., Grillot, D. A., Merino, R., and Nunez, G. (1996) Bax can antagonize Bcl-XL during etoposide and cisplatin-induced cell death independently of its heterodimerization with Bcl-x$_L$. *J. Biol. Chem.* **271**, 22,764–22,772.
16. Zha, H., Aime-Sempe, C., Sato, T., and Reed, J. C. (1996) Proapoptotic protein Bax heterodimerizes with Bcl-2 and homodimerizes with Bax via a novel domain (BH3) distinct from BH1 and BH2. *J. Biol. Chem.* **271**, 7440–7444.
17. Oltvai, Z. N. and Korsmeyer, S. J. (1994) Checkpoints of dueling dimers foil death wishes. *Cell* **79**, 189–192.
18. Adams, J. M. and Cory, S. (1998) The Bcl-2 protein family: arbiters of cell survival. *Science* **281**, 1322–1326.
19. Pan, G., O'Rourke, K., and Dixit, V. M. (1998) Caspase-9, Bcl-x$_L$, and Apaf-1 form a ternary complex. *J. Biol. Chem.* **273**, 5841–5845.
20. Nechushtan, A., Smith, C. L., Hsu, Y. T., and Youle, R. J. (1999) Conformation of the Bax c-terminus regulates subcellular location and cell death. *EMBO J.* **18**, 2330–2341.
21. Alvarez, R. D., Gomez-Navarro, J., Wang, M., et al. (2000) Adenoviral-mediated suicide gene therapy for ovarian cancer. *Mol. Ther.* **2**, 524–530.

22. Tsuruta, Y., Mandai, M., Konishi, I., et al. (2001) Combination effect of adenovirus-mediated pro-apoptotic bax gene transfer with cisplatin or paclitaxel treatment in ovarian cancer cell lines. *Eur. J. Cancer* **37,** 531–541.
23. Lowe, S. L., Rubinchik, S., Honda, T., McDonnell, T. J., Dong, J. Y., and Norris, J. S. (2001) Prostate-specific expression of Bax delivered by an adenoviral vector induces apoptosis in LNCaP prostate cancer cells. *Gene Ther.* **8,** 1363–1371.
24. Norris, J. S., Hyer, M. L., Voelkel-Johnson, C., Lowe, S. L., Rubinchik, S., and Dong, J. Y. (2001) The use of Fas Ligand, TRAIL and Bax in gene therapy of prostate cancer. *Curr. Gene Ther.* **1,** 123–136.
25. Marcelli, M., Cunningham, G. R., Walkup, M., et al. (1999) Signaling pathway activated during apoptosis of the prostate cancer cell line LNCaP: overexpression of caspase-7 as a new gene therapy strategy for prostate cancer. *Cancer Res.* **59,** 382–390.
26. Boyd, J. M., Gallo, G. J., Elangovan, B., et al. (1995) Bik, a novel death-inducing protein shares a distinct sequence motif with Bcl-2 family proteins and interacts with viral and cellular survival-promoting proteins. *Oncogene* **11,** 1921–1928.
27. Zou, Y., Peng, H., Zhou, B., et al. (2002) Systemic tumor suppression by the proapoptotic gene bik. *Cancer Res.* **62,** 8–12.
28. Hegde, R., Srinivasula, S. M., Ahmad, M., Fernandesalnemri, T., and Alnemri, E. S. (1998) Blk, a bhs-containing mouse protein that interacts with bcl-2 and bcl-xl, is a potent death agonist. *J. Biol. Chem.* **273,** 7783–7786.
29. Pataer, A., Fang, B. L., Yu, R., et al. (2000) Adenoviral Bak overexpression mediates caspase-dependent tumor killing. *Cancer Res.* **60,** 788–792.
30. Cuconati, A., Degenhardt, K., Sundararajan, R., Anschel, A., and White, E. (2002) Bak and Bax function to limit adenovirus replication through apoptosis induction. *J. Virol.* **76,** 4547–4558.
31. Pataer, A., Fang, B., Yu, R., et al. (2000) Adenoviral Bak overexpression mediates caspase-dependent tumor killing. *Cancer Res.* **60,** 788–792.
32. Roucou, X., Montessuit, S., Antonsson, B., and Martinou, J. C. (2002) Bax oligomerization in mitochondrial membranes requires tBid (caspase-8-cleaved Bid) and a mitochondrial protein. *Biochem. J.* **368,** 915–921.
33. Inohara, N., Ding, L. Y., Chen, S., and Nunez, G. (1997) Harakiri, a novel regulator of cell death, encodes a protein that activates apoptosis and interacts selectively with survival-promoting proteins bcl-2 and bcl-x-l. *EMBO J.* **16,** 1686–1694.
34. Ealovega, M. W., McGinnis, P. K., Sumantran, V. N., Clarke, M. F., and Wicha, M. S. (1996) Bcl-x(s) gene therapy induces apoptosis of human mammary tumors in nude mice. *Cancer Res.* **56,** 1965–1969.
35. Ashkenazi, A. and Dixit, V. M. (1998) Death receptors: signaling and modulation. *Science* **281,** 1305–1308.
36. Hyer, M. L., Voelkel-Johnson, C., Rubinchik, S., Dong, J., and Norris, J. S. (2000) Intracellular Fas ligand expression causes Fas-mediated apoptosis in human prostate cancer cells resistant to monoclonal antibody-induced apoptosis. *Mol. Ther.* **2,** 348–358.
37. Hedlund, T. E., Meech, S. J., Srikanth, S., et al. (1999) Adenovirus-mediated expression of Fas ligand induces apoptosis of human prostate cancer cells. *Cell Death Differ.* **6,** 175–182.
38. Rubinchik, S., Wang, D., Yu, H., et al. (2001) A complex adenovirus vector that delivers FASL-GFP with combined prostate-specific and tetracycline-regulated expression. *Mol. Ther.* **4,** 416–426.
39. Shinoura, N., Yoshida, Y., Sadata, A., et al. (1998) Apoptosis by retrovirus- and adenovirus-mediated gene transfer of Fas ligand to glioma cells: implications for gene therapy. *Hum. Gene Ther.* **9,** 1983–1993.
40. Wu, X., He, Y., Falo, L. D. Jr., Hui, K. M., and Huang, L. (2001) Regression of human mammary adenocarcinoma by systemic administration of a recombinant gene encoding the hFlex-TRAIL fusion protein. *Mol. Ther.* **3,** 368–374.
41. Kagawa, S., He, C., Gu, J., et al. (2001) Antitumor activity and bystander effects of the tumor necrosis factor-related apoptosis-inducing ligand (TRAIL) gene. *Cancer Res.* **61,** 3330–3338.
42. Voelkel-Johnson, C., King, D. L., and Norris, J. S. (2002) Resistance of prostate cancer cells to soluble TNF-related apoptosis-inducing ligand (TRAIL/Apo2L) can be overcome by doxorubicin or adenoviral delivery of full-length TRAIL. *Cancer Gene Ther.* **9,** 164–172.
43. Kondo, S., Ishizaka, Y., Okada, T., et al. (1998) FADD gene therapy for malignant gliomas in vitro and in vivo. *Hum. Gene Ther.* **9,** 1599–1608.
44. Ambar, B. B., Frei, K., Malipiero, U., et al. (1999) Treatment of experimental glioma by administration of adenoviral vectors expressing Fas ligand. *Hum. Gene Ther.* **10,** 1641–1648.
45. Keane, M. M., Ettenberg, S. A., Nau, M. M., Russell, E. K., and Lipkowitz, S. (1999) Chemotherapy augments TRAIL-induced apoptosis in breast cell lines. *Cancer Res.* **59,** 734–741.
46. Hedlund, T. E., Duke, R. C., Schleicher, M. S., and Miller, G. J. (1998) Fas-mediated apoptosis in seven human prostate cancer cell lines: correlation with tumor stage. *Prostate* **36,** 92–101.
47. Rokhlin, O. W., Bishop, G. A., Hostager, B. S., et al. (1997) Fas-mediated apoptosis in human prostatic carcinoma cell lines. *Cancer Res.* **57,** 1758–1768.
48. Hyer, M. L., Sudarshan, S., Kim, Y., et al. (2002) Downregulation of c-FLIP sensitizes DU145 prostate cancer cells to fas-mediated apoptosis. *Cancer Biol. Ther.* **1,** 401–406.

49. Kelly M, Hoel, B. D., and Voelkel-Johnson C. (2002) Doxorubicin pretreatment sensitizes prostate cancer cell lines to TRAIL induced apoptosis, which correlates with the loss of c-FLIP expression. *Cancer Biol. Ther.* **1,** 520–527.

50. Kim, Y., Suh, N., Sporn, M., and Reed, J. C. (2002) An inducible pathway for degradation of FLIP protein sensitizes tumor cells to TRAIL-induced apoptosis. *J. Biol. Chem.* **277,** 22,320–22,329.

51. Hyer, M. L., Sudarshan, S., Schwartz, D. A., Hannun, Y. A., Dong, J.-Y., and Norris, J. S. (2003) Quantification and characterization of the bystander effect in prostate cancer cells following adenovirus-mediated FasL expression. *Cancer Gene Ther.* **10,** 330–339.

52. Tepper, C. G., Jayadev, S., Liu, B., et al. (1995) Role for ceramide as an endogenous mediator of Fas-induced cytotoxicity. *Proc. Natl. Acad. Sci. USA* **92,** 8443–8447.

53. Kolesnick, R. (2002) The therapeutic potential of modulating the ceramide/sphingomyelin pathway. *J. Clin. Invest.* **110,** 3–8.

54. Ng, C. P., Zisman, A., and Bonavida, B. (2002) Synergy is achieved by complementation with Apo2L/TRAIL and actinomycin D in Apo2L/TRAIL-mediated apoptosis of prostate cancer cells: role of XIAP in resistance. *Prostate* **53,** 286–299.

55. Shinoura, N., Koike, H., Furitu, T., et al. (2000) Adenovirus-mediated transfer of caspase-8 augments cell death in gliomas: implication for gene therapy. *Hum. Gene Ther.* **11,** 1123–1137.

56. Yamabe, K., Shimizu, S., Ito, T., et al. (1999) Cancer gene therapy using a pro-apoptotic gene, caspase-3. *Gene Ther.* **6,** 1952–1959.

57. Koga, S., Hirohata, S., Kondo, Y., et al. (2000) A novel telomerase-specific gene therapy: gene transfer of caspase-8 utilizing the human telomerase catalytic subunit gene promoter. *Hum. Gene Ther.* **11,** 1397–1406.

58. Xie, X., Zhao, X., Liu, Y., et al. (2001) Adenovirus-mediated tissue-targeted expression of a caspase-9-based artificial death switch for the treatment of prostate cancer. *Cancer Res.* **61,** 6795–6804.

59. Shariat, S. F., Desai, S., Song, W., et al. (2001) Adenovirus-mediated transfer of inducible caspases: a novel "death switch" gene therapeutic approach to prostate cancer. *Cancer Res.* **61,** 2562–2571.

60. Komata, T., Kondo, Y., Kanzawa, T., et al. (2001) Treatment of malignant glioma cells with the transfer of constitutively active caspase-6 using the human telomerase catalytic subunit (human telomerase reverse transcriptase) gene promoter. *Cancer Res.* **61,** 5796–5802.

61. Chin, L., Pomerantz, J., and DePinho, R. A. (1998) The INK4a/ARF tumor suppressor: one gene—two products—two pathways. *Trends Biochem. Sci.* **23,** 291–296.

62. Yap, D. B., Hsieh, J. K., Chan, F. S., and Lu, X. (1999) mdm2: a bridge over the two tumour suppressors, p53 and Rb. *Oncogene* **18,** 7681–7689.

63. Friedman, T. (1989) Progress toward human gene therapy. *Science* **244,** 1275–1281.

64. Friedman, T. (1992) Gene therapy of cancer through restoration of tumor-suppressor functions. *Cancer* **70(Suppl.),** 1810–1817.

65. Lane, D. P. and Lain, S. (2002) Therapeutic exploitation of the p53 pathway. *Trends Mol. Med.* **8(4, Suppl.),** S38–S42.

66. Roth, J. A., Swisher, S. G., and Meyn, R. E. (1999) p53 tumor suppressor gene therapy for cancer. *Oncology (Huntingt.)* **13,** 148–154.

67. Swisher, S. G., Roth, J. A., Nemunaitis, J., et al. (1999) Adenovirus-mediated p53 gene transfer in advanced non-small-cell lung cancer. *J. Natl. Cancer Inst.* **91,** 763–771.

68. Nielsen, L. L., Dell, J., Maxwell, E., Armstrong, L., Maneval, D., and Catino, J. J. (1997) Efficacy of p53 adenovirus-mediated gene therapy against human breast cancer xenografts. *Cancer Gene Ther.* **4,** 129–138.

69. Nielsen, L. L., Lipari, P., Dell, J., Gurnani, M., and Hajian, G. (1998) Adenovirus-mediated p53 gene therapy and paclitaxel have synergistic efficacy in models of human head and neck, ovarian, prostate, and breast cancer. *Clin. Cancer Res.* **4,** 835–846.

70. Abe, T., Wakimoto, H., Bookstein, R., et al. (2002) Intra-arterial delivery of p53-containing adenoviral vector into experimental brain tumors. *Cancer Gene Ther.* **9,** 228–235.

71. Shono, T., Tofilon, P. J., Schaefer, T. S., Parikh, D., Liu, T. J., and Lang, F. F. (2002) Apoptosis induced by adeno-virus-mediated p53 gene transfer in human glioma correlates with site-specific phosphorylation. *Cancer Res.* **62,** 1069–1076.

72. Ko, S. C., Gotoh, A., Thalmann, G. N., et al. (1996) Molecular therapy with recombinant p53 adenovirus in an androgen-independent, metastatic human prostate cancer model. *Hum. Gene Ther.* **7,** 1683–1691.

73. Schumacher, G., Bruckheimer, E. M., Beham, A. W., et al. (2001) Molecular determinants of cell death induction following adenovirus-mediated gene transfer of wild-type p53 in prostate cancer cells. *Int. J. Cancer* **91,** 159–166.

74. Cowen, D., Salem, N., Ashoori, F., et al. (2000) Prostate cancer radiosensitization in vivo with adenovirus-mediated p53 gene therapy. *Clin. Cancer Res.* **6,** 4402–4408.

75. Spitz, F. R., Nguyen, D., Skibber, J. M., Meyn, R. E., Cristiano, R. J., and Roth, J. A. (1996) Adenoviral-mediated wild-type p53 gene expression sensitizes colorectal cancer cells to ionizing radiation. *Clin. Cancer Res.* **2,** 1665–1671.

76. Waku, T., Fujiwara, T., Shao, J., et al. (2000) Contribution of CD95 ligand-induced neutrophil infiltration to the bystander effect in p53 gene therapy for human cancer. *J. Immunol.* **165,** 5884–5890.

77. Ghaneh, P., Greenhalf, W., Humphreys, M., et al. (2001) Adenovirus-mediated transfer of p53 and p16(INK4a) results in pancreatic cancer regression in vitro and in vivo. *Gene Ther.* **8,** 199–208.

78. Imanishi, R., Ohtsuru, A., Iwamatsu, M., et al. (2002) A histone deacetylase inhibitor enhances killing of undifferentiated thyroid carcinoma cells by p53 gene therapy. *J. Clin. Endocrinol. Metab.* **87,** 4821–4824.

79. Ramondetta, L., Mills, G. B., Burke, T. W., and Wolf, J. K. (2000) Adenovirus-mediated expression of p53 or p21 in a papillary serous endometrial carcinoma cell line (SPEC-2) results in both growth inhibition and apoptotic cell death: potential application of gene therapy to endometrial cancer. *Clin. Cancer Res.* **6,** 278–284.

80. Kirn, D., Niculescu-Duvaz, I., Hallden, G., and Springer, C. J. (2002) The emerging fields of suicide gene therapy and virotherapy. *Trends Mol. Med.* **8(4, Suppl.),** S68–S73.

81. Gunzburg, W. H. and Salmons, B. (2001) Novel clinical strategies for the treatment of pancreatic carcinoma. *Trends Mol. Med.* **7,** 30–37.

82. Dix, B. R., Edwards, S. J., and Braithwaite, A. W. (2001) Does the antitumor adenovirus ONYX-015/dl1520 selectively target cells defective in the p53 pathway? *J. Virol.* **75,** 5443–5447.

83. Edwards, S. J., Dix, B. R., Myers, C. J., et al. (2002) Evidence that replication of the antitumor adenovirus ONYX-015 is not controlled by the p53 and p14^{ARF} tumor suppressor genes. *J. Virol.* **76,** 12,483–12,490.

84. Geoerger, B., Grill, J., Opolon, P., et al. (2002) Oncolytic activity of the E1B-55 kDa-deleted adenovirus ONYX-015 is independent of cellular p53 status in human malignant glioma xenografts. *Cancer Res.* **62,** 764–772.

85. Hickman, E. S., Moroni, M. C., and Helin, K. (2002) The role of p53 and pRB in apoptosis and cancer. *Curr. Opin. Genet. Dev.* **12,** 60–66.

86. Riley, D. J., Nikitin, A. Y., and Lee, W. H. (1996) Adenovirus-mediated retinoblastoma gene therapy suppresses spontaneous pituitary melanotroph tumors in Rb+/– mice. *Nat. Med.* **2,** 1316–1321.

87. Nikitin, A. Y., Juarez-Perez, M. I., Li, S., Huang, L., and Lee, W. H. (1999) RB-mediated suppression of spontaneous multiple neuroendocrine neoplasia and lung metastases in Rb+/– mice. *Proc. Natl. Acad. Sci. USA* **96,** 6571.

88. Chang, M. W., Barr, E., Seltzer, J., et al. (1995) Cytostatic gene therapy for vascular proliferative disorders with a constitutively active form of the retinoblastoma gene product. *Science* **267,** 518–522.

89. Steiner, M. S., Zhang, X., Wang, Y., and Lu, Y. (2000) Growth inhibition of prostate cancer by an adenovirus expressing a novel tumor suppressor gene, pHyde. *Cancer Res.* **60,** 4419–4425.

90. Zhang, X., Steiner, M. S., Rinaldy, A., and Lu, Y. (2001) Apoptosis induction in prostate cancer cells by a novel gene product, pHyde, involves caspase-3. *Oncogene* **20,** 5982–5990.

91. Serrano, M., Hannon, G. J., and Beach, D. (1993) A new regulatory motif in cell-cycle control causing specific inhibition of cyclin D/CDK4. *Nature* **366,** 704–707.

92. Nobori, T., Miura, K., Wu, D. J., Lois, A., Takabayashi, K., and Carson, D. A. (1994) Deletions of the cyclin-dependent kinase-4 inhibitor gene in multiple human cancers. *Nature* **368,** 753–756.

93. Kamb, A., Gruis, N. A., Weaver-Feldhaus, J., et al. (1994) A cell cycle regulator potentially involved in genesis of many tumor types. *Science* **264,** 436–440.

94. Bates, S., Bonetta, L., MacAllan, D., et al. (1994) CDK6 (PLSTIRE) and CDK4 (PSK-J3) are a distinct subset of the cyclin-dependent kinases that associate with cyclin D1. *Oncogene* **9,** 71–79.

95. Robles, S. J. and Adami, G. R. (1998) Agents that cause DNA double strand breaks lead to p16INK4a enrichment and the premature senescence of normal fibroblasts. *Oncogene* **16,** 1113–1123.

96. Serrano, M., Lin, A. W., McCurrach, M. E., Beach, D., and Lowe, S. W. (1997) Oncogenic ras provokes premature cell senescence associated with accumulation of p53 and p16INK4a. *Cell* **88,** 593–602.

97. Harada, H., Nakagawa, K., Iwata, S., et al. (1999) Restoration of wild-type p16 down-regulates vascular endothelial growth factor expression and inhibits angiogenesis in human gliomas. *Cancer Res.* **59,** 3783–3789.

98. Chintala, S. K., Fueyo, J., Gomez-Manzano, C., et al. (1997) Adenovirus-mediated p16/CDKN2 gene transfer suppresses glioma invasion in vitro. *Oncogene* **15,** 2049–2057.

99. Wieser, R. J., Faust, D., Dietrich, C., and Oesch, F. (1999) p16INK4 mediates contact-inhibition of growth. *Oncogene* **18,** 277–281.

100. Schreiber, M., Muller, W. J., Singh, G., and Graham, F. L. (1999) Comparison of the effectiveness of adenovirus vectors expressing cyclin kinase inhibitors p16INK4A, p18INK4C, p19INK4D, p21(WAF1/CIP1) and p27KIP1 in inducing cell cycle arrest, apoptosis and inhibition of tumorigenicity. *Oncogene* **18,** 1663–1676.

101. Naruse, I., Heike, Y., Hama, S., Mori, M., and Saijo, N. (1998) High concentrations of recombinant adenovirus expressing p16 gene induces apoptosis in lung cancer cell lines. *Anticancer Res.* **18,** 4275–4282.

102. Lukas, J., Parry, D., Aagaard, L., et al. (1995) Retinoblastoma-protein-dependent cell-cycle inhibition by the tumour suppressor p16. *Nature* **375,** 503–506.

103. Diaz, M. O., Rubin, C. M., Harden, A., et al. (1990) Deletions of interferon genes in acute lymphoblastic leukemia. *N. Engl. J. Med.* **322,** 77–82.

104. Orlow, I., Lacombe, L., Hannon, G. J., et al. (1995) Deletion of the p16 and p15 genes in human bladder tumors. *J. Natl. Cancer Inst.* **87,** 1524–1529.

105. James, C. D., He, J., Collins, V. P., Allalunis-Turner, M. J., and Day, R. S. 3rd. (1993) Localization of chromosome 9p homozygous deletions in glioma cell lines with markers constituting a continuous linkage group. *Cancer Res.* **53,** 3674–3676.

106. Fountain, J. W., Karayiorgou, M., Ernstoff, M. S., et al. (1992) Homozygous deletions within human chromosome band 9p21 in melanoma. *Proc. Natl. Acad. Sci. USA* **89,** 10,557–10,561.

107. Hussussian, C. J., Struewing, J. P., Goldstein, A. M., et al. (1994) Germline p16 mutations in familial melanoma. *Nat. Genet.* **8,** 15–21.

108. Jen, J., Harper, J. W., Bigner, S. H., et al. (1994) Deletion of p16 and p15 genes in brain tumors. *Cancer Res.* **54,** 6353–6358.

109. Li, Y. J., Hoang-Xuan, K., Delattre, J. Y., Poisson, M., Thomas, G., and Hamelin, R. (1995) Frequent loss of heterozygosity on chromosome 9, and low incidence of mutations of cyclin-dependent kinase inhibitors p15 (MTS2) and p16 (MTS1) genes in gliomas. *Oncogene* **11,** 597–600.

110. Hatta, Y., Hirama, T., Miller, C. W., Yamada, Y., Tomonaga, M., and Koeffler, H. P. (1995) Homozygous deletions of the p15 (MTS2) and p16 (CDKN2/MTS1) genes in adult T-cell leukemia. *Blood* **85,** 2699–2704.

111. Takeuchi, S., Bartram, C. R., Seriu, T., et al. (1995) Analysis of a family of cyclin-dependent kinase inhibitors: p15/MTS2/INK4B, p16/MTS1/INK4A, and p18 genes in acute lymphoblastic leukemia of childhood. *Blood* **86,** 755–760.

112. Xiao, S., Li, D., Corson, J. M., Vijg, J., and Fletcher, J. A. (1995) Codeletion of p15 and p16 genes in primary non-small cell lung carcinoma. *Cancer Res.* **55,** 2968–2971.

113. Xio, S., Li, D., Vijg, J., Sugarbaker, D. J., Corson, J. M., and Fletcher, J. A. (1995) Codeletion of p15 and p16 in primary malignant mesothelioma. *Oncogene* **11,** 511–515.

114. Cairns, P., Polascik, T. J., Eby, Y., et al. (1995) Frequency of homozygous deletion at p16/CDKN2 in primary human tumours. *Nat. Genet.* **11,** 210–212.

115. Chen, Z. H., Zhang, H., and Savarese, T. M. (1996) Gene deletion chemoselectivity: codeletion of the genes for p16(INK4), methylthioadenosine phosphorylase, and the alpha- and beta-interferons in human pancreatic cell carcinoma lines and its implications for chemotherapy. *Cancer Res.* **56,** 1083–1090.

116. Jin, X., Nguyen, D., Zhang, W. W., Kyritsis, A. P., and Roth, J. A. (1995) Cell cycle arrest and inhibition of tumor cell proliferation by the p16INK4 gene mediated by an adenovirus vector. *Cancer Res.* **55,** 3250–3253.

117. Fu, X., Zhang, S., and Ran, R. (1999) [Effect of exogenous p16 gene on the growth of wild-type p53 human lung adenocarcinoma cells]. *Chin. J. Oncol.* **21,** 102–104.

118. Bai, J., Zhu, X., Zheng, X., and Wu, Y. (2001) Retroviral vector containing human p16 gene and its inhibitory effect on Bcap-37 breast cancer cells. *Chin. Med. J.* **114,** 497–501.

119. Campbell, I., Magliocco, A., Moyana, T., Zheng, C., and Xiang, J. (2000) Adenovirus-mediated p16INK4 gene transfer significantly suppresses human breast cancer growth. *Cancer Gene Ther.* **7,** 1270–1278.

120. Modesitt, S. C., Ramirez, P., Zu, Z., Bodurka-Bevers, D., Gershenson, D., and Wolf, J. K. (2001) In vitro and in vivo adenovirus-mediated p53 and p16 tumor suppressor therapy in ovarian cancer. *Clin. Cancer Res.* **7,** 1765–1772.

121. Murphy, M. E. (2001) The battle between tumor suppressors: is gene therapy using p16(INK4a) more efficacious than p53 for treatment of ovarian carcinoma? [letter; comment]. *Clin. Cancer Res.* **7,** 1487–1489.

122. Steiner, M. S., Zhang, Y., Farooq, F., Lerner, J., Wang, Y., and Lu, Y. (2000) Adenoviral vector containing wild-type p16 suppresses prostate cancer growth and prolongs survival by inducing cell senescence. *Cancer Gene Ther.* **7,** 360–372.

123. Wang, M., Wei, J., and Zhang, J. (2001) Replacement of the p16 gene in human ovarian cancer cells. *Chin. Med. J.* **114,** 857–859.

124. Allay, J. A., Steiner, M. S., Zhang, Y., Reed, C. P., Cockroft, J., and Lu, Y. (2000) Adenovirus p16 gene therapy for prostate cancer. *World J. Urol.* **18,** 111–120.

125. Calbo, J., Marotta, M., Cascallo, M., et al. (2001) Adenovirus-mediated wt-p16 reintroduction induces cell cycle arrest or apoptosis in pancreatic cancer. *Cancer Gene Ther.* **8,** 740–750.

126. Wang, T. J., Huang, M. S., Hong, C. Y., Tse, V., Silverberg, G. D., and Hsiao, M. (2001) Comparisons of tumor suppressor p53, p21, and p16 gene therapy effects on glioblastoma tumorigenicity in situ. *Biochem. Biophys. Res. Commun.* **287,** 173–180.

127. Yarbrough, W. (2002) The ARF-p16 gene locus in cacinogenesis and therapy of head and neck squamous cell carcinoma. *Laryngoscope* **112,** 2114–2128.

128. Cheng, J., Lin, C., and Xing, R. (1999) [Apoptosis of human melanoma cell line WM-983A by p16 gene transduction]. *Chin. J. Oncol.* **21,** 89–92.

129. Harper, J., Adami, G., Wie, N., Keyomarsi, K., and Elledge, S. (1993) the p21 cdk-interacting protein Cip1 is a potent inhibitor of G1 cyclin-dependent kinases. *Cell* **75,** 805–816.

130. El-Deiry, W., Tokino, T., Velculescu, V., et al. (1993) WAF1, a potential mediator of p53 tumor suppressor. *Cell* **75,** 817–825.

131. Polyak, K., Kato, J. Y., Solomon, M. J., et al. (1994) p27Kip1, a cyclin-Cdk inhibitor, links transforming growth factor-beta and contact inhibition to cell cycle arrest. *Genes Dev.* **8,** 9–22.

132. Toyoshima, H. and Hunter, T. (1994) p27, a novel inhibitor of G1 cyclin-Cdk protein kinase activity, is related to p21. *Cell* **78**, 67–74.

133. Lee, M. H., Reynisdottir, I., and Massague, J. (1995) Cloning of p57KIP2, a cyclin-dependent kinase inhibitor with unique domain structure and tissue distribution. *Genes Dev.* **9**, 639–649.

134. Harper, J. W., Elledge, S. J., Keyomarsi, K., et al. (1995) Inhibition of cyclin-dependent kinases by p21. *Mol. Biol. Cell* **6**, 387–400.

135. Johnson, M., Dimitrov, D., Vojta, P. J., et al. (1994) Evidence for p53-independent pathway for upregulation of SDI1/CIP1/WAF1/p21 RNA in human cells. *Mol. Carcinog.* **11**, 59–64.

136. el-Deiry, W. S., Harper, J. W., O'Connor, P. M., et al. (1994) WAF1/CIP1 is induced in p53-mediated G1 arrest and apoptosis. *Cancer Res.* **54**, 1169–1174.

137. Eastham, J. A., Hall, S. J., Sehgal, I., et al. (1995) In vivo gene therapy with p53 or p21 adenovirus for prostate cancer. *Cancer Res.* **55**, 5151–5155.

138. Chen, J., Willingham, T., Shuford, M., et al. (1996) Effects of ectopic overexpression of p21(WAF1/CIP1) on aneuploidy and the malignant phenotype of human brain tumor cells. *Oncogene* **13**, 1395–1403.

139. Kadowaki, Y., Fujiwara, T., Fukazawa, T., et al. (1999) Induction of differentiation-dependent apoptosis in human esophageal squamous cell carcinoma by adenovirus-mediated p21sdi1 gene transfer. *Clin. Cancer Res.* **5**, 4233–4241.

140. Chen, Y. Q., Cipriano, S. C., Arenkiel, J. M., and Miller, F. R. (1995) Tumor suppression by p21WAF1. *Cancer Res.* **55**, 4536–4539.

141. Kondo, S., Barna, B. P., Kondo, Y., et al. (1996) WAF1/CIP1 increases the susceptibility of p53 non-functional malignant glioma cells to cisplatin-induced apoptosis. *Oncogene* **13**, 1279–1285.

142. Lincet, H., Poulain, L., Remy, J. S., et al. (2000) The p21(cip1/waf1) cyclin-dependent kinase inhibitor enhances the cytotoxic effect of cisplatin in human ovarian carcinoma cells. *Cancer Lett.* **161**, 17–26.

143. Kang, K. H., Kim, W. H., and Choi, K. H. (1999) p21 promotes ceramide-induced apoptosis and antagonizes the antideath effect of Bcl-2 in human hepatocarcinoma cells. *Exp. Cell Res.* **253**, 403–412.

144. Tsao, Y. P., Huang, S. J., Chang, J. L., Hsieh, J. T., Pong, R. C., and Chen, S. L. (1999) Adenovirus-mediated p21(WAF1/SDII/CIP1) gene transfer induces apoptosis of human cervical cancer cell lines. *J. Virol.* **73**, 4983–4990.

145. Hingorani, R., Bi, B., Dao, T., Bae, Y., Matsuzawa, A., and Crispe, I. N. (2000) CD95/Fas signaling in T lymphocytes induces the cell cycle control protein p21cip-1/WAF-1, which promotes apoptosis. *J. Immunol.* **164**, 4032–4036.

146. Shinoura, N., Yoshida, Y., Asai, A., Kirino, T., and Hamada, H. (2000) Adenovirus-mediated transfer of p53 and Fas ligand drastically enhances apoptosis in gliomas. *Cancer Gene Ther.* **7**, 732–738.

147. Xie, Y., Gilbert, J. D., Kim, J. H., and Freytag, S. O. (1999) Efficacy of adenovirus-mediated CD/5-FC and HSV-1 thymidine kinase/ganciclovir suicide gene therapies concomitant with p53 gene therapy. *Clin. Cancer Res.* **5**, 4224–4232.

148. Mohiuddin, I., Cao, X., Fang, B., Nishizaki, M., and Smythe, W. R. (2001) Significant augmentation of pro-apoptotic gene therapy by pharmacologic bcl-xl down-regulation in mesothelioma. *Cancer Gene Ther.* **8**, 547–554.

149. Pulkkanen, K. J., Laukkanen, J. M., Fuxe, J., et al. (2002) The combination of HSV-tk and endostatin gene therapy eradicates orthotopic human renal cell carcinomas in nude mice. *Cancer Gene Ther.* **9**, 908–916.

150. Tanaka, M., Fraizer, G. C., De La Cerda, J., Cristiano, R. J., Liebert, M., and Grossman, H. B. (2001) Connexin 26 enhances the bystander effect in HSVtk/GCV gene therapy for human bladder cancer by adenovirus/PLL/DNA gene delivery. *Gene Ther.* **8**, 139–148.

151. Brockstedt, D. G., Diagana, M., Zhang, Y., et al. (2002) Development of anti-tumor immunity against a non-immunogenic mammary carcinoma through in vivo somatic GM-CSF, IL-2, and HSVtk combination gene therapy. *Mol. Ther.* **6**, 627–636.

152. Benedetti, S., Dimeco, F., Pollo, B., et al. (1997) Limited efficacy of the HSV-TK/GCV system for gene therapy of malignant gliomas and perspectives for the combined transduction of the interleukin-4 gene. *Hum. Gene Ther.* **8**, 1345–1353.

153. Hall, S. J., Canfield, S. E., Yan, Y., Hassen, W., Selleck, W. A., and Chen, S. H. (2002) A novel bystander effect involving tumor cell-derived Fas and FasL interactions following Ad.HSV-tk and Ad.mIL-12 gene therapies in experimental prostate cancer. *Gene Ther.* **9**, 511–517.

154. Lee, A., DeJong, G., Guo, J., Bu, X., and Jia, W. W. (2000) Bax expressed from a herpes viral vector enhances the efficacy of N,N'-bis(2-hydroxyethyl)-N-nitrosourea treatment in a rat glioma model. *Cancer Gene Ther.* **7**, 1113–1119.

155. Zhang, Y., Yu, J., Unni, E., et al. (2002) Monogene and polygene therapy for the treatment of experimental prostate cancers by use of apoptotic genes bax and bad driven by the prostate-specific promoter ARR_2PB. *Hum. Gene Ther.* **13**, 2051–2064.

156. Frost, P. J., Belldegrun, A., and Bonavida, B. (1999) Sensitization of immunoresistant prostate carcinoma cell lines to Fas/Fas ligand-mediated killing by cytotoxic lymphocytes: independence of de novo protein synthesis. *Prostate* **41**, 20–30.

157. Micheau, O., Solary, E., Hammann, A., Martin, F., and Dimanche-Boitrel, M. T. (1997) Sensitization of cancer cells treated with cytotoxic drugs to fas-mediated cytotoxicity. *J. Natl. Cancer Inst.* **89**, 783–789.

158. Beltinger, C., Fulda, S., Walczak, H., and Debatin, K. M. (2002) TRAIL enhances thymidine kinase/ganciclovir gene therapy of neuroblastoma cells. *Cancer Gene Ther.* **9**, 372–381.

159. Nagane, M., Pan, G., Weddle, J. J., Dixit, V. M., Cavenee, W. K., and Huang, H. J. (2000) Increased death receptor 5 expression by chemotherapeutic agents in human gliomas causes synergistic cytotoxicity with tumor necrosis factor-related apoptosis-inducing ligand in vitro and in vivo. *Cancer Res.* **60,** 847–853.
160. Roth, J. A., Nguyen, D., Lawrence, D. D., et al. (1996) Retrovirus-mediated wild-type p53 gene transfer to tumors of patients with lung cancer. *Nat. Med.* **2,** 985–991.
161. Pisters, L., McDonnell, T., Troncoso, P., et al. (2001) Intraprostatic Ad-p53 gene therapy induces apoptosis in locally advanced adenocarcinoma of the prostate [abstract 699]. *Proc. Am. Soc. Clin. Oncol.* **20,** 175a.
162. Nemunaitis, J., Swisher, S. G., Timmons, T., et al. (2000) Adenovirus-mediated p53 gene transfer in sequence with cisplatin to tumors of patients with non-small-cell lung cancer. *J. Clin. Oncol.* **18,** 609–622.
163. Vorburger, S. A. and Hunt, K. K. (2002) Adenoviral gene therapy. *Oncologist* **7,** 46–59.

Duen-Hwa Yan, Kung-Ming Rau, and Mien-Chie Hung

1. INTRODUCTION

Metastasis is the major cause of death for cancer patients. The presence of metastatic tumors often indicates the late stage of the disease progression in which the tumor cells have undergone multiple genetic changes that may have contributed to resistance to radiation and chemotherapy treatment. To treat the elusive metastatic tumors, an efficient systemic delivery system that carries the therapeutic payload to multiple tumor targets in a patient would be needed. The therapeutic agent has to be powerful enough to inhibit the tumor growth or to eliminate it. In this chapter, we focus the discussion on our experience using adenovirus *E1A* (Ad.*E1A*) as a therapeutic gene in cancer gene therapy treatment for metastatic tumors. Finally, we describe our findings that show the antitumor and antimetastasis activities of a novel therapeutic gene, *p202*, and its potential use against metastatic tumors.

2. *E1A* AS ANTIMETASTASIS GENE

2.1. E1A *as a Metastasis Suppressor Gene*

Ad.*E1A* is a multifunctional protein that has a wide range of effects on transformation, deoxyribonucleic acid (DNA) synthesis, apoptosis, differentiation, and tumor suppression *(1–3)*. *E1A* was initially characterized as an oncogene mainly because of its ability to promote growth and immortalization of quiescent rodent cells *(4,5)* and to cooperate with ras oncogene to transform these cells *(6)*. However, *E1A* has not been associated with human malignancies despite extensive studies to look for such a link. Rather, *E1A* was shown to suppress experimental metastasis of rodent cells transformed by the ras oncogene *(7–9)* and by the neu oncogene *(10)*. *E1A* was also shown to suppress metastasis of certain human tumor cell lines *(11)*.

Metastasis is a complex, multistep process in which tumor cells must interact with extracellular matrix and stroma cells to initiate and finish the metastatic process. Therefore, it is not surprising to find the relationship between *E1A*-mediated suppression of metastasis and the upregulation of metastasis suppressor genes such as E-cadherins *(12,13)*, a nucleoside diphosphate kinase (*NM23*) *(8)*, and tissue inhibitors of metalloproteinase (*TIMPs*) *(14)* and the downregulation of metastasis-promoting genes such as matrix metalloproteinases (*MMPs*) like *MMP-1 (11)*, *MMP-3 (15,16)*, *MMP-9 (10,11,17–20)*, urokinase-type plasminogen activator *(11)*, adhesion molecules (e.g., *CD44s*) *(21)*, and *HER-2 (10,22)*.

Although *E1A* was reported initially not to have the tumor suppressor activity *(11)*, increasing experimental data point to the ability of *E1A* to suppress tumorigenesis, as illustrated by the observations that *E1A* was able to inhibit the tumorigenicity of the transformed rodent cells *(22–25)* and of

From: *Contemporary Cancer Research*
Cancer Gene Therapy
Edited by: D. T. Curiel and J. T. Douglas © Humana Press Inc., Totowa, NJ

the human cancer cell lines *(26–29)*. Therefore, based on its ability to suppress both tumorigenicity and metastasis, *E1A* has been considered a tumor suppressor gene *(2,30–34)*.

The above-mentioned experiments primarily used the *E1A* stable transfectants to define the tumor suppressor activity of E1A. These experiments provide proof of principle for *E1A*-associated tumor suppression activity, but are not "therapy" *per se*. To translate *E1A* into an effective therapeutic gene, we have developed several gene therapy strategies using liposome and viral vectors as gene delivery systems. We demonstrated that *E1A*-based gene therapy treatments could indeed yield therapeutic efficacies in human xenograft mouse models that mimic breast *(35)*, ovarian *(36,37)*, and lung *(38)* cancers.

With these encouraging preclinical studies, the safety issue remained a serious concern for moving *E1A* to clinical trials because the prevailing conception was that *E1A* was an oncogene *(39,40)*. In 1995, we proposed to the Food and Drug Administration and the Recombinant DNA Advisory Committee of the National Institutes of Health a phase I clinical trial of *E1A* treatment targeting only patients with HER-2-overexpressing tumors. At the time, our proposal provided the only available gene therapy data with the clear mechanism that E1A transcriptionally downregulates HER-2 oncogene, leading to suppression of tumorigenicity and metastasis. In this section, we focus the discussion on our experience regarding how the laboratory findings were translated into clinical trials.

2.2. E1A *Suppression of* HER-2 *Overexpression-Mediated Tumorigenesis and Metastasis*

2.2.1. HER-2 *Overexpression and Metastasis*

Amplification/overexpression of the *HER-2* proto-oncogene was found in approx 30% of human breast *(41–44)* and ovarian *(45–47)* cancers. Significantly, patients with breast and ovarian cancer with HER-2 overexpression in their tumors often have a poor overall survival rate and shorter time to relapse compared with other patients without HER-2 overexpression. Thus, HER-2 overexpression has been a useful pathological marker for poor prognosis *(41,45,46)*. HER-2 overexpression was also found with high frequency in lung *(48,49)*, gastric *(50)*, bladder *(51)*, and oral cancers *(52–54)*, suggesting that HER-2 overexpression likely plays a critical role in the development of human malignancies.

Clinically, HER-2 overexpression is also associated with disease progression and metastasis *(55)*. HER-2 overexpression is correlated with early metastasis as well as with increased incidence of metastasis *(56,57)*. In experimental systems, for example, enforced HER-2 overexpression in the non-small lung cancer cell line NCI-H460, which expresses a very low level of HER-2, enhances metastatic potential *(58)*. More important, all of the HER-2-overexpressing NCI-H460 transfectants developed extrapulmonary metastases (in the ribs, mesentery, ovary, and stomach). Formation of extrapulmonary metastasis requires tumor cells to grow in a less-favorable nonorthotopic microenvironment; therefore, the HER-2-overexpressing transfectants may have gained the ability to overcome organ selectivity of growth. Enforced HER-2 expression also partially restored the metastatic potential of the otherwise less-metastatic breast cancer cells in vitro and in vivo *(59)*, confirming that HER-2 overexpression is one of the causes for the metastatic phenotype.

Because HER-2 is expressed at low levels in normal tissues, HER-2-based cancer drugs should have selective therapeutic effects against HER-2-overexpressing tumors. Based on this idea, many therapeutic strategies have been developed to target HER-2-overexpressing tumors *(60–62)*. One of them is E1A-based gene therapy treatment for HER-2-overexpressing tumors.

2.2.2. E1A *Suppression of* HER-2 *Overexpression-Mediated Metastasis*

E1A represses the expression of steady-state *HER-2* messenger ribonucleic acid (RNA) and protein by downregulating *HER-2* promoter activity *(63,64)*. Because HER-2 overexpression enhances the metastatic potential of the cancer cell *(10,58)*, it is conceivable that E1A may downregulate HER-2 expression, leading to suppression of metastasis. Indeed, E1A expression in HER-2-overexpressing cancer cells rendered the cells less metastatic *(10,22)*. However, E1A could suppress metastasis regard-

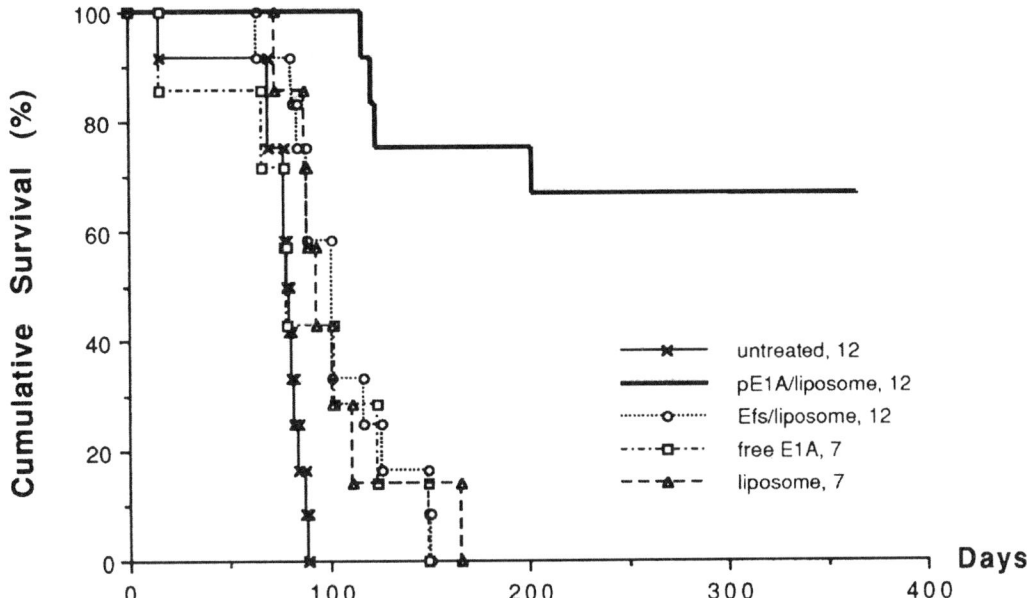

Fig. 1. Mice treated with wild-type *E1A*: Liposome complexes (heavy solid line) survived longer than untreated mice (solid line with crosses) or mice treated with wild-type *E1A* DNA alone, with liposome alone, or with liposome plus *E1A* frame-shift DNA (*Efs*) ($p < 0.01$). Mice were given intraperitoneal injections of 2×10^6 viable SKOV-3 human ovarian cancer cells 5 days before treatment. In two experiments, a total of 7 or 12 mice made up each experimental group (as indicated in the figure key). Mice were examined for tumor symptoms and were killed when they appeared moribund. Similar results were obtained from these experiments, and results were combined for analysis. The survival curves were obtained by recording the total survival days for each mouse in different groups from the day of injection with SKOV-3 cells (day 1, 100% survival) to the day they died. (Excerpt from Fig. 2 in ref. *37*. The permission to use this figure was granted by Nature Publishing Group.)

less of HER-2 expression level. This idea is supported by the observation that, although reexpressing HER-2 in E1A-expressing cancer cells could restore their tumorigenicity, it failed to restore the metastatic potential or the MMP expression *(22)*. This result is consistent with earlier reports that indicated E1A is associated with metastasis suppression activity *(7,11)* and further suggests that E1A mediates metastasis suppression by targeting the downstream molecules of the HER-2-induced metastasis-signaling pathway.

2.3. E1A *Gene Therapy*

2.3.1. *Preclinical Studies*

To test the efficacy of an *E1A*-based gene therapy in mice bearing human HER-2-overexpressing tumors, three orthotopic cancer xenograft models (i.e., ovarian, breast, and lung) were established, and two E1A delivery systems were used: a cationic liposome 3β[*N*-(*N'*-dimethylaminoethane)-carbamoyl] cholesterol:dioleoylphatidylethanolamine (3:2) (DC-Chol):DOPE *(65)* and Ad.*E1A (64)*.

2.3.1.1. OVARIAN CANCER MODEL

The orthotopic ovarian cancer model was established by injecting human HER-2-overexpressing ovarian cancer cells (i.e., SKOV3) intraperitoneally into female nu/nu mice (Fig. 1). The implanted ovarian tumors obtained from the mesentery and inside the peritoneal cavity showed HER-2-positive staining *(37)*. The tumor-bearing mice received intraperitoneal injection of either *E1A* expression vector complex with DC-Chol (DCC-*E1A*) *(37)* or Ad.*E1A* *(36)*.

Necropsy analysis showed that some of *E1A*/DC-Chol-treated mice, although they died of tumor-related symptoms, had no detectable tumor invasion and metastasis as commonly seen in mice in the control groups, (i.e., no treatment, mutant *E1A*/DC-Chol, *E1A* alone, or DC-Chol alone) *(37)*. When examined, tumor tissues excised from the *E1A*/DC-Chol-treated mice, it was clear that *E1A* expression correlated well with downregulation of HER-2 protein, but there was no decrease in HER-2 protein level in the tumors obtained from the control groups. Remarkably, 70% of the *E1A*/DC-Chol-treated mice survived more than a year; the controls all died within 200 days *(37)*. The surviving mice appeared normal and healthy because there were no detectable tumors inside the mice or any obvious side effect associated with the treatment. These results showed that (1) by intraperitoneal injection, *E1A*/DC-Chol complex is a useful vehicle to transduce *E1A* into ovarian cancer cells in vivo, and (2) *E1A*/DC-Chol treatment could repress HER-2 expression, suppress tumor growth, reduce metastasis, increase survival, and have no obvious side effect. This observation was among the first evidence to indicate the efficacy and the feasibility of using *E1A*/DC-Chol-based gene therapy to treat ovarian cancer effectively in a xenograft model.

The efficacy of using Ad.*E1A* in the above orthotopic ovarian cancer model appeared similar to that obtained from the *E1A*/DC-Chol treatment *(36,37)*. In addition to SKOV3, the Ad.*E1A* study included a low HER-2-expressing human ovarian cancer cell line, 2774. Intriguingly, although Ad.*E1A* could effectively increase survival in the SKOV3 tumor model, it failed to do so in the 2774 tumor model *(36,66)*. This result was not caused by a difference of viral infection efficiency between SKOV3 and 2774 cell lines because both could be infected equally, as determined by adenovirus-carrying β-galactosidase gene (Ad.*LacZ*) *(36)*.

This observation raises a possibility that E1A may mediate a preferential antitumor effect on HER-2-overexpressing ovarian cancer cells, but not on ovarian cancer cells with low HER-2 expression. Alternatively, a more rigorous treatment may be needed for such low HER-2-expressing cancer cells as 2774 to achieve a similar efficacy seen in treating the HER-2-overexpressing cancer cells. SKOV3 tumors excised from Ad.*E1A*-infected mice showed positive staining for E1A proteins and concurrent reduction of HER-2 protein expression on the same tumor samples. This result therefore confirms in vivo a causal relationship between E1A expression and HER-2 downregulation. Using Ad.*LacZ* to monitor the E1A expression spectrum in SKOV3 tumor model, it is encouraging to know that high LacZ expression was found in malignant ascites and tumors compared with that in other tissues and organs, suggesting that Ad.*E1A* may preferentially target these tumor sites *(36)*.

2.3.1.2. Breast Cancer Model

Ad.*E1A* infection preferentially inhibited the growth of HER-2-overexpressing breast cancer cells (e.g., MDA-MB-361 and SKBR3), whereas there was little or no E1A-mediated growth-inhibitory effect on the low HER-2-expressing cancer cells (e.g., MDA-MB-435 and MDA-MB-231) *(35)*. Based on this observation, both Ad.*E1A* and *E1A*/DC-Chol were used to assess the potential efficacy in an orthotopic, HER-2-overexpressing breast cancer model.

MDA-MB-361 cells were transplanted into the mammary fat pads of female nu/nu mice. The mammary tumors usually become palpable about 45 days after implantation. Ad.*E1A* or *E1A*/DC-Chol was intratumorally injected. Six months of *E1A* treatment by either Ad.*E1A* or *E1A*/DC-Chol prolonged survival (the mean survival was longer than 2 years, as opposed to less than 15 months in the control groups) and inhibited tumor growth. The Ad.E1A treatment appeared slightly better than *E1A*/DC-Chol treatment. Remarkably, no metastasis was found in intraperitoneal organs, such as liver, intestine, spleen, and kidney *(35)*.

These results are consistent with the ability of *E1A* to inhibit metastasis and are reminiscent of the E1A-mediated antitumor effect on the HER-2-overexpressing ovarian cancer model, in which no detectable metastasis was found in *E1A*-treated mice *(37)*. The mammary tumor suppression correlated well with the expression of E1A and the downregulation of HER-2 protein as determined by Western blot and immunohistochemical analysis on the tumor samples *(35)*. The data suggest the feasibility of an *E1A*-based gene therapy (either by Ad.*E1A* or by *E1A*/DC-Chol) against HER-2-over-expressing breast cancer in vivo.

A toxicity study was subsequently conducted in immunocompetent mice to ensure the safety of the procedure and the minimum side effects associated with the *E1A* gene therapy treatment *(66,67)*.

2.3.2. Clinical Trials

2.3.2.1. PHASE I BREAST AND OVARIAN CANCER

2.3.2.1.1. Intracavity Administration. To evaluate the feasibility of using *E1A* gene therapy for patients with HER-2-overexpressing cancer, a phase I clinical trial was conducted in a group of patients with advanced breast and ovarian cancer. E1A/DC-Chol cationic liposome complex (DCC-*E1A*) was injected into the thoracic or peritoneal cavity. These results obtained from the phase I studies demonstrated limited toxicity (may be because of DCC-*E1A* rather than E1A expression), efficient *E1A* gene transfer (indicated by the *E1A* messenger RNA expression in tumors as well as in certain distant organs), and downregulation of HER-2. DCC-*E1A* treatment was also associated with decreased tumor clumps and proliferating cell population and increased apoptotic cells. Interestingly, the increase of apoptotic cells correlates well with an increase of tumor necrosis factor-α (TNF-α) level. Because E1A inactivates NF-κB *(68)*, an antiapoptotic molecule induced by TNF-α, it is likely that the increase of apoptotic cells is because of the sensitization to TNF-α-induced apoptosis by E1A. Overall, of 18 patients with advanced cancer of the breast ($n = 6$) or ovary ($n = 12$) treated with DCC-E1A, at least 1 patient with breast cancer had no pathological evidence of tumor; 2 patients had minor responses; 8 had stable disease; and 6 had progressive disease *(69)*. These results suggest the feasibility of the DCC-*E1A* trial.

2.3.2.1.2. Intratumoral Administration. In a phase I trial, nine patients with recurrent and unresectable breast tumors were treated with DCC-*E1A* through intratumoral injection. There were no dose-limiting drug-related toxicities, and no drug-related adverse effects were observed. E1A expression was readily detectable in tumor samples after DCC-*E1A* treatment. In one patient with breast cancer, no apparent pathological evidence of tumor at the tumor site of treatment was observed *(70)*.

2.3.2.2. PHASE II HEAD AND NECK CANCER WITH INTRATUMORAL ADMINISTRATION

A phase I study of DCC-*E1A* treatment with 9 patients with head and neck cancers has been completed *(70)*. The results of this study indicated no dose-limiting toxicity, and doses used were below the maximally tolerated dose. E1A expression and HER-2 downregulation were seen in DCC-*E1A*-treated tumor biopsies. After the successful phase I study, a multicenter phase II study was completed *(71)*. DCC-*E1A* was used as a single agent and was administered by intratumoral injection. Among 24 patients with recurrent, unresectable, head and neck cancer treated, 4.2% (1 of 24) showed a complete response, and 37.5% (9 out of 24) showed an objective response or reached a state of stable disease. The most common side effect was pain at the injection site, but there were no serious adverse events related to DCC-*E1A* administration.

These results suggest that intratumoral injection of DCC-*E1A* is safe and well tolerated. Based on the encouraging results of the phase II trials, a possible combined DCC-*E1A* therapy with ionizing radiation and/or chemotherapy should be feasible in the near future.

3. *p202* AS ANTIMETASTASIS GENE

3.1. p202

The p202 protein is encoded by one of the six or more murine interferon-inducible genes of the gene 200 cluster on chromosome 1q21–23 *(72)*. This family of proteins shares, close to their carboxyl termini, partially homologous segments 200 amino acids long. So far, *p202* is the best-characterized member of this family, which includes *p203*, *p204*, and *D3* in the mouse *(72)* and *MNDA, IFI 16*, and *AIM2* in human *(73)*. The pathological relevance of *p202* was realized by the identification of *p202* as a candidate gene using a mouse model for systemic lupus erythematosus *(74)*. The human counterpart of *p202*, however, has not been identified.

p202 is primarily a nuclear, chromatin-associated 52-kDa phosphoprotein and is primarily involved in protein–protein interactions. Notably, several important transcriptional regulators, including retinoblastoma gene (Rb) *(75)*, E2F-1 *(76)*, E2F-4, p107 and p130 *(77)*, Fos/Jun (AP-1), a p53-binding protein (53BP-1) *(78)*, c-Myc *(79)*, MyoD, and myogenin *(80)* were physically associated with p202 in vitro and in vivo. These observations strongly suggest a functional significance of p202 in cell cycle regulation, signal transduction, apoptosis, and differentiation. The p202-associated protein–protein interactions generally result in inhibition of the promoter activities *(76,77,79,80–83)*. In most cases, direct blocking of the transcriptional factor binding to its cognate DNA element by p202 is responsible for the transcription repression.

Similar to the interferon-induced growth inhibition, persistent expression of p202 was shown to be growth inhibitory in rodent cells *(76–78,81,84,85)* and human cancer cells *(82,83,86,87)*. The p202-mediated growth inhibition was associated with attenuation at the G1/S cell cycle transition. Although the molecular mechanism of p202-mediated growth inhibition is not well understood, the observation that p202 binds to several important cell cycle regulatory molecules in vitro and in vivo, such as Rb, p107, p130, E2F-1, E2F-4, and c-Myc, has shed light on the p202 action in cell cycle regulation *(75–77,79)*. For example, p202 interacts with E2F-1 and abrogates E2F-1-mediated transcriptional activation of certain S-phase genes, such as *DHFR*, *b-Myb*, and *PCNA*, resulting in attenuation of S-phase entry *(76)*. p202 also suppresses transformation, as indicated by the inability of p202-expressing cancer cells to grow in soft agar *(82,83,86)*.

In addition to growth inhibition, we recently showed that p202 expression promotes apoptosis *(87)*. The p202-mediated apoptosis appears to be dependent on the activation of caspases. Based on the growth-inhibitory and proapoptotic activities of p202, we performed preclinical studies to evaluate the feasibility of using *p202* in gene therapy treatment of experimental tumors.

3.2. p202 *in Preclinical Gene Therapy Studies*

3.2.1. Breast Cancer Model

Metastatic breast cancer is a deadly disease. Conventional treatments using chemotherapy and radiation with or without surgical intervention have yielded limited success. We have shown ex vivo antitumor activity using *p202* expression vector and polyethylenimine complex in an orthotopic breast cancer xenograft model *(83)*. Because breast cancer is a metastatic disease, it is critical to develop a systemic delivery system that would allow delivery of *p202* gene through intravenous injection to the primary and metastasized tumor sites.

To this end, we undertook two approaches and compared the efficacy of systemic *p202* gene therapy treatment using either a p202-expressing recombinant adenovirus (Ad-*p202*) or CMV-*p202*/SN2 liposome complex in an orthotopic breast cancer xenograft model. CMV-*p202* is a p202 expression vector driven by cytomegalovirus (CMV) promoter. SN2 liposome formulation has been tested and showed high gene delivery efficiency in systemic gene therapy animal models *(88)*. We found that tumor growth was significantly reduced in both Ad-*p202* and CMV-*p202*/SN2 treatment groups *(87)* (Y. Wen and M.-C. Hung, unpublished data).

These data are highly significant because CMV-*p202*/SN2 and Ad-*p202* had to overcome many immunological, physiological, and structural barriers inside and outside the blood vessels to reach tumor cells and release their therapeutic effect as compared with other experimental therapy models, such as intratumoral injection *(89)*. These results strongly suggest the feasibility of a systemic *p202*-based gene therapy treatment for breast cancer.

On examining the tumor treated with Ad-*p202* or CMV-*p202*/SN2 by immunohistochemical assays, we found that the level of p202 protein correlated well with the extent of apoptosis in tumors in both models as determined by terminal deoxynucleotide transferase-mediated dUTP nick end labeling assay that stains the ends of DNA fragments. This observation is in agreement with our in vitro data that showed Ad-*p202* infection induces apoptosis *(87)*. Thus, the p202-induced apoptosis contributed to the overall antitumor activities in vivo.

In addition, we observed a much reduced level of an angiogenic factor, vascular endothelial growth factor (VEGF), in breast tumors treated with either CMV-*p202*/SN2 or Ad-*p202* compared with that of the control treatments. This result is consistent with our previous observation that p202 expression suppressed metastasis and angiogenesis in pancreatic tumors *(82)* (discussed in the next section). Thus, our data strongly suggested *p202* is a potent therapeutic gene suitable for breast cancer gene therapy.

3.2.2. Pancreatic Cancer Model

Pancreatic cancer is highly aggressive and is a leading cause of cancer death in Western countries. The deadliness of this disease is illustrated by the prediction in 1999 that 28,600 new cases would be diagnosed, and most cases would be fatal *(90)*. The main reason for the extremely poor prognosis is that patients often present with advanced stage at the time of diagnosis. The median survival varies between 4 and 6 months, and the 5-year survival rate is less than 2% *(91)*. Currently, there is no effective treatment for this deadly disease because conventional chemotherapy and radiation treatments have had very limited success in improving patient survival *(92)*. Therefore, novel treatment strategies against this disease are urgently needed.

We showed previously that p202 is able to suppress the transformation phenotype (e.g., inhibition of growth in soft agar) of pancreatic cancer cells (Panc-1) in vitro *(82)*. It is possible that p202 could suppress tumorigenicity in vivo. To test the therapeutic effect of *p202* in pancreatic cancer xenograft models, we performed tumorigenicity assays using both subcutaneous and orthotopic mouse models. We showed that, in either model, the tumorigenicity of p202-expressing Panc-1 cells was greatly reduced compared with that of the parental pancreatic cancer cells. In particular, we found that, in the orthotopic model, the p202-expressing Panc-1 cells not only formed tumors at a lower frequency, but also that those mice with tumors had a significantly longer survival rate compared with the mice bearing Panc-1 tumors. These results clearly demonstrated that p202 possesses potent antitumor activity in vivo *(82)*.

3.2.2.1. P202 SUPPRESSION OF METASTASIS

On examining the orthotopic pancreatic tumor growth in mice, we noticed 40% of Panc-1 tumor-bearing mice and 20% of vector control tumor-bearing mice with liver metastasis. In contrast, there was no detectable liver metastasis in mice with p202-expressing tumors. This result suggested that p202 may have an antimetastasis activity in vivo.

To test this hypothesis in vitro, we employed a double-chamber assay *(58)* in which the test cells were grown in the top chamber, and the bottom chamber was filled with the conditioned media containing chemoattractant (e.g., laminin). A Matrigel-coated membrane was used to separate the two chambers. To migrate from the top chamber to the bottom chamber, cells must digest the barrier (i.e., the reconstituted basement membrane matrix) by producing secretory proteases such as MMPs before they penetrate the pores on the membrane. Thus, this assay somewhat mimics the metastatic process, and the number of cells found in the bottom chamber therefore is indicative of the metastatic potential of the test cells.

Based on this criterion, we found that p202-expressing Panc-1 cells were less able to penetrate the membrane than the parental Panc-1 cells and thus were less metastatic. This in vitro observation is consistent with the in vivo data and lends support to the hypothesis that p202 suppresses metastasis. Consistent with the antimetastasis activity of p202, we also showed the activity of MMP-2, a metastasis promoter, is reduced in p202-expressing Panc-1 cells *(82)*.

3.2.2.2. P202 SUPPRESSION OF ANGIOGENESIS

It has been well documented that tumor growth and metastasis require persistent growth of new blood vessels (neovasculature) (reviewed in ref. *93*). To examine further the p202-mediated antitumor activity in pancreatic tumor, we analyzed the formation of neovasculature in p202-expressing tumors and Panc-1 tumors. We found that the number of blood vessels (as stained by antibody against a blood vessel marker, i.e., CD31; *94*) was significantly reduced in p202-expressing tumor compared with Panc-1 tumor *(82)*. Consistent with the reduced angiogenesis, we also found, using immunohistochemical analysis, the expression of angiogenic factors such as interleukin 8 (IL-8) and VEGF (reviewed in ref. *93*) are reduced in p202-expressing tumors *(82)*.

Because p202 is generally known as a negative transcriptional regulator, we tested if the repression of IL-8 or VEGF protein in p202-1 tumor is because of transcriptional repression by p202. We performed a reporter assay by cotransfecting p202 expression vector with a luciferase reporter driven by either IL-8 or VEGF promoter into Panc-1 cells. Interestingly, we found p202 transfection resulted in an inhibition of both IL-8 and VEGF promoter activities (Y. Wen and M.-C. Hung, unpublished results). Thus, this observation suggested that p202 suppresses IL-8 and VEGF expression on the transcriptional level. Taken together, our data strongly indicate that p202 expression is associated with reduced angiogenesis, which may contribute in part to the reduced tumor growth and metastatic potential of the p202-expressing tumors.

3.2.2.3. P202/LIPOSOME ADMINISTRATION SUPPRESSION OF TUMOR GROWTH IN HUMAN PANCREATIC CANCER XENOGRAFT MODEL

To test the therapeutic effect of a *p202*-based treatment in a preclinical gene therapy model, we treated the subcutaneous Panc-1 tumors via intratumoral injection of CMV-*p202* using a nonviral delivery system, SN2. We showed that CMV-*p202*/SN2 treatment resulted in significant tumor growth inhibition compared with the control treatments. On examining the tumor biopsies by immunohistochemical methods, we found that the level of p202 protein expression correlated well with the extent of apoptosis in CMV-*p202*/liposome-treated tumors by terminal deoxynucleotide transferase-mediated dUTP nick end labeling. Again, this result is consistent with the idea that the p202-mediated apoptosis contributes to the overall antitumor activities *(87)*. This result provides a scientific basis for further investigation into the utility of *p202*-based gene therapy in pancreatic cancer treatment.

4. FUTURE DIRECTION

In this chapter, we summarized our findings related to suppression of metastasis by two therapeutic genes, *E1A* and *p202*. Both are potent in suppressing tumorigenesis, metastasis, and angiogenesis. *E1A* is in phase II clinical trials, and the preliminary data obtained have been encouraging *(95)*. Both *E1A* and *p202* could sensitize cancer cells to apoptosis induced by TNF-α or γ-irradiation *(68,83,87,96)*. Mechanistic studies suggested that E1A and p202 inactivate NF-κ *(97)*, an antiapoptotic factor induced by TNF-α or γ-irradiation, leading to enhanced apoptosis. These data provide a rationale to develop the combined therapy of *E1A* (or *p202*) and TNF-α (or γ-irradiation), which should yield a better therapeutic effect than using a single agent. It is also likely that *E1A* or *p202* combined with chemotherapeutic agents *(98)*, which activate NF-κB, may enhance the effectiveness of tumor killing.

Furthermore, because systemic treatment is imperative for treating metastatic tumors, the targeting specificity should be of concern for minimizing potential side effects. One way to overcome this drawback is to express *E1A* or *p202* gene under the control of a tumor-specific promoter or by delivery by a tumor-specific gene delivery system. By the specific expression of E1A or p202 at tumor sites combined with appropriate chemotherapeutic agents that sensitize cancer cells to apoptosis, we would expect much effective killing of metastatic tumors.

REFERENCES

1. Ben-Israel, H. and Kleinberger, T. (2002) Adenovirus and cell cycle control. *Front. Biosci.* **7**, d1369–1395.
2. Frisch, S. M. and Mymryk, J. S. (2002) Adenovirus-5 E1A: paradox and paradigm. *Nat. Rev. Mol. Cell Biol.* **3**, 441–452.
3. Frisch, S. M. (1996) Reversal of malignancy by the adenovirus E1a gene. *Mutat. Res.* **350**, 261–266.
4. Houweling, A., van den Elsen, P. J., and van der Eb, A. J. (1980) Partial transformation of primary rat cells by the leftmost 4.5% fragment of adenovirus 5 DNA. *Virology* **105**, 537–550.
5. Howe, J. A., Mymryk, J. S., Egan, C., Branton, P. E., and Bayley, S. T. (1990) Retinoblastoma growth suppressor and a 300-kDa protein appear to regulate cellular DNA synthesis. *Proc. Natl. Acad. Sci. USA* **87**, 5883–5887.
6. Ruley, H. E. (1983) Adenovirus early region 1A enables viral and cellular transforming genes to transform primary cells in culture. *Nature* **304**, 602–606.
7. Pozzatti, R., McCormick, M., Thompson, M. A., and Khoury, G. (1988) The E1a gene of adenovirus type 2 reduces the metastatic potential of ras-transformed rat embryo cells. *Mol. Cell. Biol.* **8**, 2984–2988.
8. Steeg, P. S., Bevilacqua, G., Pozzatti, R., Liotta, L. A., and Sobel, M. E. (1988) Altered expression of NM23, a gene associated with low tumor metastatic potential, during adenovirus 2 E1a inhibition of experimental metastasis. *Cancer Res.* **48**, 6550–6554.
9. Pozzatti, R., McCormick, M., Thompson, M. A., Garbisa, S., Liotta, L., and Khoury, G. (1988) Regulation of the metastatic phenotype by the E1A gene of adenovirus-2. *Adv. Exp. Med. Biol.* **233**, 293–301.
10. Yu, D., Hamada, J., Zhang, H., Nicolson, G. L., and Hung, M. C. (1992) Mechanisms of c-erbB2/neu oncogene-induced metastasis and repression of metastatic properties by adenovirus 5 E1A gene products. *Oncogene* **7**, 2263–2270.
11. Frisch, S. M., Reich, R., Collier, I. E., Genrich, L. T., Martin, G., and Goldberg, G. I. (1990) Adenovirus E1A represses protease gene expression and inhibits metastasis of human tumor cells. *Oncogene* **5**, 75–83.
12. Frisch, S. M. (1994) E1a induces the expression of epithelial characteristics. *J. Cell Biol.* **127**, 1085–1096.
13. Hennig, G., Behrens, J., Truss, M., Frisch, S., Reichmann, E., and Birchmeier, W. (1995) Progression of carcinoma cells is associated with alterations in chromatin structure and factor binding at the E-cadherin promoter in vivo. *Oncogene* **11**, 475–484.
14. Santoro, M., Battaglia, C., Zhang, L., et al. (1994) Cloning of the rat tissue inhibitor of metalloproteinases type 2 (TIMP-2) gene: analysis of its expression in normal and transformed thyroid cells. *Exp. Cell Res.* **213**, 398-403.
15. Offringa, R., Smits, A. M., Houweling, A., Bos, J. L., and van der Eb, A. J. (1988) Similar effects of adenovirus E1A and glucocorticoid hormones on the expression of the metalloprotease stromelysin. *Nucleic Acids Res.* **16**, 10,973–10,984.
16. Linder, S., Popowicz, P., Svensson, C., Marshall, H., Bondesson, M., and Akusjarvi, G. (1992) Enhanced invasive properties of rat embryo fibroblasts transformed by adenovirus E1A mutants with deletions in the carboxy-terminal exon. *Oncogene* **7**, 439–443.
17. Garbisa, S., Pozzatti, R., Muschel, R. J., et al. (1987) Secretion of type IV collagenolytic protease and metastatic phenotype: induction by transfection with c-Ha-ras but not c-Ha-ras plus Ad2-E1a. *Cancer Res.* **47**, 1523–1528.
18. Offringa, R., Gebel, S., van Dam, H., et al. (1990) A novel function of the transforming domain of E1a: repression of AP-1 activity. *Cell* **62**, 527–538.
19. Bernhard, E. J., Muschel, R. J., and Hughes, E. N. (1990) Mr 92,000 gelatinase release correlates with the metastatic phenotype in transformed rat embryo cells. *Cancer Res.* **50**, 3872–3877.
20. Bernhard, E. J., Hagner, B., Wong, C., Lubenski, I., and Muschel, R. J. (1995) The effect of E1A transfection on MMP-9 expression and metastatic potential. *Int. J. Cancer* **60**, 718–724.
21. Hofmann, M., Rudy, W., Gunthert, U., et al. (1993) A link between ras and metastatic behavior of tumor cells: ras induces CD44 promoter activity and leads to low-level expression of metastasis-specific variants of CD44 in CREF cells. *Cancer Res.* **53**, 1516–1521.
22. Yu, D., Shi, D., Scanlon, M., and Hung, M. C. (1993) Reexpression of neu-encoded oncoprotein counteracts the tumor-suppressing but not the metastasis-suppressing function of E1A. *Cancer Res.* **53**, 5784–5790.
23. Yu, D. H., Scorsone, K., and Hung, M. C. (1991) Adenovirus type 5 E1A gene products act as transformation suppressors of the neu oncogene. *Mol. Cell. Biol.* **11**, 1745–1750.
24. Chen, H., Yu, D., Chinnadurai, G., Karunagaran, D., and Hung, M. C. (1997) Mapping of adenovirus 5 E1A domains responsible for suppression of neu-mediated transformation via transcriptional repression of neu. *Oncogene* **14**, 1965–1971.
25. Deng, J., Xia, W., and Hung, M. C. (1998) Adenovirus 5 E1A-mediated tumor suppression associated with E1A-mediated apoptosis in vivo. *Oncogene* **17**, 2167–2175.
26. Frisch, S. M. (1991) Antioncogenic effect of adenovirus E1A in human tumor cells. *Proc. Natl. Acad. Sci. USA* **88**, 9077–9081.
27. Yu, D., Wolf, J. K., Scanlon, M., Price, J. E., and Hung, M. C. (1993) Enhanced c-erbB-2/neu expression in human ovarian cancer cells correlates with more severe malignancy that can be suppressed by E1A. *Cancer Res.* **53**, 891–898.
28. Frisch, S. M. and Dolter, K. E. (1995) Adenovirus E1a-mediated tumor suppression by a c-erbB-2/neu-independent mechanism. *Cancer Res.* **55**, 5551–5555.

29. Dickopp, A., Esche, H., Swart, G., Seeber, S., Kirch, H. C., and Opalka, B. (2000) Transformation-defective adenovirus 5 E1A mutants exhibit antioncogenic properties in human BLM melanoma cells. *Cancer Gene Ther.* **7,** 1043–1050.

30. Chinnadurai, G. (1992) Adenovirus E1a as a tumor-suppressor gene. *Oncogene* **7,** 1255–1258.

31. Mymryk, J. S. (1996) Tumour suppressive properties of the adenovirus 5 E1A oncogene. *Oncogene* **13,** 1581–1589.

32. Yu, D. and Hung, M. C. (1998) The erbB2 gene as a cancer therapeutic target and the tumor- and metastasis-suppressing function of E1A. *Cancer Metastasis Rev.* **17,** 195–202.

33. Yan, D.-H., Shao, R., and Hung, M.-C. (2001) E1A cancer gene therapy. In *Gene Therapy of Cancer*, 2nd ed. (Lattime, E. C. and Gerson, S. L., eds.), Academic Press, San Diego, CA, 2001.

34. Ueno, N. T., Yu, D., and Hung, M. C. (2001) E1A: tumor suppressor or oncogene? Preclinical and clinical investigations of E1A gene therapy. *Breast Cancer* **8,** 285–293.

35. Chang, J. Y., Xia, W., Shao, R., et al. (1997) The tumor suppression activity of E1A in HER-2/neu-overexpressing breast cancer. *Oncogene* **14,** 561–568.

36. Zhang, Y., Yu, D., Xia, W., and Hung, M. C. (1995) HER-2/neu-targeting cancer therapy via adenovirus-mediated E1A delivery in an animal model. *Oncogene* **10,** 1947–1954.

37. Yu, D., Matin, A., Xia, W., Sorgi, F., Huang, L., and Hung, M. C. (1995) Liposome-mediated in vivo E1A gene transfer suppressed dissemination of ovarian cancer cells that overexpress HER-2/neu. *Oncogene* **11,** 1383–1388.

38. Chang, J. Y., Xia, W., Shao, R., and Hung, M. C. (1996) Inhibition of intratracheal lung cancer development by systemic delivery of E1A. *Oncogene* **13,** 1405–1412.

39. Nevins, J. R., Imperiale, M. J., Feldman, L. T., and Kao, H. T. (1984) Role of the adenovirus transforming gene (E1A) in the general control of gene expression. *Transplant. Proc.* **16,** 438–440.

40. Nevins, J. R. (1995) Adenovirus E1A: transcription regulation and alteration of cell growth control. *Curr. Top. Microbiol. Immunol.* **199,** 25–32.

41. Slamon, D. J., Clark, G. M., Wong, S. G., Levin, W. J., Ullrich, A., and McGuire, W. L. (1987) Human breast cancer: correlation of relapse and survival with amplification of the HER-2/neu oncogene. *Science* **235,** 177–182.

42. Slamon, D. J. and Clark, G. M. (1988) Amplification of c-erbB-2 and aggressive human breast tumors? *Science* **240,** 1795–1798.

43. McCann, A. H., Dervan, P. A., O'Regan, M., et al. (1991) Prognostic significance of c-erbB-2 and estrogen receptor status in human breast cancer. *Cancer Res.* **51,** 3296–3303.

44. Gusterson, B. A., Gelber, R. D., Goldhirsch, A., et al. (1992) Prognostic importance of c-erbB-2 expression in breast cancer. International (Ludwig) Breast Cancer Study Group. *J. Clin. Oncol.* **10,** 1049–1056.

45. Slamon, D. J., Godolphin, W., Jones, L. A., et al. (1989) Studies of the HER-2/neu proto-oncogene in human breast and ovarian cancer. *Science* **244,** 707–712.

46. Berchuck, A., Kamel, A., Whitaker, R., et al. (1990) Overexpression of Her-2/neu is associated with poor survival in advanced epithelial ovarian cancer. *Cancer Res.* **50,** 4087–4091.

47. Zhang, X., Silva, E., Gershenson, D., and Hung, M. C. (1989) Amplification and rearrangement of c-erb B proto-oncogenes in cancer of human female genital tract. *Oncogene* **4,** 985–989.

48. Schneider, P. M., Hung, M. C., Chiocca, S. M., et al. (1989) Differential expression of the c-erbB-2 gene in human small cell and non-small cell lung cancer. *Cancer Res.* **49,** 4968–4971.

49. Weiner, D. B., Nordberg, J., Robinson, R., et al. (1990) Expression of the neu gene-encoded protein (p185neu) in human non-small cell carcinomas of the lung. *Cancer Res.* **50,** 421–425.

50. Yokota, J., Yamamoto, T., Miyajima, N., et al. (1988) Genetic alterations of the c-erbB-2 oncogene occur frequently in tubular adenocarcinoma of the stomach and are often accompanied by amplification of the v-erbA homologue. *Oncogene* **2,** 283–287.

51. Zhau, H. E., Zhang, X., von, E. A., Scorsone, K., Babaian, R. J., Ro, J. Y., and Hung, M. C. (1990) Amplification and expression of the c-erb B-2/neu proto-oncogene in human bladder cancer. *Mol. Carcinog.* **3,** 254–257.

52. Hou, L., Shi, D., Tu, S. M., Zhang, H. Z., Hung, M. C., and Ling, D. (1992) Oral cancer progression and c-erbB-2/neu proto-oncogene expression. *Cancer Lett.* **65,** 215–220.

53. Xia, W. Y., Lau, Y. K., Zhang, H. Z., et al. (1997) Strong correlation between c-Erbb-2 overexpression and overall survival of patients with oral squamous cell carcinoma. *Clin. Cancer Res.* **3,** 3–9.

54. Xia, W., Lau, Y. K., Zhang, H. Z., et al. (1999) Combination of EGFR, HER-2/neu, and HER-3 is a stronger predictor for the outcome of oral squamous cell carcinoma than any individual family members. *Clin. Cancer Res.* **5,** 4164–4174.

55. Eccles, S. A. (2001) The role of c-erbB-2/HER2/neu in breast cancer progression and metastasis. *J. Mammary Gland Biol. Neoplasia* **6,** 393–406.

56. Menard, S., Tagliabue, E., Campiglio, M., and Pupa, S. M. (2000) Role of HER2 gene overexpression in breast carcinoma. *J. Cell. Physiol.* **182,** 150–162.

57. Revillion, F., Bonneterre, J., and Peyrat, J. P. (1998) ERBB2 oncogene in human breast cancer and its clinical significance. *Eur. J. Cancer* **34,** 791–808.

58. Yu, D., Wang, S. S., Dulski, K. M., Tsai, C. M., Nicolson, G. L., and Hung, M. C. (1994) c-erbB-2/neu overexpression enhances metastatic potential of human lung cancer cells by induction of metastasis-associated properties. *Cancer Res.* **54,** 3260–3266.

59. Tan, M., Yao, J., and Yu, D. (1997) Overexpression of the c-erbB-2 gene enhanced intrinsic metastasis potential in human breast cancer cells without increasing their transformation abilities. *Cancer Res.* **57,** 1199–1205.
60. Hung, M.-C., Wang, S.-C., and Hortobagyi, G. (1999) Targeting HER-2/neu-overexpressing cancer cells with transcriptional repressor genes delivered by cationic liposome. In *Nonviral Vectors for Gene Therapy* (Hung, M.-C., Huang, L., and Wagner, E., eds.), Academic Press, New York, pp. 357–375.
61. Yu, D. and Hung, M.-C. (2000) Therapeutic resistance of *erb*B-2-overexpressing cancers and strategies to overcome this resistance. In *DNA Alterations in Cancer* (Ehrlich, M., ed.), Eaton, Natick, MA, pp. 457–470.
62. Slamon, D., Leyland-Jones, B., Shak, S., et al. (1998) Addition of Herceptin™ (humanized anti-HER2 antibody) to first line chemotherapy for HER2 overexpressing metastatic breast cancer (HER2+/MBC) markedly increase anticancer activity: a randomized, multinational controlled phase III trial. *Proc. Annu. Meet. Am. Soc. Clin. Oncol.,* 376.
63. Yu, D., Suen, T. C., Yan, D. H., Chang, L. S., and Hung, M. C. (1990) Transcriptional repression of the neu protooncogene by the adenovirus 5 E1A gene products. *Proc. Natl. Acad. Sci. USA* **87,** 4499–4503.
64. Yan, D. H., Chang, L. S., and Hung, M. C. (1991) Repressed expression of the HER-2/c-erbB-2 proto-oncogene by the adenovirus E1a gene products. *Oncogene* **6,** 343–345.
65. Gao, X. and Huang, L. (1991) A novel cationic liposome reagent for efficient transfection of mammalian cells. *Biochem. Biophys. Res. Commun.* **179,** 280–285.
66. Xing, X., Zhang, S., Chang, J. Y., et al. (1998) Safety study and characterization of E1A-liposome complex gene delivery in an ovarian cancer model. *Gene Ther.* **5,** 1538–1544.
67. Xing, X., Liu, V., Xia, W., et al. (1997) Safety studies of the intraperitoneal injection of E1A—liposome complex in mice. *Gene Ther.* **4,** 238–243.
68. Shao, R., Hu, M. C., Zhou, B. P., et al. (1999) E1A sensitizes cells to tumor necrosis factor-induced apoptosis through inhibition of IkappaB kinases and nuclear factor kappaB activities. *J. Biol. Chem.* **274,** 21,495–21,498.
69. Hortobagyi, G. N., Ueno, N. T., Xia, W., et al. (2001) Cationic liposome-mediated E1A gene transfer to human breast and ovarian cancer cells and its biologic effects: a phase I clinical trial. *J. Clin. Oncol.* **19,** 3422–3433.
70. Yoo, G. H., Hung, M. C., Lopez-Berestein, G., et al. (2001) Phase I trial of intratumoral liposome E1A gene therapy in patients with recurrent breast and head and neck cancer. *Clin. Cancer Res.* **7,** 1237–1245.
71. Villaret, D., Glisson, B., Kenady, D., et al. (2002) A multicenter phase II study of tgDCC-E1A for the intratumoral treatment of patients with recurrent head and neck squamous cell carcinoma. *Head Neck* **24,** 661–669.
72. Lengyel, P., Choubey, D., Li, S.-J., and Datta, B. (1995) The interferon-activatable gene 200 cluster: from structure toward function. *Semin. Virol.* **6,** 203–213.
73. Landolfo, S., Gariglio, M., Gribaudo, G., and Lembo, D. (1998) The Ifi 200 genes: an emerging family of IFN-inducible genes. *Biochimie* **80,** 721–728.
74. Rozzo, S. J., Allard, J. D., Choubey, D., et al. (2001) Evidence for an interferon-inducible gene, Ifi202, in the susceptibility to systemic lupus. *Immunity* **15,** 435–443.
75. Choubey, D. and Lengyel, P. (1995) Binding of an interferon-inducible protein (p202) to the retinoblastoma protein. *J. Biol. Chem.* **270,** 6134–6140.
76. Choubey, D., Li, S.-J., Datta, B., Gutterman, J. U., and Lengyel, P. (1996) Inhibition of E2F-mediated transcription by p202. *EMBO J.* **15,** 5668–5678.
77. Choubey, D. and Gutterman, J. U. (1997) Inhibition of E2F-4/DP-1-stimulated transcription by p202. *Oncogene* **15,** 291–301.
78. Datta, B., Li, B., Choubey, D., Nallur, G., and Lengyel, P. (1996) p202, an interferon-inducible modulator of transcription, inhibits transcriptional activation by the p53 tumor suppressor protein, and a segment from the p53-binding protein 1 that binds to p202 overcomes this inhibition. *J. Biol. Chem.* **271,** 27,544–27,555.
79. Wang, H., Liu, C., Lu, Y., et al. (2000) The interferon- and differentiation-inducible p202a protein inhibits the transcriptional activity of c-Myc by blocking its association with Max. *J. Biol. Chem.* **275,** 27,377–27,385.
80. Datta, B., Min, W., Burma, S., and Lengyel, P. (1998) Increase in p202 expression during skeletal muscle differentiation: inhibition of MyoD protein expression and activity by p202. *Mol. Cell. Biol.* **18,** 1074–1083.
81. Min, W., Ghosh, S., and Lengyel, P. (1996) The interferon-inducible p202 protein as a modulator of transcription: inhibition of NFkB, c-Fos, and c-Jun activities. *Mol. Cell. Biol.* **16,** 359–368.
82. Wen, Y., Yan, D.-H., Wang, B., et al. (2001) p202, an interferon-inducible protein, mediates multiple anti-tumor activities in human pancreatic cancer xenograft models. *Cancer Res.* **61,** 7142–7147.
83. Wen, Y., Yan, D. H., Spohn, B., Deng, J., Lin, S. Y., and Hung, M. C. (2000) Tumor suppression and sensitization to tumor necrosis factor alpha-induced apoptosis by an interferon-inducible protein, p202, in breast cancer cells. *Cancer Res.* **60,** 42–46.
84. Choubey, D. and Gutterman, J. U. (1996) The interferon-inducible growth-inhibitory p202 protein: DNA binding properties and identification of a DNA binding domain. *Biochem. Biophys. Res. Commun.* **221,** 396–401.
85. Gutterman, J. U. and Choubey, D. (1999) Retardation of cell proliferation after expression of p202 accompanies an increase in p21(WAF1/CIP1). *Cell Growth Differ.* **10,** 93–100.
86. Yan, D.-H., Wen, Y., Spohn, B., Choubey, D., Gutterman, J. U., and Hung, M.-C. (1999) Reduced growth rate and transformation phenotype of the prostate cancer cells by an interferon-inducible protein, p202. *Oncogene* **18,** 807–811.

87. Ding, Y., Wen, Y., Spohn, B., et al. (2002) Pro-apoptotic and anti-tumor activities of adenovirus-mediated p202 gene transfer. *Clin. Cancer Res.* **8,** 3290–3297.
88. Zou, Y., Peng, H., Zhou, B., et al. (2002) Systemic tumor suppression by the proapoptotic gene bik. *Cancer Res.* **62,** 8–12.
89. Nishikawa, M. and Huang, L. (2001) Nonviral vectors in the new millennium: delivery barriers in gene transfer. *Hum. Gene Ther.* **12,** 861–870.
90. Landis, S. H., Murray, T., Bolden, S., and Wingo, P. A. (1999) Cancer statistics, 1999. *CA Cancer J. Clin.* **49,** 8–31.
91. Rosewicz, S. and Wiedenmann, B. (1997) Pancreatic carcinoma. *Lancet* **349,** 485–489.
92. Staley, C. A., Lee, J. E., Cleary, K. R., et al. (1996) Preoperative chemoradiation, pancreaticoduodenectomy, and intraoperative radiation therapy for adenocarcinoma of the pancreatic head. *Am. J. Surg.* **171,** 118–124; discussion, 124–115.
93. Hanahan, D. and Folkman, J. (1996) Patterns and emerging mechanisms of the angiogenic switch during tumorigenesis. *Cell* **86,** 353–364.
94. DeLisser, H. M., Newman, P. J., and Albelda, S. M. (1993) Platelet endothelial cell adhesion molecule (CD31). *Curr. Top. Microbiol. Immunol.* **184,** 37–45.
95. Reynolds, T. C., Alberts, D., Gershenson, D., et al. (2000) Activity of E1A in human clinical trials. In *ASCO*, abstract no. 1809.
96. Shao, R., Karunagaran, D., Zhou, B. P., et al. (1997) Inhibition of nuclear factor-kappaB activity is involved in E1A-mediated sensitization of radiation-induced apoptosis. *J. Biol. Chem.* **272,** 32,739–32,742.
97. Baldwin, A. S. J. (1996) The NF-kB and IkB proteins: new discoveries and insights. *Annu. Rev. Immunol.* **14,** 649–681.
98. Pahl, H. L. (1999) Activators and target genes of Rel/NF-kappaB transcription factors. *Oncogene* **18,** 6853–6866.

20

Antimetastatic Gene Therapy

Prostate Cancer Theory to Therapy

Thomas A. Gardner, Juan Antonio Jiménez, Leland W. K. Chung, and Chinghai Kao

1. INTRODUCTION: UNIQUE OBSTACLES IN ATTACKING METASTATIC PROSTATE CANCER

The treatment of disseminated cancer remains a great challenge for the urologists, oncologists, radiation therapists, and, more importantly, the patients and families affected by the devastating diagnosis and various treatments. At the time of initial diagnosis, individuals will have a 7 to 55% incidence of metastases, depending on the site of the initial tumor *(1)*. The ideal therapy is one that will destroy the cancer cells, but spare the patient's normal cells. Chemotherapy, the most common therapy for metastases or systemic cancer, is targeted at the growth differential between normal and cancer cells. Unfortunately, normal cells attempting division will often be inadvertently targeted, resulting in toxicities. The dose-limiting toxicities associated with classical cancer chemotherapies limit the amount of drug that can be delivered to the tumor and often allow the tumor to survive and cause failure of the chemotherapy.

Gene therapy provides a novel vantage point to overcome this formidable challenge. If the ideal treatment provides cure without additional suffering, then gene therapy may become the ideal treatment. It is a "silver bullet" created to seek out a cancer cell and alter its internal functions to arrest its further growth or its further existence. This chapter describes the approaches used for developing gene therapy strategies based on transcriptional targeting for a series of metastatic cancers.

Localized and locally advanced cancer can cause great suffering, but are not generally the cause of death in patients with cancer. Mortality is usually secondary to the inability to inhibit metastatic cancer growth. The systemic spread of cancer cells to multiple organs throughout the body provides a significant obstacle to effective therapy. In addition, the metastatic cancer cell often possesses the ability to interact with its surroundings and establish new sites of metastasis.

Investigations over the past several decades have led to the elucidation of the molecular mechanisms that enable the epithelial and stromal interactions. For instance, the interactions of prostate cancer cells with bone stromal cells have been well established and have begun to provide molecular targets for gene therapy, that is, specific targets for prostate osseous metastasis *(2–8)*. Molecular understanding of prostate cancer cells and the supportive noncancerous cells of a metastasis is the critical step in the successful development of a gene therapy strategy against metastatic prostate cancer. Fortunately, the past several decades have provided an explosion of information that has allowed several novel approaches to be developed using gene therapy for prostate cancer *(9)*.

From: *Contemporary Cancer Research*
Cancer Gene Therapy
Edited by: D. T. Curiel and J. T. Douglas © Humana Press Inc., Totowa, NJ

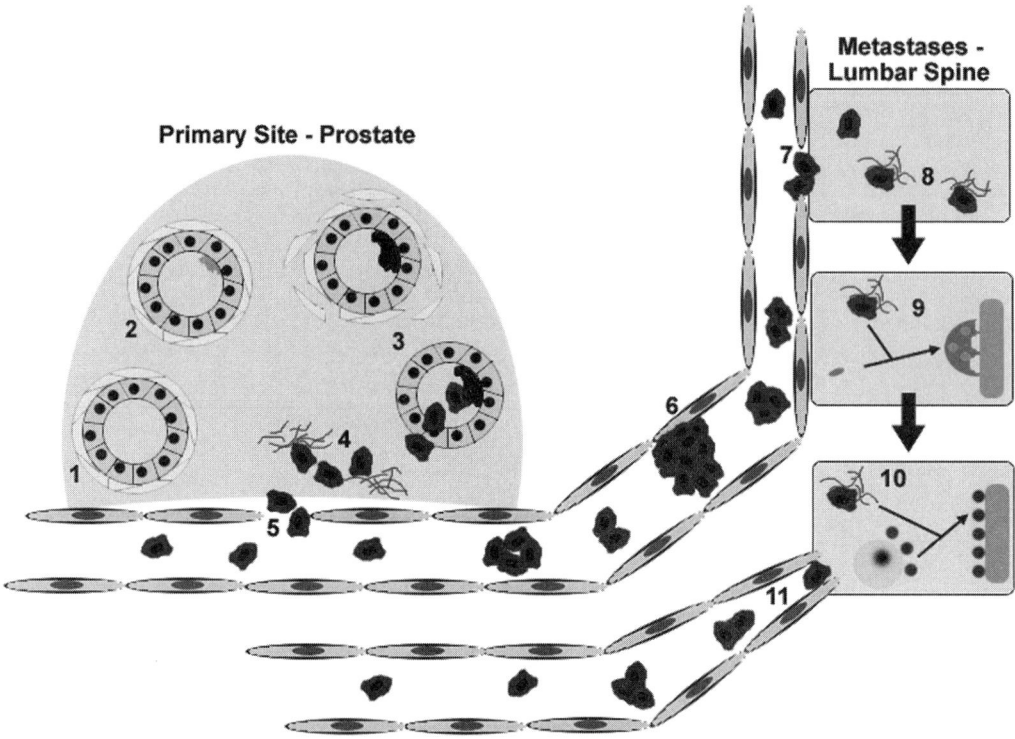

Fig. 1. Progression of prostate cancer from primary lesion to osseous metastasis: (1) normal prostate acinar gland with basal and luminal layers; (2) development of prostate intraepithelial neoplasia (PIN) within the lumen; (3) development of prostate cancer occurs with loss of the basal layer; (4) migration of prostate cancer cells and attachment to extracellular matrix (ECM); (5) intravasation of tumor cells into blood vessel; (6) embolization of cancer cells and endothelial–epithelial interactions leading to attachment of cancer cells to the vessel wall; (7) extravasation of cancer cells at the metastatic site; (8) interaction with ECM components; (9) prostate cancer cell binding to osteoclasts mediated by RANK ligand; (10) prostate cancer cells accommodated within bone pits leads to proliferation and metastatic colonization; (11) angiogenesis and intravasation leads to further dissemination of the cancer.

2. DISSECTING THE COMPONENTS OF A METASTASIS: ELUCIDATION OF POTENTIAL TARGETS

Tumor development and progression are a highly regulated and coordinated cascade of multistage molecular processes in which cancer cells undergo genetic changes that lead to phenotypic alterations, including the capacity to metastasize. *Metastasis* is defined as the formation of progressively growing secondary tumor foci at distant sites discontinuous with the primary tumor *(10)*. Each metastatic focus is clonal in nature because it originates from a single tumor cell. For a cell to form a clinically significant metastasis, it must complete a series of well-defined steps collectively known as the *metastasis cascade*.

The act of metastasis generally involves the following stages (Fig. 1):

1. Activation of the oncogene, causing genetic alteration and transformation of the target cell.
2. Proliferation of the transformed cells and the shift in the balance with cell death.
3. The ability of the transformed cells to avoid destruction by the immune surveillance mechanisms.
4. Stimulation of the proangiogenic factors and ingrowth of new blood vessels from the preexisting ones (angiogenesis/neovascularization).

5. Localized invasion and destruction of extracellular matrix components and parenchymal cells.
6. Migration of the tumor cells away from the primary tumor mass.
7. Penetration of the tumor cells through the blood vessel wall (intravasation).
8. Embolization of cancer cells to distant organs.
9. Molecular interaction of cancer cells with erythrocytes, neutrophils, platelets, and components of coagulation factors within the bloodstream.
10. Arrest of cancer cells within the lumen of small blood vessels or lymphatics and adhesion to endothelial cells.
11. Reverse penetration of the cancer cells through the blood vessels at the metastatic site (extravasation).
12. Proliferation of cancer cells, resulting in the formation of secondary tumors and metastatic colonization.

The failure of the cancer cell to complete any one of the steps in the metastatic cascade eventually results in its failure to form clinically significant metastasis. Several metastasis-associated genes have been identified that play a critical role either in progression or metastasis of the carcinoma cells *(11–22)*. Each of these many steps may provide targets for gene therapy strategies and possible escape routes for prostate cancer cells. Thus, targeting several key steps may provide the best approach.

The components of a prostate cancer metastasis can be separated into three main function groups: seed, soil, and irrigation system (prostate cancer cell, supportive bone environment, and angiogenesis, respectively). Each process described above is a potential step for interference in the metastatic cascade, and each of the proteins discussed next provides a target to inhibit the transition from one or several of the steps described.

2.1. Prostate Cancer Epithelial Cell Component (Seed)

The prostate cancer epithelial cell component provides excellent targets for gene therapy. Because the prostate gland becomes a vestigial structure for men after their reproductive years, prostate-specific proteins present good prostate cancer targets. For example, several proteins (prostate-specific antigen [PSA], prostate-specific membrane antigen [PSMA], and prostatic acid phosphatase [PAP]) are prostate-specific proteins used in immune therapy against prostate cancer via a variety of gene transfer approaches. These and several other proteins produced are detailed next in the context of transcriptional regulation.

2.1.1. Tumor Metastasis Suppressors

Tumor metastasis suppressors such as KAI1 and MKK4/SEK1 as well as cell surface protein alterations (i.e., CD44, integrins, selectins, cadherins, and the immunoglobulin superfamily) permit the metastasis to occur and survive. They are a few of the numerous potential targets for gene therapy.

The localization of metastasis suppressor activity to rat chromosome 2 prompted the search for homologous metastasis suppressor genes in prostate cancer. Microcell-mediated chromosomal transfer of human chromosome 11 into Dunning AT6.1 and AT3.1 rat prostate cancer cells and the analysis of the resulting microcell hybrids for metastasis suppression in immunodeficient mice led to the identification of KAI1 (also known as CD82), which maps to 11p11.2–p13 *(19,23)*. KAI1 contains peptide motifs that place it in the tetraspanin family of proteins, which function as membrane adaptors that organize large oligomeric complexes containing other tetraspanins, integrins, cell adhesion molecules (CAMs), kinases, GTPases, and phosphatases. Ectopic expression of KAI1 in AT6.1 Dunning rat prostate cancer cells reduced the number of overt lung metastases by 66% compared with parental AT6.1 controls *(19)*. KAI1 expression had no effect on primary tumor growth, meeting the criteria of a metastasis suppressor gene. KAI1 expression is downregulated in metastatic and high-grade prostate tumors as well as in 100% of lymph node metastases *(24,25)*. Studies indicated that KAI1 forms complexes with E-cadherin, β_1 integrins, and epidermal growth factor receptor (EGFR), which have been implicated in metastasis progression *(19)*. Expression of KAI1 decreases both the invasiveness and motility of cells in vitro and alters cell–cell interactions *(19,26)*. Lowered KAI1 expression has also been associated with progression in a wide variety of cancers, including pancreatic, hepatocellular, bladder, breast, and non-small cell lung cancers *(27–31)*.

2.1.2. MKK4/SEK1

MKK4/SEK1 is a metastasis suppressor when transfected into metastatic prostate and ovarian cancer cell lines. Immunohistochemical studies indicated that MKK4 expression is reduced in primary prostate tumors and in metastatic ovarian carcinomas *(32,33)*. MKK4 occupies the mitogen-activated protein kinase position upstream of JUN-terminal kinase and p38 and has been mapped at the chromosomal location 17p11.2 *(34,35)*. Upstream of MEKK4/SEK1 is MEKK1 *(36)*. Although originally named because of its ability to activate MEK1, MEKK1 is a much more specific activator of MKK4/SEK1 than it is of MEK1 *(37)*. Expression of human MKK4 in AT6.1 cells has been shown to reduce the number of spontaneous metastases by approx 77% without affecting the primary tumor growth *(35)*. MKK4-mediated suppression occurs by inhibiting the growth of disseminated cancer cells after their arrival at the secondary site *(35,38)*.

2.1.3. CD44

To allow and encourage the epithelial–stomal interaction described in Section 2.2 to occur, several cell surface proteins have been implicated. CD44, integrins, cadherins, selectins, and the immunoglobulin super family each facilitate the cell-to-cell interactions and provide potential targets for transductional targeting. For instance, the main form of CD44 (CD44H), a transmembrane 80-kDa glycoprotein, is widely expressed in a variety of lymphoid and epithelial cells and in malignant tumors. CD44 has many variant forms generated by alternative splicing. The expression of certain variant CD44 isoforms has been correlated with the degree of tumor differentiation, tumor cell invasion, and metastatic potential *(39,40)*. In fact, CD44 was identified as another prostate cancer metastasis suppressor gene *(41)*.

Ectopic expression of the standard isoform (CD44-s) in AT3.1 Dunning rat prostate cancer cells leads to more than 60% reduction in the number of spontaneous lung metastases without affecting the primary tumor growth. Several clinical studies strongly supported the role of CD44 in the suppression of human prostate cancer metastasis. There is an inverse correlation between the expression of CD44 and the grade and metastatic stage of prostate tumors *(42–46)*. In addition, CD44 expression is either lost or very weak in all prostate cancer metastases *(43–47)*; CD44-s loss predicts poor prognosis after radical prostatectomy independent of stage and grade *(42,45,47)*.

The precise mechanism by which CD44 suppresses metastasis is not clear. It has been speculated that CD44-mediated metastasis suppression may occur through contact inhibition of cancer cell growth within micrometastatic foci at the secondary site. Consistent with such a model, CD44 downregulation has been observed in experimental models during the outgrowth of micrometastasis into overt metastatic lesions *(48)*. The association of CD44-merlin/ezrin/radixin/meosin complexes with osteopontin, a bone matrix remodeling protein, is thought to promote the metastasis of several cancers, including cancer of the prostate *(49)*.

2.1.4. Integrins

Integrins are a diverse family of transmembrane glycoproteins that mediate cell–matrix and cell–cell interactions *(50,51)*. Integrins consist of an α- and a β-subunit; so far, 18 α- and 8 β-subunits have been identified that can associate in a variety of combinations to give rise to 25 distinct heterodimers, with each specific for a unique ligand *(52)*. Each integrin consists of a noncovalently linked α- and β-subunit, with each subunit having a large extracellular domain, a single membrane-spanning domain, and a short, noncatalytic cytoplasmic tail. Several studies have demonstrated the association between the regulation of integrin expression and cancer *(53)*.

Changes in the integrin pattern during malignant transformation are highly dependent on the type of cancer. An altered integrin expression pattern allows the cancer cells to recognize variable matrices, but it may also lead to altered signaling and changes in gene expression. The action of integrins has been extensively studied in melanoma, breast cancer, and prostate cancer.

The integrin $\alpha_v\beta_3$ is strongly expressed at the invasive front of malignant melanoma cells and angiogenic blood vessels, but weakly expressed on preneoplastic melanomas and quiescent blood vessels *(54)*.

The increase in its expression correlates with the conversion of melanoma growth from radial to vertical *(55)*. However, there are metastatic melanoma cells that express little or no $\alpha_v\beta_3$ integrin on their surface *(56,57)*, suggesting that no single adhesion receptor is irreplaceable in melanoma progression. Integrins $\alpha_2\beta_1$ and $\alpha_3\beta_1$ have been found to play a role in melanoma cell migration, and their expression was increased in metastatic cells compared to the cells in the primary tumor *(58–63)*.

The expression of β_1 integrin in primary melanoma facilitates the emergence of regional lymph node metastasis *(64)*; the expression of β_1 integrins in metastasis of melanoma has been shown to predict a longer disease-free survival period *(65)*. The expression of integrin β_3 has been reported to correlate positively to lung metastasis and is associated with poor survival rates *(66)*.

The laminin receptors, especially $\alpha_6\beta_1$, are involved in metastatic processes, possibly during extravasation. Multiple binding epitopes on $\alpha_6\beta_1$ may contribute to the migratory and adhesive properties mediated by this integrin *(62,67)*. In contrast to α_6 integrins, the expression of laminin receptor $\alpha_7\beta_1$ has been shown to inhibit malignant features like cell growth and metastasis in mouse melanoma cell lines *(68)*.

Fibronectin-binding integrin $\alpha_5\beta_1$ has a stimulatory effect on the growth of quiescent human melanoma cells; another fibronectin receptor, $\alpha_4\beta_1$, has been found to facilitate melanoma cell migration *(69,70)*. The $\alpha_{IIb}\beta_3$ integrin, which is typically found in platelets, may also occur on metastatic murine and human melanoma cells and may contribute to invasion *(72,72)*.

Several studies have reported on the alteration in the expression pattern of integrins in breast cancer. Immunohistochemical analyses of poorly differentiated breast adenocarcinomas have shown significant decrease in integrin $\alpha_2\beta_1$ and slight decrease in $\alpha_5\beta_1$ and $\alpha_v\beta_3$ integrin expression levels *(73)*. In the case of breast cancer, the interactions between bone matrix proteins and invading breast cancer cells are pivotal because bone is a typical site of breast cancer metastasis. Integrins $\alpha_v\beta_3$ and $\alpha_v\beta_5$ are involved in bone sialoprotein-induced cancer cell adhesion, proliferation, and migration. However, the function of these integrins differs, so that $\alpha_v\beta_3$, with expression that is involved in metastasis, participates in cell migration, whereas $\alpha_v\beta_5$ is likely to facilitate cell adhesion and proliferation *(74,75)*. In highly invasive mammary epithelial cells, the process of osteopontin-induced migration is dependent on $\alpha_v\beta_3$ integrin and involves the activation of the hepatocyte growth factor receptor (Met) *(76)*. Integrin $\alpha_3\beta_1$ is involved in breast cancer cell migration and invasion by regulating the production of matrix metalloproteinase 2 (MMP-2) *(76)* and is related to the metastatic capacity of breast cancer cells by increasing the activity of MMP-9 *(77)*.

Immunostaining of breast cancer tissue specimens has indicated that the loss of $\alpha_1\beta_1$, $\alpha_2\beta_1$, $\alpha_3\beta_1$, $\alpha_6\beta_1$, and $\alpha_v\beta_5$ integrins is associated with the formation of axillary metastases *(78)*. The expression of $\alpha_6\beta_4$ integrin inhibits malignant properties of breast cancer cells by inducing apoptosis via activation of p53. However, the expression of this integrin may facilitate carcinoma progression if p53 is in a mutated, inactive form *(79,80)*. It has also been suggested that integrin $\alpha_6\beta_4$-mediated invasion occurs through PI3-kinase signaling *(81)*.

The studies on integrin expression patterns in prostate cancer are limited. According to one report, all primary and metastatic carcinomas expressed $\alpha_2\beta_1$ and α_6 integrins. The expression level of $\alpha_2\beta_1$ was downregulated in grade I and II prostate tumors; in grade III tumors, the expression was heterogeneous, but in lymph node metastasis, $\alpha_2\beta_1$ expression was upregulated *(81)*. The increased expression of α_6 integrin may contribute to the invasive capacity of prostate cancer cells *(53,82)*.

On the other hand, the loss of β_4 integrin has been reported to occur in prostate cancer progression concomitantly with the loss of its ligand, laminin 5 *(83)*. The malignant prostate cancer cells may lose their ability to polarize and regulate a normal acinar morphogenesis because of decrease or change in the distribution of $\alpha_6\beta_1$ integrin *(84,85)*. The decrease in $\alpha_6\beta_4$ integrin expression may occur because of androgen regulation in androgen-sensitive cancer cells. In contrast, androgen-independent prostate cancer cells may maintain their expression of $\alpha_6\beta_4$, which supports their high invasion capacity, whereas $\alpha_6\beta_1$ and $\alpha_3\beta_1$ expression may be related to less-invasive phenotypes *(86,87)*. Transforming growth factor-$\beta1$ has been shown to upregulate the integrin $\alpha_2\beta_1$- and $\alpha_3\beta_1$-mediated adhesion of prostate cancer cells to type I collagen *(3,88)*. Similarly, in studies on the adhesion of prostate epithelial cells or human prostate carcinoma cells to type I collagen or to the stroma of human bone marrow, it has been clear that the interactions are predominantly mediated by $\alpha_2\beta_1$ integrin *(88–90)*. Integrin $\alpha_{IIb}\beta_3$ has also been implicated as having a role in the metastasis of prostate cancer *(91,92)*.

2.1.5. Cancer Cell Component

CAMs facilitate communication between the tumor cells and the extracellular environment *(93,94)*. A wide variety of CAMs with distinctive structural and functional features have been identified. They can be broadly classified into four different categories: selectins, cadherins, immunoglobulin superfamily, and integrins.

2.1.5.1. SELECTINS

Selectins are a class of calcium-dependent transmembrane glycoproteins that can specifically bind to many carbohydrate moieties *(95)*. Selectins have a conserved structural motif with an N-terminal calcium-dependent lectinlike domain, an EGF-like domain, multiple complement regulatorylike regions, a transmembrane domain, and a short cytoplasmic tail *(95)*. The E, P, and L selectins are the best-characterized members and are involved in weak cell–cell interactions and leukocyte rolling *(96)*. Many epithelial tumors express high levels of sialyl Lewis X antigen and exhibit enhanced tumor growth and metastasis in vivo *(97–100)*. The selectins can bind specifically to many carbohydrate moieties, including sialyl Lewis X, and may play a role in mediating tumor cell interactions with the microvasculature, thereby contributing to the metastatic cascade *(99)*. Monoclonal antibodies and peptidomimetics directed against selectins have been shown to block tumor cell metastasis in vivo *(99,101)*.

2.1.5.2. CADHERINS

Calcium adhesion molecules of the cadherin family (E-cadherin, P-cadherin, and N-cadherin) mediate cell–cell binding and generally display an inhibitory effect on the metastatic process. Cadherin proteins are diminished in cancer cells. Cadherins contain a large extracellular region composed of at least five ectodomains, a transmembrane domain, and a cytoplasmic tail *(102,103)*. The intracellular domain of cadherins is connected to catenins, which function as a link to the actin cytoskeleton. The functional cadherin-catenin complexes have been implicated in tumor invasion and metastasis. Transfection of E-cadherin-negative cells with E-cadherin complementary DNA resulted in inhibition of motility and invasion *(104,105)*. In contrast, the transfected cancer cells expressing both E- and N-cadherin display enhanced migration, invasion, growth factor-induced MMP-9 synthesis, and metastatic potential *(106)*. Taken together, these findings indicate that cadherins may regulate tumor cell metastasis by a variety of mechanisms, including altering tight cell–cell interactions and sensitizing tumor cells to growth factor-induced upregulation of proteolytic enzymes.

2.1.5.3. IMMUNOGLOBULIN SUPERFAMILY

Besides selectins and cadherins, the members of the immunoglobulin superfamily are involved in mediating homotypic cell–cell interactions *(107)*. Members of the immunoglobulin superfamily have an extracellular domain composed of immunoglobulin homology units stabilized by disulfide bonds. Some members, such as NCAM, have a transmembrane domain and a cytoplasmic tail; others are anchored to the cell surface through lipid interactions. The immunoglobulin superfamily includes well-characterized members like ICAM-1, VCAM, NCAM, carcinoembryonic antigen, DCC, and MUC18 *(93,94,107–109)*.

Many of these molecules are involved in immune cell recognition, leukocyte trafficking, and neural development *(100,107,109)*. Several studies have implicated members of the immunoglobulin superfamily in the regulation of metastasis. For example, immunohistochemical studies have revealed that ICAM-1 expression levels are elevated in metastatic hepatocarcinomas compared to more benign tumors *(110)*, and ICAM-1 knockout mice have demonstrated a resistance to T-cell lymphoma metastasis *(111)*. Other studies have shown a positive correlation between expression of carcinoembryonic antigen in colon carcinoma progression and upregulation of MUC18 in malignant melanomas *(93, 110,112,113)*. These findings strongly suggest that the members of the immunoglobulin superfamily play an important role in the regulation of tumor invasion and metastasis.

Each the proteins and protein families above are directly or indirectly involved in enhancing cancer cell survival or its ability to interact with the stromal cells at the site of a metastasis. The summation of functions of the above proteins allows a prostate cancer cell, as well as other tumor types, to develop independent growth and to communicate with the stromal cells of a potential metastatic site, establishing the epithelial–stromal interraction described in Section 2.2.

2.2. Epithelial–Stromal Cell Interaction Component (Soil)

The osseous metastasis is a rich environment that supports the establishment of a metastatic focus of prostate cancer and, via cell-to-cell interactions, promotes sustained growth. For the prostate cancer epithelial cell to survive in the bone marrow, it needs to mimic the activities of the supportive stoma (i.e., osteoblasts, osteoclasts, and osteocytes) *(114)*. Prostate cancer cells obtain the ability to mimic the activities of bone cells by producing several proteins necessary for skeletal homeostasis, such as osteocalcin, osteopontin, osteonectin, and bone sialoproteins.

We have hypothesized that this transformation of prostate epithelial cells is a critical step and as such provides a significant target. Normal prostate epithelial cells do not make typical bone proteins, but when they acquire the ability to form a tumor and metastasize, the bonelike nature of these tumor cells is readily apparent. We have termed this capacity the *osteomimetic property* or *osteomimicry* of prostate cancer cells. Osteomimetic properties are also typical for breast cancer cells, which have the propensity to metastasize to bone. The exact mechanisms leading to the overt manifestation of this ability remain to be elucidated.

The osteocalcin protein under the transcriptional control of the osteocalcin promoter is one of the osteomimetic mechanisms investigated by our laboratory. Through transcription factor switching, transacting factors in AI prostate cancer cells may be upregulated so that they are capable of recruiting critical transcription factors to *cis*-elements residing within the human OC (hOC) promoter for enhanced gene transcription *(115)*. These findings have led hypothesis-driven investigations and clinical trials to confirm this hypothesis.

The metastatic cascade represented in Fig. 1 illustrates the critical communication between the cancer cell and the extracellular matrix and stromal cells of a future osseous metastasis. Once the prostate cancer cells have migrated to the bone marrow, the osteomimetic properties of these cells both aid in obscuring these cells from immune surveillance and recruit resident cells such as osteoclasts to prepare the bone matrix for further prostate cell growth. For example, the metastatic cells secrete RANK ligand (RANKL), a ligand for RANK (receptor activator of NF(B). RANKL is a regulator of bone resorption and remodeling *(116)*.

The prostate cancer cells will then bind to RANK on the osteoclasts. This binding allows for osteoclast activation, "pit" development of the bone matrix, and eventual accommodation of the prostate cancer cell. A publication demonstrated that invading prostate cancer cells not only express soluble RANKL, but also develop other mineralizing characteristics of an osteoblastic phenotype, including production of alkaline phosphatase, osteocalcin, osteonectin, bone sialoprotein, osteoprotegerin, and most crucially for mineralization, formation of hydroxyapatite *(117)*.

2.3. Angiogenic Component (Irrigation System)

To metastasize, a tumor cell must overcome a series of physical barriers. Usually, less than 1 cell in approx 100,000 has all the attributes to produce a successful metastasis *(118)*. Folkman first put forward the hypothesis that the growth of solid tumors is angiogenesis dependent *(119,120)*. It is now widely accepted that tumor growth and metastasis require vascularization to provide both nourishment and a route for tumor cell extravasation *(121)*.

This has led to the consideration that angiogenesis is a viable target for antitumor therapy *(122)*. The angiogenic process consists of a series of interactive events: Quiescent endothelial cells are stimulated by angiogenic factors to degrade the underlying basement membrane, to migrate within the interstitial matrix, to proliferate, and to organize themselves into tubular structures, which in turn become mature blood vessels. During angiogenesis, the endothelial cells undergo functional changes and show molecular features that are different from normal, quiescent endothelium.

These differences can be exploited to target tumor endothelium selectively and to prevent neovascularization. A diverse array of multifunctional cytokines from multiple cellular sources are involved in sustaining the growth and progression of tumors through neovascularization. The angiogenic process reflects a competition among cytokines that, on one hand, functions to promote angiogenesis and, on the other hand, suppresses the angiogenic response. Tumor neovascularization occurs when the dynamic equilibrium that governs the orderly production of proangiogenic and angiostatic molecules becomes disrupted in favor of those members that promote angiogenesis *(123–127)*. In a pioneering study, O'Rielly et al. showed that a disruption in the net balance between positive and negative regulators of angiogenesis can have a profound effect on tumor growth and metastasis *(128)*.

Many molecules influence the various components of the angiogenic response *(129–131)*. Some of the most extensively studied mediators shown to stimulate tumor angiogenesis include basic fibroblast growth factor *(132–135)*, vascular endothelial cell growth factor or vascular permeability factor *(115,136–138)*, interleukin-8, angiogenin, platelet-derived endothelial cell growth factor, platelet-derived growth factor, hepatocyte growth factor, transforming growth factor-α and -β, and tumor necrosis factor-α, a TIE-2 receptor ligand called angiopoietin *(139)*. The negative regulators so far identified include thrombospondin *(140)*, the 16-kDa N-terminal fragment of prolactin *(141)*, angiostatin *(128)*, endostatin *(141)*, and tumstatin *(143)*.

3. IDENTIFICATION OF TRANSCRIPTION TARGETS OF PROSTATE CANCER METASTASIS

Investigations into the molecular attributes of prostate cancer led to the elucidation of several prostate cancer-specific proteins. Several of these proteins have stimulated investigations into the regulatory elements and have led to transcriptional-targeted therapies. Several of the more interesting proteins and regulatory elements are described in this section and in other reviews *(144,145)*.

3.1. Osteocalcin Promoter

Osteocalcin (bone γ-carboxyglutamic acid)-containing protein (BGP) is a 50-amino acid, 5.8-kDa, major noncollagenous protein found in adult bone and has been shown to be transcriptionally regulated by 1,25-dihydroxyvitamin D_3 *(146,147)*. The human, rat, and murine osteocalcin genes have been cloned, and each consists of 4 exons and 3 introns *(148–151)*. Interestingly, the human and rat promoter are positively regulated by 1,25-dihydroxyvitamin D; the mouse OC promoter is negatively regulated by1,25-dihydroxyvitamin D_3.

Montecino et al. *(152)* reported that the key promoter elements are located in two DNase I hypersensitive sites. The proximal hypersensitive site (–170 to –70) includes sequence motifs that specifically interact with basal transcription factors such as Msx *(153–155)*, HLH protein Id-1 *(156)*, AP-1 *(157)*, a bone-specific nuclear matrix associated protein NMP-2 *(158)*, and a member of the AML family of transcription factors *(159,160)*. The distal hypersensitive domain (–600 to –400) contains the vitamin D-responsive element (–465 to –437), which interacts with the VDR-RXRα complex in a ligand-dependent manner. Others *(161–164)* demonstrated that the promoter segment –343 to –108 is critical for inducing both proximal nuclease hypersensitivity and basal transcriptional activity, and the DNase I hypersensitivity at –600 is not essential for vitamin D-dependent transcriptional upregulation.

The stimulation of osteocalcin gene expression by 1,25-dihydroxyvitamin D_3 is associated with sequence-specific binding of nuclear factors to a 26-bp sequence 5'-CTGGGTGAATGAGGACATT

ACTGACC-3' located between −462 and −437. This sequence contains a region of hyphenated dyad symmetry and shares homology with consensus steroid-responsive elements The promoter region has been shown to contain two sites of an E-box motif (a consensus binding site for HLH proteins) termed OCE1 (CACATG at −102) and OCE2 (CAGCTG at −149) *(156)*.

Mutagenesis studies have indicated that osteoblastic-specific gene transcription is regulated via the interaction between certain E-box binding transcription factors in osteoblasts and the OCE1 sequence in the promoter region of the osteocalcin gene. Banerjee et al. *(157)* demonstrated that an AML-1 binding sequence within the proximal promoter (nucleotides −138 to −130) contributes to 75% of the level of osteocalcin gene expression. The promoter region is not GC rich and does not contain a consensus sequence for the SP1-binding site *(165)*.

Regarding in vitro and in vivo experiments, Ko et al. *(166)* developed an osteocalcin promoter-driven thymidine kinase (TK)-expressing recombinant adenoviral vector to achieve tissue-specific killing of osteosarcoma cells in an experimental animal model. Administration of this vector followed by acyclovir treatment led to significant growth inhibition of osteosarcoma in the experimental animal model.

Cheon et al. *(167)* used a chemogene therapy approach by combining OC promoter-driven TK expression and acyclovir plus methotrexate treatment regimen in nude mice bearing either subcutaneous human osteosarcoma (MG-63) or rat osteosarcoma. Their results indicated that osteosarcoma tumor growth was more efficiently inhibited because of synergistic effects of combined methotrexate and acyclovir treatment.

Shirakawa et al. *(168)* further demonstrated the potential utility of an adenoviral osteocalcin promoter-mediated suicide gene therapy for osteosarcoma pulmonary metastasis in nude mice. Hou et al. *(169)* demonstrated osteoblast-specific gene expression in adherent bone marrow cells using a 1.7-kb rat OC-CAT gene. Recipient mice were positive for osteoblast-specific expression following bone marrow transplantation.

3.2. PSA Promoter

3.2.1. Protein and Promoter

The gene for PSA, a member of the glandular kallikrein family, was independently characterized by Riegman and colleagues *(170,171)* and Lundwall *(172)*. The gene is 7130 bp long, includes 633 bp of 5' and 639 bp of 3' flanking untranslated sequence, contains five exons, and is located on the long arm of chromosome 19, in the region q13.3-qter *(171)*. The promoter contains a variant TATA box (TTTATA) at position −28 to −23, a GC box at −53 to −48, and a CACCC box at −129 to −125. An imperfect palindromic sequence AGAACAGCAAGTGCT is found at position −170 to −156; GGGAGGG and CAGCCTC repeats are located in the region −123 to −72. The expression of PSA is only detected in human prostate *(173–175)* and has been shown to be androgen responsive *(176)*. This is achieved by several transcription factors involved in regulating PSA gene.

Two functionally active androgen receptor-binding sites or androgen response elements have been identified at positions −170 (ARE-I) and −394 (ARE-II) *(176–180)*. Cleutjens et al. *(178)* identified a complex, androgen-regulated, 440-bp enhancer (−4366 to −3874) that contains a high-affinity, AR-binding site ARE-III 5'-GGAGGAACATATTGTATCGAT-3' at position −4200. In subsequent studies, a 6-kb PSA promoter fragment was shown to confer prostate-specific and androgen-regulated expression of β-galactosidase in transgenic mice *(181)*.

Pang et al. *(182)* identified an 822-bp PSA gene regulatory sequence PSAR that, when combined with the PSA promoter (PCPSA-P), exhibited enhanced luciferase activity in LNCaP cells. On stimulation with 10 to 100 nM dihydrotestosterone, a more than 1000-fold increase in expression was observed compared to androgen-negative controls. Their studies further suggested that this 822-bp sequence alone could serve as a promoter, thereby indicating that the complete PSA promoter contains two functional domains: A proximal promoter and a distal promoter, which can also function as an enhancer.

Yeung et al. *(183)* identified two *cis*-acting elements within the 5.8-kb PSA promoter that are essential for the androgen-independent activity of PSA promoter in prostate cancer cells. Their studies provided evidence that androgen-independent activation of PSA promoter in androgen-independent prostate cancer cell line C4-2 involves two distinct regions, a 440-bp AREc and a 150-bp pN/H, responsible for upregulation of the PSA promoter activity by employing two different pathways. AREc confers high basal PSA promoter activity in C4-2 cells; pN/H is a strong, AR-independent, positive-regulatory element of the PSA promoter in both LNCaP and C4-2 cells. Further, a 17-bp RI fragment within the pN/H region was identified as the key *cis*-element that interacts with a 45-kDa prostate cancer cell-specific transcription factor to mediate androgen and AR-independent transcriptional activation of the PSA promoter. By juxtaposing AREc and pN/H, a chimeric PSA promoter has been created that exhibits two- to threefold higher activity than wild-type PSA promoter in both LNCaP and C4-2 cells.

Oettgen et al. *(184)* identified a novel prostate epithelial-specific Ets transcription factor PDEF that is involved in PSA gene regulation and acts as a coregulator of AR. PDEF acts as an androgen-independent transcriptional activator of the PSA promoter. It also directly interacts with the DNA-binding domain of AR and enhances androgen-mediated activation of the PSA promoter. Thus, strong tissue specificity of the PSA promoter makes it an ideal candidate for prostate cancer gene therapy.

Latham et al. *(185)* compared tissue-specific expression of luciferase reporter vectors by employing PSA, human glandular kallikrein (hKLK2), and cytomegalovirus (CMV) promoters in PSA-positive LNCaP and PSA-negative CoLo320, DG75, A2780, and Jurkat cells. Their studies revealed that minimal 628-bp PSA and hKLK2 promoters showed only low-level androgen-independent expression in both PSA-positive and PSA-negative cell lines. Tandem duplication of the PSA promoter slightly increased expression in LNCaP cells. Addition of CMV enhancer upstream of the PSA or hKLK2 promoter led to substantially enhanced and nonspecific luciferase expression in all the cell lines. By placing a 1455-bp PSA enhancer sequence upstream of either the PSA or hKLK2 promoter, a 20-fold increase in tissue-specific luciferase expression was observed. Tandem duplication of the PSA enhancer increased the expression 50-fold higher than either promoter and retained tissue specificity. The expression from all the enhancer constructs was 100-fold above the basal levels on induction with androgen dihydrotestosterone.

3.2.2. In Vitro and In Vivo Experiments

These prostate-specific enhancer sequences were incorporated in adenoviral vectors to express EGFP and nitroreductase. The results indicated low-level expression of EGFP by PSA enhancer/promoter in LNCaP and no expression in non-PSA-producing EJ cells when compared with CMV promoter-driven EGFP. However, PSA enhancer/promoter was able to express comparable levels of nitroreductase in a tissue-specific manner in LNCaP cells alone. These transduced LNCaP cells, on treatment with CB1954, exhibited cytotoxicity. The replication-competent adenoviral vector CN706, in which the E1A gene is under the transcriptional control of the PSA enhancer/promoter, has been shown to exhibit selective toxicity toward PSA-expressing prostate cancer cells *(186)*.

Martiniello-Wilks et al. *(187)* examined the efficacy of adenoviral vectors with 630-bp PSA promoter-driven herpes simplex virus (HSV)-TK and *Escherichia coli* PNP genes for their ability to kill AI prostate cancer cell line PC-3 tumor xenografts in a nude mouse model. Both HSV-TK- and *E. coli* PNP-expressing adenoviral vectors were able to achieve significant tumor regression in vivo following ganciclovir or 6MPDR treatment.

Gotoh et al. *(188)* developed transcriptionally targeted recombinant adenoviral vectors by incorporating either 5837-bp long or 642-bp short PSA promoter elements to drive the expression of HSV-TK. The long PSA promoter had superior activity over the short promoter and was more active in C4-2 cells than in LNCaP cells. In vitro expression of TK conferred marked killing of C4-2 cells on acyclovir treatment. Administration of this virus in an in vivo subcutaneous C4-2 tumor model followed by acyclovir treatment revealed significant reduction in tumor burden.

Lee et al. *(189)* demonstrated tissue-specific growth suppression of PSA-positive and PSA-negative cell lines by transfecting PSA promoter/enhancer-driven p53 tumor suppressor gene. Human prostate cancer- and tissue-specific genes P503, P540S, and P510S have been identified using a combination of complementary DNA library subtraction and high-throughput microarray screening *(190)*. It would be interesting to characterize the promoter regions of these genes and use them in developing transcriptionally targeted adenoviral vectors.

3.3. PSMA Promoter

PSMA, a 100-kDa type II membrane glycoprotein, was originally identified as an antigen interacting with a prostate-specific monoclonal antibody, 7E11-C5.3, raised against an insoluble fraction of the LNCaP prostate cancer cell line *(191)*. A variety of approaches, such as immunohistochemical staining, reverse transcriptase polymerase chain reaction, and *in situ* hybridization, demonstrated that PSMA is expressed predominantly in prostate tissue and tumor neovasculature, with low levels of expression detected in several other tissues; the highest expression was in prostate cancer and tumor neovasculature, with expression decreasing in order as follows: Prostate, proximal gastrointestinal tract, salivary glands, kidney, and brain *(192)*. Northern blot analysis and affinity column purification detected two different forms of PSMA, full length and an alternatively spliced variant PSM, which lacks the first 57 amino acids. The physiological substrates of PSMA and its variant in the prostate remain unknown, but PSMA and PSM have the following enzymatic activities: Folate hydrolase activity *(193)*, *N*-acetylated-linked acidic dipeptidase (NAALADase) activity *(194)*, and dipeptidyl peptidase IV activity *(195)*. Interestingly, a PSMA enzymatic inhibitor (quisqualate) and antisense RNA-to-PSMA delay the growth of LNCaP *(192)*, suggesting that PSMA may have an important role in prostate cancer (Pca) growth.

The gene encoding PSMA, called *FOLH1*, is located at chromosome 11p11–p12, containing 19 exons *(196)*. Further study mapped a PSMA-like gene to another chromosomal region, 11q14. It was suspected that the PSMA gene was duplicated (exons 2–19) from the PSMA-like gene an estimated 20 million years ago *(196,197)*. Mice harbor only PSMA-like gene, which is expressed mainly (in decreasing order) in kidney, brain, testis, and salivary gland, but not in prostate *(198)*. There is a strong likelihood that PSMA expressions detected in some human tissues are the result of expression of PSMA-like gene *(192)*.

PSMA has drawn attention for clinical use because of its expression patterns. Serum PSMA in patients with prostate cancer is significantly higher than in normal men and patients with benign prostate hyperplasia, suggesting that PSMA can be a marker protein for prostate cancer diagnosis. Because the level of PSMA expression is downregulated by androgen, patients undergoing hormone ablation therapy exhibit increasing serum PSMA expression. Consistently, its expression is further elevated in patients with more malignant bone and lymph node metastatic prostate cancers *(199,200)*, suggesting enhanced expression of PSMA as prostate cancer progresses *(201,202)*.

Such expression patterns have led to several studies using PSMA for prostate cancer diagnosis and therapy. Currently, the PSA level in serum is a widespread diagnostic marker for prostate cancer, but PSA is limited in its usefulness *(203)* to predict tumor burden and metastatic potential. Furthermore, PSA levels in serum are unable to differentiate between prostate cancer and benign prostatic hyperplasia. These limitations require other marker proteins for diagnostic purposes. Reports indicated that PSMA could be an alternative or complementary marker for prostate cancer progression *(204–206)*.

PSMA is a marker protein for prostate cancer, and its almost-exclusive, prostate-restricted expression enabled several studies using PSMA as a target protein for prostate cancer therapy. Primary T lymphocytes expressing artificial T-cell receptor-zeta-CD28 fusion protein, which recognizes PSMA, effectively lysed tumor cells expressing PSMA *(207)*. Warren et al. *(208)* used the enzymatic activity of PSMA to convert a synthetic amoebapore helix 3 peptide to cytolytic peptide directed against PSMA-expressing cells. Antibodies against PSMA have been developed for diagnostic purposes and for targeting the prostate. Despite these promising beginnings, study of the regulation of PSMA expression is far from complete.

A 1.2-kb PSMA promoter upstream of *FOLH1* gene mediating high reporter activity has been cloned *(196)*. However, we and others have observed significant activity of this 1.2-kb PSMA promoter in several PSMA-negative cells, such as PC-3, HEK293, HeLa, and MCF-7 cells *(209,210*; Kao, C., 2003, unpublished data). This leaky activity of the 1.2-kb PSMA promoter might contribute to the weak expression of PSMA in organs other than the prostate. Unlike 1.2-kb PSMA promoter, the PSMA enhancer core (PSME) residing in intron 3 of PSMA gene *(FOLH1)* exhibited very strong prostate-specific activity only in PSMA-positive LNCaP, C4-2, CWR22rv, and MDA Pca 2b cells, with very low activity in PC-3 cells and no activity in other PSMA-negative cells tested *(211)*.

Like PSMA expression, PSME is negatively regulated by androgens, so it exhibits much higher activity at low levels or in the absence of androgens *(200–211)*. The PSME enhancer element can be functionally split into three regions: an upstream region, a direct repeat region, and a partial *Alu* repeat sequence, which is a member of the SINE (short interspersed element). We believe that the direct repeat region is the main element that controls the prostate-specific activity of PSME.

3.4. Chimeric Promoter PSES

Unlike probasin and OC, PSA and PSMA are well-characterized human PSAs. We are actively investigating the regulatory mechanism of PSA and PSMA expression in AI prostate cancers to achieve better control of E1a and E1b expression. We found that the main prostate-specific enhancer activity of PSA enhancer core is located in a 189-bp region called AREc3. The main prostate-specific enhancer activity of the PSMA enhancer core is located in a 331-bp region called PSME(del2). A combination of AREc3 and PSME(del2), called PSES, showed much stronger transcriptional activity than either AREc3 or PSME(del2) alone in the presence or absence of androgen and retained tight prostate-specific activity in cell lines *(211)*. Patients with AI tumors are still in androgen ablation therapy, for which only low levels of androgen will be present. Overexpressed or mutated AR in AI prostate cancer together with low levels of residual androgen in the patient might weakly activate AREc3 and slightly suppress PSME(del2), so both AREc3 and PSME(del2) are likely to have weak activity in AI prostate cancers under androgen ablation therapy. On the other hand, PSES will have high activity in these AI prostate cancers, so it is an attractive tool for developing a prostate-restricted, replication-competent adenovirus for patients with AI cancers.

4. PROSTATE CANCER ANTIMETASTATIC CLINICAL TRIALS: THEORY TRANSLATES INTO THERAPY

Prostate cancer has been a target for investigators interested in gene therapy. There are 50 gene transfer protocols registered with the Office of Biologic Activities (OAB; http://www4.od.nih.gov/oba/rac/PROTOCOL.pdf). These protocols range from vaccine approaches to oncolytic adenoviral approaches and comprise 15% of the 357 cancer therapy protocols. A majority of the clinical protocols toward metastatic prostate cancer involve vaccine-based approaches to engage and stimulate the immune system to combat sites of metastases. Several of the nonvaccine approaches targeting metastatic prostate cancer demonstrate the ability to translate the basic understanding of the prostate cancer cell to a clinical trial. The three clinical trials discussed next are based on the theory described throughout this chapter demonstrating that these basic investigations in biology of prostate cancer metastasis can be translated to the clinic and confirm the hypothesis proposed in the introduction.

4.1. Phase I Study of Ad-OC-TK Plus Valacyclovir for the Treatment of Metastatic or Recurrent Prostate Cancer

Using the principles outlined in this chapter, we designed, preclinically tested, and clinically verified the phase I study of Ad-OC-TK plus valacyclovir for the treatment of metastatic or recurrent prostate cancer (OBA 9812-276). We designed a clinical protocol to test the hypothesis that the osteocalcin promoter can transcriptionally regulate HSV-TK production specifically within a prostate cancer cell and the supportive cells of a bone metastasis *(212)*. The protocol and patients enrolled are described in ref. *8*. The clinical results and laboratory correlates are fully outlined in ref. *213*. This clinical trial represents the ability to develop a hypothesis, design a gene therapy approach, and validate this approach in vitro and in vivo and in the clinic. The hypothesis was that the osteocalcin promoter could transcriptionally regulate HSV-TK production when delivered to osseous metastases by an adenoviral vector and kill prostate cancer cells with acyclovir administration. Table 6 of ref. *213* summarizes that this trial's laboratory correlates validate the hypothesis put forth at the onset of the trial. Immunohistochemical analysis of the specimens before, during, and after therapy revealed that prostate cancer has sufficient coxsackie-adenovirus receptor and osteocalcin expression and that exposure to Ad-OC-TK resulted in TK production and decreased proliferation (ki-67) and increased apoptosis (apotag) with valacyclovir administration.

4.2. Phase I/II Dose-Finding Trial of the Intravenous Injection of Calydon CV787, a PSA Cytolytic Adenovirus, in Patients With Hormone-Refractory Metastatic Prostate Cancer

The ongoing phase I/II dose-finding trial (OBA 9910-345) of the intravenous injection of calydon CV787 harnesses the oncolytic potential of the adenovirus under the transcriptional regulation of the PSA and probasin promoters. This trial was designed with systemic administration of the cytolytic virus in men with hormone-refractory metastatic prostate cancer. The preliminary results are that the transcriptional targeting provides the safety of a systemic adenovirus, with viremia occurring at the time of injection and several days after the injection. Limited information on the clinical results of this trial is available, but the safety profile is supportive of this approach.

4.3. Phase I Study of Intratumoral Injections of Ad-OC-E1a for Metastatic or Locally Recurrent Prostate Cancer, Part 1: Dose Finding; Part 2: Index Lesion Escalation

The proposed phase I trial (OBA 0010-426) builds on the OC-TK trial in Section 4.2. by harnessing the oncolytic potential of the adenovirus Ad-OC-E1a via direct injection into bone metastases. Matsubara et al. validated this approach preclinically *(214)*. The enhanced strength of the oncolytic approach should lead to improved clinical responses.

5. SUMMARY

Antimetastatic gene therapy for prostate cancer remains a formidable challenge. Thorough bench investigations followed by clinical trials supported by extensive laboratory correlates should allow for the ultimate development of a gene therapy.

REFERENCES

1. Jemal, A., Murray, T., Samuels, A., Ghafoor, A., Ward, E., and Thun, M. J. (2003) Cancer statistics, 2003. *CA Cancer J. Clin.* **53**, 5–26.
2. Gleave, M., Hsieh, J. T., Gao, C. A., von Eschenbach, A. C., and Chung, L. W. K. (1991) Acceleration of human prostate cancer growth in vivo by factors produced by prostate and bone fibroblasts. *Cancer Res.* **51**, 3753–3761.
3. Festuccia, C., Bologna, M., Gravina, G. L., et al. (1999) Osteoblast conditioned media contain TGF-beta1 and modulate the migration of prostate tumor cells and their interactions with extracellular matrix components. *Int. J. Cancer* **81**, 395–403.
4. Wu, H. C., Hsieh, J. T., Gleave, M. E., Brown, N. M., Pathak, S., and Chung, L. W. K. (1994) Derivation of androgen-independent human LNCaP prostatic cancer cell sublines: role of bone stromal cells. *Int. J. Cancer* **57**, 406–417.
5. Thalmann, G. N., Anizinis, P. E., Chang, S. M., et al. (1994) Androgen-independent cancer progression and bone metastasis in the LNCaP model of human prostate cancer. *Cancer Res.* **54**, 2577–2581.
6. Chung, L. W. K. (1995) The role of stroma-epithelial interaction in normal and malignant growth. *Cancer Surveys* **23**, 33–42.

7. Rhee, H. W., Zhau, H. E., Pathak, S., et al. (2001) Permanent phenotypic and genotypic changes of prostate cancer cells cultured in a three-dimensional rotating-wall vessel. *In Vitro Cell Dev. Biol. Anim.* **37,** 127–140.

8. Koeneman, K. S., Kao, C., Ko, S. C., et al. (2000) Osteocalcin-directed gene therapy for prostate-cancer bone metastasis. *World J. Urol.* **18,** 102–110.

9. Gardner, T. A., Sloan, J., Raikwar, S. P., and Kao, C. (2002) Prostate cancer gene therapy: past experiences and future promise. *Cancer Metastasis Rev.* **21,** 137–145.

10. Welch, D. R. and Rinker-Schaeffer, C. W. (1999) What defines a useful marker of metastasis in human cancer? *J. Natl. Cancer Inst.* **91,** 1351–1353.

11. Moustafa, A. S. and Nicolson, G. L. (1997) Breast cancer metastasis-associated genes: prognostic significance and therapeutic implications. *Oncol. Res.* **9,** 505–525.

12. Welch, D. R., Steeg, P. S., and Rinker-Schaeffer, C. W. (2000) Molecular biology of breast cancer metastasis. Genetic regulation of human breast carcinoma metastasis. *Breast Cancer Res.* **2,** 408–416.

13. Steeg, P. S., Bevilacqua, G., Kopper, L., et al. (1988) Evidence for a novel gene associated with low tumor metastatic potential. *J. Natl. Cancer Inst.* **80,** 200–204.

14. Ebralidze, A., Tulchinsky, E., Grigorian, M., et al. (1989) Isolation and characterization of a gene specifically expressed in different metastatic cells and whose deduced gene product has a high degree of homology to a Ca^{2+}-binding protein family. *Genes Dev.* **3,** 1086–1093.

15. Dear, T. N., Ramshaw, I. A., and Kefford, R. F. (1988) Differential expression of a novel gene, WDNM1, in nonmetastatic rat mammary adenocarcinoma cells. *Cancer Res.* **48,** 5203–5209.

16. Dear, T. N., McDonald, D. A., and Kefford, R. F. (1989) Transcriptional down-regulation of a rat gene, WDNM2, in metastatic DMBA-8 cells. *Cancer Res.* **49,** 5323–5328.

17. Phillips, S. M., Bendall, A. J., and Ramshaw, I. A. (1990) Isolation of gene associated with high metastatic potential in rat mammary adenocarcinomas. *J. Natl. Cancer Inst.* **82,** 199–203.

18. Basset, P., Bellocq, J. P., Wolf, C., et al. (1990) A novel metalloproteinase gene specifically expressed in stromal cells of breast carcinomas. *Nature* **348,** 699–704.

19. Dong, J. T., Lamb, P. W., Rinker-Schaeffer, C. W., et al. (1995) KAI1, a metastasis suppressor gene for prostate cancer on human chromosome 11p11.2. *Science* **268,** 884–886.

20. Seraj, M. J., Samant, R. S., Verderame, M. F., and Welch, D. R. (2000) Functional evidence for a novel human breast carcinoma metastasis suppressor, BRMS1, encoded at chromosome 11q13. *Cancer Res.* **60,** 2764–2769.

21. Steeg, P. S. (2003) Metastasis suppressors alter the signal transduction of cancer cells. *Nat. Rev. Cancer* **3,** 55–63.

22. Kauffman, E. C., Robinson, V. L., Stadler, W. M., Sokoloff, M. H., and Rinker-Schaeffer, C. W. (2003) Metastasis suppression: the evolving role of metastasis suppressor genes for regulating cancer cell growth at the secondary site. *J. Urol.* **169,** 1122–1133.

23. Ichikawa, T., Ichikawa, Y., Dong, J., et al. (1992) Localization of metastasis suppressor gene(s) for prostatic cancer to the short arm of human chromosome 11. *Cancer Res.* **52,** 3486–3490.

24. Dong, J. T., Suzuki, H., Pin, S. S., et al. (1996) Down-regulation of the KAI1 metastasis suppressor gene during the progression of human prostatic cancer infrequently involves gene mutation or allelic loss. *Cancer Res.* **56,** 4387–4390.

25. Ueda, T., Ichikawa, T., Tamaru, J., et al. (1996) Expression of the KAI1 protein in benign prostatic hyperplasia and prostate cancer. *Am. J. Pathol.* **149,** 1435–1440.

26. Takaoka, A., Hinoda, Y., Satoh, S., et al. (1998) Suppression of invasive properties of colon cancer cells by a metastasis suppressor KAI1 gene. *Oncogene* **16,** 1443–1453.

27. Yang, X., Welch, D. R., Phillips, K. K., Weissman, B. E., and Wei, L. L. (1997) KAI1, a putative marker for metastatic potential in human breast cancer. *Cancer Lett.* **119,** 149–155.

28. Guo, X., Friess, H., Graber, H. U., et al. (1996) KAI1 expression is up-regulated in early pancreatic cancer and decreased in the presence of metastases. *Cancer Res.* **56,** 4876–4880.

29. Guo, X. Z., Friess, H., Di Mola, F. F., et al. (1998) KAI1, a new metastasis suppressor gene, is reduced in metastatic hepatocellular carcinoma. *Hepatology* **28,** 1481–1488.

30. Yu, Y., Yang, J. L., Markovic, B., et al. (1997) Loss of KAI1 messenger RNA expression in both high-grade and invasive human bladder cancers. *Clin. Cancer Res.* **3,** 1045–1049.

31. Adachi, M., Taki, T., Ieki, Y., Huang, C. L., Higashiyama, M., and Miyake, M. (1996) Correlation of KAI1/CD82 gene expression with good prognosis in patients with non-small cell lung cancer. *Cancer Res.* **56,** 1751–1755.

32. Kim, H. L., Vander Griend, D. J., Yang, X., et al. (2001) Mitogen-activated protein kinase kinase 4 metastasis suppressor gene expression is inversely related to histological pattern in advancing human prostatic cancers. *Cancer Res.* **61,** 2833–2837.

33. Yamada, S. D., Hickson, J. A., Hrobowski, Y., et al. (2002) Mitogen-activated protein kinase kinase 4 (MKK4) acts as a metastasis suppressor gene in human ovarian carcinoma. *Cancer Res.* **62,** 6717–6723.

34. White, R. A., Hughes, R. T., Adkison, L. R., Bruns, G., and Zon, L. I. (1996) The gene encoding protein kinase SEK1 maps to mouse chromosome 11 and human chromosome 17. *Genomics* **34,** 430–432.

35. Yoshida, B. A., Dubauskas, Z., Chekmareva, M. A., Christiano, T. R., Stadler, W. M., and Rinker-Schaeffer, C. W. (1999) Mitogen-activated protein kinase kinase 4/stress-activated protein/Erk kinase 1 (MKK4/SEK1), a prostate cancer metastasis suppressor gene encoded by human chromosome 17. *Cancer Res.* **59,** 5483–5487.

36. Lange-Carter, C. A. and Johnson, G. L. (1994) Ras-dependent growth factor regulation of MEK kinase in PC12 cells. *Science* **265,** 1458–1461.

37. Yan, M., Dai, T., Deak, J. C., et al. (1994) Activation of stress-activated protein kinase by MEKK1 phosphorylation of its activator SEK1. *Nature* **372,** 798–800.

38. Chekmareva, M. A., Kadkhodaian, M. M., Hollowell, C. M., et al. (1998) Chromosome 17-mediated dormancy of AT6.1 prostate cancer micrometastases. *Cancer Res.* **58,** 4963–4969.

39. Kuryu, M., Ozaki, T., Nishida, K., Shibahara, M., Kawai, A., and Inoue, H. (1999) Expression of CD44 variants in osteosarcoma. *J. Cancer Res. Clin. Oncol.* **125,** 646–652.

40. Ladeda, V., Aguirre Ghiso, J. A., and Bal de Kier Joffe, E. (1998) Function and expression of CD44 during spreading, migration, and invasion of murine carcinoma cells. *Exp. Cell Res.* **242,** 515–527.

41. Gao, A. C., Lou, W., Dong, J. T., and Isaacs, J. T. (1997) CD44 is a metastasis suppressor gene for prostatic cancer located on human chromosome 11p13. *Cancer Res.* **57,** 846–849.

42. Kallakury, B. V., Sheehan, C. E., Ambros, R. A., et al. (1998) Correlation of p34cdc2 cyclin-dependent kinase overexpression, CD44s downregulation, and HER-2/neu oncogene amplification with recurrence in prostatic adenocarcinomas. *J. Clin. Oncol.* **16,** 1302–1309.

43. Nagabhushan, M., Pretlow, T. G., Guo, Y. J., Amini, S. B., Pretlow, T. P., and Sy, M. S. (1996) Altered expression of CD44 in human prostate cancer during progression. *Am. J. Clin. Pathol.* **106,** 647–651.

44. Takahashi, S., Kimoto, N., Orita, S., Cui, L., Sakakibara, M., and Shirai, T. (1998) Relationship between CD44 expression and differentiation of human prostate adenocarcinomas. *Cancer Lett.* **129,** 97–102.

45. Noordzij, M. A., van Steenbrugge, G. J., Verkaik, N. S., Schroder, F. H., and van der Kwast, T. H. (1997) The prognostic value of CD44 isoforms in prostate cancer patients treated by radical prostatectomy. *Clin. Cancer Res.* **3,** 805–815.

46. De Marzo, A. M., Bradshaw, C., Sauvageot, J., Epstein, J. I., and Miller, G. J. (1998) CD44 and CD44v6 downregulation in clinical prostatic carcinoma: relation to Gleason grade and cytoarchitecture. *Prostate* **34,** 162–168.

47. Noordzij, M. A., van Steenbrugge, G. J., Schroder, F. H., and Van der Kwast, T. H. (1999) Decreased expression of CD44 in metastatic prostate cancer. *Int. J. Cancer* **84,** 478–483.

48. Kogerman, P., Sy, M. S., and Culp, L. A. (1998) Over-expression of human CD44s in murine 3T3 cells: selection against during primary tumorigenesis and selection for during micrometastasis. *Clin. Exp. Metastasis* **16,** 83–93.

49. Tozawa, K., Yamada, Y., Kawai, N., Okamura, T., Ueda, K., and Kohri, K. (1999) Osteopontin expression in prostate cancer and benign prostatic hyperplasia. *Urol. Int.* **62,** 155–158.

50. Ruoslahti, E. (1991) Integrins. *J. Clin. Invest.* **87,** 1–5.

51. Hynes, R. O. (1992) Integrins: versatility, modulation, and signaling in cell adhesion. *Cell* **69,** 11–25.

52. van der Flier, A. and Sonnenberg, A. (2001) Function and interactions of integrins. *Cell Tissue Res.* **305,** 285–298.

53. Edlund, M., Miyamoto, T., Sikes, R. A., et al. (2001) Integrin expression and usage by prostate cancer cell lines on laminin substrata. *Cell Growth Differ.* **12,** 99–107.

54. Brooks, P. C., Clark, R. A., and Cheresh, D. A. (1994) Requirement of vascular integrin alpha v beta 3 for angiogenesis. *Science* **264,** 569–571.

55. Hsu, M. Y., Shih, D. T., Meier, F. E., et al. (1998) Adenoviral gene transfer of beta3 integrin subunit induces conversion from radial to vertical growth phase in primary human melanoma. *Am. J. Pathol.* **153,** 1435–1442.

56. Danen, E. H., Jansen, K. F., Van Kraats, A. A., Cornelissen, I. M., Ruiter, D. J., and Van Muijen, G. N. (1995) Alpha v-integrins in human melanoma: gain of alpha v beta 3 and loss of alpha v beta 5 are related to tumor progression in situ but not to metastatic capacity of cell lines in nude mice. *Int. J. Cancer* **61,** 491–496.

57. Marshall, J. F., Rutherford, D. C., Happerfield, L., et al. (1998) Comparative analysis of integrins in vitro and in vivo in uveal and cutaneous melanomas. *Br. J. Cancer* **77,** 522–529.

58. Klein, C. E., Dressel, D., Steinmayer, T., et al. (1991) Integrin alpha 2 beta 1 is upregulated in fibroblasts and highly aggressive melanoma cells in three-dimensional collagen lattices and mediates the reorganization of collagen I fibrils. *J. Cell Biol.* **115,** 1427–1436.

59. Natali, P. G., Nicotra, M. R., Bartolazzi, A., Cavaliere, R., and Bigotti, A. (1993) Integrin expression in cutaneous malignant melanoma: association of the alpha 3/beta 1 heterodimer with tumor progression. *Int. J. Cancer* **54,** 68–72.

60. Yoshinaga, I. G., Vink, J., Dekker, S. K., Mihm, M. C. Jr., and Byers, H. R. (1993) Role of alpha 3 beta 1 and alpha 2 beta 1 integrins in melanoma cell migration. *Melanoma Res.* **3,** 435–441.

61. Etoh, T., Thomas, L., Pastel-Levy, C., Colvin, R. B., Mihm, M. C. Jr., and Byers, H. R. (1993) Role of integrin alpha 2 beta 1 (VLA-2) in the migration of human melanoma cells on laminin and type IV collagen. *J. Invest. Dermatol.* **100,** 640–647.

62. Danen, E. H., van Muijen, G. N., van de Wiel-van Kemenade, E., Jansen, K. F., Ruiter, D. J., and Figdor, C. G. (1993) Regulation of integrin-mediated adhesion to laminin and collagen in human melanocytes and in non-metastatic and highly metastatic human melanoma cells. *Int. J. Cancer* **54,** 315–321.

63. Melchiori, A., Mortarini, R., Carlone, S., et al. (1995) The alpha 3 beta 1 integrin is involved in melanoma cell migration and invasion. *Exp. Cell Res.* **219,** 233–242.

64. Hieken, T. J., Ronan, S. G., Farolan, M., Shilkaitis, A. L., and Das Gupta, T. K. (1996) Beta 1 integrin expression: a marker of lymphatic metastases in cutaneous malignant melanoma. *Anticancer Res.* **16,** 2321–2324.

65. Vihinen, P., Nikkola, J., Vlaykova, T., et al. (2000) Prognostic value of beta1 integrin expression in metastatic melanoma. *Melanoma Res.* **10,** 243–251.

66. Hieken, T. J., Ronan, S. G., Farolan, M., Shilkaitis, A. L., and Das Gupta, T. K. (1999) Molecular prognostic markers in intermediate-thickness cutaneous malignant melanoma. *Cancer* **85,** 375–382.

67. Hangan, D., Morris, V. L., Boeters, L., von Ballestrem, C., Uniyal, S., and Chan, B. M. (1997) An epitope on VLA-6 (alpha6beta1) integrin involved in migration but not adhesion is required for extravasation of murine melanoma B16F1 cells in liver. *Cancer Res.* **57,** 3812–3817.

68. Ziober, B. L., Chen, Y. Q., Ramos, D. M., Waleh, N., and Kramer, R. H. (1999) Expression of the alpha7beta1 laminin receptor suppresses melanoma growth and metastatic potential. *Cell Growth Differ.* **10,** 479–490.

69. Mortarini, R., Gismondi, A., Santoni, A., Parmiani, G., and Anichini, A. (1992) Role of the alpha 5 beta 1 integrin receptor in the proliferative response of quiescent human melanoma cells to fibronectin. *Cancer Res.* **52,** 4499–4506.

70. Mould, A. P., Askari, J. A., Craig, S. E., Garratt, A. N., Clements, J., and Humphries, M. J. (1994) Integrin alpha 4 beta 1-mediated melanoma cell adhesion and migration on vascular cell adhesion molecule-1 (VCAM-1) and the alternatively spliced IIICS region of fibronectin. *J. Biol. Chem.* **269,** 27,224–27,230.

71. Timar, J., Bazaz, R., Kimler, V., et al. (1995) Immunomorphological characterization and effects of 12-(S)-HETE on a dynamic intracellular pool of the alpha IIb beta 3-integrin in melanoma cells. *J. Cell Sci.* **108(Pt. 6),** 2175–2186.

72. Trikha, M., Timar, J., Lundy, S. K., et al. (1997) The high affinity alphaIIb beta3 integrin is involved in invasion of human melanoma cells. *Cancer Res.* **57,** 2522–2528.

73. Zutter, M. M., Mazoujian, G., and Santoro, S. A. (1990) Decreased expression of integrin adhesive protein receptors in adenocarcinoma of the breast. *Am. J. Pathol.* **137,** 863–870.

74. Sung, V., Stubbs, J. T. 3rd, Fisher, L., Aaron, A. D., and Thompson, E. W. (1998) Bone sialoprotein supports breast cancer cell adhesion proliferation and migration through differential usage of the alpha(v)beta3 and alpha(v)beta5 integrins. *J. Cell. Physiol.* **176,** 482–494.

75. Wong, N. C., Mueller, B. M., Barbas, C. F., et al. (1998) Alphav integrins mediate adhesion and migration of breast carcinoma cell lines. *Clin. Exp. Metastasis* **16,** 50–61.

76. Tuck, A. B., Elliott, B. E., Hota, C., Tremblay, E., and Chambers, A. F. (2000) Osteopontin-induced, integrin-dependent migration of human mammary epithelial cells involves activation of the hepatocyte growth factor receptor (Met). *J. Cell. Biochem.* **78,** 465–475.

77. Morini, M., Mottolese, M., Ferrari, N., et al. (2000) The alpha 3 beta 1 integrin is associated with mammary carcinoma cell metastasis, invasion, and gelatinase B (MMP-9) activity. *Int. J. Cancer* **87,** 336–342.

78. Gui, G. P., Wells, C. A., Browne, P. D., et al. (1995) Integrin expression in primary breast cancer and its relation to axillary nodal status. *Surgery* **117,** 102–108.

79. Jones, J. L., Royall, J. E., Critchley, D. R., and Walker, R. A. (1997) Modulation of myoepithelial-associated alpha6 beta4 integrin in a breast cancer cell line alters invasive potential. *Exp. Cell Res.* **235,** 325–333.

80. Bachelder, R. E., Marchetti, A., Falcioni, R., Soddu, S., and Mercurio, A. M. (1999) Activation of p53 function in carcinoma cells by the alpha6beta4 integrin. *J. Biol. Chem.* **274,** 20,733–20,737.

81. O'Connor, K. L., Shaw, L. M., and Mercurio, A. M. (1998) Release of cAMP gating by the alpha6beta4 integrin stimulates lamellae formation and the chemotactic migration of invasive carcinoma cells. *J. Cell Biol.* **143,** 1749–1760.

82. Rabinovitz, I., Nagle, R. B., and Cress, A. E. (1995) Integrin alpha 6 expression in human prostate carcinoma cells is associated with a migratory and invasive phenotype in vitro and in vivo. *Clin. Exp. Metastasis* **13,** 481–491.

83. Davis, T. L., Cress, A. E., Dalkin, B. L., and Nagle, R. B. (2001) Unique expression pattern of the alpha6beta4 integrin and laminin-5 in human prostate carcinoma. *Prostate* **46,** 240–248.

84. Knox, J. D., Cress, A. E., Clark, V., et al. (1994) Differential expression of extracellular matrix molecules and the alpha 6-integrins in the normal and neoplastic prostate. *Am. J. Pathol.* **145,** 167–174.

85. Bello-DeOcampo, D., Kleinman, H. K., Deocampo, N. D., and Webber, M. M. (2001) Laminin-1 and alpha6beta1 integrin regulate acinar morphogenesis of normal and malignant human prostate epithelial cells. *Prostate* **46,** 142–153.

86. Dedhar, S., Saulnier, R., Nagle, R., and Overall, C. M. (1993) Specific alterations in the expression of alpha 3 beta 1 and alpha 6 beta 4 integrins in highly invasive and metastatic variants of human prostate carcinoma cells selected by in vitro invasion through reconstituted basement membrane. *Clin. Exp. Metastasis* **11,** 391–400.

87. Bonaccorsi, L., Carloni, V., Muratori, M., et al. (2000) Androgen receptor expression in prostate carcinoma cells suppresses alpha6beta4 integrin-mediated invasive phenotype. *Endocrinology* **141,** 3172–3182.

88. Kostenuik, P. J., Singh, G., and Orr, F. W. (1997) Transforming growth factor beta upregulates the integrin-mediated adhesion of human prostatic carcinoma cells to type I collagen. *Clin. Exp. Metastasis* **15,** 41–52.

89. Kostenuik, P. J., Sanchez-Sweatman, O., Orr, F. W., and Singh, G. (1996) Bone cell matrix promotes the adhesion of human prostatic carcinoma cells via the alpha 2 beta 1 integrin. *Clin. Exp. Metastasis* **14,** 19–26.

90. Lang, S. H., Clarke, N. W., George, N. J., and Testa, N. G. (1997) Primary prostatic epithelial cell binding to human bone marrow stroma and the role of alpha2beta1 integrin. *Clin. Exp. Metastasis* **15**, 218–227.

91. Trikha, M., Timar, J., Lundy, S. K., et al. (1996) Human prostate carcinoma cells express functional alphaIIb(beta)3 integrin. *Cancer Res.* **56**, 5071–5078.

92. Trikha, M., Raso, E., Cai, Y., et al. (1998) Role of alphaII(b)beta3 integrin in prostate cancer metastasis. *Prostate* **35**, 185–192.

93. Albelda, S. M. (1993) Role of integrins and other cell adhesion molecules in tumor progression and metastasis. *Lab. Invest.* **68**, 4–17.

94. Johnson, J. P. (1999) Cell adhesion molecules in the development and progression of malignant melanoma. *Cancer Metastasis Rev.* **18**, 345–357.

95. Kansas, G. S. (1996) Selectins and their ligands: current concepts and controversies. *Blood* **88**, 3259–3287.

96. Somers, W. S., Tang, J., Shaw, G. D., and Camphausen, R. T. (2000) Insights into the molecular basis of leukocyte tethering and rolling revealed by structures of P- and E-selectin bound to SLe(X) and PSGL-1. *Cell* **103**, 467–479.

97. Stanford, D. R., Starkey, J. R., and Magnuson, J. A. (1986) The role of tumor-cell surface carbohydrate in experimental metastasis. *Int. J. Cancer* **37**, 435–444.

98. Kishimoto, T., Ishikura, H., Kimura, C., Takahashi, T., Kato, H., and Yoshiki, T. (1996) Phenotypes correlating to metastatic properties of pancreas adenocarcinoma in vivo: the importance of surface sialyl Lewis(a) antigen. *Int. J. Cancer* **69**, 290–294.

99. Fukuda, M. N., Ohyama, C., Lowitz, K., et al. (2000) A peptide mimic of E-selectin ligand inhibits sialyl Lewis X-dependent lung colonization of tumor cells. *Cancer Res.* **60**, 450–456.

100. Matsushita, Y., Cleary, K. R., Ota, D. M., Hoff, S. D., and Irimura, T. (1990) Sialyl-dimeric Lewis-X antigen expressed on mucin-like glycoproteins in colorectal cancer metastases. *Lab. Invest.* **63**, 780–791.

101. Kobayashi, K., Matsumoto, S., Morishima, T., Kawabe, T., and Okamoto, T. (2000) Cimetidine inhibits cancer cell adhesion to endothelial cells and prevents metastasis by blocking E-selectin expression. *Cancer Res.* **60**, 3978–3984.

102. Nollet, F., Kools, P., and van Roy, F. (2000) Phylogenetic analysis of the cadherin superfamily allows identification of six major subfamilies besides several solitary members. *J. Mol. Biol.* **299**, 551–572.

103. Leckband, D. and Sivasankar, S. (2000) Mechanism of homophilic cadherin adhesion. *Curr. Opin. Cell Biol.* **12**, 587–592.

104. Behrens, J., Birchmeier, W., Goodman, S. L., and Imhof, B. A. (1985) Dissociation of Madin-Darby canine kidney epithelial cells by the monoclonal antibody anti-arc-1: mechanistic aspects and identification of the antigen as a component related to uvomorulin. *J. Cell Biol.* **101**, 1307–1315.

105. Behrens, J., Mareel, M. M., Van Roy, F. M., and Birchmeier, W. (1989) Dissecting tumor cell invasion: epithelial cells acquire invasive properties after the loss of uvomorulin-mediated cell-cell adhesion. *J. Cell Biol.* **108**, 2435–2447.

106. Hazan, R. B., Phillips, G. R., Qiao, R. F., Norton, L., and Aaronson, S. A. (2000) Exogenous expression of N-cadherin in breast cancer cells induces cell migration, invasion, and metastasis. *J. Cell Biol.* **148**, 779–790.

107. Williams, A. F. and Barclay, A. N. (1988) The immunoglobulin superfamily—domains for cell surface recognition. *Annu. Rev. Immunol.* **6**, 381–405.

108. Johnson, J. P. (1991) Cell adhesion molecules of the immunoglobulin supergene family and their role in malignant transformation and progression to metastatic disease. *Cancer Metastasis Rev.* **10**, 11–22.

109. Gonzalez-Amaro, R., Diaz-Gonzalez, F., and Sanchez-Madrid, F. (1998) Adhesion molecules in inflammatory diseases. *Drugs* **56**, 977–988.

110. Sun, J. J., Zhou, X. D., Liu, Y. K., et al. (1999) Invasion and metastasis of liver cancer: expression of intercellular adhesion molecule 1. *J. Cancer Res. Clin. Oncol.* **125**, 28–34.

111. Aoudjit, F., Potworowski, E. F., Springer, T. A., and St-Pierre, Y. (1998) Protection from lymphoma cell metastasis in ICAM-1 mutant mice: a posthoming event. *J. Immunol.* **161**, 2333–2338.

112. Denton, K. J., Stretch, J. R., Gatter, K. C., and Harris, A. L. (1992) A study of adhesion molecules as markers of progression in malignant melanoma. *J. Pathol.* **167**, 187–191.

113. Lehmann, J. M., Riethmuller, G., and Johnson, J. P. (1989) MUC18, a marker of tumor progression in human melanoma, shows sequence similarity to the neural cell adhesion molecules of the immunoglobulin superfamily. *Proc. Natl. Acad. Sci. USA* **86**, 9891–9895.

114. Koeneman, K. S., Yeung, F., and Chung, L. W. (1999) Osteomimetic properties of prostate cancer cells: a hypothesis supporting the predilection of prostate cancer metastasis and growth in the bone environment. *Prostate* **39**, 246–261.

115. Yeung, F., Law, W. K., Yeh, C. H., et al. (2002) Regulation of human osteocalcin promoter in hormone-independent human prostate cancer cells. *J. Biol. Chem.* **277**, 2468–2476.

116. Brown, J. M., Corey, E., Lee, Z. D., et al. (2001) Osteoprotegerin and rank ligand expression in prostate cancer. *Urology* **57**, 611–616.

117. Lin, D. L., Tarnowski, C. P., Zhang, J., et al. (2001) Bone metastatic LNCaP-derivative C4-2B prostate cancer cell line mineralizes in vitro. *Prostate* **47**, 212–221.

118. Fidler, I. J., Gersten, D. M., and Hart, I. R. (1978) The biology of cancer invasion and metastasis. *Adv. Cancer Res.* **28**, 149–250.

119. Folkman, J. (1971) Tumor angiogenesis: therapeutic implications. *N. Engl. J. Med.* **285,** 1182–1186.
120. Folkman, J. (1972) Anti-angiogenesis: new concept for therapy of solid tumors. *Ann. Surg.* **175,** 409–416.
121. Folkman, J. (1996) Tumor angiogenesis and tissue factor. *Nat. Med.* **2,** 167–168.
122. Folkman, J. (1996) Fighting cancer by attacking its blood supply. *Sci. Am.* **275,** 150–154.
123. Folkman, J. (1985) Toward an understanding of angiogenesis: search and discovery. *Perspect. Biol. Med.* **29,** 10–36.
124. Rastinejad, F., Polverini, P. J., and Bouck, N. P. (1989) Regulation of the activity of a new inhibitor of angiogenesis by a cancer suppressor gene. *Cell* **56,** 345–355.
125. Bouck, N. (1990) Tumor angiogenesis: the role of oncogenes and tumor suppressor genes. *Cancer Cells* **2,** 179–185.
126. Liotta, L. A., Steeg, P. S., and Stetler-Stevenson, W. G. (1991) Cancer metastasis and angiogenesis: an imbalance of positive and negative regulation. *Cell* **64,** 327–336.
127. Hanahan, D. and Folkman, J. (1996) Patterns and emerging mechanisms of the angiogenic switch during tumorigenesis. *Cell* **86,** 353–364.
128. O'Reilly, M. S., Holmgren, L., Shing, Y., et al. (1994) Angiostatin: a novel angiogenesis inhibitor that mediates the suppression of metastases by a Lewis lung carcinoma. *Cell* **79,** 315–328.
129. Folkman, J. and Klagsbrun, M. (1987) Angiogenic factors. *Science* **235,** 442–447.
130. Klagsbrun, M. and D'Amore, P. A. (1991) Regulators of angiogenesis. *Annu. Rev. Physiol.* **53,** 217–239.
131. Moses, M. A. and Langer, R. (1991) Inhibitors of angiogenesis. *Biotechnology (NY)* **9,** 630–634.
132. Basilico, C. and Moscatelli, D. (1992) The FGF family of growth factors and oncogenes. *Adv. Cancer Res.* **59,** 115–165.
133. Gualandris, A., Urbinati, C., Rusnati, M., Ziche, M., and Presta, M. (1994) Interaction of high-molecular-weight basic fibroblast growth factor with endothelium: biological activity and intracellular fate of human recombinant M(r) 24,000 bFGF. *J. Cell. Physiol.* **161,** 149–159.
134. Montesano, R., Vassalli, J. D., Baird, A., Guillemin, R., and Orci, L. (1986) Basic fibroblast growth factor induces angiogenesis in vitro. *Proc. Natl. Acad. Sci. USA* **83,** 7297–7301.
135. Bussolino, F., Albini, A., Camussi, G., et al. (1996) Role of soluble mediators in angiogenesis. *Eur. J. Cancer* **32A,** 2401–2412.
136. Lloyd, R. V., Vidal, S., Horvath, E., Kovacs, K., and Scheithauer, B. (2003) Angiogenesis in normal and neoplastic pituitary tissues. *Microsc. Res. Tech.* **60,** 244–250.
137. Shweiki, D., Itin, A., Soffer, D., and Keshet, E. (1992) Vascular endothelial growth factor induced by hypoxia may mediate hypoxia-initiated angiogenesis. *Nature* **359,** 843–845.
138. Plate, K. H., Breier, G., Weich, H. A., and Risau, W. (1992) Vascular endothelial growth factor is a potential tumour angiogenesis factor in human gliomas in vivo. *Nature* **359,** 845–848.
139. Bouck, N., Stellmach, V., and Hsu, S. C. (1996) How tumors become angiogenic. *Adv. Cancer Res.* **69,** 135–174.
140. Good, D. J., Polverini, P. J., Rastinejad, F., et al. (1990) A tumor suppressor-dependent inhibitor of angiogenesis is immunologically and functionally indistinguishable from a fragment of thrombospondin. *Proc. Natl. Acad. Sci. USA* **87,** 6624–6628.
141. Ferrara, N., Clapp, C., and Weiner, R. (1991) The 16K fragment of prolactin specifically inhibits basal or fibroblast growth factor stimulated growth of capillary endothelial cells. *Endocrinology* **129,** 896–900.
142. O'Reilly, M. S., Boehm, T., Shing, Y., et al. (1997) Endostatin: an endogenous inhibitor of angiogenesis and tumor growth. *Cell* **88,** 277–285.
143. Sudhakar, A., Sugimoto, H., Yang, C., Lively, J., Zeisberg, M., and Kalluri, R. (2003) Human tumstatin and human endostatin exhibit distinct antiangiogenic activities mediated by alpha v beta 3 and alpha 5 beta 1 integrins. *Proc. Natl. Acad. Sci. USA* **100,** 4766–4771.
144. Gardner, T. A. (2002) Transcriptional targeting of adenoviral vectors. *Sci. Med.* **8,** 124–125.
145. Gardner, T. A., Raikwar, S. P., and Kao, C. (2002) Transcriptional targeting. In *Adenoviral Vectors for Gene Therapy* (Curiel, D. T. and Douglas, J. T., eds.), Academic Press, New York, chap. 9, pp. 247–286.
146. Pan, L. C. and Price, P. A. (1984) The effect of transcriptional inhibitors on the bone gamma-carboxyglutamic acid protein response to 1,25-dihydroxyvitamin D3 in osteosarcoma cells. *J. Biol. Chem.* **259,** 5844–5847.
147. Price, P. A. and Williamson, M. K. (1985) Primary structure of bovine matrix Gla protein, a new vitamin K-dependent bone protein. *J. Biol. Chem.* **260,** 14,971–14,975.
148. Kerner, S. A., Scott, R. A., and Pike, J. W. (1989) Sequence elements in the human osteocalcin gene confer basal activation and inducible response to hormonal vitamin D3. *Proc. Natl. Acad. Sci. USA* **86,** 4455–4459.
149. Lian, J., Stewart, C., Puchacz, E., et al. (1989) Structure of the rat osteocalcin gene and regulation of vitamin D-dependent expression. *Proc. Natl. Acad. Sci. USA* **86,** 1143–1147.
150. Desbois, C., Hogue, D. A., and Karsenty, G. (1994) The mouse osteocalcin gene cluster contains three genes with two separate spatial and temporal patterns of expression. *J. Biol. Chem.* **269,** 1183–1190.
151. Desbois, C., Seldin, M. F., and Karsenty, G. (1994) Localization of the osteocalcin gene cluster on mouse chromosome 3. *Mamm. Genome* **5,** 321–322.
152. Montecino, M., Pockwinse, S., Lian, J., Stein, G., and Stein, J. (1994) DNase I hypersensitive sites in promoter elements associated with basal and vitamin D dependent transcription of the bone-specific osteocalcin gene. *Biochemistry* **33,** 348–353.

153. Hoffmann, H. M., Catron, K. M., van Wijnen, A. J., et al. (1994) Transcriptional control of the tissue-specific, developmentally regulated osteocalcin gene requires a binding motif for the Msx family of homeodomain proteins. *Proc. Natl. Acad. Sci. USA* **91**, 12,887–12,891.

154. Towler, D. A., Bennett, C. D., and Rodan, G. A. (1994) Activity of the rat osteocalcin basal promoter in osteoblastic cells is dependent upon homeodomain and CP1 binding motifs. *Mol. Endocrinol.* **8**, 614–624.

155. Towler, D. A., Rutledge, S. J., and Rodan, G. A. (1994) Msx-2/Hox 8.1: a transcriptional regulator of the rat osteocalcin promoter. *Mol. Endocrinol.* **8**, 1484–1493.

156. Tamura, M. and Noda, M. (1994) Identification of a DNA sequence involved in osteoblast-specific gene expression via interaction with helix-loop-helix (HLH)-type transcription factors. *J. Cell Biol.* **126**, 773–782.

157. Banerjee, C., Hiebert, S. W., Stein, J. L., Lian, J. B., and Stein, G. S. (1996) An AML-1 consensus sequence binds an osteoblast-specific complex and transcriptionally activates the osteocalcin gene. *Proc. Natl. Acad. Sci. USA* **93**, 4968–4973.

158. Merriman, H. L., van Wijnen, A. J., Hiebert, S., et al. (1995) The tissue-specific nuclear matrix protein, NMP-2, is a member of the AML/CBF/PEBP2/runt domain transcription factor family: interactions with the osteocalcin gene promoter. *Biochemistry* **34**, 13,125–13,132.

159. Geoffroy, V., Ducy, P., and Karsenty, G. (1995) A PEBP2 alpha/AML-1-related factor increases osteocalcin promoter activity through its binding to an osteoblast-specific *cis*-acting element. *J. Biol. Chem.* **270**, 30,973–30,979.

160. Banerjee, C., Stein, J. L., Van Wijnen, A. J., Frenkel, B., Lian, J. B., and Stein, G. S. (1996) Transforming growth factor-beta 1 responsiveness of the rat osteocalcin gene is mediated by an activator protein-1 binding site. *Endocrinology* **137**, 1991–2000.

161. Markose, E. R., Stein, J. L., Stein, G. S., and Lian, J. B. (1990) Vitamin D-mediated modifications in protein–DNA interactions at two promoter elements of the osteocalcin gene. *Proc. Natl. Acad. Sci. USA* **87**, 1701–1705.

162. Demay, M. B., Gerardi, J. M., DeLuca, H. F., and Kronenberg, H. M. (1990) DNA sequences in the rat osteocalcin gene that bind the 1,25-dihydroxyvitamin D3 receptor and confer responsiveness to 1,25-dihydroxyvitamin D3. *Proc. Natl. Acad. Sci. USA* **87**, 369–373.

163. Breen, E. C., van Wijnen, A. J., Lian, J. B., Stein, G. S., and Stein, J. L. (1994) In vivo occupancy of the vitamin D responsive element in the osteocalcin gene supports vitamin D-dependent transcriptional upregulation in intact cells. *Proc. Natl. Acad. Sci. USA* **91**, 12,902–12,906.

164. Montecino, M., Frenkel, B., Lian, J., Stein, J., and Stein, G. (1996) Requirement of distal and proximal promoter sequences for chromatin organization of the osteocalcin gene in bone-derived cells. *J. Cell. Biochem.* **63**, 221–228.

165. Briggs, M. R., Kadonaga, J. T., Bell, S. P., and Tjian, R. (1986) Purification and biochemical characterization of the promoter-specific transcription factor, Sp1. *Science* **234**, 47–52.

166. Ko, S. C., Cheon, J., Kao, C., et al. (1996) Osteocalcin promoter-based toxic gene therapy for the treatment of osteosarcoma in experimental models. *Cancer Res.* **56**, 4614–4619.

167. Cheon, J., Ko, S. C., Gardner, T. A., et al. (1997) Chemogene therapy: osteocalcin promoter-based suicide gene therapy in combination with methotrexate in a murine osteosarcoma model. *Cancer Gene Ther.* **4**, 359–365.

168. Shirakawa, T., Ko, S. C., Gardner, T. A., et al. (1998) In vivo suppression of osteosarcoma pulmonary metastasis with intravenous osteocalcin promoter-based toxic gene therapy. *Cancer Gene Ther.* **5**, 274–280.

169. Hou, Z., Nguyen, Q., Frenkel, B., et al. (1999) Osteoblast-specific gene expression after transplantation of marrow cells: implications for skeletal gene therapy. *Proc. Natl. Acad. Sci. USA* **96**, 7294–7299.

170. Riegman, P. H., Vlietstra, R. J., van der Korput, J. A., Romijn, J. C., and Trapman, J. (1989) Characterization of the prostate-specific antigen gene: a novel human kallikrein-like gene. *Biochem. Biophys. Res. Commun.* **159**, 95–102.

171. Riegman, P. H., Vlietstra, R. J., Klaassen, P., et al. (1989) The prostate-specific antigen gene and the human glandular kallikrein-1 gene are tandemly located on chromosome 19. *FEBS Lett.* **247**, 123–126.

172. Lundwall, A. (1989) Characterization of the gene for prostate-specific antigen, a human glandular kallikrein. *Biochem. Biophys. Res. Commun.* **161**, 1151–1159.

173. Wang, M. C., Valenzuela, L. A., Murphy, G. P., and Chu, T. M. (1979) Purification of a human prostate specific antigen. *Invest. Urol.* **17**, 159–163.

174. Wang, M. C., Papsidero, L. D., Kuriyama, M., Valenzuela, L. A., Murphy, G. P., and Chu, T. M. (1981) Prostate antigen: a new potential marker for prostatic cancer. *Prostate* **2**, 89–96.

175. Gallee, M. P., van Vroonhoven, C. C., van der Korput, H. A., et al. (1986) Characterization of monoclonal antibodies raised against the prostatic cancer cell line PC-82. *Prostate* **9**, 33–45.

176. Riegman, P. H., Vlietstra, R. J., van der Korput, H. A., Romijn, J. C., and Trapman, J. (1991) Identification and androgen-regulated expression of two major human glandular kallikrein-1 (hGK-1) mRNA species. *Mol. Cell. Endocrinol.* **76**, 181–190.

177. Cleutjens, K. B., van Eekelen, C. C., van der Korput, H. A., Brinkmann, A. O., and Trapman, J. (1996) Two androgen response regions cooperate in steroid hormone regulated activity of the prostate-specific antigen promoter. *J. Biol. Chem.* **271**, 6379–6388.

178. Cleutjens, K. B., van der Korput, H. A., van Eekelen, C. C., van Rooij, H. C., Faber, P. W., and Trapman, J. (1997) An androgen response element in a far upstream enhancer region is essential for high, androgen-regulated activity of the prostate-specific antigen promoter. *Mol. Endocrinol.* **11**, 148–161.

179. Cleutjens, C. B., Steketee, K., van Eekelen, C. C., van der Korput, J. A., Brinkmann, A. O., and Trapman, J. (1997) Both androgen receptor and glucocorticoid receptor are able to induce prostate-specific antigen expression, but differ in their growth- stimulating properties of LNCaP cells. *Endocrinology* **138,** 5293–5300.

180. Wang, Y., Xu, J., Pierson, T., O'Malley, B. W., and Tsai, S. Y. (1997) Positive and negative regulation of gene expression in eukaryotic cells with an inducible transcriptional regulator. *Gene Ther.* **4,** 432–441.

181. Cleutjens, K. B., van der Korput, H. A., Ehren-van Eekelen, C. C., et al. (1997) A 6-kb promoter fragment mimics in transgenic mice the prostate-specific and androgen-regulated expression of the endogenous prostate-specific antigen gene in humans. *Mol. Endocrinol.* **11,** 1256–1265.

182. Pang, S., Dannull, J., Kaboo, R., et al. (1997) Identification of a positive regulatory element responsible for tissue-specific expression of prostate-specific antigen. *Cancer Res.* **57,** 495–499.

183. Yeung, F., Li, X., Ellett, J., Trapman, J., Kao, C., and Chung, L. W. (2000) Regions of prostate-specific antigen (PSA) promoter confer androgen-independent expression of PSA in prostate cancer cells. *J. Biol. Chem.* **275,** 40,846–40,855.

184. Oettgen, P., Finger, E., Sun, Z., et al. (2000) PDEF, a novel prostate epithelium-specific Ets transcription factor, interacts with the androgen receptor and activates prostate-specific antigen gene expression. *J. Biol. Chem.* **275,** 1216–1225.

185. Latham, J. P., Searle, P. F., Mautner, V., and James, N. D. (2000) Prostate-specific antigen promoter/enhancer driven gene therapy for prostate cancer: construction and testing of a tissue-specific adenovirus vector. *Cancer Res.* **60,** 334–341.

186. Rodriguez, R., Schuur, E. R., Lim, H. Y., Henderson, G. A., Simons, J. W., and Henderson, D. R. (1997) Prostate attenuated replication competent adenovirus (ARCA) CN706: a selective cytotoxic for prostate-specific antigen-positive prostate cancer cells. *Cancer Res.* **57,** 2559–2563.

187. Martiniello-Wilks, R., Garcia-Aragon, J., Daja, M. M., et al. (1998) In vivo gene therapy for prostate cancer: preclinical evaluation of two different enzyme-directed prodrug therapy systems delivered by identical adenovirus vectors. *Hum. Gene Ther.* **9,** 1617–1626.

188. Gotoh, A., Ko, S. C., Shirakawa, T., et al. (1998) Development of prostate-specific antigen promoter-based gene therapy for androgen-independent human prostate cancer. *J. Urol.* **160,** 220–229.

189. Lee, S. E., Jin, R. J., Lee, S. G., et al. (2000) Development of a new plasmid vector with PSA-promoter and enhancer expressing tissue-specificity in prostate carcinoma cell lines. *Anticancer Res.* **20,** 417–422.

190. Xu, L. L., Srikantan, V., Sesterhenn, I. A., et al. (2000) Expression profile of an androgen regulated prostate specific homeobox gene NKX3.1 in primary prostate cancer. *J. Urol.* **163,** 972–979.

191. Landwall, A. (1989) Characterization of the gene for prostate-specific antigen, a human glandular kallikrein. *Biochem. Biophys. Res. Commun.* **161,** 1151–1159.

192. Tasch, J., Gong, M., Sadelain, M., and Heston, W. D. (2001) A unique folate hydrolase, prostate-specific membrane antigen (PSMA): a target for immunotherapy? *Crit. Rev. Immunol.* **21,** 249–261.

193. Pinto, J. T., Suffoletto, B. P., Berzin, T. M., et al. (1996) Prostate-specific membrane antigen: a novel folate hydrolase in human prostatic carcinoma cells. *Clin. Cancer Res.* **2,** 1445–1451.

194. Carter, R. E., Feldman, A. R., and Coyle, J. T. (1996) Prostate-specific membrane antigen is a hydrolase with substrate and pharmacologic characteristics of a neuropeptidase. *Proc. Natl. Acad. Sci. USA* **93,** 749–753.

195. Pangalos, M. N., Neefs, J. M., Somers, M., et al. (1999) Isolation and expression of novel human glutamate carboxypeptidases with *N*-acetylated alpha-linked acidic dipeptidase and dipeptidyl peptidase IV activity. *J. Biol. Chem.* **274,** 8470–8483.

196. O'Keefe, D. S., Su, S. L., Bacich, D. J., et al. (1998) Mapping, genomic organization and promoter analysis of the human prostate-specific membrane antigen gene. *Biochim. Biophys. Acta* **1443,** 113–127.

197. Maraj, B. H., Leek, J. P., Karayi, M., Ali, M., Lench, N. J., and Markham, A. F. (1998) Detailed genetic mapping around a putative prostate-specific membrane antigen locus on human chromosome 11p11.2. *Cytogenet. Cell Genet.* **81,** 3–9.

198. Bacich, D. J., Pinto, J. T., Tong, W. P., and Heston, W. D. (2001) Cloning, expression, genomic localization, and enzymatic activities of the mouse homolog of prostate-specific membrane antigen/NAALADase/folate hydrolase. *Mamm. Genome* **12,** 117–123.

199. Sweat, S. D., Pacelli, A., Murphy, G. P., and Bostwick, D. G. (1998) Prostate-specific membrane antigen expression is greatest in prostate adenocarcinoma and lymph node metastases. *Urology* **52,** 637–640.

200. Wright, G. L., Grob, B. M., Haley, C., et al. (1996) Upregulation of prostate-specific membrane antigen after androgen-deprivation therapy. *Urology* **48,** 326–334.

201. Stamey, T. A., Yang, N., Hay, A. R., McNeal, J. E., Feiha, F. S., and Redwine, E. (1987) Prostate-specific antigen as a serum marker for adenocarcinoma of the prostate. *N. Engl. J. Med.* **317,** 909–916.

202. Oesterling, J. E. (1991) Prostate-specific antigen: a valuable clinical tool. *Oncology* **5,** 107–122.

203. Cookson, M. S., Floyd, M. K., Ball, T. P. Jr., Miller, E. K., and Sarosdy, M. F. (1995) The lack of predictive value of prostate specific antigen density in the detection of prostate cancer in patients with normal rectal examinations and intermediate prostate specific antigen levels. *J. Urol.* **154,** 1070–1073.

204. Burger, M. J., Tebay, M. A., Keith, P. A., et al. (2002) Expression analysis of delta-catenin and prostate-specific membrane antigen: their potential as diagnostic markers for prostate cancer. *Int. J. Cancer* **100,** 228–237.

205. Hara, N., Kasahara, T., Kawasaki, T., et al. (2002) Reverse transcription-polymerase chain reaction detection of prostate-specific antigen, prostate-specific membrane antigen, and prostate stem cell antigen in 1 mL of peripheral blood: value for the staging of prostate cancer. *Clin. Cancer Res.* **8,** 1794–1799.
206. Xiao, Z., Adam, B. L., Cazares, L. H., et al. (2001) Quantitation of serum prostate-specific membrane antigen by a novel protein biochip immunoassay discriminates benign from malignant prostate disease. *Cancer Res.* **61,** 6029–6033.
207. Maher, J., Brentjens, R. J., Gunset, G., Riviere, I., and Sadelain, M. (2002) Human T-lymphocyte cytotoxicity and proliferation directed by a single chimeric TCRzeta/CD28 receptor. *Nat. Biotechnol.* **20,** 70–75.
208. Warren, P., Li, L., Song, W., et al. (2001) In vitro targeted killing of prostate tumor cells by a synthetic amoebapore helix 3 peptide modified with two gamma-linked glutamate residues at the COOH terminus. *Cancer Res.* **61,** 6783–6787.
209. Good, D., Schwarzenberger, P., Eastham, J. A., et al. (1999) Cloning and characterization of the prostate-specific membrane antigen promoter. *J. Cell. Biochem.* **74,** 395–405.
210. Watt, F., Martorana, A., Brookes, D. E., et al. (2001) A tissue-specific enhancer of the prostate-specific membrane antigen gene, FOLH1. *Genomics* **73,** 243–254.
211. Lee, S. J., Kim, H. S., Yu, R., et al. (2002) Novel prostate-specific promoter derived from PSA and PSMA enhancers. *Mol. Ther.* **6,** 415–421.
212. Lee, S.-J., Kim, H.-S., Yu, R., et al. (2002) Novel prostate-specific promoter derived from PSA and PSMA enhancers. *Mol. Ther.* **6,** 415–421.
213. Gardner, T. A., Ko, S. C., Kao, C., et al. (1998) Exploiting stromal-epithelial interaction for model development and new strategies of gene therapy for prostate cancer and osteosarcoma metastases. *Gene Ther. Mol. Biol.* **2,** 41–58.
214. Kubo, H., Gardner, T. A., Wada, Y., et al. (2003) Phase I dose escalation clinical trial of adenovirus vector carrying osteocalcin promoter-driven herpes simplex virus thymidine kinase in localized and metastatic hormone-refractory prostate cancer. *Hum. Gene Ther.* **14,** 227–241.
215. Matsubara, S., Wada, Y., Gardner, T. A., et al. (2001) A conditional replication-competent adenoviral vector, Ad-OC-E1a, to cotarget prostate cancer and bone stroma in an experimental model of androgen-independent prostate cancer bone metastasis. *Cancer Res.* **61,** 6012–6019.

21

Drug Resistance Gene Transfer as an Antitumor Strategy

Colin L. Sweeney and R. Scott McIvor

1. INTRODUCTION

The application of gene transfer techniques holds great promise for improved antitumor therapy. The overall goal of gene transfer in the treatment of neoplastic disease is either to augment the body's ability to eliminate the tumor or to somehow specifically weaken the tumor, in each case relative to other, normal tissues in the body. Other chapters in this volume describe direct molecular, immunological, prodrug activation, and antiangiogenic approaches as genetic antitumor therapeutic strategies. Another approach that has been explored is the introduction of genes conferring resistance to chemotherapeutic agents into normal cells and tissues as a means of protection from the toxic side effects of cancer chemotherapy. The systems that have been the most extensively studied for this purpose are the P-glycoprotein or multidrug resistance (MDR) system, drug-resistant forms of dihydrofolate reductase (DHFR), and O^6-alkylguanine-DNA alkyltransferase (AGT), although other systems have emerged as well.

In general, the therapeutic strategy involves the introduction and expression of a drug resistance gene in hematopoietic cell populations, thereby rendering the chemotherapeutic agent less toxic for the recipient and allowing more effective antitumor chemotherapy either through more aggressive drug administration or by reduced side effects at an unescalated dose. A related application of drug resistance gene transfer is for the purpose of achieving in vivo selection.

This chapter reviews the molecular basis of these drug resistance systems, preclinical and clinical evidence for their effectiveness in supporting improved antitumor chemotherapy, and the prospects and challenges for future development and application of drug resistance gene transfer. In general, these drug resistance systems were first characterized in cultured mammalian cells, sometimes as dominant selectable and amplifiable markers, providing some of the first molecular and pharmacological insights into their potential for in vivo application. Application of germline and somatic cell gene transfer technologies allowed the evaluation of these systems in the in vivo setting (in mice and, in some cases, larger animals). These applications have progressed to clinical trials, with several reports of clinical MDR gene transfer and with several other drug resistance gene transfer trials pending. In reviewing the status of these different systems as adjuncts for improved chemotherapy, we emphasize the key goal of increased dose tolerance in these studies and its subsequent application to antitumor effectiveness either in the preclinical or in the clinical setting.

2. DRUG RESISTANCE SYSTEMS

2.1. Multidrug Resistance (MDR)

The human *mdr-1* gene encodes P-glycoprotein, an efflux pump that recognizes a variety of substrates, including a number of anticancer drugs, such as paclitaxel (Taxol), vincristine, doxorubicin,

From: *Contemporary Cancer Research*
Cancer Gene Therapy
Edited by: D. T. Curiel and J. T. Douglas © Humana Press Inc., Totowa, NJ

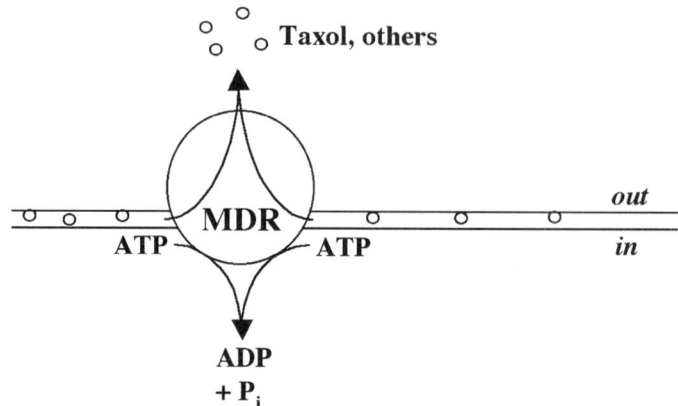

Fig. 1. MDR activity. MDR is a membrane glycoprotein that mediates the ATP-dependent efflux of numerous toxic drugs (small circles), such as Taxol, accumulating in the cell membrane.

etoposide, and actinomycin D, for elimination from cells. The gene product is a 170-kDa membrane glycoprotein that mediates efflux in an reaction dependent on adenosine triphosphate (ATP) *(1,2)*. P-glycoprotein contains 12 transmembrane regions and 2 ATP-binding domains *(3)*.

The mechanism of drug efflux by MDR is not clear, but appears to involve removal of lipophilic drugs from within the plasma membrane (Fig. 1) *(4,5)*. The role of MDR in the development of resistance to these agents was observed in the emergence of drug-resistant tumors that overexpress MDR *(6–8)*. MDR expression has also been observed in hematopoietic cells, particularly in CD34+ precursors *(9,10)*. MDR was subsequently shown to be an effective tool as a dominant and amplifiable selectable marker in cultured mammalian cells, supporting the concept of its use for protection from drug toxicity *(11–13)*. The MDR phenotype has also been associated with the *MRP* gene *(14)*, which encodes multi-drug resistance protein, a membrane glycoprotein exhibiting a partial overlap in drug resistance with MDR *(15,16)*. However, the use of *MRP* as a selectable drug resistance gene has not been as extensively characterized.

2.2. O^6-Alkylguanine-DNA Alkyltransferase (AGT)

Deoxyribonucleic acid (DNA)-methylating agents such as temozolomide and chloroethylating agents such as 1,3-bis(2-chloroethyl)-1-nitrosourea (BCNU) and mitozolomide cause alkylation at the O^6 position of guanine in DNA and have been used as chemotherapeutic agents for treatment of a variety of tumors. Treatment with chloroethylating agents results in cytotoxicity because of rapid formation of a DNA interstrand crosslink between the modified guanine and the complementary strand cytosine.

The mechanism of toxicity of methylating agents appears to involve chromosomal breaks induced by abortive mismatch repair following replication (reviewed in ref. *17*). AGT, also known as O^6-methylguanine-DNA methyltransferase (MGMT), is a protein that repairs damage caused by DNA-alkylating agents. Mammalian AGT repairs O^6-methylguanine adducts in double-stranded DNA, but can also act on other alkyl groups at the O^6 position of guanine and can repair O^4-methylthymine. AGT repairs alkylated DNA by direct stoichiometric transfer of the alkyl adduct to an internal cysteine residue (Fig. 2) (reviewed in ref. *17*). This transfer is irreversible, resulting in inactivation of the alkylated AGT protein in what has been termed a "suicide" process.

Human AGT is a 207-amino acid, 21-kDa protein for which the crystal structure has been solved *(18,19)*. Human bone marrow and hematopoietic progenitor cells have a low level of endogenous AGT expression *(20)*, explaining the dose-limiting myelosuppression for alkylating agents in chemotherapy. In addition, many tumors exhibit high levels of AGT activity, rendering them more resistant to alkylating agents *(21,22)*.

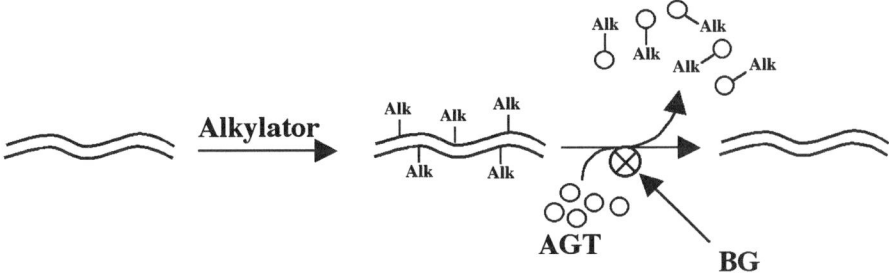

Fig. 2. AGT activity. Agents such as BCNU modify DNA (double wavy lines) by alkylating guanine bases (Alk–). AGT (small circles) removes these alkyl adducts in a stoichiometric fashion, a process inhibited by O^6-benzylguanine (BG), unless the AGT is a mutant form resistant to BG.

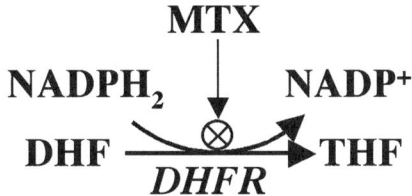

Fig. 3. DHFR activity. DHFR converts dihydrofolate (DHF) to tetrahydrofolate (THF) in the presence of the reduced form (NADPH$_2$) of nicotinamide adenine dinucleotide phosphate (NADP$^+$). The reaction is inhibited by antifolates such as methotrexate (MTX).

DNA repair by mammalian AGT can be inhibited by free-base substrates such as O^6-benzylguanine (BG). BG directly competes with alkylated DNA for binding to AGT, permanently inactivating human AGT through transfer of the benzyl adduct of BG to the cysteine acceptor site of the protein (reviewed in ref. *17*). In conjunction with alkylating agents, BG has been shown to increase cytotoxicity in human tumor cell lines in vitro *(23,24)* and decrease tumor growth in xenograft models *(25–27)*; it is under testing in clinical trials *(28–31)*.

A number of mutant AGT proteins have been established that exhibit increased resistance to BG *(32,33)*. These mutations are located near the cysteine acceptor site at amino acid 145 of human AGT. In particular, mutations at positions 140 and 156 have been extensively studied. Mutation of proline at position 140 to alanine (P140A) or lysine (P140K) results in a 25-fold or greater than 6000-fold increase, respectively, in resistance to BG compared to wild-type AGT *(33)*. A glycine-to-alanine substitution at position 156 (G156A) results in a 240-fold increase in resistance; a double mutation of proline to alanine at position 140 and glycine to alanine at position 156 (P140A/G156A) results in a greater than 1200-fold increase *(32)*. Introduction of mutant AGT genes into cell lines has been shown to provide protection from cytotoxicity caused by the combination of BG and DNA-alkylating agents *(34,35)*.

2.3. Dihydrofolate Reductase (DHFR)

A third drug resistance system that has been developed is that of mutant, drug-resistant forms of DHFR. This enzyme catalyzes the nicotinamide adenine dinucleotide phosphate-dependent conversion of dihydrofolate to tetrahydrofolate (Fig. 3), an immediate precursor to numerous folate metabolites that serve as one-carbon donors in cellular metabolism, including *de novo* purine biosynthesis and thymidylate synthesis *(36)*. Antifolates such as methotrexate (MTX) and trimetrexate are tight-binding, substrate analog inhibitors of DHFR, and treatment of cells with these drugs results in profound inhibition of cellular metabolism and a subsequent antiproliferative effect. MTX has been used as an effective antitumor agent, most notably in the treatment of acute lymphocytic leukemia, osteosarcoma, Ewing's sarcoma, and choriocarcinoma *(37,38)*. However, there are significant toxicities associated with the administration of MTX, particularly myelosuppression and gastrointestinal toxicity.

Cellular resistance to MTX has been associated with *DHFR* gene amplification, reduced drug transport, and alterations in intracellular glutamylation or deglutamylation of the drug (discussed in ref. *39*). Coamplification of genes along with DHFR has been used extensively as a means of engineering cells to express high levels of proteins in mammalian cells. The existence of drug-resistant forms of DHFR as another mechanism by which cells become resistant to antifolates was suggested early on by kinetic inhibition studies of enzyme extracted from several different cell lines adapted to grow at high concentrations of MTX (*see* ref. *39*). The mutation hypothesis was subsequently verified by the sequencing of a DHFR complementary DNA (cDNA) clone encoding a leucine-to-arginine substitution at codon position 22, isolated from a MTX-resistant 3T6 cell line expressing drug-resistant DHFR *(40)*. That this mutation in the *DHFR* gene conferred resistance to MTX was confirmed by transfection of expression plasmids into numerous cultured mammalian cell lines, demonstrating that the modified sequence functioned as a dominant selectable marker similar to the microbial *NEO* and *EcoGPT* genes characterized at around the same time.

Since the original isolation of the murine L22R mutation, there have been numerous studies of the generation and characterization of drug-resistant DHFRs, with implications for the application of these drug resistance genes both in vitro and in vivo. These reports have included the isolation of cDNA clones from drug-resistant cell lines, screening for drug-resistant forms in *Escherichia coli*, and site-directed mutagenesis (reviewed in ref. *39*). Our laboratory used a polymerase chain reaction-based saturation mutagenesis strategy coupled with MTX selection in mammalian cells to isolate a series of 13 recombinants at positions 22 and 31 of the murine *DHFR* gene conferring drug resistance *(41)*.

Rational design of substitutions at several positions in the DHFR active site has also generated numerous forms that confer substantial resistance to antifolates, including the study of double mutants *(39)*. Generation of these variants and characterization of their kinetic inhibition properties have provided insight into the relationship between the structure and the function of the DHFR active site and have provided tools for conferring drug resistance and for selection of target cell populations in gene transfer studies.

In general, there is a trade-off between the degree of drug resistance and the level of retained catalytic activity exhibited by any particular DHFR variant. The originally isolated L22R mutant, for example, is characterized by a high degree of resistance to MTX (for us, the 50% inhibitory concentration [IC_{50}] increased by 2000-fold compared to wild type), but is catalytically impaired, exhibiting only 1 to 2% of the wild-type level of activity *(41)*.

The mutagenesis studies described here generated several mutant forms that exhibited an improved combination of drug resistance and catalytic activity (reviewed in ref. *39*), such as the human and murine L22Y variants. In general, examination of the kinetic inhibition character of these variant enzymes and the associated cellular resistance conferred by their expression has provided an essential basis for their application in chemoprotection and in vivo selection, as described next.

3. IN VIVO PROTECTION OF ANIMALS FROM DRUG TOXICITY: STUDIES IN THE MOUSE

The MDR, AGT, and DHFR systems have been examined extensively in the mouse as a small animal model system for the potential of drug resistance gene expression in hematopoietic cells to allow rescue from the toxicity associated with chemotherapeutic drug administration. These studies have employed transgenic animals expressing drug resistance genes and retrovirally transduced marrow transplanted into normal recipients to target drug resistance genes for expression in hematopoietic cells. Results from these studies provided considerable proof of principle for the concept of drug resistance gene expression providing increased resistance of animals to chemotherapeutic agents, with implications for the application of this approach in dose intensification strategies or to achieve reduced toxicity at currently applied doses of antitumor agents.

The use of MDR for chemoprotection was first demonstrated in experiments in which the gene was expressed in transgenic mice *(42,43)*; resistance to a number of agents, including Taxol and daunomycin, was observed not only in the transgenics, but also in animals that had been transplanted with marrow obtained from MDR transgenics *(44)*. Retroviral transduction strategies emerging at the time were then used to demonstrate that transduction and expression of MDR in mouse marrow conferred significant resistance to hematological toxicity in animals administered Taxol or bisantrene *(45,46)*.

Hanania et al. *(45)* demonstrated gene transfer into hematopoietic stem cells in serial transplant experiments in which expression of the transduced gene was maintained through multiple serial marrow transplants in mice over a 17-month period. Transduction studies have been hampered by decreased MDR expression because of aberrant splicing from MDR cDNA in retroviral vectors *(47–49)*. Transplant with MDR-transduced marrow has also been associated with a myeloproliferative disorder in some animals *(50,51)*.

In the AGT system, compared to mice transplanted with *lacZ*-transduced marrow, Davis et al. *(52)* reported significantly improved survival in lethally irradiated mice transplanted with bone marrow progenitors transduced with a retrovirus encoding G156A AGT and treated with BG and BCNU. In addition, BG and BCNU treatment increased the percentage of bone marrow cells expressing G156A AGT at 13 weeks posttransplant from 30 to 60% and increased BG/BCNU resistance of G156A-transduced colony-forming cells collected at 23 weeks posttransplant compared to *lacZ*-transduced cells or untreated mice, demonstrating in vivo selection of bone marrow progenitor cells expressing a drug-resistant AGT *(see* Section 5.).

Protection from a potential mutagenic effect of treatment with BG and temozolomide was demonstrated by Chinnasamy et al. *(53)* using the P140A/G156A mutant AGT. Decreased micronucleus formation in bone marrow was observed in drug-treated mice following transplant with transduced marrow.

Relevant to human applications, transduction of primary human CD34$^+$ cells with a retroviral vector encoding the G156A mutant AGT resulted in increased resistance to BG plus BCNU in methylcellulose colony-forming assays compared to untransduced cells *(54)* and in more primitive long-term culture-initiating cells compared to cells transduced with a control *lacZ* vector *(55)*.

Early transgenic work was conducted by Isola and Gorden in the DHFR system *(56)*, establishing animals bearing the L22R murine *DHFR* transgene. *DHFR* gene transfer into hematopoietic cells was demonstrated by Hock and Miller in in vitro analyses *(57)*, with subsequent demonstration of protection from lethal doses of MTX by engraftment with *DHFR*-transduced marrow by Williams et al. *(58)*. Corey et al. demonstrated the maintenance of drug resistance in serially transplanted marrow cells, confirming retroviral transduction and drug resistance of long-term repopulating hematopoietic stem cells *(59)*. Numerous drug-resistant DHFRs have subsequently been tested and found to confer protection from the toxicity of MTX or trimetrexate by expression in hematopoietic cells *(39)*.

Studies in our laboratory utilized a transgenic model system on a syngeneic background, allowing conditions that can be highly controlled with respect to the frequency and character of drug-resistant cells introduced into recipient animals *(60,61)*. Although highly artificial in the sense that all of the DHFR-expressing cells contain the identical transgene, this system provides considerable reproducibility between groups and between experiments, which has greatly facilitated hematological and pharmacological characterization of the drug resistance conferred in recipient animals.

We initially demonstrated drug resistance in FVB/N recipient animals transplanted with syngeneic L22R and L22Y *DHFR* transgenic marrow *(61,62)*. Transplantation with L22R transgenic marrow conferred resistance to MTX administered daily at a dose of 4 mg/kg, which was surprising because this dose causes not only myelosuppression, but also substantial gastrointestinal toxicity in mice *(62)*. Chemoprotection under these conditions was not associated with reduced drug levels, assessed in pharmacokinetic experiments *(63)*. We found that there was a significant increase in villus length in animals protected by transplantation with L22R *DHFR* transgenic marrow *(62)*, and that there was substantial infiltration of donor *DHFR* transgenic cells into the small intestine of engrafted animals

(61). An intriguing possibility that arises from these results is that engraftment with drug-resistant marrow also protects recipients from the gastrointestinal toxicity of MTX administration. The cellular and molecular mechanisms by which this cross-protection occurs is currently under investigation.

Use of the transgenic system subsequently allowed us to demonstrate the importance of more committed drug-resistant progenitors in mediating drug resistance soon after transplant *(64)* and allowed us to obtain a precise determination of the increase in maximum tolerated dose conferred by engraftment with L22R and L22Y DHFR transgenic marrow (a two- to threefold increase) *(61,65)*. We also observed significant drug resistance in animals transplanted after nonmyeloablative conditioning subsequently engrafted at a level as low as 1% donor DHFR transgenic cells *(66)*. Although the mechanism by which such low-level engraftment confers drug resistance on recipient animals has yet to be determined, these results indicate that only a moderate level of gene transfer (greater than 1%) will be necessary to confer protection from antifolate toxicity.

4. APPLICATION OF DRUG RESISTANCE
GENE TRANSFER FOR IMPROVED ANTITUMOR THERAPY

One of the primary purposes of drug resistance gene transfer is to improve dose tolerance in the subject, thus providing either reduced toxicity at existing doses of antitumor chemotherapy or allowing dose intensification. Although there has been much accomplished in experimental animals demonstrating reduced toxicity after drug resistance gene transfer (described in Section 3.), studies testing the applicability of this increased drug resistance for improved antitumor therapy have been limited.

Zhao et al. demonstrated improved survivability of mice bearing EO771 mammary adenocarcinoma tumors when transplanted with marrow exposed to a variant serine-31 DHFR retrovirus and subsequently administered MTX *(67)*. Hanania and Deisseroth demonstrated more effective treatment with Taxol of 11A1 mammary tumors transduced with a p53 chemosensitization vector in mice transplanted with MDR-transduced marrow *(68)*. The efficacy of mutant AGT for improved tumor chemotherapy was tested by Koç et al. in a BCNU-resistant SW480 human colon cancer xenograft model in mice transplanted with marrow transduced with the G156A mutant AGT *(69)*. Multiple rounds of administration of BG and BCNU resulted in selection for transduced G156A marrow and consequently improved drug tolerance in mice and significantly delayed tumor growth at high doses of BG plus BCNU that were lethal to mice lacking G156A marrow.

In our laboratory, we have utilized the predictable increase in MTX dose tolerance in recipients of L22Y DHFR transgenic marrow to test its utility in the treatment of several tumors of varying antifolate sensitivity. In this system, escalated doses of MTX were not found to be effective against the 32Dp210 murine model of chronic myeloid leukemia (CML); in fact, MTX exacerbated tumorigenicity *(70)*. However, administration of an increased trimetrexate dose significantly delayed tumor onset, and tumor did not emerge when trimetrexate was coadministered with the nucleoside transport inhibitor prodrug nitrobenzyl-mercaptopurine-riboside phosphate (NBMPR-P), which inhibits salvage of thymidine and purine nucleosides, thereby increasing antifolate potency *(71–73)*. Although tumor did emerge after withdrawal of drug administration, these experiments demonstrated the potential usefulness of antifolates against CML in this model system when administered at the increased doses affordable by expression of drug-resistant DHFR. This, in combination with an antisense approach targeting the breakpoint of the *BCR/ABL* oncogene in CML *(74)*, is under exploration as a therapeutic approach at the University of Minnesota.

We also established FVB/N mammary carcinoma (FMC), a new mammary adenocarcinoma maintained as a subcutaneous, transplantable tumor line in FVB/N mice, for testing in combination with the syngeneic transplant system established as described using *DHFR* transgenic marrow. The FMC tumor did not exhibit appreciable sensitivity to MTX, even at the higher doses achieved in animals engrafted with *DHFR* transgenic marrow or in *DHFR* transgenic animals *(75)*. Improved antitumor activity was observed, however, when animals were treated with trimetrexate, particularly when administered in combination with NBMPR-P *(76)*. Our work with the 32Dp210 and FMC tumors indicated that, for tumors that do not exhibit sensitivity to MTX, use of an alternate antifolate such as trimetrexate in combination with a nucleoside transport inhibitor can be an effective antitumor approach, particularly when a more aggressive regimen can be administered as a result of drug-resistant DHFR expression. It is anticipated that MTX dose escalation will be more effective against tumors exhibiting greater sensitivity to this drug, and these studies are currently under way in the transgenic model system.

5. IN VIVO SELECTION OF HEMATOPOIETIC CELLS EXPRESSING DRUG RESISTANCE GENES

The anticipated effectiveness of therapeutic gene transfer into hematopoietic cells is currently limited by the efficiency of the process in large animals and humans. There is great hope for improved gene transfer efficiency through the use of alternate vectors, such as lentivirus vectors *(77)* or foamy virus vectors *(78)*, or through alternate exposure and cell-processing procedures *(79)*. Another approach for increasing the representation of transduced cells in the circulation is by in vivo selection through the application of some pharmacological selection pressure. All three of the major drug resistance systems have been tested for this purpose, generating varying results with respect to the stability of enriched engraftment levels and the extent of enrichment from low initial levels of engrafted cells containing the drug resistance gene.

In independent studies in the MDR system, Sorrentino et al. *(80)* and Podda et al. *(81)* found an increase in MDR-transduced peripheral blood leukocytes after administration of Taxol, demonstrating the usefulness of drug selection in achieving increased representation of cells expressing the drug resistance gene. However, selection at the level of hematopoietic stem cells capable of stable, long-term engraftment was not conclusively demonstrated in these studies. One potential explanation for the lack of selectivity at the stem cell level is the relatively high level of endogenous MDR expression in more primitive hematopoietic cells *(9,10)*. Such expression could make it difficult to achieve conditions of differential survivability between endogenous stem cells and newly introduced stem cells transduced with an MDR-encoding vector. Introduction of mutant MDRs resistant to inhibitors of wild-type P-glycoprotein *(82,83)* may allow selection of transduced stem cells over endogenous cells expressing only wild-type MDR.

Use of the *DHFR* gene for in vivo selection was anticipated for many years, but the approach was not brought to fruition until the problem was addressed and solved by Allay et al., who demonstrated that exposure to antifolate (trimetrexate, in this case) was not by itself effective in mediating stem cell toxicity, and that stem cell toxicity required coadministration of NBMRP-P to prevent nucleoside salvage and rescue from antifolate toxicity *(72)*. Allay et al. then went on to demonstrate the utility of this pharmacological approach in expanding *DHFR* (human L22Y)-transduced cells in a way that was stable in long-term primary recipients and in secondary transplant recipients as well *(84)*. Our laboratory corroborated the selectivity of DHFR-expressing stem cells using the transgenic model system under similar pharmacological conditions as those described by Allay et al. *(85,86)*. However, reliable conditions for in vivo selection of DHFR-expressing stem cells from an initial low level of engraftment (from 0.1 to 1.0%) have yet to be established.

The AGT system has emerged as the most successful with respect to the goal of achieving effective conditions for in vivo selection. Drug-resistant AGT was demonstrated to allow for up to 940-fold enrichment of limiting numbers of G156A-transduced marrow progenitors transplanted into nonmyeloablated mice following administration of BG and BCNU *(87)*, a level of in vivo selection greater than that observed using other drug resistance genes. Ragg et al. *(88)* and Sawai et al. *(89)* reported, based on subsequent hematopoietic reconstitution of secondary transplant recipients, in vivo selection at the hematopoietic stem cell level by drug treatment in mice transplanted with P140K-transduced marrow. Drug administration in these studies consisted of BG and BCNU once a week for 4–5 weeks *(88)* or BG and temozolomide five times a week every 3–4 weeks *(89)*.

In contrast with the AGT system, stem cell selection in the DHFR system has required daily administration of trimetrexate plus NBMPR-P for up to 2 weeks and for several rounds of treatment over an extended period of time. The difference between these two systems most likely lies in their very different mechanisms of action. For the antifolates, selection is based on the antiproliferative effect resulting from depleted pools of purine and thymidine nucleotides, requiring continued presence of the drug during the selection process. For alkylators such as BCNU, a single exposure results in DNA modification, such that subsequent proliferation in the absence of drug triggers an apoptotic signal and cell death unless the damage has been repaired by AGT.

6. STUDIES IN LARGE ANIMALS AND HUMAN TRIALS

Studies of drug resistance gene transfer and expression in large animals to date have been limited, but nonetheless instructive, with respect to the cellular, genetic, and pharmacological challenges of gene transfer in an expanded setting. Stead et al. reported early ex vivo retroviral *DHFR* gene transfer studies in dogs, in which interpretability was limited because of low-efficiency gene transfer *(90)*. In an *MDR* gene transfer study in marmosets, Hibino et al. reported detection of transduced hematopoietic cells up to 400 days posttransplant, but the low levels (less than 1%) of transduced peripheral blood granulocytes did not protect animals against docetaxel-induced neutropenia *(91)*. Long-term low-level engraftment was observed in rhesus macaques infused with MDR-transduced marrow; there was an initial high level of transduced cells that subsequently dropped to low levels despite cytokine administration *(92)*. A report of ex vivo MDR gene transfer in dogs documented the emergence of transduced peripheral blood cells after Taxol administration, but after the drug was withdrawn, the level of transduced cells subsided, although it remained detectable for 16 months *(93)*.

These results indicate that, although successful transduction of primitive hematopoietic stem cells has been achieved, selective outgrowth is occurring primarily in more differentiated cell populations, among which nontransduced cells appear to be more sensitive to drug administration than more primitive cells, so the selective benefit is lost on drug withdrawal. An exception to this trend in large animals has been observed in the AGT system, in which a stable increase in AGT-positive cells was observed in dogs after administration of BCNU plus BG *(94)*. These results provide hope for the application of drug resistance gene transfer and expression as a means of conferring in vivo selection pressure to increase the representation of gene-transduced cells in vivo.

The success of *MDR* gene transfer studies in animals provided preclinical support for several human trials of *MDR* gene transfer (Table 1). These trials were designed to test first for the effectiveness of retroviral transduction conditions in mediating gene transfer into hematopoietic cell populations, then to determine whether the treatment would confer protection of patients from myelosuppression should they relapse at some time posttransplant and thus require chemotherapy.

Hanania et al. *(95)* reported a high level of transduction in granulocyte-macrophage colony-forming units (CFU-GM) that did not appear to contribute to engraftment posttransplant because the presence of MDR-marked cells was not detected in patients. Cowan et al. *(96)* reported that relatively high levels (9%) of MDR-marked granulocytes were maintained during multiple rounds of paclitaxel administration in one patient transplanted with MDR-transduced marrow, but these levels eventually declined.

Low-to-undetectable cell marking in patients has also been reported in several studies *(48,96–98)*. Using improved retroviral transduction procedures, Abonour et al. *(49)* achieved a higher level of *MDR* gene transfer in hematopoietic cells and reported a transient increase in transduced cell representation on administration of Taxol. This study has been widely regarded as providing evidence for the feasibility of gene transfer into human hematopoietic stem cells and extended the concept of in vivo selection to the human setting.

Of all the drug resistance systems discussed in this chapter, MDR has advanced the furthest in clinical application. However, even for MDR, the primary purpose of the genetic manipulation (i.e.,

Table 1
Human Clinical Chemoprotection Protocols[a]

OBA number	Principal investigator	Disease	Gene	Agent	Reference
9306-044	Deisseroth	Ovarian cancer	*MDR-1*	Paclitaxel	*95*
9306-051	Hesdorffer	Advanced cancer	*MDR-1*	Paclitaxel	*97,98*
9309-054	O'Shaughnessy	Breast cancer	*MDR-1*	Paclitaxel	*48,96*
9406-077	Deisseroth	Breast cancer	*MDR-1*	Paclitaxel	
9601-143	Cowan	Breast cancer	*MDR-1*	Paclitaxel	*96*
9701-172	Cornetta	Germ cell tumors	*MDR-1*	Paclitaxel	*49*
9701-173	Croop	Brain tumors	*MGMT*	CCNU[b]	
9705-187	Verfaillie	Chronic myeloid leukemia	*DHFR*	Methotrexate	
9809-265	Gerson	Advanced solid tumors	*MGMT*	BG, BCNU[c]	
0001-376	Bertino	Lymphoma	*DHFR-CD*[d]	Methotrexate/Ara-C	
0005-400	Becker	Lymphoma	*MDR-1*	Paclitaxel	
0104-466	Belani	Lung cancer	*MnSOD*[e]	Radiation	

[a]Listed by the Office of Biotechnology Activities as of April 16, 2003 (http://www4.od.nih.gov/oba/).
[b]CCNU, lomustine.
[c]BG, BCNU; *see* Section 2.2.
[d]CD, cytidine deaminase, conferring resistance to Ara-C, arabinosyl-cytosine.
[e]MnSOD, manganese superoxide dismutase, conferring protection from radiation-induced inflammation.

to allow more aggressive antitumor chemotherapy or reduced toxicity at an unescalated dose) has yet to be addressed in the human clinical setting.

7. CONCLUSION AND FUTURE STUDIES

Hematopoietic cells have long been considered a key target population for therapeutic gene transfer, and the introduction of drug resistance genes is a major strategy by which gene transfer into hematopoietic cells might be applied in the treatment of cancer. Advances in the field as summarized in this chapter demonstrate the potential of this strategy in preclinical model systems and in early human clinical trials. The ability to render animals less sensitive to drug toxicity is apparent for several combinations of chemotherapeutic agents and drug resistance genes, indicating the potential for reducing the severity of toxic responses associated with cancer chemotherapy. The extent to which dose escalation might be applied for improved antitumor therapy will depend on the actual increase in dose tolerance achieved through drug resistance gene expression *(61,62,65)*. Applicability of increased dose tolerance can then be tested directly in tumor-bearing animals for improved antitumor effect at the higher doses tolerated by drug resistance gene expression *(71,75,76)*.

Drug resistance genes may also be applied for the purpose of in vivo selection, expanding the population of cells expressing the drug resistance gene by administration of the selective agent *(52,80,81, 84–89)*. Applicability of this approach will depend on the degree to which expansion of cells expressing the drug resistance gene can be achieved, starting from the relatively low frequencies of gene transfer currently feasible in large animals and humans. Such selectivity would extend the utility of drug resistance gene transfer to the treatment of inherited diseases and other conditions in addition to cancer.

REFERENCES

1. Juliano, R. L. and Ling, V. (1976) A surface glycoprotein modulating drug permeability in Chinese hamster ovary cell mutants. *Biochim. Biophys. Acta* **455,** 152–162.
2. Horio, M., Gottesman, M. M., and Pastan, I. (1988) ATP-dependent transport of vinblastine in vesicles from human multidrug-resistant cells. *Proc. Natl. Acad. Sci. USA* **85,** 3580–3584.

3. Chen, C. J., Chin, J. E., Ueda, K., et al. (1986) Internal duplication and homology with bacterial transport proteins in the mdr1 (P-glycoprotein) gene from multidrug-resistant human cells. *Cell* **47**, 381–389.

4. Raviv, Y., Pollard, H. B., Bruggemann, E. P., Pastan, I., and Gottesman, M. M. (1990) Photosensitized labeling of a functional multidrug transporter in living drug-resistant tumor cells. *J. Biol. Chem.* **265**, 3975–3980.

5. Higgins, C. F. and Gottesman, M. M. (1992) Is the multidrug transporter a flippase? *Trends Biochem. Sci.* **17**, 18–21.

6. Kartner, N., Riordan, J. R., and Ling, V. (1983) Cell surface P-glycoprotein associated with multidrug resistance in mammalian cell lines. *Science* **221**, 1285–1288.

7. Fojo, A. T., Ueda, K., Slamon, D. J., Poplack, D. G., Gottesman, M. M., and Pastan, I. (1987) Expression of a multi-drug-resistance gene in human tumors and tissues. *Proc. Natl. Acad. Sci. USA* **84**, 265–269.

8. Goldstein, L. J., Galski, H., Fojo, A., et al. (1989) Expression of a multidrug resistance gene in human cancers. *J. Natl. Cancer Inst.* **81**, 116–124.

9. Chaudhary, P. M. and Roninson, I. B. (1991) Expression and activity of P-glycoprotein, a multidrug efflux pump, in human hematopoietic stem cells. *Cell* **66**, 85–94.

10. Drach, D., Zhao, S., Drach, J., et al. (1992) Subpopulations of normal peripheral blood and bone marrow cells express a functional multidrug resistant phenotype. *Blood* **80**, 2729–2734.

11. Ueda, K., Cardarelli, C., Gottesman, M. M., and Pastan, I. (1987) Expression of a full-length cDNA for the human "MDR1" gene confers resistance to colchicine, doxorubicin, and vinblastine. *Proc. Natl. Acad. Sci. USA* **84**, 3004–3008.

12. Kane, S. E., Troen, B. R., Gal, S., Ueda, K., Pastan, I., and Gottesman, M. M. (1988) Use of a cloned multidrug resistance gene for coamplification and overproduction of major excreted protein, a transformation-regulated secreted acid protease. *Mol. Cell. Biol.* **8**, 3316–3321.

13. Kane, S. E., Reinhard, D. H., Fordis, C. M., Pastan, I., and Gottesman, M. M. (1989) A new vector using the human multidrug resistance gene as a selectable marker enables overexpression of foreign genes in eukaryotic cells. *Gene* **84**, 439–446.

14. Cole, S. P., Bhardwaj, G., Gerlach, J. H., et al. (1992) Overexpression of a transporter gene in a multidrug-resistant human lung cancer cell line. *Science* **258**, 1650–1654.

15. Cole, S. P., Sparks, K. E., Fraser, K., et al. (1994) Pharmacological characterization of multidrug resistant MRP-transfected human tumor cells. *Cancer Res.* **54**, 5902–5910.

16. Zaman, G. J., Flens, M. J., van Leusden, M. R., et al. (1994) The human multidrug resistance-associated protein MRP is a plasma membrane drug-efflux pump. *Proc. Natl. Acad. Sci. USA* **91**, 8822–8826.

17. Pegg, A. E. (2000) Repair of O^6-alkylguanine by alkyltransferases. *Mutat. Res.* **462**, 83–100.

18. Wibley, J. E., Pegg, A. E., and Moody, P. C. (2000) Crystal structure of the human O^6-alkylguanine-DNA alkyltransferase. *Nucleic Acids Res.* **28**, 393–401.

19. Daniels, D. S., Mol, C. D., Arvai, A. S., Kanugula, S., Pegg, A. E., and Tainer, J. A. (2000) Active and alkylated human AGT structures: a novel zinc site, inhibitor and extrahelical base binding. *EMBO J.* **19**, 1719–1730.

20. Gerson, S. L., Phillips, W., Kastan, M., Dumenco, L. L., and Donovan, C. (1996) Human CD34+ hematopoietic progenitors have low, cytokine-unresponsive O^6-alkylguanine-DNA alkyltransferase and are sensitive to O^6-benzylguanine plus BCNU. *Blood* **88**, 1649–1655.

21. Gerson, S. L. and Trey, J. E. (1988) Modulation of nitrosourea resistance in myeloid leukemias. *Blood* **71**, 1487–1494.

22. Gerson, S. L., Berger, N. A., Arce, C., Petzold, S. J., and Willson, J. K. (1992) Modulation of nitrosourea resistance in human colon cancer by O^6-methylguanine. *Biochem. Pharmacol.* **43**, 1101–1107.

23. Dolan, M. E., Moschel, R. C., and Pegg, A. E. (1990) Depletion of mammalian O^6-alkylguanine-DNA alkyltransferase activity by O^6-benzylguanine provides a means to evaluate the role of this protein in protection against carcinogenic and therapeutic alkylating agents. *Proc. Natl. Acad. Sci. USA* **87**, 5368–5372.

24. Dolan, M. E., Mitchell, R. B., Mummert, C., Moschel, R. C., and Pegg, A. E. (1991) Effect of O^6-benzylguanine analogues on sensitivity of human tumor cells to the cytotoxic effects of alkylating agents. *Cancer Res.* **51**, 3367–3372.

25. Dolan, M. E., Stine, L., Mitchell, R. B., Moschel, R. C., and Pegg, A. E. (1990) Modulation of mammalian O^6-alkylguanine-DNA alkyltransferase in vivo by O^6-benzylguanine and its effect on the sensitivity of a human glioma tumor to 1-(2-chloroethyl)-3-(4-methylcyclohexyl)-1-nitrosourea. *Cancer Commun.* **2**, 371–377.

26. Friedman, H. S., Dolan, M. E., Moschel, R. C., et al. (1992) Enhancement of nitrosourea activity in medulloblastoma and glioblastoma multiforme. *J. Natl. Cancer Inst.* **84**, 1926–1931.

27. Mitchell, R. B., Moschel, R. C., and Dolan, M. E. (1992) Effect of O6-benzylguanine on the sensitivity of human tumor xenografts to 1,3-bis(2-chloroethyl)-1-nitrosourea and on DNA interstrand cross-link formation. *Cancer Res.* **52**, 1171–1175.

28. Friedman, H. S., Kokkinakis, D. M., Pluda, J., et al. (1998) Phase I trial of O^6-benzylguanine for patients undergoing surgery for malignant glioma. *J. Clin. Oncol.* **16**, 3570–3575.

29. Spiro, T. P., Gerson, S. L., Liu, L., et al. (1999) O^6-benzylguanine: a clinical trial establishing the biochemical modulatory dose in tumor tissue for alkyltransferase-directed DNA repair. *Cancer Res.* **59**, 2402–2410.

30. Friedman, H. S., Pluda, J., Quinn, J. A., et al. (2000) Phase I trial of carmustine plus O^6-benzylguanine for patients with recurrent or progressive malignant glioma. *J. Clin. Oncol.* **18**, 3522–3528.

31. Quinn, J. A., Pluda, J., Dolan, M. E., et al. (2002) Phase II trial of carmustine plus O^6-benzylguanine for patients with nitrosourea-resistant recurrent or progressive malignant glioma. *J. Clin. Oncol.* **20**, 2277–2283.

32. Crone, T. M., Goodtzova, K., Edara, S., and Pegg, A. E. (1994) Mutations in human O^6-alkylguanine-DNA alkyltransferase imparting resistance to O^6-benzylguanine. *Cancer Res.* **54**, 6221–6227.

33. Xu-Welliver, M., Kanugula, S., and Pegg, A. E. (1998) Isolation of human O^6-alkylguanine-DNA alkyltransferase mutants highly resistant to inactivation by O^6-benzylguanine. *Cancer Res.* **58**, 1936–1945.

34. Hickson, I., Fairbairn, L. J., Chinnasamy, N., Dexter, T. M., Margison, G. P., and Rafferty, J. A. (1996) Protection of mammalian cells against chloroethylating agent toxicity by an O^6-benzylguanine-resistant mutant of human O^6-alkylguanine-DNA alkyltransferase. *Gene Ther.* **3**, 868–877.

35. Loktionova, N. A. and Pegg, A. E. (1996) Point mutations in human O^6-alkylguanine-DNA alkyltransferase prevent the sensitization by O^6-benzylguanine to killing by *N,N'*-bis (2-chloroethyl)-*N*-nitrosourea. *Cancer Res.* **56**, 1578–1583.

36. Blakley, R. L. (1995) Eukaryotic dihydrofolate reductase. *Adv. Enzymol. Relat. Areas Mol. Biol.* **70**, 23–102.

37. Jolivet, J., Cowan, K. H., Curt, G. A., Clendeninn, N. J., and Chabner, B. A. (1983) The pharmacology and clinical use of methotrexate. *N. Engl. J. Med.* **309**, 1094–1104.

38. Schornagel, J. H. and McVie, J. G. (1983) The clinical pharmacology of methotrexate. *Cancer Treat. Rev.* **10**, 53–75.

39. McIvor, R. S. (2002) Protection from antifolate toxicity by expression of drug-resistant dihydrofolate reductase. In *Gene Therapy of Cancer*, 2nd ed. (Lattime, E. C. and Gerson, S. L., eds.), Academic Press, San Diego, CA, pp. 383–392.

40. Simonsen, C. C. and Levinson, A. D. (1983) Isolation and expression of an altered mouse dihydrofolate reductase cDNA. *Proc. Natl. Acad. Sci. USA* **90**, 2495–2499.

41. Morris, J. A. and McIvor, R. S. (1994) Saturation mutagenesis at dihydrofolate reductase codons 22 and 31. A variety of amino acid substitutions conferring methotrexate resistance. *Biochem. Pharmacol.* **47**, 1207–1220.

42. Galski, H., Sullivan, M., Willingham, M. C., et al. (1989) Expression of a human multidrug resistance cDNA (MDR1) in the bone marrow of transgenic mice: resistance to daunomycin-induced leukopenia. *Mol. Cell. Biol.* **9**, 4357–4363.

43. Mickisch, G. H., Licht, T., Merlino, G. T., Gottesman, M. M., and Pastan, I. (1991) Chemotherapy and chemosensitization of transgenic mice which express the human multidrug resistance gene in bone marrow: efficacy, potency, and toxicity. *Cancer Res.* **51**, 5417–5424.

44. Mickisch, G. H., Aksentijevich, I., Schoenlein, P. V., et al. (1992) Transplantation of bone marrow cells from transgenic mice expressing the human MDR1 gene results in long-term protection against the myelosuppressive effect of chemotherapy in mice. *Blood* **79**, 1087–1093.

45. Hanania, E. G., Fu, S., Roninson, I., Zu, Z., and Deisseroth, A. B. (1995) Resistance to taxol chemotherapy produced in mouse marrow cells by safety-modified retroviruses containing a human MDR-1 transcription unit. *Gene Ther.* **2**, 279–284.

46. Aksentijevich, I., Cardarelli, C. O., Pastan, I., and Gottesman, M. M. (1996) Retroviral transfer of the human MDR1 gene confers resistance to bisantrene-specific hematotoxicity. *Clin. Cancer Res.* **2**, 973–980.

47. Sorrentino, B. P., McDonagh, K. T., Woods, D., and Orlic, D. (1995) Expression of retroviral vectors containing the human multidrug resistance 1 cDNA in hematopoietic cells of transplanted mice. *Blood* **86**, 491–501.

48. Moscow, J. A., Huang, H., Carter, C., et al. (1999) Engraftment of MDR1 and NeoR gene-transduced hematopoietic cells after breast cancer chemotherapy. *Blood* **94**, 52–61.

49. Abonour, R., Williams, D. A., Einhorn, L., et al. (2000) Efficient retrovirus-mediated transfer of the multidrug resistance 1 gene into autologous human long-term repopulating hematopoietic stem cells. *Nat. Med.* **6**, 652–658.

50. Bunting, K. D., Galipeau, J., Topham, D., Benaim, E., and Sorrentino, B. P. (1999) Effects of retroviral-mediated MDR1 expression on hematopoietic stem cell self-renewal and differentiation in culture. *Ann. NY Acad. Sci.* **872**, 125–140.

51. Bunting, K. D., Zhou, S., Lu, T., and Sorrentino, B. P. (2000) Enforced P-glycoprotein pump function in murine bone marrow cells results in expansion of side population stem cells in vitro and repopulating cells in vivo. *Blood* **96**, 902–909.

52. Davis, B. M., Reese, J. S., Koç, O. N., Lee, K., Schupp, J. E., and Gerson, S. L. (1997) Selection for G156A O^6-methylguanine DNA methyltransferase gene-transduced hematopoietic progenitors and protection from lethality in mice treated with O^6-benzylguanine and 1,3-bis(2-chloroethyl)-1-nitrosourea. *Cancer Res.* **57**, 5093–5099.

53. Chinnasamy, N., Rafferty, J. A., Hickson, I., et al. (1998) Chemoprotective gene transfer II: multilineage in vivo protection of haemopoiesis against the effects of an antitumour agent by expression of a mutant human O^6-alkyl-guanine-DNA alkyltransferase. *Gene Ther.* **5**, 842–847.

54. Reese, J. S., Koç, O. N., Lee, K. M., et al. (1996) Retroviral transduction of a mutant methylguanine DNA methyltransferase gene into human CD34 cells confers resistance to O^6-benzylguanine plus 1,3-bis(2-chloroethyl)-1-nitrosourea. *Proc. Natl. Acad. Sci. USA* **93**, 14,088–14,093.

55. Koç, O. N., Reese, J. S., Szekely, E. M., and Gerson, S. L. (1999) Human long-term culture initiating cells are sensitive to benzylguanine and 1,3-bis(2-chloroethyl)-1-nitrosourea and protected after mutant (G156A) methylguanine methyltransferase gene transfer. *Cancer Gene Ther.* **6**, 340–348.

56. Isola, L. M. and Gordon, J. W. (1986) Systemic resistance to methotrexate in transgenic mice carrying a mutant dihydrofolate reductase gene. *Proc. Natl. Acad. Sci. USA* **83**, 9621–9625.

57. Hock, R. A. and Miller, A. D. (1986) Retrovirus-mediated transfer and expression of drug resistance genes in human haematopoietic progenitor cells. *Nature* **320,** 275–277.
58. Williams, D. A., Hsieh, K., DeSilva, A., and Mulligan, R. C. (1987) Protection of bone marrow transplant recipients from lethal doses of methotrexate by the generation of methotrexate-resistant bone marrow. *J. Exp. Med.* **166,** 210–218.
59. Corey, C. A., DeSilva, A. D., Holland, C. A., and Williams, D. A. (1990) Serial transplantation of methotrexate-resistant bone marrow: protection of murine recipients from drug toxicity by progeny of transduced stem cells. *Blood* **75,** 337–343.
60. Morris, J. A., May, C., Kim, H. S., et al. (1996) Comparative methotrexate resistance of transgenic mice expressing two distinct dihydrofolate reductase variants. *Transgenics* **2,** 53–67.
61. James, R. I., May, C., Vagt, M. D., Studebaker, R., and McIvor, R. S. (1997) Transgenic mice expressing the tyr22 variant of murine DHFR: protection of transgenic marrow transplant recipients from lethal doses of methotrexate. *Exp. Hematol.* **25,** 1286–1295.
62. May, C., Gunther, R., and McIvor, R. S. (1995) Protection of mice from lethal doses of methotrexate by transplantation with transgenic marrow expressing drug-resistant dihydrofolate reductase activity. *Blood* **86,** 2439–2448.
63. Belur, L. R., Boelk-Galvan, D., Diers, M. D., McIvor, R. S., and Zimmerman, C. L. (2001) Methotrexate accumulates to similar levels in animals transplanted with normal vs drug-resistant transgenic marrow. *Cancer Res.* **61,** 1522–1526.
64. James, R. I., May, C., Vagt, M., Wagner, J. E., and McIvor, R. S. (1999) Methotrexate resistance conferred by transplantation with drug-resistant transgenic marrow cells fractionated by counterflow elutriation. *Bone Marrow Transplant.* **24,** 815–821.
65. May, C., James, R. I., Gunther, R., and McIvor, R. S. (1996) Methotrexate dose-escalation studies in transgenic mice and marrow transplant recipients expressing drug-resistant dihydrofolate reductase activity. *J. Pharmacol. Exp. Ther.* **278,** 1444–1451.
66. James, R. I., Warlick, C. A., Diers, M. D., Gunther, R., and McIvor, R. S. (2000) Mild preconditioning and low-level engraftment confer methotrexate resistance in mice transplanted with marrow expressing drug-resistant dihydrofolate reductase activity. *Blood* **96,** 1334–1341.
67. Zhao, S. C., Banerjee, D., Mineishi, S., and Bertino, J. R. (1997) Post-transplant methotrexate administration leads to improved curability of mice bearing a mammary tumor transplanted with marrow transduced with a mutant human dihydrofolate reductase cDNA. *Hum. Gene Ther.* **8,** 903–909.
68. Hanania, E. G. and Deisseroth, A. B. (1997) Simultaneous genetic chemoprotection of normal marrow cells and genetic chemosensitization of breast cancer cells in a mouse cancer gene therapy model. *Clin. Cancer Res.* **3,** 281–286.
69. Koç, O. N., Reese, J. S., Davis, B. M., Liu, L., Majczenko, K. J., and Gerson, S. L. (1999) DMGMT-transduced bone marrow infusion increases tolerance to O6-benzylguanine and 1,3-bis(2-chloroethyl)-1-nitrosourea and allows intensive therapy of 1,3-bis(2-chloroethyl)-1-nitrosourea-resistant human colon cancer xenografts. *Hum. Gene Ther.* **10,** 1021–1030.
70. Sweeney, C. L., Diers, M. D., Frandsen, J. L., Gunther, R., Verfaillie, C. M., and McIvor, R. S. (2002) Methotrexate exacerbates tumor progression in a murine model of chronic myeloid leukemia. *J. Pharmacol. Exp. Ther.* **300,** 1075–1084.
71. Sweeney, C. L., Frandsen, J. L., Verfaillie, C. M., and McIvor, R. S. (2003) Trimetrexate inhibits progression of the murine 32Dp210 model of chronic myeloid leukemia in animals expressing drug-resistant dihydrofolate reductase. *Cancer Res.* **63,** 1304–1310.
72. Allay, J. A., Spencer, H. T., Wilkinson, S. L., Belt, J. A., Blakley, R. L., and Sorrentino, B. P. (1997) Sensitization of hematopoietic stem and progenitor cells to trimetrexate using nucleoside transport inhibitors. *Blood* **90,** 3546–3554.
73. Warlick, C. A., Sweeney, C. L., and McIvor, R. S. (2000) Maintenance of differential methotrexate toxicity between cells expressing drug-resistant and wild-type dihydrofolate reductase activities in the presence of nucleosides through nucleoside transport inhibition. *Biochem. Pharmacol.* **59,** 141–151.
74. Zhao, R. C., McIvor, R. S., Griffin, J. D., and Verfaillie, C. M. (1997) Gene therapy for chronic myelogenous leukemia (CML): a retroviral vector that renders hematopoietic progenitors methotrexate-resistant and CML progenitors functionally normal and nontumorigenic in vivo. *Blood* **90,** 4687–4698.
75. McIvor, R. S., Weigel, B., Gunther, R., Diers, M. D., and Frandsen, J. (2000) Methotrexate chemotherapy of a murine mammary adenocarcinoma in animals expressing drug-resistant dihydrofolate reductase activity. *Mol. Ther.* **1,** S166.
76. Frandsen, J. L., Sweeney, C. L., Gunther, R., and McIvor, R. S. (2001) Trimetrexate chemotherapy of a murine mammary adenocarcinoma in animals expressing drug-resistant dihydrofolate reductase. *Mol. Ther.* **3,** S387.
77. Naldini, L., Blomer, U., Gallay, P., et al. (1996) In vivo gene delivery and stable transduction of nondividing cells by a lentiviral vector. *Science* **272,** 263–267.
78. Vassilopoulos, G., Trobridge, G., Josephson, N. C., and Russell, D. W. (2001) Gene transfer into murine hematopoietic stem cells with helper-free foamy virus vectors. *Blood* **98,** 604–609.
79. Liu, H., Hung, Y., Wissink, S. D., and Verfaillie, C. M. (2000) Improved retroviral transduction of hematopoietic progenitors by combining methods to enhance virus-cell interaction. *Leukemia* **14,** 307–311.

80. Sorrentino, B. P., Brandt, S. J., Bodine, D., et al. (1992) Selection of drug-resistant bone marrow cells in vivo after retroviral transfer of human MDR1. *Science* **257**, 99–103.

81. Podda, S., Ward, M., Himelstein, A., et al. (1992) Transfer and expression of the human multiple drug resistance gene into live mice. *Proc. Natl. Acad. Sci. USA* **89**, 9676–9680.

82. Cardarelli, C. O., Aksentijevich, I., Pastan, I., and Gottesman, M. M. (1995) Differential effects of P-glycoprotein inhibitors on NIH3T3 cells transfected with wild-type (G185) or mutant (V185) multidrug transporters. *Cancer Res.* **55**, 1086–1091.

83. Hafkemeyer, P., Licht, T., Pastan, I., and Gottesman, M. M. (2000) Chemoprotection of hematopoietic cells by a mutant P-glycoprotein resistant to a potent chemosensitizer of multidrug-resistant cancers. *Hum. Gene Ther.* **11**, 555–565.

84. Allay, J. A., Persons, D. A., Galipeau, J., et al. (1998) In vivo selection of retrovirally transduced hematopoietic stem cells. *Nat. Med.* **4**, 1136–1143.

85. Warlick, C. A., Diers, M. D., Wagner, J. E., and McIvor, R. S. (2002) In vivo selection of antifolate-resistant transgenic hematopoietic stem cells in a murine bone marrow transplant model. *J. Pharmacol. Exp. Ther.* **300**, 50–56.

86. McIvor, R. S., Warlick, C. A., Swanson, D. L., and Frandsen, J. L. (2001) In vivo selection of transgenic hematopoietic stem cells expressing drug-resistant dihydrofolate reductase. *Mol. Ther.* **3**, S245.

87. Davis, B. M., Koç, O. N., and Gerson, S. L. (2000) Limiting numbers of G156A O^6-methylguanine-DNA methyltransferase-transduced marrow progenitors repopulate nonmyeloablated mice after drug selection. *Blood* **95**, 3078–3084.

88. Ragg, S., Xu-Welliver, M., Bailey, J., et al. (2000) Direct reversal of DNA damage by mutant methyltransferase protein protects mice against dose-intensified chemotherapy and leads to in vivo selection of hematopoietic stem cells. *Cancer Res.* **60**, 5187–5195.

89. Sawai, N., Zhou, S., Vanin, E. F., Houghton, P., Brent, T. P., and Sorrentino, B. P. (2001) Protection and in vivo selection of hematopoietic stem cells using temozolomide, O^6-benzylguanine, and an alkyltransferase-expressing retroviral vector. *Mol. Ther.* **3**, 78–87.

90. Stead, R. B., Kwok, W. W., Storb, R., and Miller, A. D. (1988) Canine model for gene therapy: inefficient gene expression in dogs reconstituted with autologous marrow infected with retroviral vectors. *Blood* **71**, 742–747.

91. Hibino, H., Tani, K., Ikebuchi, K., et al. (1999) The common marmoset as a target preclinical primate model for cytokine and gene therapy studies. *Blood* **93**, 2839–2848.

92. Sellers, S. E., Tisdale, J. F., Agricola, B. A., et al. (2001) The effect of multidrug-resistance 1 gene vs neo transduction on ex vivo and in vivo expansion of rhesus macaque hematopoietic repopulating cells. *Blood* **97**, 1888–1891.

93. Licht, T., Haskins, M., Henthorn, P., et al. (2002) Drug selection with paclitaxel restores expression of linked IL-2 receptor gamma-chain and multidrug resistance (MDR1) transgenes in canine bone marrow. *Proc. Natl. Acad. Sci. USA* **99**, 3123–3128.

94. Neff, T., Horn, P. A., Peterson, L. J., et al. (2002) BCNU-mediated in vivo selection of MGMT-transduced allogeneic hematopoietic cells in a large animal model. *Blood* **100**, 689.

95. Hanania, E. G., Giles, R. E., Kavanagh, J., et al. (1996) Results of MDR-1 vector modification trial indicate that granulocyte/macrophage colony-forming unit cells do not contribute to posttransplant hematopoietic recovery following intensive systemic therapy. *Proc. Natl. Acad. Sci. USA* **93**, 15,346–15,351.

96. Cowan, K. H., Moscow, J. A., Huang, H., et al. (1999) Paclitaxel chemotherapy after autologous stem-cell transplantation and engraftment of hematopoietic cells transduced with a retrovirus containing the multidrug resistance complementary DNA (MDR1) in metastatic breast cancer patients. *Clin. Cancer Res.* **5**, 1619–1628.

97. Devereux, S., Corney, C., Macdonald, C., et al. (1998) Feasibility of multidrug resistance (MDR-1) gene transfer in patients undergoing high-dose therapy and peripheral blood stem cell transplantation for lymphoma. *Gene Ther.* **5**, 403–408.

98. Hesdorffer, C., Ayello, J., Ward, M., et al. (1998) Phase I trial of retroviral-mediated transfer of the human MDR1 gene as marrow chemoprotection in patients undergoing high-dose chemotherapy and autologous stem-cell transplantation. *J. Clin. Oncol.* **16**, 165–172.

22

Chemosensitization

Per Eystein Lønning

1. BACKGROUND

With a few important exceptions like dysgerminomas, some lymphoproliferative states, and childhood malignancies, chemotherapy for advanced cancer offers temporary relief only because of development of drug resistance. Although adjuvant endocrine as well as chemotherapy may improve long-term survival in breast cancer *(1,2)* and probably other solid tumors like bowel cancer *(3)*, the modest improvements indicate that only a minor fraction of those exposed to such therapy benefits. Accordingly, drug resistance is the main cause of therapy failure, and subsequent death, in malignant diseases.

The key problem is the lack of understanding of the mechanisms of drug resistance. This relates not only to cytotoxic compounds, but also to other forms of treatment, including endocrine agents as well as novel "targeted" compounds (*see* Section 5.). Taking breast cancer, the malignancy most extensively studied so far, as an example, the literature provides a list of prognostic factors; however, predictive factors, indicating which patients may actually benefit from a certain therapy, are few (*see* ref. *4* for a detailed discussion of the difference between the parameters "prognostic" and "predictive" factors). Although studies have analyzed the biology of different cancers like tumors of the breast, lung, prostate, and the nervous system using microarray techniques *(5–12)*, so far the results have improved prognostication only; understanding of the mechanisms of resistance is no closer.

Defining *sensitization* as any strategy aimed at modulating the activity of cytotoxics, the term includes not only different forms of gene therapy (including viral vectors, ribozymes, and small interfering ribonucleic acids), but also administration of different compounds, like monoclonal antibodies and small molecules. Notably, proof-of-concept results achieved with such strategies may suggest that, in some cases, the pathways outlined could be attached by even more effective strategies involving viral transfections as well as use of genetically engineered cells. Thus, at this stage, it is important to consider results achieved through all these alternative strategies to explore directions for future studies in gene therapy.

In theory, sensitization could be divided into two major categories, those aimed at restoring an abnormal or defect function in the tumor cell (like inhibiting overexpressed P-glycoprotein or erbB-2, repairing gene defects in the apoptotic pathway, and so on) and those aimed at introducing a "second antitumor strategy" (like inhibiting the insulinlike growth-factor receptor I, commonly expressed in all tissues with exception of the liver) that could potentiate, for example, the effect of a chemotherapeutic compound. In practice, many strategies, like antiangiogenetic therapy, could be grouped under both headings, depending on whether vessel growth in malignant tissue is considered a physiological process in response to cancer growth or a key factor involved in the pathological process itself.

In practice, sensitization to chemotherapy or radiotherapy may be achieved by different approaches (Fig. 1; Table 1), like manipulating local blood flow or blood gas tension *(13–15)*, modulating drug

From: *Contemporary Cancer Research*
Cancer Gene Therapy
Edited by: D. T. Curiel and J. T. Douglas © Humana Press Inc., Totowa, NJ

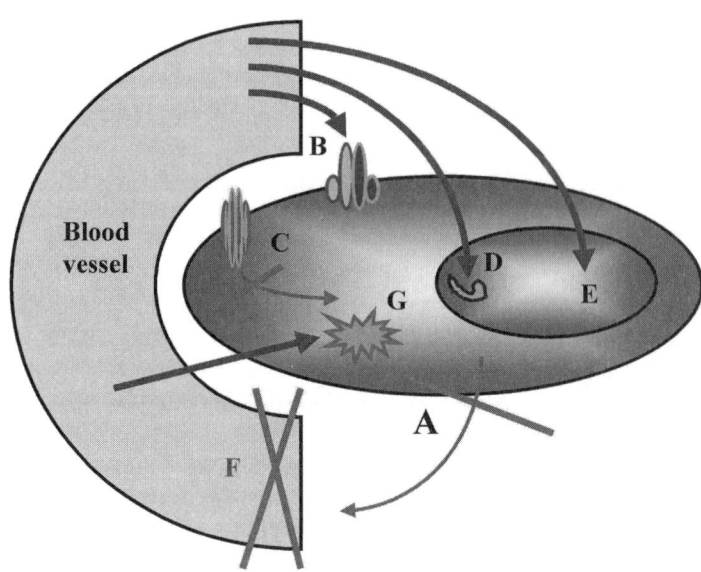

Fig. 1. Potential mechanisms of sensitization: A, blocking membrane pumps extruding drugs from the cell (e.g., P-glycoprotein); B, blocking growth receptors, like the erbB-2 heterodimer with trastuzumab; C, inhibiting different tyrosine kinases; D, stimulating (retinoic acid) or blocking (antiestrogens) steroid receptors; E, repairing gene defects in the apoptotic/growth arrest pathway or inhibiting cyclines; F, depriving tumors of their blood supply (oxygen and nutrients); G, oncolytic viruses.

Table 1
Potential Targets for Chemosensitization Based on Contemporary Knowledge

Manipulating drug disposition	*p*-glycoprotein?
	Other membrane pumps?
Blocking "upstream" targets in tumors expressing	erbB-2
proto-oncogenes/particular translocations	EGF-R
	Retinoic acid receptor
	p210[BCR-ABL]
	KIT protein
Reparing defects in the apoptotic/growth arrest pathway	Repair defect p53
	Other genes?
	Cycline inhibition?
	Fas/DR4/5 system?
Inhibiting angiogenesis?	Vascular endothelial growth factor
	Other factors
Oncolytic viruses	*See* Chapters 13–16

disposition by inhibiting membrane pumps or conjugating enzymes *(16,17)* or attacking oncogenes (like erbB-2) as well as cyclins *(18–20)*. Another important approach may be repair of defects in over-expressed genes involved in growth arrest or apoptosis that may be inactivated through mutations *(21)*, hypermethylations *(22,23)*, or dominant negative splice proteins *(24,25)*. In addition to restoring gene defects, an approach may be to overexpress a gene expressed as wild-type in the tumor cell to achieve a pharmacological effect *(26)*.

Considering gene products to act in activating or inhibiting cascades and the likelihood that different tumors may express defects in different genes involved in such pathways, an alternative approach here could be to transfect a "common downstream target," like a caspase, to all tumors. However, as discussed in Section 4., although such an approach may have a potential as monotherapy, it would probably increase toxicity if combined with cytotoxic drugs. For some genes, like *TP53*, gene function may be enhanced directly not only by transfecting the gene itself, but also by transfecting gene fragments coding a truncated protein that may activate an otherwise defect amino acid-substituted protein *(27)*.

Importantly, it is not known whether restoration of sensitivity in the bulk of the tumor cells (but leaving small clones of resistant cells intact) may cure the patient or if every cell needs to be killed. Evidence from adjuvant therapy in breast cancer that revealed chemotherapy *(1)* as well as endocrine treatment *(2)* to improve long-term survival (understood as killing of micrometastases) despite noncurability in the metastatic setting may be consistent with the concept that the "last tumor cell" may be killed by alternative mechanisms (like by the immune system). Notably, the finding that genetic disturbances like *TP53* mutations are seen in small primary tumors *(28,29)* makes it likely that most patients suffering from micrometastases may harbor small subfractions of resistant cells.

2. CHEMORESISTANCE

Potential mechanisms of drug resistance are discussed in Chapter 8 and are only mentioned briefly here. Although different mechanisms such as overexpression of membrane pumps like P-glycoprotein, multidrug-resistance protein (MRP), and others *(16,30)*; alterations in drug-modulating enzymes like the glutathione sulfotransferases *(31,32)*; overexpression of proto-oncogenes *(33)*; deletion or amplification of topoisomerase II *(34–36)*; and disturbances in the apoptotic function *(37,38)* have been shown to cause drug resistance in different experimental systems, evidence linking the different mechanisms to drug resistance in vivo is limited. Looking at one of the mechanisms most extensively studied in vivo, overexpression of the P-glycoprotein, there is little evidence supporting a major role for this mechanism in solid tumors; first, it has been difficult to correlate protein overexpression or gene amplification with chemo-resistance in different tumors *(39)*; second, the therapeutic efficiency of P-glycoprotein inhibitors in sensitizing solid tumors to chemotherapy remains to be proven *(40–43)*.

Considering treatment options like endocrine manipulation or therapies targeting growth factor receptors or oncogenes, it is likely that most of the potential mechanisms of resistance to cytotoxic compounds (like defects in the apoptotic machinery) may be involved here as well. However, in addition, there is the possibility of defects in the upstream pathways involving the receptor/targets and their downstream pathways. Taking endocrine therapy of breast cancer as an example, resistance to hormonal manipulation in tumors expressing the estrogen receptor may involve different mechanisms, like defect receptor coactivator function, receptor phosphorylation status, as well as several other potential mechanisms (*see* ref. *44* for references). However, as all forms of effective therapy are likely to depend on intact growth arrest and/or apoptosis, this issue should be a main topic for any discussion of sensitization.

Notably, there are several pitfalls in the study of drug resistance in vivo. A major issue is optimal design of clinical studies. Studying the effects of therapy in early cancer, end points like overall and relapse-free survival may not necessarily reflect sensitivity to therapy; these outcomes are influenced by tumor growth rate and metastatic potential in addition to the effect of therapy. Further, an improved relapse-free survival could be because of durable growth arrest and may not necessarily reflect death of micrometastatic cells. Finally, it is not known whether the bulk of the cells in the primary tumor and the micrometastatic cells express similar biological characteristics, creating uncertainties about the validity of correlating pathological findings from the primary tumor to outcomes like relapse and cancer death (*see* ref. *45* for a detailed discussion of these issues). Although novel molecular techniques may allow assessment of the different mechanisms, there is a need for clinical studies designed especially to address these questions in vivo.

In the following sections, potential mechanisms of drug sensitizing are reviewed together with evidence linking potential mechanisms to drug resistance in vivo.

3. ATTACHING THE P-GLYCOPROTEIN AND RELATED CELLULAR DRUG EXTRUSION MECHANISMS

The substantial number of elegant preclinical studies reporting correlations between expression of the P-glycoprotein pump protein or amplification of its multidrug resistance gene on the one hand and lack of drug sensitivity on the other (*see* references in ref. *16*) suggested drug expulsion could play a key role in depriving chemosensitivity. Based on the finding that P-glycoprotein pump function could be inhibited by different conventional pharmacological compounds (*40,46–52*), clinical trials were implemented to test inhibitory compounds like tamoxifen given in high doses (480–720 mg daily for 5 days; regular dose 20 mg daily) in concert with the P-glycoprotein substrate etoposide (*40,53*). Based on the finding that P-glycoprotein could also be inhibited with cyclosporine (*42*), cyclosporine derivatives designed to inhibit P-glycoprotein in a specific manner have been implemented (*41,43,54,55*).

So far, the results from trials evaluating these compounds have been disappointing, revealing few clinical effects but significant toxicity problems, mostly related to the fact that these pumps are likely to play a key role in the excretory functions of visceral organs and probably the blood–brain barrier (*56,57*). These effects may cause alterations in the pharmacokinetics of many compounds (*58*). The negative findings of these studies with respect to antitumor effects questions a major role for such mechanisms in chemoresistance and makes targeting of the P-glycoprotein or the multidrug resistance gene by transfecting methods an unlikely mechanism for sensitization.

Yet, caution needs to be taken in abandoning cellular drug extrusion as a potential mechanism of drug resistance at this stage (*59*). The lack of correlation between P-glycoprotein expression and drug resistance detected in many solid tumors like breast cancer may be because of technical problems assessing the parameter (*39*). Although this precludes patients from selection for studies based on individual tumor characteristics, the possibility may still exist that a modest overexpression could be biologically important; thus, a subfraction of patients could benefit from such therapies. However, taking into account the number of pharmacological agents shown to inhibit the pump, if better predictive factors and biological evidence support the case for future trials, these could probably be done using classical pharmacological agents with little need for novel transfection strategies.

4. TARGETING DEFECTS IN THE APOPTOTIC/CELL CYCLE PATHWAYS

One of the few factors for which there is substantial evidence linking lack of function to chemoresistance to certain drugs is the *TP53* gene, which codes for the p53 protein. In addition to several studies revealing an association between disturbances in p53 function and a poor prognosis in many malignancies (*see* references in ref. *29*), mutations in the *TP53* gene have been linked to drug resistance in preclinical models (*37,38*) and, most important, to drug resistance in different human cancers, like hematological malignancies (*60–62*) and breast cancers in vivo (*21,63*). Because mutated p53 often has an extended cellular half-life caused by its defect in MDM2 binding, ubiquination, and subsequent degradation (*29,64*) overexpression of the p53 protein has been used as a surrogate marker for mutation status. However, many mutations (in breast cancer, about 30%), particularly of the nonsense type but also some point mutations (probably because of defect folding or enhanced degradation), do not stain (*65,66*), and use of protein immunostaining as a surrogate parameter is no longer recommended (*29*).

The finding that mutations in the *TP53* gene predict drug resistance to certain regimens for particular tumors makes this an interesting target for gene therapy, as does the evidence that its function may be restored not only by transfecting the whole gene, but also by transfecting gene fragments coding for particular fragments (*27,67*). Yet, there are three important problems. First, lack of cross-resistance to different regimens and the observation that *TP53* mutations may predict resistance to

Table 2
Responses to Doxorubicin Administered as Primary Monotherapy
to Patients Suffering From Advanced Breast Cancer *(65)*

	Response to therapy	
TP53 status	Response/stable disease	Progressive disease
Wild-type *TP53* or mutations not affecting the L2/L3 domains	67	4
TP53 mutations affecting the L2 or L3 domains	14	5

Although we observed a significant correlation between chemoresistance and *TP53* mutations affecting the L2 or L3 loops of the protein ($p = 0.008$), notably there were patients expressing wild-type *TP53* or *TP53* mutations not affecting these loops that did not respond to therapy; other patients harboring L2/L3 mutations responded.

anthracyclines but not, for example, the taxanes *(63)* illustrates that the mechanisms of resistance may differ among different compounds; thus, it is likely that any mechanism defined may predict only for resistance to a limited number of drugs. Second, even when *TP53* mutations have been found to pre-dict resistance (such as for the anthracyclines in breast cancer), we are left with the finding that some tumors express drug resistance despite harboring wild-type *TP53*. It is not known whether these tumors may harbor gene defects located up- or downstream in the *TP53* pathway or whether mechanisms totally different may be involved. Third, the finding that, in the same setting *(66)*, several tumors harboring *TP53* mutations may respond to the therapy (Table 2) suggests redundant mechanisms may be involved, compensating for the loss.

One explanation for these observations may be that apoptoses in response to genotoxicity may be executed by redundant "cascades" (Fig. 2A). According to this hypothesis, the observations mentioned may be explained by postulating that apoptosis in response to anthracycline treatment may be executed through (at least) two different pathways, one involving p53. If both of these pathways are disturbed, the cell becomes resistant to therapy. Thus, drug resistance in tumors harboring wild-type *TP53* may be because of dysfunctions of genes acting up- or downstream of the p53 (Fig. 2A); apoptosis in tumors harboring mutated *TP53* could be executed through the "redundant" pathway.

Actually, such a model may be consistent with several observations in the literature. Tumor types known to express poor sensitivity to anthracyclines but harboring wild-type *TP53* in general (like melanomas) may have disturbances in other genes involved in the same pathway, like Apaf-1 *(68)*. However, this model also illustrates what could be a substantial problem; although we may restore a defect p53 function and restore sensitivity in the bulk of the cells, the likelihood is high that the tumor may harbor cellular subclones that escape therapy because of defects in other genes involved in the same pathway. Cell clones harboring defects in one of the two "redundant" pathways may create a hazard; despite therapy sensitivity, the fact that they already harbor one of two events necessary for resistance put them into a high-risk category (analogous to the Knutson "double-hit theory" *(69)*, with the exception that this deals with two, and not a single, gene).

These considerations may illustrate an important principle that distinguishes drug resistance in vivo from preclinical models; although preclinical experiments assess the effects of combined gene defects by knocking out two or more distinct genes *(70)*, in vivo resistance may be characterized by defects in different genes acting up- or downstream in networks. One problem here may be that, apart from acting in a "key" pathway, each gene probably influences the function of numerous additional genes *(71,72)*, as may be illustrated using p53 as an example. Although defects in different genes involved in a particular cascade could have the same biological effect on that particular function, the fact that each gene also may activate multiple additional pathways suggests such mutations may create a different gene profile on microarrays *(72)*, preventing a uniform clustering profile of the resistant tumor phenotype (depicted in Fig. 2B). Thus, to assess defects in the apoptotic machinery, a detailed

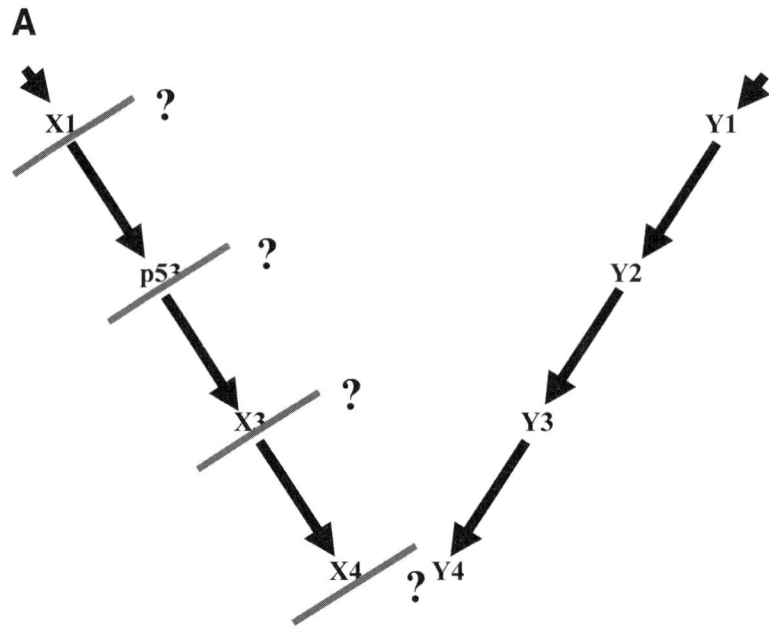

Fig. 2. (A) Illustration of the hypothesis that mutations affecting different genes located up- or downstream of each other may have similar effects on a genetic pathway.

assessment of the function not only of single genes, but also of several genes working within the same network, based on an up-front hypothesis, is needed to diagnose the defects.

Considering gene therapy, restoration of gene function in tumors harboring a particular defect leading to restoration of drug sensitivity would be the ultimate proof for a key biological function of that factor in the drug response. Direct injections of retroviral- and adenoviral vectors carrying wild-type *TP53* into nonsmall cell lung cancers (NSCLC) harboring *TP53* defects have shown antitumor effects as monotherapy as well as sensitization of tumors to treatment with platinum drugs *(73,74)*. Pending on strategies for successful systemic administration, the effect of such therapy on relapse rate and long-term survival will address the value of such a single-gene strategy or provide evidence whether we need to go for multiple-gene transfection strategies. Interestingly, in vitro experiments on NSCLC-derived cell lines indicated transfection of *CDKN2A* to restore radiation sensitivity in cell lines lacking p16 expression, but only when they expressed a normal p53 function *(75)*.

A second strategy could be to go for particular downstream targets. The caspases represent the ultimate downstream executors *(76)*; thus, one approach could be to adapt a strategy stimulating the downstream caspase 3 in concert with administration of chemotherapy. However, such a strategy may be detrimental; first, it actually may not represent "sensitization" in response to therapy because the pathway linking the genotoxic damage caused by the cytotoxic drug to caspase activation would be disrupted; therefore, the two mechanisms may not act in concert (Fig. 2C). Although it may be argued that this could strengthen the effects of redundant pathways (the Y pathway in Fig. 2C), based on the assumptions discussed above, it is likely that such pathways may also be inactivated in resistant cells. The effect of coadministration of a cytotoxic agent and gene transfection could be an additive effect of the mechanisms in cells harboring an intact apoptotic cascade, but no effect of the chemotoxic agent compared to transfection with the caspase gene alone in tumors with upstream defects disconnecting the signaling pathway between genotoxic damage and caspase activation. The paradoxical effect therefore could be to increase the toxic effects on normal cells compared to the drug resis-

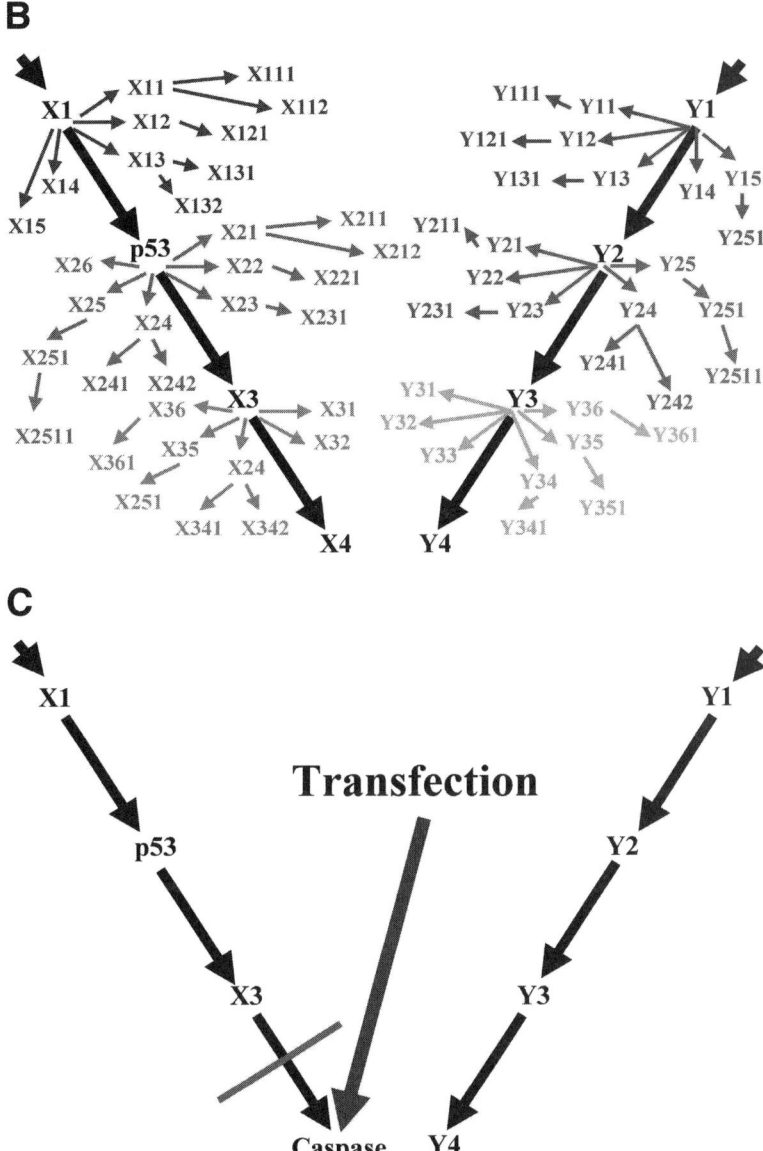

Fig. 2. (B) Although blocking different genes in a cascade may have similar effects on a particular pathway, because of redundant pathways activated by the different genes such mutations may be expected to cause a different gene expression profile on microarrays. **(C)** Transfection of a downstream gene like a caspase could be detrimental in tumors expressing a transmission block between the sensitizer triggering apoptosis and the downstream target because it may sensitize normal cells, but not those harboring such mutations, to the apoptotic signal triggered by cytotoxic compounds.

tant ones. In theory, it may be concluded that transfection of downstream genes to achieve pharmacological effects could be a treatment option as monotherapy; as a way to sensitize the effects of chemotherapeutics, it probably may be detrimental.

An interesting option may be transfection of genes like *TP53* in pharmacological doses. Thus, two studies revealed transfection of an additional copy of the full *TP53* gene *(26)* or a truncated mutant

(77) activating the wild-type p53 protein to enhance response to DNA damage and inhibit tumor development in murine models. Although transfection of the normal *TP53* copy did not cause detectable side effects, transfection of the hyperactive truncated mutant was associated with early aging. This illustrates potential detrimental effects of inducing hyperactivity of particular genes in normal cells.

5. TARGETING PROTO-ONCOGENES OR GROWTH FACTOR RECEPTORS

Many tumors reveal overexpression/gene amplification of oncogenes, growth factors, or their receptors; examples include the epidermal growth factor receptor (EGFR) or erbB-2. Although the incidence of alterations may vary between different tumor groups, EGFR and erbB-2 overexpression/ amplification represent general disturbances detected in several different tumor forms *(78–83)*.

The finding that expression of many factors may correlate with prognosis *(84,85)* is suggestive of, but does not define, a specific biological role of a factor; thus, an individual parameter may be a covariate to other mechanisms, or it could be a marker of tumor growth rate or metastatic potential, but not be related to drug sensitivity. Expression of the estrogen receptor may serve as an example; despite being the receptor for one of the most potent growth-stimulatory ligands to breast cancer cells, receptor expression is also associated with a good short-term prognosis in patients not exposed to antihormonal therapy *(86,87)*. The most likely explanation is that receptor expression is a covariate of other prognostic factors, such as tumor cell differentiation and proliferation *(88)*.

Of particular interest is the proto-oncogene erbB-2, which has been extensively studied in breast cancer. Although overexpression of erbB-2 has been associated with chemoresistance to anthracyclines *(89)*, data from our group suggest erbB-2 expression could be a covariate of *TP53* mutations *(66)*. Thus, for metastatic tumors overexpressing this proto-oncogene (+++), about 25% will achieve an objective response to treatment with the humanized antibody trastuzumab *(90–92)*. Despite the fact that the minority of these patients reveal an objective response and nearly all relapse in less than 2 years, it reveals a proof of principle that such a strategy may influence tumor growth in vivo. Importantly, combining trastuzumab with chemotherapy improved the response rate as well as the time to progression in patients with breast cancer *(93)*.

Yet, such an observation may have several explanations. On the one hand, administration of trastuzumab could influence chemosensitivity by interacting with the mechanisms of resistance; on the other hand, there may be two independent mechanisms, with the total effect observed just the sum of these effects. In vitro experiments support the view that expression of erbB-2 may induce more rapid regrowth of resistant cells and not be the cause of resistance by itself *(94)*. Evidence suggested that the combined effects of trastuzumab and chemotherapy are additive; however, for some drugs like docetaxel, they seem to be synergistic *(95)*. Whatever the mechanism, the result is increased response to combined therapy, and the potential of exploring sensitization through alternative strategies targeting the erbB-2 pathway should be explored further.

Gefitinib (ZD1839; Iressa) is a small molecular compound that inhibits the EGFR tyrosine kinase *(96)*. This receptor is known to be overexpressed in many malignancies, particularly lung cancer *(97)*, but also is associated with poor prognosis in malignancy *(98,99)*. A phase I trial recorded stable disease in few patients suffering from different tumors, like NSCLC, hormone-refractory prostatic cancer, and ovarian and colorectal cancers *(100)*. Although most phase I/II studies in NSCLC reported response rates in the range of 10–20%, administering the compound in concert with chemotherapy did not improve outcome *(96)*. Although an explanation for these findings is lacking *(101)*, the fact that patients were not assessed for EGFR expression may have diluted the result.

Other growth factors, like the IGF system, may be of interest, despite the fact that the IGF type I receptor is expressed in most normal tissues, and its ligand, the IGF-I, is the effector of growth hormone actions in normal tissue. Thus, the IGF type I receptor has been found expressed in different malignancies, such as cancer of the breast, large bowel, lung, ovary, and prostate and gliomas *(102)*.

Experimental evidence has provided an important role of the IGF system in growth of different tumor-derived cell lines and xenografts (*see* ref. *103* for references), and the key IGF-binding protein, IGF-binding protein 3, seems to have a ligand-independent role in the apoptotic process *(104)*. High plasma levels of IGF-I have been related to subsequent risk of breast cancer in premenopausal women *(105)*. Notably, although manipulation of the IGF system (by interacting with IGF-I, its receptor, or the binding proteins) may be an interesting approach to sensitize tumor cells to other therapies, evidence so far has not suggested antitumor effects of suppressing the synthesis of IGF-I through administration of somatostatin analogues either as monotherapy or in concert with tamoxifen *(106–109)*. Considering the important role of the IGF system not only with respect to growth hormone effects, but also to glucose homeostasis *(110)*, obviously attempts to manipulate this system may be limited by toxicity problems.

A second group of targets is specific genetic disturbances occurring in particular tumor forms. Thus, some tumors, particularly hematological malignancies, may harbor particular genetic mutations/translocations, suggesting specific strategies of value. Acute promyelocytic leukemia is a rare variant of acute myelogenic leukemia characterized by the (15:17) reciprocal chromosomal translocation, causing a fusion between the retinoic acid receptor alpha gene and the promyelocytic leukemia gene *(111)*. Thus, treatment with retinoic acid may cause temporary complete remission in the majority of patients and improve long-term outcome when administered in concert with chemotherapy *(112)*. In another leukemia variant, the chronic myeloid form, about 90% are characterized by the (9:20) reciprocal translocation (detectable as the so-called Philadelphia chromosome), causing a fusion protein (p210$^{BCR-ABL}$) with dysregulated tyrosine kinase activity *(113–118)*. Imitamib mesylate (Gleevec) inhibits this enzyme as well as several other kinases, including C-KIT, frequently revealing hyperactivity in gastrointestinal stromal tumors through gain-of-function mutations *(119–121)*. Thus, treatment of chronic myeloid leukemia as well as gastrointestinal stromal tumors with imitamib has been associated with dramatic remissions *(122,123)*. However, the long-term effects as well as potential sensitization to treatment with chemotherapy remain to be elucidated.

In conclusion, targeted therapy with different compounds directed toward particular oncogenes has provided mixed results. Based on current knowledge, it is likely that a limited number of tumors may be successful candidates for such approaches in the future. However, for those found to be sensitive, factors like improved delivery (e.g., by installing genetically engineered cells) could be explored as an approach to improve delivery.

6. ANGIOGENESIS

Much knowledge has been gained concerning the importance of angiogenesis to tumor growth. Thus, different growth factors known to stimulate/inhibit angiogenesis have been characterized *(124, 125)*, and the aim of preventing tumor growth by depriving the cells of their oxygen and energy supply is tempting. However, although factors like vascular density have been correlated with prognosis in different malignancies *(126)*, the role of antiangiogenetic therapy remains to be settled.

7. CYTOLYTIC VIRUSES

Gene therapy using cytolytic viruses is addressed in Chapters 13–16; only the issue of combining such agents with cytotoxics in an attempt to sensitize tumor cells is addressed here. Thus, animal models have suggested improved efficacy from administering the E1B 55-kDa gene-deleted adenovirus dl1520 (ONYX-015) in concert with cytotoxics compared to what was achieved by any agent alone *(127)*. This agent has been studied in several trials and has been administered by different routes as monotherapy and in concert with chemotoxic agents *(128)*. However, although the results from recent studies administering the viral agent in concert with different cytostatics to patients suffering from different malignancies considered nonsensitive to cytotoxic therapy have suggested some therapeutic efficacy of combined treatment *(129–134)*, this needs to be confirmed in larger clinical studies before any definite conclusion may be drawn.

8. SUMMARY AND CONCLUSIONS

Sensitizing as an approach to improve anticancer treatment is just beginning. Although targeted therapy has been successful against some agents, the results for others have been disappointing, underlining the problem of predicting effect from preclinical data. Although some of the unsuccessful approaches could be caused by lack of selection of appropriate patients, lack of compound efficacy, or inefficient delivery strategies, the limited understanding of the mechanisms causing drug failure in vivo still represents a key problem preventing effective strategies. Thus, translational research exploring the mechanisms of drug resistance is highly warranted. Similarly, although studies correlating particular molecular alterations to drug failure may outline therapeutic strategies, research in gene therapy (as well as other mechanisms) aiming at restoring chemosensitivity by antagonizing oncogenes or restoring defective gene function may provide the ultimate proof whether a particular mechanism is the cause of drug resistance or a statistical correlate only.

REFERENCES

1. Abe, O., Abe, R., Enomoto, K., et al. (1998) Polychemotherapy for early breast cancer: an overview of the randomised trials. *Lancet* **352,** 930–942.
2. Clarke, M., Collins, R., Davies, C., Godwin, J., Gray, R., and Peto, R. (1998) Tamoxifen for early breast cancer: an overview of the randomised trials. *Lancet* **351,** 1451–1467.
3. Taal, B. G., Van Tinteren, H., and Zoetmulder, F. (2001) Adjuvant 5FU plus levamisole in colonic or rectal cancer: improved survival in stage II and III. *Br. J. Cancer* **85,** 1437–1443.
4. Henderson, I. C. and Patek, A. J. (1998) The relationship between prognostic and predictive factors in the management of breast cancer. *Breast Cancer Res. Treat.* **52,** 261–288.
5. Ahr, A., Karn, T., Solbach, C., et al. (2002) Identification of high risk breast-cancer patients by gene expression profiling. *Lancet* **359,** 131–132.
6. Beer, D., Kardia, S., Huang, C.-C., et al. (2002) Gene-expression profiles predict survival of patients with lung adenocarcinoma. *Nat. Med.* **8,** 816–824.
7. van de Vijver, M. J., He, Y. D., van 't Veer, L. J., et al. (2002) A gene-expression signature as a predictor of survival in breast cancer. *N. Engl. J. Med.* **347,** 1999–2009.
8. Dhanasekaran, S. M., Barrette, T. R., Ghosh, D., et al. (2001) Delineation of prognostic biomarkers in prostate cancer. *Nature* **412,** 822–826.
9. Pomeroy, S. L., Tamayo, P., Gaasenbeek, M., et al. (2002) Prediction of central nervous system embryonal tumour outcome based on gene expression. *Nature* **415,** 436–442.
10. Shipp, M. A., Ross, K. N., Tamayo, P., et al. (2002) Diffuse large B-cell lymphoma outcome prediction by gene-expression profiling and supervised machine learning. *Nat. Med.* **8,** 68–74.
11. Singh, D., Febbo, P. G., Ross, K., et al. (2002) Gene expression correlates of clinical prostate cancer behavior. *Cancer Cell* **1,** 203–209.
12. Sørlie, T., Perou, C. M., Tibshirani, R., et al. (2001) Gene expression patterns of breast carcinomas distinguish tumor subclasses with clinical implications. *Proc. Nat. Acad. Sci. USA* **98,** 10,869–10,874.
13. Jain, R. K. (1996) Delivery of molecular medicine to solid tumors. *Science* **271,** 1079–1080.
14. Stohrer, M., Boucher, Y., Stangassinger, M., and Jain, R. K. (2002) Oncotic pressure in solid tumors is elevated. *Cancer Res.* **60,** 4251–4255.
15. Vaupel, P., Thews, O., and Hoeckel, M. (2001) Treatment resistance of solid tumors—role of hypoxia and anemia. *Med. Oncol.* **18,** 243–259.
16. Ling, V. (1992) P-Glycoprotein and resistance to anticancer drugs. *Cancer* **69,** 2603–2609.
17. Dirven, H. A. A. M., Ommen, B. V., and Bladeren, P. J. V. (1994) Involvement of human glutathione S-transferase isoenzymes in the conjugation of cyclophosphamide metabolites with glutathione. *Cancer Res.* **54,** 6215–6220.
18. Pegram, M. D. and Slamon, D. J. (1999) Combination therapy with trastuzumab (Herceptin) and cisplatin for chemoresistant metastatic breast cancer: evidence for receptor-enhanced chemosensitivity. *Semin. Oncol.* **26,** 89–95.
19. Sauter, E. R., Yeo, U. C., von Stemm, A., et al. (2002) Cyclin D1 is a candidate oncogene in cutaneous melanoma. *Cancer Res.* **62,** 3200–3206.
20. Grant, S. and Roberts, J. D. (2003) The use of cyclin-dependent kinase inhibitors alone or in combination with established cytotoxic drugs in cancer chemotherapy. *Drug Resist. Updat.* **6,** 15–26.

21. Aas, T., Børresen, A.-L., Geisler, S., et al. (1996) Specific P53 mutations are associated with *de novo* resistance to doxorubicin in breast cancer patients. *Nat. Med.* **2**, 811–814.

22. Baylin, S. B. and Herman, J. G. (2000) DNA hypermethylation in tumorigenesis—epigenetics joins genetics. *Trends Genet.* **16**, 168–174.

23. Herman, J. G. (1999) Hypermethylation of tumor suppressor genes in cancer. *Semin. Cancer Biol.* **9**, 359–367.

24. Fillippovich, I., Sorokina, N., Gatei, M., et al. (2001) Transactivation-deficient p73 alpha (P73 Delta exon2) inhibits apoptosis and competes with p53. *Oncogene* **20**, 514–522.

25. O'Nions, J., Brooks, L. A., Sullivan, A., et al. (2001) p73 is over-expressed in vulval cancer principally as the Delta 2 isoform. *Br. J. Cancer* **85**, 1551–1556.

26. Garcia-Cao, I., Garcia-Cao, M., Martin-Caballero, J., et al. (2002) "Super p53" mice exhibit enhanced DNA damage response, are tumor resistant and age normally. *EMBO J.* **21**, 6225–6235.

27. deFromentel, C. C., Gruel, N., Venot, C., et al. (1999) Restoration of transcriptional activity of p53 mutants in human tumour cells by intracellular expression of anti-p53 single chain Fv fragments. *Oncogene* **18**, 551–557.

28. Andersen, T. I., Holm, R., Nesland, J. M., Heimdal, K. R., Ottestad, L., and Børresen, A. L. (1993) Prognostic significance of TP53 alterations in breast carcinoma. *Br. J. Cancer* **68**, 540–548.

29. Soussi, T. and Beroud, C. (2001) Assessing TP53 status in human tumours to evaluate clinical outcome. *Nat. Rev. Cancer* **1**, 233–240.

30. Borst, P., Evers, R., Kool, M., and Wijnholds, J. (2000) A family of drug transporters: the multidrug resistance-associated proteins. *J. Natl. Cancer Inst.* **92**, 1295–1302.

31. Ban, N., Takahashi, Y., Takayama, T., et al. (1996) Transfection of glutathione S-transferase (GST)-pi antisense complementary DNA increases the sensitivity of a colon cancer cell line to adriamycin, cisplatin, melphalan, and etoposide. *Cancer Res.* **56**, 3577–3582.

32. Schröder, C. P., Godwin, A. K., O'Dwyer, P. J., Tew, K. D., Hamilton, T. C., and Ozols, R. F. (1996) Glutathione and drug resistance. *Cancer Invest.* **14**, 158–168.

33. Baselga, J., Norton, L., Albanell, J., Kim, Y. M., and Mendelsohn, J. (1998) Recombinant humanized anti-HER2 antibody (Herceptin™) enhances the antitumor activity of paclitaxel and doxorubicin against HER2/neu overexpressing human breast cancer xenografts. *Cancer Res.* **58**, 2825–2831.

34. Withoff, S., Keith, W. N., Knol, A. J., et al. (1996) Selection of a subpopulation with fewer DNA topoisomerase II alpha gene copies in a doxorubicin-resistant cell line panel. *Br. J. Cancer* **74**, 502–507.

35. Järvinen, T. A. H., Holli, K., Kuukasjarvi, T., and Isola, J. J. (1998) Predictive value of topoisomerase II alpha and other prognostic factors for epirubicin chemotherapy in advanced breast cancer. *Br. J. Cancer* **77**, 2267–2273.

36. Tanner, M., Jarvinen, P., and Isola, J. (2001) Amplification of HER-2/neu and topoisomerase II alpha in primary and metastatic breast cancer. *Cancer Res.* **61**, 5345–5348.

37. Lowe, S. W., Ruley, H. E., Jacks, T., and Housman, D. E. (1993) p53-dependent apoptosis modulates the cytotoxicity of anticancer agents. *Cell* **74**, 957–967.

38. Lowe, S. W., Bodis, S., McClatchey, A., et al. (1994) p53 status and the efficacy of cancer therapy in vivo. *Science* **266**, 807–810.

39. Broxterman, H. J., Lankelma, J., and Pinedo, H. M. (1996) How to probe clinical tumour samples for P-glycoprotein and multidrug resistance-associated protein. *Eur. J. Cancer* **32A**, 1024–1033.

40. Stuart, N. S. A., Philip, P., Harris, A. L., et al. (1992) High-dose tamoxifen as an enhancer of etoposide cytotoxicity. Clinical effects and in vitro assessment in P-glycoprotein expressing cell lines. *Br. J. Cancer* **66**, 833–839.

41. Baekelandt, M., Lehne, G., Trope, C. G., et al. (2001) Phase I/II trial of the multidrug-resistance modulator valspodar combined with cisplatin and doxorubicin in refractory ovarian cancer. *J. Clin. Oncol.* **19**, 2983–2993.

42. Bartlett, N. L., Lum, B. L., Fisher, G. A., et al. (1994) Phase I trial of doxorubicin with cyclosporine as a modulator of multidrug resistance. *J. Clin. Oncol.* **12**, 835–842.

43. Peck, R. A., Hewett, J., Harding, M. W., et al. (2001) Phase I and pharmacokinetic study of the novel MDR1 and MRP1 inhibitor biricodar administered alone and in combination with doxorubicin. *J. Clin. Oncol.* **19**, 3130–3141.

44. Geisler, J. and Lønning, P. (2001) Resistance to endocrine therapy of breast cancer: recent advances and tomorrows challenges. *Clin. Breast Cancer* **1**, 297–308.

45. Lønning, P. (2003) Study of suboptimum treatment response: lessons from breast cancer. *Lancet Oncol.* **4**, 177–185.

46. Fleming, G. F., Amato, J. M., Agresti, M., and Safa, A. R. (1992) Megestrol acetate reverses multidrug resistance and interacts with P-glycoprotein. *Cancer Chemother. Pharmacol.* **29**, 445–449.

47. Chen, G., Ramachandran, C., and Krishan, A. (1993) Thaliblastine, a plant alkaloid, circumvents multidrug resistance by direct binding to P-glycoprotein. *Cancer Res.* **53**, 2544–2547.

48. Speicher, L. A., Barone, L. R., Chapman, A. E., et al. (1994) P-Glycoprotein binding and modulation of the multidrug-resistant phenotype by estramustine. *J. Natl. Cancer Inst.* **86**, 688–694.

49. Callaghan, R. and Higgins, C. F. (1995) Interaction of tamoxifen with the multidrug resistance P-glycoprotein. *Br. J. Cancer* **71**, 294–299.

50. Schlemmer, S. R., Yang, C.-H., and Sirotnak, F. M. (1995) Functional modulation of multidrug resistance-related P-glycoprotein by Ca^{2+}-calmodulin. *J. Biol. Chem.* **270**, 11,040–11,042.

51. DiDiodato, G. and Sharom, F. J. (1997) Interaction of combinations of drugs, chemosensitisers, and peptides with the P-glycoprotein multidrug transporter. *Biochem. Pharmacol.* **53**, 1789–1797.

52. Germann, U. A., Ford, P. J., Shlyakhter, D., Mason, V. S., and Harding, M. W. (1997) Chemosensitization and drug accumulation effects of VX-710, verapamil, cyclosporin A, MS-209 and GF120918 in multidrug resistant HL60/ADR cells expressing the multidrug resistance-associated protein MRP. *Anticancer Drug* **8**, 141–155.

53. Kirk, J., Syed, S. K., Harris, A. L., et al. (1994) Reversal of P-glycoprotein-mediated multidrug resistance by pure anti-oestrogens and novel tamoxifen derivatives. *Biochem. Pharmacol.* **48**, 277–285.

54. Chico, I., Kang, M. H., Bergan, R., et al. (2001) Phase I study of infusional paclitaxel in combination with the P-glycoprotein antagonist PSC 833. *J. Clin. Oncol.* **19**, 832–842.

55. Rowinsky, E. K., Smith, L., Wang, Y. M., et al. (1998) Phase I and pharmacokinetic study of paclitaxel in combination with biricodar, a novel agent that reverses multidrug resistance conferred by overexpression of both MDR1 and MRP. *J. Clin. Oncol.* **16**, 2964–2976.

56. Hunter, J. and Hirst, B. H. (1997) Intestinal secretion of drugs. The role of P-glycoprotein and related drug efflux systems in limiting oral drug absorption. *Adv. Drug Deliv. Rev.* **25**, 129–157.

57. Tsuji, A. and Tamai, I. (1997) Blood–brain barrier function of P-glycoprotein. *Adv. Drug Deliv. Rev.* **25**, 287–298.

58. Levêque, D. and Jehl, F. (1995) P-Glycoprotein and pharmacokinetics. *Anticancer Res.* **15**, 331–336.

59. Leonessa, F. and Clarke, R. (2003) ATP binding cassette transporters and drug resistance in breast cancer. *Endocr. Relat. Cancer* **10**, 43–73.

60. Wattel, E., Preudhomme, C., Hecquet, B., et al. (1994) p53 mutations are associated with resistance to chemotherapy and short survival in hematologic malignancies. *Blood* **84**, 3148–3157.

61. Preudhomme, C. and Fenaux, P. (1997) The clinical significance of mutations of the P53 tumour suppressor gene in haematological malignancies. *Br. J. Haematol.* **98**, 502–511.

62. Ichikawa, A., Kinoshita, T., Watanabe, T., et al. (1997) Mutations of the p53 gene as a prognostic factor in aggressive B-cell lymphoma. *N. Engl. J. Med.* **337**, 529–534.

63. Kandioler-Eckersberger, D., Ludwig, C., Rudas, M., et al. (2000) TP53 mutation and p53 overexpression for prediction of response to neoadjuvant treatment in breast cancer patients. *Clin. Cancer Res.* **6**, 50–56.

64. Gu, J. J., Kawai, H., Nie, L. G., et al. (2002) Mutual dependence of MDM2 and MDMX in their functional inactivation of p53. *J. Biol. Chem.* **277**, 19,251–19,254.

65. Sjögren, S., Inganäs, M., Norberg, T., et al. (1996) The p53 gene in breast cancer: prognostic value of complementary DNA sequencing vs immunohistochemistry. *J. Natl. Cancer Inst.* **88**, 173–182.

66. Geisler, S., Lønning, P. E., Aas, T., et al. (2001) Influence of TP53 gene alterations and c-erbB-2 expression on the response to treatment with doxorubicin in locally advanced breast cancer. *Cancer Res.* **61**, 2505–2512.

67. Selivanova, G., Iotsova, V., Okan, I., et al. (1997) Restoration of the growth suppression function of mutant p53 by a synthetic peptide derived from the p53 C-terminal domain. *Nat. Med.* **3**, 632–638.

68. Soengas, M. S., Capodieci, P., Polsky, D., et al. (2001) Inactivation of the apoptosis effector apaf-1 in malignant melanoma. *Nature* **409**, 207–211.

69. Knudson, A. G. (1971) Mutation and cancer: statistical study of retinoblastoma. *Proc. Natl. Acad. Sci. USA* **68**, 820–823.

70. Flores, E. R., Tsai, K. Y., Crowley, D., et al. (2002) p63 and p73 are required for p53-dependent apoptosis in response to DNA damage. *Nature* **416**, 560–564.

71. Kannan, K., Amariglio, N., Rechavi, G., et al. (2001) DNA microarrays identification of primary and secondary target genes regulated by p53. *Oncogene* **20**, 2225–2234.

72. Lønning, P. E. (2004) Genes causing inherited cancer as beacons identifying the mechanisms of chemoresistance. *Trends Mol. Med.* **10**, 113–118.

73. Roth, J. A., Nguyen, D., Lawrence, D. D., et al. (1996) Retrovirus-mediated wild-type p53 gene transfer to tumors of patients with lung cancer. *Nat. Med.* **2**, 985–991.

74. Weill, D., Mack, M., Roth, J., et al. (2002) Adenoviral-mediated p53 gene transfer to non-small cell lung cancer through endobronchial injection. *Chest* **118**, 966–970.

75. Kawabe, S., Roth, J. A., Wilson, D. R., and Meyn, R. E. (2002) Adenovirus-mediated p16(INK4a) gene expression radiosensitizes non-small cell lung cancer cells in a p53-dependent manner. *Oncogene* **19**, 5359–5366.

76. Hussein, M. R., Haemel, A. K., and Wood, G. S. (2003) Apoptosis and melanoma: molecular mechanisms. *J. Pathol.* **199**, 275–288.

77. Tyner, S. D., Venkatachalam, S., Choi, J., et al. (2002) p53 mutant mice that display early ageing-associated phenotypes. *Nature* **415**, 45–53.

78. Slamon, D. J., Godolphin, W., Jones, L. A., et al. (1989) Studies of the HER-2/neu proto-oncogene in human breast and ovarian cancer. *Science* **244**, 707–712.

79. Kruger, S., Weitsch, G., Buttner, H., et al. (2002) Overexpression of c-erbB-2 oncoprotein in muscle-invasive bladder carcinoma: relationship with gene amplification, clinicopathological parameters and prognostic outcome. *Int. J. Oncol.* **21**, 981–987.

80. Shi, Y., Brands, F. H., Chatterjee, S., et al. (2001) HER-2/neu expression in prostate cancer: high level of expression associated with exposure to hormone therapy and androgen independent disease. *J. Urol.* **166**, 1514–1519.

81. Shackney, S. E., Smith, C. A., Pollice, A., et al. (1999) Genetic evolutionary staging of early non-small cell lung cancer: the p53 → Her-2/neu → ras sequence. *J. Thorac. Cardiovasc. Surg.* **118**, 259–267.

82. Ciardiello, F. and Tortora, G. (2002) Anti-epidermal growth factor receptor drugs in cancer therapy. *Exp. Opin. Investig. Drugs* **11**, 755–768.

83. Ferrero, J. M., Ramaioli, A., Largillier, R., et al. (2001) Epidermal growth factor receptor expression in 780 breast cancer patients: a reappraisal of the prognostic value based on an 8-year median follow-up. *Ann. Oncol.* **12**, 841–846.

84. Foekens, J. A., Portengen, H., Putten, W. L. J. V., et al. (1989) Prognostic value of receptors for insulin-like growth factor I, somatostatin, and epidermal growth factor in human breast cancer. *Cancer Res.* **49**, 7002–7009.

85. Slamon, D. J., Clark, G. M., Wong, S. G., Levin, W. J., Ullrich, A., and McGuire, W. L. (1987) Human breast cancer: correlation of relapse and survival with amplification of the HER-2/neu oncogene. *Science* **235**, 177–182.

86. Hähnel, R., Woodings, T., and Vivian, A. B. (1979) Prognostic value of estrogen receptors in primary breast cancer. *Cancer* **44**, 671–675.

87. Vollenweider-Zerargui, L., Barrelet, L., Wong, Y., Lemarchand-Béraud, T., and Gómez, F. (1986) The predictive value of estrogen and progesterone receptors' concentrations on the clinical behavior of breast cancer in women. Clinical correlation on 547 patients. *Cancer* **57**, 1171–1180.

88. Skinner, J. R., Wanebo, H. J., Betsill, W. L., Wilhelm, M. C., Drake, C. R., and Macleod, R. M. (1982) Evaluation of the pathologic and prognostic correlates of estrogen receptors in primary breast cancer. *Ann. Surg.* **196**, 636–641.

89. Thor, A. D., Berry, D. A., Budman, D. R., et al. (1998) erbB-2, p53, and efficacy of adjuvant therapy in lymph node-positive breast cancer. *J. Natl. Cancer Inst.* **90**, 1346–1360.

90. Cobleigh, M. A., Vogel, C. L., Tripathy, D., et al. (1999) Multinational study of the efficacy and safety of humanized anti-HER2 monoclonal antibody in women who have HER2-overexpressing metastatic breast cancer that has progressed after chemotherapy for metastatic disease. *J. Clin. Oncol.* **17**, 2639–2648.

91. Vogel, C., Cobleigh, M. A., Tripathy, D., et al. (2001) First-line, single-agent Herceptin® (Trastuzumab) in metastatic breast cancer: a preliminary report. *Eur. J. Cancer* **37**, S25–S29.

92. Baselga, J. (2000) Clinical trials of single-agent trastuzumab (Herceptin). *Semin. Oncol.* **27**, 20–26.

93. Slamon, D. J., LeylandJones, B., Shak, S., et al. (2001) Use of chemotherapy plus a monoclonal antibody against HER2 for metastatic breast cancer that overexpresses HER2. *N. Engl. J. Med.* **344**, 783–792.

94. Pegram, M. D., Finn, R. S., Arzoo, K., Beryt, M., Pietras, R. J., and Slamon, D. J. (1997) The effect of HER-2/neu overexpression on chemotherapeutic drug sensitivity in human breast and ovarian cancer cells. *Oncogene* **15**, 537–547.

95. Pegram, M., Hsu, S., Lewis, G., et al. (1999) Inhibitory effects of combinations of HER-2/neu antibody and chemotherapeutic agents used for treatment of human breast cancers. *Oncogene* **18**, 2241–2251.

96. Culy, C. R. and Faulds, D. (2002) Gefitinib. *Drugs* **62**, 2237–2248.

97. Salomon, D. S., Brandt, R., Ciardiello, F., and Normanno, N. (1995) Epidermal growth factor-related peptides and their receptors in human malignancies. *Crit. Rev. Oncol./Hematol.* **19**, 183–232.

98. Sainsbury, J. R., Farndon, J. R., Needham, G. K., Malcolm, A. J., and Harris, A. L. (1987) Epidermal-growth-factor receptor status as predictor of early recurrence of and death from breast cancer. *Lancet* **1**, 1398–1402.

99. Spyratos, F., Delarue, J. C., Andrieu, C., et al. (1990) Epidermal growth factor receptors and prognosis in primary breast cancer. *Breast Cancer Res.* **17**, 83–89.

100. Baselga, J., Rischin, D., Ranson, M., et al. (2002) Phase I safety, pharmacokinetic, and pharmacodynamic trial of ZD1839, a selective oral epidermal growth factor receptor tyrosine kinase inhibitor, in patients with five selected solid tumor types. *J. Clin. Oncol.* **20**, 4292–4302.

101. Burton, A. (2002) What went wrong with Iressa? *Lancet Oncol.* **3**, 708.

102. Macaulay, V. M. (1992) Insulin-like growth factors and cancer. *Br. J. Cancer* **65**, 311–320.

103. Helle, S. I. and Lønning, P. E. (1995) Insulin-like growth factors in breast and prostatic cancer. *Endocr. Relat. Cancer* **2**, 153–169.

104. Butt, A. J. and Williams, A. C. (2001) IGFBP-3 and apoptosis—a licence to kill? *Apoptosis* **6**, 199–205.

105. Hankinson, S. E., Willett, W. C., Colditz, G. A., et al. (1998) Circulating concentrations of insulin-like growth factor-I and risk of breast cancer. *Lancet* **351**, 1393–1396.

106. Canobbio, L., Cannata, D., Miglietta, L., and Boccardo, F. (1993) Somatuline and tamoxifen in postmenopausal breast cancer patients. *Ann. NY Acad. Sci.* **698**, 362–366.

107. Ingle, J. N., Suman, V. J., Kardinal, C. G., et al. (1999) A randomized trial of tamoxifen alone or combined with octreotide in the treatment of women with metastatic breast carcinoma. *Cancer* **85**, 1284–1292.

108. Helle, S. I., Geisler, J., Poulsen, J. P., et al. (1998) Microencapsulated octreotide pamoate in advanced breast cancer: a phase I study. *Br. J. Cancer* **78**, 14–20.

109. Cascinu, S., Ferro, E. D., and Catalano, G. (1995) A randomised trial of octreotide vs best supportive care only in advanced gastrointestinal cancer patients refractory to chemotherapy. *Br. J. Cancer* **71**, 97–101.

110. Zenobi, P. D., JaeggiGroisman, S. E., Riesen, W. F., Røder, M. E., and Froesch, E. R. (1992) Insulin-like growth factor-I improves glucose and lipid metabolism in type 2 diabetes mellitus. *J. Clin. Invest.* **90,** 2234–2241.

111. Zelent, A., Guidez, F., Melnick, A., Waxman, S., and Licht, J. D. (2001) Translocations of the RARa gene in acute promyelocytic leukemia. *Oncogene* **20,** 7186–7203.

112. Degos, L. and Wang, Z. Y. (2001) All *trans* retinoic acid in acute promyelocytic leukemia. *Oncogene* **20,** 7140–7145.

113. Rowley, J. D. (1973) New consistent chromosomal abnormality in chronic myelogenous leukemia identified by quinacrine fluorescence and giemsa staining. *Nature* **243,** 290–293.

114. Groffen, J., Stephenson, J. R., Heisterkamp, N., Deklein, A., Bartram, C. R., and Grosveld, G. (1984) Philadelphia chromosomal breakpoints are clustered within a limited region, Bcr, on chromosome-22. *Cell* **36,** 93–99.

115. Bartram, C. R., Deklein, A., Hagemeijer, A., et al. (1983) Translocation of C-Abl oncogene correlates with the presence of a Philadelphia-chromosome in chronic myelocytic-leukemia. *Nature* **306,** 277–280.

116. Shtivelman, E., Lifshitz, B., Gale, R. P., and Canaani, E. (1985) Fused transcript of Abl and Bcr genes in chronic myelogenous leukemia. *Nature* **315,** 550–554.

117. Heisterkamp, N., Stephenson, J. R., Groffen, J., et al. (1983) Localization of the C-Abl oncogene adjacent to a translocation break point in chronic myelocytic-leukemia. *Nature* **306,** 239–242.

118. Lugo, T. G., Pendergast, A. M., Muller, A. J., and Witte, O. N. (1990) Tyrosine kinase-activity and transformation potency of Bcr-Abl oncogene products. *Science* **247,** 1079–1082.

119. Buchdunger, E., Cioffi, C. L., Law, N., et al. (2000) Abl protein-tyrosine kinase inhibitor STI571 inhibits in vitro signal transduction mediated by c-Kit and platelet-derived growth factor receptors. *J. Pharmacol. Exp. Ther.* **295,** 139–145.

120. Heinrich, M. C., Griffith, D. J., Druker, B. J., Wait, C. L., Ott, K. A., and Zigler, A. J. (2000) Inhibition of c-kit receptor tyrosine kinase activity by STI 571, a selective tyrosine kinase inhibitor. *Blood* **96,** 925–932.

121. Hirota, S., Isozaki, K., Moriyama, Y., et al. (1998) Gain-of-function mutations of c-kit in human gastrointestinal stromal tumors. *Science* **279,** 577–580.

122. O'Brien, S. G., Guilhot, F., Larson, R. A., et al. (2003) Imatinib compared with interferon and low-dose cytarabine for newly diagnosed chronic-phase chronic myeloid leukemia. *N. Engl. J. Med.* **348,** 994–1004.

123. Joensuu, H., Fletcher, C., Dimitrijevic, S., Silberman, S., Roberts, P., and Demetri, G. (2002) Management of malignant gastrointestinal stromal tumours. *Lancet Oncol.* **3,** 655–664.

124. Friesel, R. E. and Maciag, T. (1995) Molecular mechanisms of angiogenesis: fibroblast growth factor signal transduction. *FASEB J.* **9,** 919–925.

125. Folkman, J. (1998) Antiangiogenic gene therapy. *Proc. Natl. Acad. Sci. USA* **95,** 9064–9066.

126. Straume, O., Chappuis, P. O., Salvesen, H. B., et al. (2002) Prognostic importance of glomeruloid microvascular proliferation indicates an aggressive angiogenic phenotype in human cancers. *Cancer Res.* **62,** 6808–6811.

127. Heise, C., Lemmon, M., and Kirn, D. (2000) Efficacy with a replication-selective adenovirus plus cisplatin-based chemotherapy: dependence on sequencing but not p53 functional status or route of administration. *Clin. Cancer Res.* **6,** 4908–4914.

128. Kirn, D. (2001) Clinical research results with dl1520 (ONYX-015), a replication-selective adenovirus for the treatment of cancer: what have we learned? *Gene Ther.* **8,** 89–98.

129. Khuri, F. R., Nemunaitis, J., Ganly, I., et al. (2000) A controlled trial of intratumoral ONYX-015, a selectively-replicating adenovirus, in combination with cisplatin and 5-fluorouracil in patients with recurrent head and neck cancer. *Nat. Med.* **6,** 879–885.

130. Lamont, J. P., Nemunaitis, J., Kuhn, J. A., Landers, S. A., and McCarty, T. M. (2000) A prospective phase II trial of ONYX-015 adenovirus and chemotherapy in recurrent squamous cell carcinoma of the head and neck (the Baylor experience). *Ann. Surg. Oncol.* **7,** 588–592.

131. Wen, S. F., Mahavni, V., Quijano, E., et al. (2003) Assessment of p53 gene transfer and biological activities in a clinical study of adenovirus-p53 gene therapy for recurrent ovarian cancer. *Cancer Gene Ther.* **10,** 224–238.

132. Freytag, S. O., Khil, M., Stricker, H., et al. (2002) Phase I study of replication-competent adenovirus-mediated double suicide gene therapy for the treatment of locally recurrent prostate cancer. *Cancer Res.* **62,** 4968–4976.

133. Reid, T., Galanis, E., Abbruzzese, J., et al. (2002) Hepatic arterial infusion of a replication-selective oncolytic adenovirus (dl1520): phase II viral, immunologic, and clinical endpoints. *Cancer Res.* **62,** 6070–6079.

134. Hecht, J. R., Bedford, R., Abbruzzese, J. L., et al. (2003) A phase I/II trial of intratumoral endoscopic ultrasound injection of ONYX-015 with intravenous gemcitabine in unresectable pancreatic carcinoma. *Clin. Cancer Res.* **9,** 555–561.

23
Radiosensitization by Gene Therapy

Steven J. Chmura, Michael Garofalo, and Ralph R. Weichselbaum

1. INTRODUCTION

1.1. Radiation Therapy: An Evolving, Technologically Driven Field

Since 1895, ionizing radiation (IR), delivered by either linear accelerators or brachytherapy implants, has been used to treat and cure numerous human malignancies (1,2). Advances in linear accelerator technology allow the delivery of radiation in the form of high-energy photons (X-rays) or charged particles (electrons). Although radiotherapy is used as a sole modality for cancer therapy in many malignancies, it is increasingly employed as part of a multimodality approach in cancer treatment. The balance between tumor cell killing and normal tissue toxicity defines the therapeutic ratio and ultimately limits the probability of cure.

Radiation therapy is normally given in small daily doses (1.8–2.0 Gy) over 6–7 weeks to cure epithelial tumors smaller than 1 cm. The tumorcidal doses of 65–70 Gy are delivered in a fractionated manner to reduce the normal tissue toxicity by taking advantage of the ability of nontumor tissues to repair themselves more efficiently than tumor cells. Efforts to improve radiotherapy primarily focus on (1) optimizing the delivery of IR through new advances in hardware and software technologies and (2) modifying the biological response of both normal and tumor tissues to IR. The utilization of gene therapy as part of the latter strategy is the focus of this chapter.

The addition of concurrent chemotherapy to IR has proven to have potent radiosensitizing effects in a number of cancer sites, including head and neck (3,4), cervix (5,6), and lung, with randomized studies demonstrating improvements in local tumor control and survival (7,8). Concern over normal tissue toxicity, following both dose escalation attempts and concurrent chemotherapy strategies, has prompted investigation into radioprotection agents (9). The aminothiol amifostine (Ethyol) reduces toxicity to normal tissues without altering the probability of cure with radiotherapy. Amifostine and similar agents are currently the subject of research and clinical trials. However, to develop more selective radiosensitizing strategies and improved radioprotection agents, understanding the basis of radiation-induced cell death in tumors and normal tissues is important.

1.2. IR-Induced Gene Expression and Cell Death

IR kills both tumor and normal tissues through several mechanisms. Tumor cell death is either postmitotic (necrotic) or apoptotic (10,11). IR interacts both directly with deoxyribonucleic acid (DNA) and indirectly through the hydrolysis of water and other cellular targets. Single- and double-stranded DNA breaks occur through both direct interaction with radiation and reactive oxygen intermediates, resulting in a host of transcriptional events that may alter the cell cycle, induce DNA repair, or trigger apoptosis (12,13). In addition to the effects of IR on DNA and transcriptional events, membrane-bound receptors or cellular membranes themselves initiate second-messenger cascades

From: *Contemporary Cancer Research*
Cancer Gene Therapy
Edited by: D. T. Curiel and J. T. Douglas © Humana Press Inc., Totowa, NJ

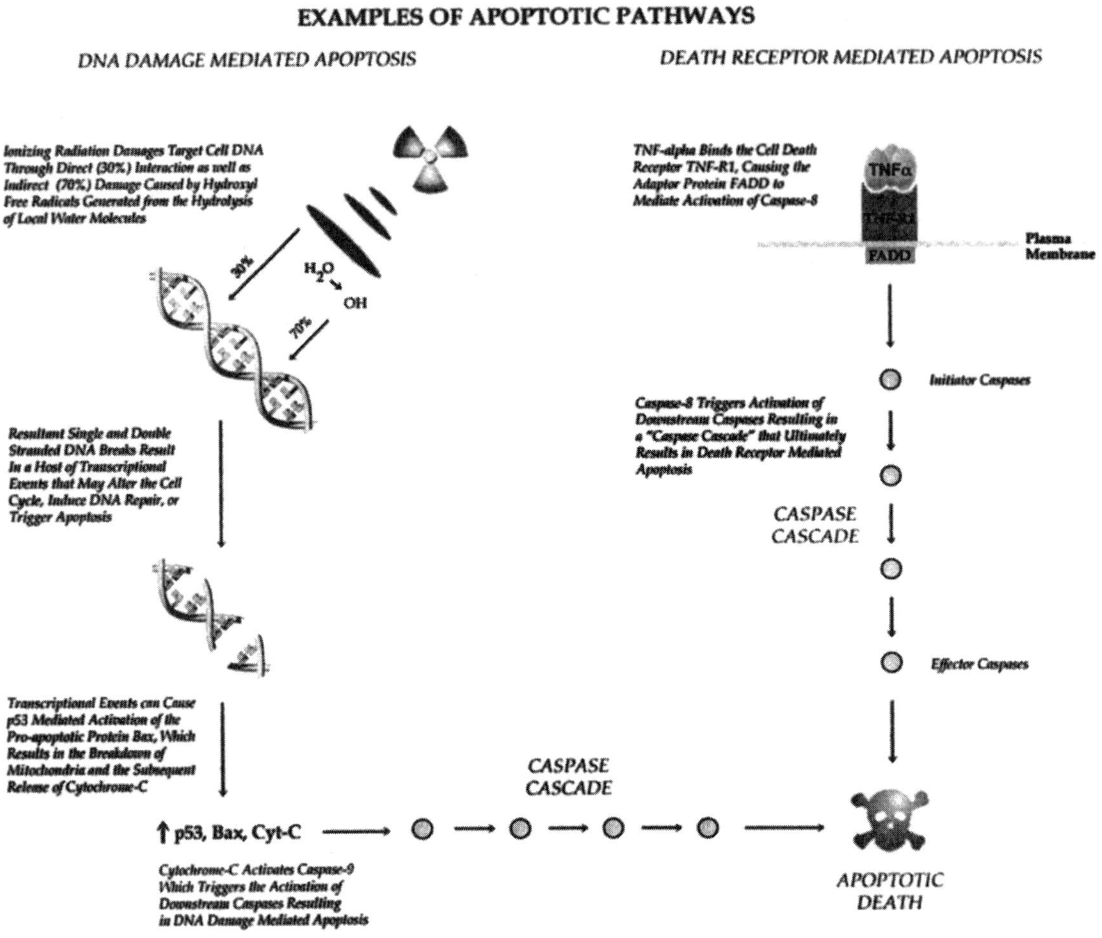

EXAMPLES OF APOPTOTIC PATHWAYS

DNA DAMAGE MEDIATED APOPTOSIS   *DEATH RECEPTOR MEDIATED APOPTOSIS*

Ionizing Radiation Damages Target Cell DNA Through Direct (30%) Interaction as well as Indirect (70%) Damage Caused by Hydroxyl Free Radicals Generated from the Hydrolysis of Local Water Molecules

TNF-alpha Binds the Cell Death Receptor TNF-R1, Causing the Adaptor Protein FADD to Mediate Activation of Caspase-8

TNFα

FADD

Plasma Membrane

Initiator Caspases

Resultant Single and Double Stranded DNA Breaks Result In a Host of Transcriptional Events that May Alter the Cell Cycle, Induce DNA Repair, or Trigger Apoptosis

Caspase-8 Triggers Activation of Downstream Caspases Resulting in a "Caspase Cascade" that Ultimately Results in Death Receptor Mediated Apoptosis

CASPASE CASCADE

Transcriptional Events can Cause p53 Mediated Activation of the Pro-apoptotic Protein Bax, Which Results in the Breakdown of Mitochondria and the Subsequent Release of Cytochrome-C

Effector Caspases

CASPASE CASCADE

↑ p53, Bax, Cyt-C ⟶ ○ ⟶ ○ ⟶ ○ ⟶ ○ ⟶

APOPTOTIC DEATH

Cytochrome-C Activates Caspase-9 Which Triggers the Activation of Downstream Caspases Resulting in DNA Damage Mediated Apoptosis

Fig. 1. Ionizing radiation initiates signal transduction.

that can mediate cell death *(14–17)*. IR initiates a cascade of second messengers through both direct DNA damage and the production of reactive oxygen intermediaries, which results in loss of reproductive integrity or apoptosis (Fig. 1).

1.3. A New Radiosensitizing Strategy: Enhancement of the Therapeutic Ratio Through Gene Therapy

Theoretical and experimental data exist to suggest that combining gene therapy with IR will improve clinical outcomes. First, both IR and gene therapy can target different, partially nonoverlapping mechanisms of tumor cell killing and normal cell toxicity. Second, gene therapy strategies combined with IR have been shown to radiosensitize tumor cells in vitro and in vivo *(18–26)*. Third, IR increases the transduction and expression of foreign genes following delivery with viral or nonviral vectors *(27,28)*. Transduction and expression of foreign genes in tumors remain a substantial obstacle to gene therapy strategies. Finally, radiation may enhance the "bystander effect" of specific gene therapy strategies, decreasing the need to transduce a large percentage of tumor cells *(29–32)*. For example, in vitro and in vivo data demonstrated that tumor cells expressing the foreign gene herpes simplex virus thymidine kinase (HSV-tk) treated with ganciclovir (GCV) transmit their toxicity to adjacent cells (which have not been transduced with HSV-tk). Therefore, the bystander effect may substantially improve the therapeutic ratio despite the fact that only a limited number of tumor cells are directly transduced.

This chapter reviews strategies that combine radiation therapy and gene therapy in an attempt to improve tumor cell killing while minimizing normal tissue toxicity. Strategies by which gene therapy has been shown to improve IR-induced tumor cell killing include (1) replacement of known mutated or deleted genes such as p53 that IR-induced tumor cell death; (2) delivery of genes encoding prodrug-converting enzymes into tumors, permitting accumulation of active toxic antitumor agents in the tumor bed while potentially minimizing systemic toxicity; (3) construction of genetically engineered viruses with therapeutic genes under the control of radiation-inducible promoters; and (4) IR enhancement of replication-competent viruses that proliferate preferentially in tumor cells following IR.

2. VIRAL VECTORS THAT DELIVER EXOGENOUS GENES

2.1. Gene Delivery Systems Employed With IR

Both viral and nonviral vectors have been employed in combination with radiation therapy *(33–35)*. Further, either replication-competent or replication-incompetent viral vectors are highly efficient at delivering therapeutic genes to tumor cells. The most commonly studied replication-deficient viral vector to date with radiotherapy in preclinical or phase I//II trials is adenovirus. Adenovirus is utilized because of its ability to transfect tumor cells independent of cell proliferation, to accommodate large inserts, and to be produced and stored efficiently. Replication-incompetent retroviral vectors have also been employed to transfect proliferating tumor cells in preclinical experiments with IR.

Replication-competent herpes simplex virus 1 (HSV-1) and adenovirus, in combination with radiotherapy, are used in clinical trials. In contrast to IR-induced cell death that results from either apoptosis or necrosis, viral replication results in oncolysis. By exploiting the nonoverlapping mechanisms of tumor cell death by IR and replication-competent viruses, the therapeutic ratio may be improved. Cell-based delivery systems have also been employed in clinical trials in combination with radiotherapy *(36,37)* with IR. Nonviral gene delivery methods employing cationic lipids complexed to DNA have been used in preclinical studies with IR *(38,39)*. The following sections highlight the vector systems currently employed to enhance the efficacy of IR.

2.2. Viral Vectors Deliver Wild-Type p53 to Tumor Cells: Gene Replacement Therapy That Enhances IR-Induced Tumor Cell Killing

Although gene replacement strategies using viral or nonviral vectors were originally envisioned to correct single gene defects in nonmalignant diseases, this strategy has evolved to treat malignant diseases as a single or multimodality approach. One of the most commonly mutated genes in human tumors is p53 *(40)*. Wild-type p53 function is involved in the cellular response to DNA-damaging events following IR or chemotherapy treatment. After treatment of tumor cells with IR, p53 promotes cell cycle arrest, initiation and transcription of DNA repair complexes, and the induction of apoptosis *(41,42)*. For example, DNA damage following IR promotes p53-dependent transcription of *p21* and arrest of cells at the G1 checkpoint *(43)*. Loss of this checkpoint has been associated with decreased tumor cell apoptosis and clinical response to IR *(44)*. DNA repair complex formation is also dependent, in part, on functional p53 in association with proliferating cell nuclear antigen, DNA-dependent protein kinase , and GADD45 *(45,46)*. Taken together, these data suggest that the restoration of wild-type p53 function within tumor cells may increase the clinical efficacy of DNA-damaging agents, including IR.

Spitz et al. demonstrated that the loss of the apoptotic response to IR could be restored by adenoviral delivery of p53 under the constitutive promoter cytomegalovirus (Ad.p53) in vitro *(47)*. The replication-defective adenovirus Ad.p53 sensitized the relatively radioresistant p53–/– SW620 colorectal cells in vitro with a 2-Gy dose, increasing the apoptotic fraction of cells. This synergistic in vitro enhancement of apoptosis resulted in improved tumor control in vivo, with tumor regrowth prolonged 2 days with 5 Gy of IR alone to 37 days in the group with combined Ad.p53 and 5 Gy *(47)*. The increase in tumor cell killing occurs through both restoration of the apoptotic response to IR and an increase in postmitotic death. These in vitro studies demonstrated that adenoviral delivery of wild-type p53 sensitized normally radioresistant cells and increased cell killing *(48–51)*.

Kawabe et al. reported that wild-type p53 would preferentially radiosensitize non-small cell lung carcinoma (NSCLC) cells compared to normal lung fibroblast cells in vitro *(51)*. Both p53+/+ and p53–/– tumor cells were sensitized, suggesting selective radiosensitization of the tumor cells compared to normal tissue irrespective of wild-type p53 expression. Similar results were seen in vivo employing prostate model systems *(52)* and in lung model systems *(53)*. Taken together, these in vivo studies using p53 gene replacement demonstrated selective radiosensitization of tumor cells compared to normal tissues and provided the basis for the human phase I/II clinical trials.

Phase I trials have demonstrated the feasibility and safety of delivering adenoviral vectors expressing p53 through repeated intratumoral injections *(49,54–56)*. Preliminary trials in NSCLC demonstrated that p53 replacement can be safely administered with a low probability of toxicity. There is also some evidence of antitumoral activity at the tumor site. The efficacy of p53 replacement therapy coupled with standard radiation therapy in NSCLC is currently in clinical trials.

2.3. Replication-Deficient Vectors Deliver Suicide Genes to Tumors That Enhance IR-Mediated Killing

Although the replacement of functionally deleted tumor suppressor genes such as p53 radiosensitizes tumor cells, this approach requires that a large percentage of tumor cells express the replacement gene to achieve a significant clinical effect. Given the relatively inefficient delivery systems available to deliver genes to tumor cells in vivo, most current therapeutic strategies attempt to transfect or transduce a few tumor cells in the hope that the gene products will radiosensitize a large number of adjacent cells through a bystander effect. Therapeutically effective converting enzyme/prodrug strategies have been identified *(57,58)*. The enzymes typically employed are nonmammalian genes isolated from viruses or bacteria that convert a systemically administered inactive prodrug to a toxic antimetabolite. Studies with IR have typically delivered the genes through adenoviral vectors or cell-based systems. By delivering a gene encoding the enzyme directly into the tumor bed, intratumoral and intracellular concentrations of the active metabolite will be increased only in the tumor bed, thereby decreasing the risk of systemic toxicity.

The two most commonly employed prodrug-converting enzymes in cancer therapy are HSV-tk and cytosine deaminase (CD). HSV-tk transfected into tumor cells converts the antiherpetic prodrugs GCV *(59)* or 5-(2-bromovinyl)-2'-deoxyuridine (BVdU) *(22)* into cytotoxic molecules. Both GCV and BVdU are nucleoside analogs that, following phosphorylation by HSV-tk, are further phosphorylated by cellular kinases to molecules that interfere with DNA replication. Pyrimidine analogs incorporated into the DNA of cycling tumor cells have been shown in vitro and in vivo to act as radiosensitizing agents, although clinical trials of these compounds delivered systemically have been disappointing *(60–62)*.

In an analogous strategy to the use of HSV-tk/GCV, the prodrug 5-fluorocytosine (5-FC) is converted by the bacterial protein CD to 5-fluorouracil (5-FU) *(63)*. Through inhibition of thymidylate synthase and incorporation into ribonucleic acid (RNA), DNA replication and protein translation are disrupted, enhancing the cytotoxicty of IR *(64–66)*. 5-FU acts as a radiosensitizer and enhances the efficacy of radiotherapy in head and neck, gastrointestinal, and gynecological malignancies *(64,67)*. By selectively increasing the intratumoral concentration of 5-FU and reducing the extratumoral concentration compared to standard systemic delivery, the severe clinical toxicities of mucositis, diarrhea, and myelosuppression may be reduced.

2.4. HSV-tk and GCV Radiosensitize Tumor Cells In Vitro and In Vivo

Animal models have shown that xenografts transduced with HSV-tk and treated with systemic BVdU or GCV in combination with IR demonstrated a two- to threefold increase in survival compared with mice treated with IR alone *(68,69)*. Chhikara et al. employed a replication-deficient adenovirus carrying HSV-tk to a mouse orthotopic prostate cancer model system to assess the potential additive benefit to IR on both local control and systemic antitumor activity *(59)*. Tumor cells (RM-1) were injected both subcutaneously and into the tail vein on the same day. Mice were treated with an intratumoral injection of adenovirus-HSV-tk (Ad.tk) once per week, followed by systemic GCV and IR, which resulted in growth delay and an increase in mean survival when compared to animals treated with IR alone. In addition to increased tumor cell killing locally, systemic antitumor activity was demonstrated, with the number of lung nodule metastasis reduced by 50%. Statistically significant increases in $CD4^+$ and $CD8^+$ cells were observed in the combined arm compared to the IR-alone arm. These data suggested that suicide gene therapy techniques may potentiate the cytotoxic effects of radiation and minimize the toxicity to tissue not infected by the vector; this ultimately led to phase I clinical trials.

The reduction in tumor size and increase in the survival of animals with tumors treated with the combination of HSV-tk/prodrug and IR is achieved despite transduction of only a fraction of the tumor cell population. Experimental evidence demonstrated that a bystander effect appears to play a significant role in the efficacy of this approach *(70,71)*. Data showed that the phosphorylated GCV nucleotides diffuse into surrounding tumor cells through gap junction channels formed by connexins not transduced with the virus *(32,72)*. Dying tumor cells may also secrete interleukin-1 and interleukin-6, which may further enhance the effects of IR.

The induction of apoptosis in neighboring cells may be the largest contributor to the bystander effect. GCV treatment of HSV-tk-transduced cells increases cell surface expression of CD95 and tumor necrosis factor (TNF) receptor, leading to death domain formations and ultimately caspase activation. The induction of apoptosis in the transduced cells appears to propagate signals to the neighboring cells, causing caspase activation *(73,74)*. When combined with IR, the bystander effect has been demonstrated in vitro to account for some of the increased cytotoxicity *(75–77)*.

A phase I trial was performed in patients with locally recurrent prostate cancer who had previously received definitive radiotherapy *(78)*. The Ad.tk vector was injected into the prostate under transrectal ultrasound guidance. Systemic GCV administration followed. With escalating viral doses from 1×10^8 to 1×10^{11} infectious units, 2/18 patients developed grade 3 or 4 toxicity, and cultures from blood and urine were negative for adenovirus, demonstrating the safety of the virus.

A second phase I/II trial is ongoing, combining IR (with or without hormonal ablation) with Ad.tk, followed by oral valacyclovir instead of GCV *(77)*. The first Ad.tk was injected 48 hours prior to the start of radiotherapy, and the second was administered 48 hours after the first treatment. With a reported median follow-up of 10 months, 15/45 patients developed flulike symptoms after the Ad.tk injection. One patient developed grade 3 liver enzyme elevations. No grade 3 or above gastrointestinal toxicity occurred. Although the follow-up time is too short to assess efficacy, initial serum prostate-specific antigen (PSA) levels dropped in all but 1 patient, suggesting that Ad.tk combined with radiotherapy is a safe strategy to enhance the efficacy of radiotherapy in patients with prostate cancer.

Rainov conducted the first phase III multicenter randomized study in 248 patients with primary glialblastoma multiforme who underwent aggressive surgical resection followed by randomization to conformal radiotherapy alone or combined with retroviral-mediated delivery of the HSV-tk gene into the tumor bed and/or remaining gross tumor *(79)*. Glialblastoma multiforme is almost universally fatal, with a median survival of 8–10 months despite aggressive surgical resection and adjuvant radiotherapy. For patients randomly assigned to receive gene therapy, vector-producing fibroblasts were injected that released replication-deficient retroviral vectors to neighboring cells along the needle track. Systemic delivery of GCV was given to the arm receiving the gene therapy. With median survival and overall survival as the end points, no significant differences were observed in the two study arms. Median survival was 1 year, and 1 year overall survival was approximately 50% in both arms. Despite the lack of clinical improvement, further studies demonstrated improved systemic immune responses in the arm receiving gene therapy *(37)*. Improvements in transduction efficiency, prodrug transcription, and noninvasive in vivo assessment of tumor responses hold significant promise.

2.5. CD Increases Intratumoral Concentrations of 5-FU and Radiosensitizes Tumor Cells

In vitro studies demonstrated that transfection of CD into tumor cells followed by 5-FC treatment radiosensitizes human tumor cells *(64,65)*. Hanna et al. employed a replication-defective adenovirus that expressed CD/5-FC (Ad.CD) injected four times throughout the treatment directly into xenograft-bearing mice. 5-FC was given daily with IR (5-Gy fractions/50 Gy total), improving both growth delay and tumor regression compared to IR alone *(80)*. Rogulski et al. constructed a replication-deficient retrovirus expressing both HSV-tk and CD *(81)*. Gliosarcoma cells were infected with this CD/HSV-1 TK fusion gene and grown as xenografts in mice. 5-FC and GCV were administered systemically and potentiated the antitumor effects of IR significantly more then either prodrug strategy alone. As seen with HSV-tk/prodrug strategies, a significant bystander effect existed when combined with IR *(82–84)*. Taken together, these preclinical studies using animal models demonstrated improved growth delay and tumor regression when CD was combined with IR compared with IR alone.

Freytag et al. constructed a replication-competent adenovirus capable of delivering both HSV-tk and CD (Ad5-CD/TKrep) *(85)*. Ad5-CD/TKrep adenovirus was injected directly into the prostate of male mice. 5-FC and GCV were delivered systemically for 4 weeks combined with 56 Gy of IR to the prostate. The combination of Ad5-CD/TKrep with IR increased tumor growth delay twofold compared with IR alone. The trimodality treatment arm demonstrated a 25–40% tumor cure rate compared with 0% for IR alone. A significant reduction in retroperitoneal lymph node metastases was also noted at 3 months. Detailed histological evaluation of the surrounding normal tissues revealed no difference in the combined-modality groups compared with the IR-alone group, suggesting that this approach significantly improved the therapeutic ratio of IR. Based on these results, phase I studies to assess toxicity in humans are planned *(85)*.

3. IR CONTROLS THE EXPRESSION OF HETEROLOGOUS GENES THROUGH RADIATION-INDUCIBLE PROMOTERS

3.1. Immediate Early Genes Are Induced by IR

The immediate early genes c-Jun and Egr-1 have been implicated as effectors of the cellular response to IR *(86)*. The identification of genes induced by IR has allowed the engineering of viral vectors capable of delivering therapeutic genes under the control of radiation-inducible promoters. Characterization of the Egr-1 promoter sequence identified an AT-rich region localized between cytosines and guanines [CC(A+T)GG] *(87–89)*. This region, the CArG element, was initially identified as IR inducible using chloramphenicol acetyl transferase reporter gene constructs *(90–92)*. Subsequent studies suggested that the activation of Egr-1 transcription was dependent on the formation of oxygen radical intermediates produced following IR and other DNA-damaging agents *(93)*. In addition, a bystander effect has also been reported by which irradiated cells secrete a diffusible factor into culture media, further enhancing the IR inducibility of the promoter *(94)*. These studies demonstrated that, following IR, cellular kinases modify transcription factors in the absence of protein synthesis, permitting binding of these factors to elements in the promoter/enhancer region of Egr-1 *(95–97)*. The widespread availability of complementary DNA microarray technology has expanded this list of IR-induced genes *(98–100)*.

3.2. TNF-α Enhances the Cytotoxic Effects of Radiotherapy
Under the Control of a Radiation-Inducible Promoter

After characterizing the radiation-responsive elements in the Egr-1 promoter region, Weichselbaum and colleagues developed a strategy aimed at cloning radiation-responsive elements upstream of potentially radiosensitizing genes and packaging them into a delivery vehicle permitting IR to induce localized transcription of the therapeutic gene *(101–103)*. TNF-α was selected as a prototypic therapeutic gene for this approach because of its previously documented spectrum of antitumor effects, including the direct induction of tumor cell apoptosis *(17)*, improvement in the systemic immunologic response to the tumor *(104,105)*, and antiangiogenic properties *(106)*.

TNF-α is a trimeric cytokine that belongs to a superfamily of genes that includes FAS, TRAIL, and CD40 ligand. The molecular mechanisms that promote cell death following TNF-α binding are now well understood. Briefly, TNF-α binds to multiple membrane receptors, including TNF-R1 and TNF-R2 *(17)*. TNF-R1 promotes the formation of the intracellular adaptors TRADD and FADD. Association of these death domains causes activation of caspases 8 and ultimately caspase 3-activating complex in both a cytochrome-*c*-dependent and -independent manner, leading to tumor cell apoptosis. However, TNF-R1 may also inhibit an apoptotic response through TRADD association with TRAF-2, which promotes activation of the transcription factors NF-κB and JNK *(107,108)*. These studies suggest that TNF-α promotes both a cell death and a proliferative response.

TNF-α enhances IR-mediated cell death in multiple tumor cell lines and in animal model systems *(101,109)*. In animal models, systemic treatment with TNF-α produces an antitumor effect, with histological studies demonstrating hemorrhagic necrosis and apoptosis *(110)*. Studies demonstrated the antitumor effects of TNF-α also involve preferential destruction of tumor microvasculature *(24,26,111)*. Based on the known single-agent activity of TNF-α and its enhancement of IR-mediated cell death, a phase I clinical trial delivered TNF-α intravenously while irradiating the tumor *(112)*. Although tumor responses were recorded, the intravenously delivered TNF-α produced fatigue, nausea, and hypotension, proving clinical intolerability for patients.

3.3. Spatial and Temporal Control
of Gene Expression With Radiation-Inducible Gene Therapy

To limit the systemic toxicity of TNF-α and increase the local tumor concentration of the cytokine, a replication-defective adenoviral vector was constructed linking the Egr-1 radiation-inducible promoter to the TNF-α gene (Ad.EGR.TNF-α). The Ad.EGR.TNF-α vector was directly injected into relatively radioresistant human epidermoid carcinoma xenografts (SQ-20B) grown in athymic nude mice *(25)*. Four intratumoral injections of Ad.EGR.TNF-α combined with a clinically relevant dose of fractionated IR (50 Gy in 5-Gy fractions) greatly increased the tumorcidal effects of IR, producing not only significant reduction in tumor volume compared to the radiation-alone group of animals, but also an increase in the number of tumors cured (Fig. 2). Twenty-one days into the fractionation scheme, an 8-fold increase in TNF-α protein levels was observed in the combined-treatment (Ad.Egr.TNF and IR) arm when compared to virus alone, demonstrating that the adenoviral vector was induced in vivo by exposure to IR. In addition, preclinical studies with dose levels proposed for clinical trials (4×10^9 and 4×10^{10} particle units [pu]) demonstrated TNF-α protein levels from tumor homogenates were approx 12-fold higher in the Ad.Egr.TNF/IR-treated animals compared to animals treated with IR alone at day 28 *(113)*.

Histologic studies of the SQ-20B xenografts following treatment with Ad.Egr.TNF and IR demonstrated intratumoral vascular thrombosis; adjacent vessels in normal tissues remained patent *(24, 114)*. Toxicity surrounding the tumor was similar to that observed in the IR-alone treated group, suggesting a favorable increase in the therapeutic ratio. Similar results were observed in other experimental

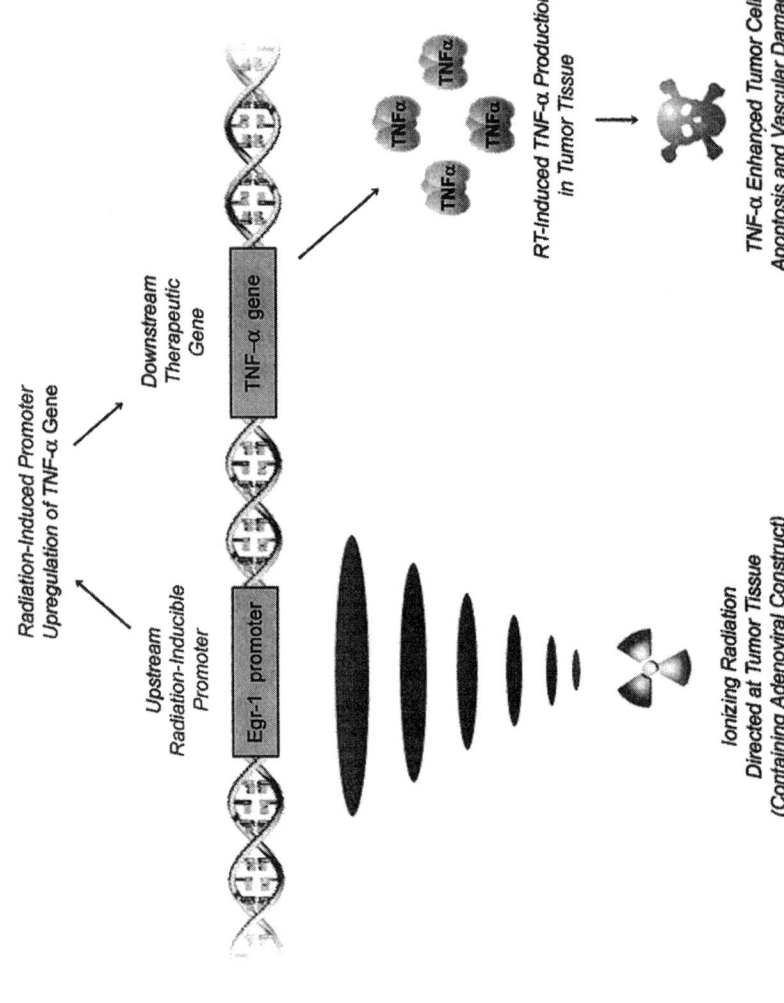

Fig. 2. Ionizing radiation induces expression of the therapeutic gene TNF-α.

animal models *(24,115,116)* and in response to DNA-damaging agents such as cisplatin *(117)*. These in vivo studies prompted phase I/II clinical trials.

The first phase I study using the Ad.Egr.TNF virus, TNFerade (GenVec) identified the maximum tolerated dose of TNFerade with daily fractionated radiotherapy in 21 patients with a wide range of solid tumors, including those of the breast, pancreas, and lung and melanoma *(118)*. TNFerade was delivered via intratumoral injections (4×10^7 to 4×10^{11} pu) eight times over the course of radiation (30–70 Gy). Plasma levels of TNF-α were less than 25 pg/mL in all patients, with no virus found in the blood or urine. No serious adverse events were reported at these doses of TNFerade. Most patients experienced NCI grade 1–2 toxicities, including fever, pain at the injection site, chills, and fatigue. Clinical complete or partial responses were demonstrated in 11/21 patients, with only 1 patient showing disease progression. Objective responses were increased in the higher dose groups, with all four complete responses reported in patients receiving $4 \times 10^{9.5}$ pu or higher.

A second phase I study was reported in patients with large-extremity soft tissue sarcomas *(119)*. TNFerade at 4×10^9 to 4×10^{11} pu was injected intratumorally twice weekly for the first week and then once per week for the remaining 4 weeks of radiotherapy. The concomitant radiation schedule was a standard preoperative dose of IR (50 Gy in 2-Gy daily fractions). Of 11 patients at the time of surgery, 10 (91%) showed a pathological complete or partial response to the combined treatment. The systemic effects of treatment were minimal. Most patients experienced flulike symptoms that improved with acetaminophen. TNF-α was not increased systemically in patients. Current clinical studies include an ongoing 17-center phase IIb randomized clinical trial of TNFerade as a first-line therapy with end points assessing overall survival, quality of life, and pathological response compared with conventional therapy.

4. REPLICATION-COMPETENT VIRUSES ENHANCE THE THERAPEUTIC RATIO OF IR

4.1. Herpes Simplex Virus 1 Alters the Cellular Context to Enhance Tumor Cell Killing

One example of an attenuated virus that has been shown to possess single-agent antitumor activity and enhance IR is HSV-1. HSV-1 is a 152-kb double-stranded DNA virus that encodes multiple proteins during its viral life cycle and produces severe clinical syndromes in an infected host. Following infection of the host through mucosal tissue, HSV-1 infects sensory neurons, replicates, and is transported to the nucleus of the neuron, in which the virus may remain quiescent for a time or replicate, lysing the neuron and producing clinical symptoms. Detailed analysis of these proteins and their function has allowed the development of attenuated, yet replication-competent, HSV-1 viruses that preferentially replicate in tumor cells (oncolysis) and further infect nearby tumor cells.

To decrease neurovirulence and permit the clinical application of HSV-1, various mutants have been engineered. The herpes gene $\gamma_1 34.5$ functionally suppresses the attempt of the host cell to terminate protein synthesis following viral infection and is a significant contributor to neurovirulence in the central nervous system (CNS). HSV-1 with deletion of both copies of the $\gamma_1 34.5$ gene (R3616) has significantly reduced neurovirulence compared to wild-type HSV-1. Animal studies demonstrated that the median lethal dose in mice infected with wild-type HSV vs R3616 is reduced from 10^2 pfu to 10^7 pfu, respectively *(120)*.

A second HSV-1 mutant (G207) is deleted in both copies of $\gamma_1 34.5$ possesses a mutation in the large subunit of ribonucleotide reductase. The dual deletion of $\gamma_1 34.5$ decreases the neurovirulence similar to that of R3616. The functional deletion of ribonucleoside reductase further restricts viral replication to proliferating tumor cells *(121,122)*. G207 has been demonstrated to be safe during intracerebral inoculations in both monkeys and humans at doses as high as 3×10^9 pfu *(122)*.

A third attenuated HSV-1 (R7020) is deleted in a single copies of $\gamma_1 34.5$, TK, and the internal repeat region (U_L). R7020 was engineered to express genes encoding HSV-2 glycoproteins to be used as a vaccine against HSV-1 and HSV-2. Despite retaining a functional copy of $\gamma_1 34.5$, it appears to be safe for non-CNS tumors, as demonstrated by both animal and human studies *(123,124)*. Studies comparing viral proliferation of R3616 and R7020 in experimental tumor systems demonstrated that R7020 is recovered 25-fold more from tumors inoculated with R7020 compared to R3616, suggesting that R7020 is a potent antitumor agent for non-CNS tumors *(124)*.

When injected into human tumor xenografts, the attenuated HSV-1 strains R3616 or G207 result in tumor growth delay. Combining radiotherapy with R3616, G207, or R7020 demonstrated a significant enhancement of the antitumor effects of radiation across a wide range of cell lines and tumor xenografts *(121,124,125)*. The combination of IR with attenuated virus resulted in recovery of 5- to 62-fold more viral particles compared to nonirradiated tumors *(124,126)*. Bradley et al. demonstrated that, in addition to improved xenograft tumor response to IR, mice bearing intracranial high-grade gliomas (U87 xenografts) inoculated with R3616 prior to standard fractionated IR demonstrated a significant improvement in overall survival compared with IR or virus alone *(127)*. The direct intracranial injection of the virus resulted in increased tumor control without evidence of increased CNS toxicity, suggesting that a true gain in the therapeutic ratio had been realized.

The mechanism by which IR increases R3616 or R7020 replication is currently under investigation. The stress response of the host cell to IR may contribute to and compliment replication of the attenuated virus in irradiated tissues. The safety of attenuated viruses in humans has recently been demonstrated. Two phase I studies have been performed with attenuated HSV variants, and there were no adverse events reported *(122,128)*. Phase I trials are beginning to characterize the safety and efficacy of a dual-modality approach combining HSV-1 (R3616) with radiotherapy (Fig. 3).

4.2. Replication-Competent Adenovirus Targets Prostate Cancer Cells and Enhances Radiotherapy

PSA is produced by both normal prostate cells, and its expression is greatly increased in patients with prostate cancer. Rodriguez et al. *(129)* constructed an attenuated, but replication-competent. adenovirus (CV706) that would preferentially replicate in PSA-producing cells. The prostate-specific enhancer element was inserted upstream of the E1A gene. In vitro studies confirmed the selective replication in PSA-producing cell lines. CV706 was effective in curing LNCaP xenograft tumors with a single intratumoral injection using 5×10^8 particles/mm^3. Using LNCaP xenografts, a single injection of CV706 combined with 10 Gy of IR was compared to IR alone and demonstrated a 6.7-fold greater antitumor effect than either therapy alone. Tumor cell necrosis and apoptosis was increased by 6- to 8-fold in the animals treated with the combined therapy. The tumor microvasculature was also decreased 12-fold in the combined group. No adverse toxicity was seen in the animals or in detailed pathological studies. These data demonstrated that CV706 acts synergistically with IR, enhancing tumor curability, and could be safely administered in the preclinical setting.

Twenty patients were enrolled in the initial phase I study. CV706 was delivered via ultrasound-guided transperineal technique in a dose escalation study from 1×10^{11} to 1×10^{13} viral particles. Of 20 patients, 15 experienced grade 2 or less fever 3–8 hours following vector injection. Patients were treated with fractionated radiotherapy to a mean dose of 68.4 Gy. With 41 months of mean follow-up data, no grade 3 or 4 toxicity was reported. Posttreatment prostatic biopsies on days 4 and 22 confirmed intraprostatic replication of CV706. Antibody titers against CV706 increased in all patients following treatment, and peak serum levels of CV706 occurred 30 minutes after injection and remained low throughout the course of treatment. All patients achieved a PSA reduction of at least 50%, and there appeared to be improved PSA response at the highest viral dose, suggesting a viral dose–response relationship. These data demonstrated that CV706 can be safely combined with IR as a neoadjuvant treatment in prostate cancer. Current clinical trials are ongoing to assess its efficacy compared to conventional radiotherapy.

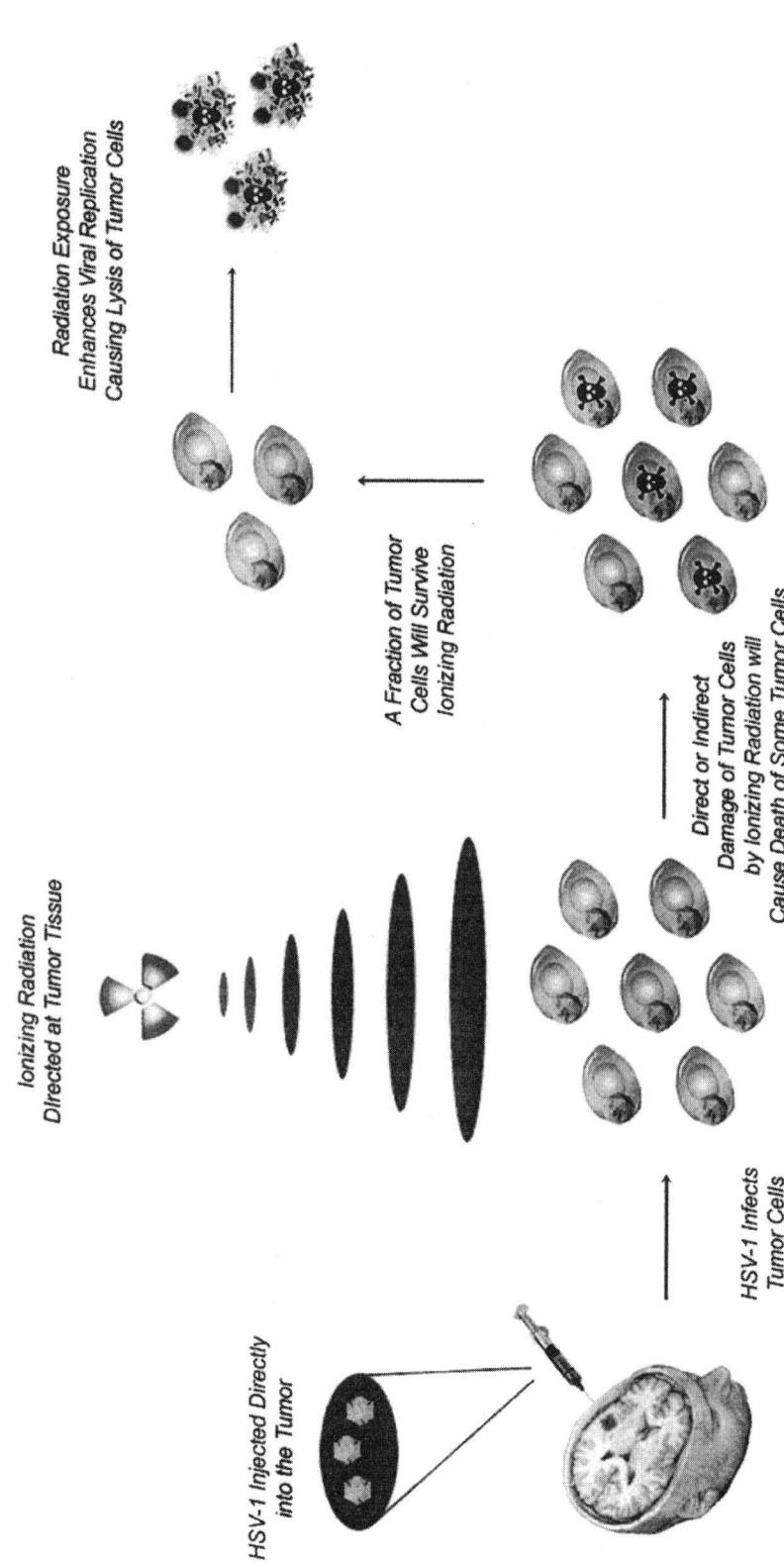

Fig. 3. Ionizing radiation increase attenuated HSV-1 viral proliferation in radioresistant tumor populations.

HSV-1 Injected Directly into the Tumor

Ionizing Radiation Directed at Tumor Tissue

Radiation Exposure Enhances Viral Replication Causing Lysis of Tumor Cells

A Fraction of Tumor Cells Will Survive Ionizing Radiation

Direct or Indirect Damage of Tumor Cells by Ionizing Radiation will Cause Death of Some Tumor Cells

HSV-1 Infects Tumor Cells

4.3. ONYX-015: *Selective Viral Replication Oncolysis* (129)

The replication-competent ONYX-015 adenovirus is well studied and is the subject of ongoing clinical trials *(130)*. Previous efforts to understand the early genes involved in human adenoviral replication demonstrated that the E1B gene encodes a 55-kDa protein that binds and suppresses wild-type p53 gene function *(131,132)*. Bischoff et al. initially demonstrated that an E1B-deleted human adenovirus mutant can preferentially replicate in and lyse p53-deficient human tumor cells *(130)*. Cells with wild-type p53, however, were spared from the viral oncolysis unless E1B was ectopically expressed. Because p53 is mutated in over 50% of human tumors, but not in normal surrounding tissues, ONYX-015 would theoretically continue to replicate throughout the tumor, destroying the p53-mutated tumor cells. Within normal tissue surrounding the tumor, viral replication would be abrogated by the functional p53 of the normal tissue. Given this approach, significant therapeutic gain could be achieved with the virus either alone or in combination with standard chemotherapy or radiotherapy.

Preclinical studies employing xenograft models demonstrated the antitumor effect of ONYX-015 *(133)*. Studies further demonstrated its significant radiosensitizing effects in animal models with multiple tumor types *(134,135)*. Current clinical trials in head and neck and ovarian cancers show encouraging tumor responses and minimal resultant toxicity when infected with ONYX-015.

Despite the promising preclinical data and current phase II/III studies under way, the selectivity of ONYX-015 for p53-mutated cells has recently been called into question *(136–139)*. Although the original studies suggested functional p53 would inhibit viral replication and oncolysis, studies suggested that other genes may be responsible for this inhibition. For example, loss of p14(ARF) disrupted the p53 signaling pathway and permitted ONYX-015 to kill multiple cell lines expressing wild-type p53 *(139,140)*. Further studies have suggested its oncolytic effects may be suppressed in multiple other cell types that express wild-type p53. Despite these in vitro findings, multiple studies have demonstrated the clinical safety and efficacy of this virus *(141–144)*. Clinical studies are also under way combining ONYX-015 with standard chemotherapy and radiation therapy *(143,145,146)*.

5. FUTURE DIRECTIONS

The gene therapy strategies discussed in this chapter rely on either direct intratumoral injection of the vector into the tumor prior to radiotherapy, or injection of the vector into the tumor bed during the time of surgical resection or biopsy. For example, the TNFerade trials for extremity sarcomas deliver the vector through multiple injection sites along the clinically palpable tumor mass. Alternatively, a computerized tomographic or ultrasound-guided approach is employed when injecting the vector into pancreatic tumors. This reliance on direct tumor injection limits the number of potential tumor sites that may be treated with the vector to clinically accessible primary tumors. In addition, the relatively low efficiency of gene transfer results not only in few tumor cells expressing the therapeutic gene, but also poor distribution of the gene throughout the tumor.

Modification of vector particles to bind and fuse with target tissue selectively may improve on nontargeted vectors currently employed in clinical trials. A targeted vector would simplify delivery through systemic administration, reduce immunogenicity, and potentially improve the distribution of the vector throughout the tumor. Although tissue-specific targeting of replication-competent HSV-1 has not yet been achieved, work has demonstrated significantly that such an approach is feasible with adenoviral vectors by ablating the native receptor binding and replacing it with tissue-specific receptors. In addition to targeting the primary tumor site, a targeted vector administered systemically would deliver the therapeutic gene to deposits of metastatic disease throughout the body. Following imaging of these metastatic deposits and delivery of the vector, conformal doses of radiation could be delivered to these sites through IMRT or other targeted technologies. By combining receptor modification strategies with improved transcriptional targeting of gene expression and conformal radiotherapy, the therapeutic ratio of radiotherapy may be further improved.

6. CONCLUSIONS

IR is an effective therapeutic modality for diverse human malignancies. Gene therapy strategies have been demonstrated in vitro and in clinical phase I/II trials to improve the tumorcidal effects of IR. The results of current clinical trials will determine if combining gene therapy with radiotherapy leads to improvement in the therapeutic ratio.

ACKNOWLEDGMENT

Ralph R. Weichselbaum is a consultant to and receives stock options and research support from GenVec and Medigene.

REFERENCES

1. Roentgen, W. C. (1959) On a new kind of x-ray [translation]. *Munch. Med. Wochenschr.* **101,** 1237–1239.
2. Curie, P., Curie, M. P., and Bemont, G. (1898) Sur une nouvelle substance fortement radioactive contenue dans la pechblende. *C. R. Acad. Sci. (Paris)* **127,** 1215–1217.
3. Argiris, A. (2002) Update on chemoradiotherapy for head and neck cancer. *Curr. Opin. Oncol.* **14,** 323–329.
4. Budach, V., Zurlo, A., and Horiot, J. C. (2002) EORTC Radiotherapy Group: achievements and future projects. European Organisation for Research and Treatment of Cancer. *Eur. J. Cancer* **38(Suppl. 4),** S134–S137.
5. Chiara, S., Bruzzone, M., Merlini, L., et al. (1994) Randomized study comparing chemotherapy plus radiotherapy vs radiotherapy alone in FIGO stage IIB-III cervical carcinoma. GONO (North-West Oncologic Cooperative Group). *Am. J. Clin. Oncol.* **17,** 294–297.
6. Souhami, L., Gil, R. A., Allan, S. E., et al. (1991) A randomized trial of chemotherapy followed by pelvic radiation therapy in stage IIIB carcinoma of the cervix. *J. Clin. Oncol.* **9,** 970–977.
7. Kim, T. Y., Yang, S. H., Lee, S. H., et al. (2002) A phase III randomized trial of combined chemoradiotherapy vs radiotherapy alone in locally advanced non-small-cell lung cancer. *Am. J. Clin. Oncol.* **25,** 238–243.
8. (1991) Induction chemotherapy plus radiation compared with surgery plus radiation in patients with advanced laryngeal cancer. The Department of Veterans Affairs Laryngeal Cancer Study Group. *N. Engl. J. Med.* **324,** 1685–1690.
9. Wasserman, T. H. and Brizel, D. M. (2001) The role of amifostine as a radioprotector. *Oncology (Huntingt.)* **15,** 1349–1354; discussion 1357–1360.
10. Reed, J. C. (1999) Mechanisms of apoptosis avoidance in cancer. *Curr. Opin. Oncol.* **11,** 68–75.
11. Dewey, W. C., Ling, C. C., and Meyn, R. E. (1995) Radiation-induced apoptosis: relevance to radiotherapy. *Int. J. Radiat. Oncol. Biol. Phys.* **33,** 781–796.
12. Dizdaroglu, M. (1992) Measurement of radiation-induced damage to DNA at the molecular level. *Int. J. Radiat. Biol.* **61,** 175–183.
13. Dizdaroglu, M. (1992) Oxidative damage to DNA in mammalian chromatin. *Mutat. Res.* **275,** 331–342.
14. Lin, X., Fuks, Z., and Kolesnick, R. (2000) Ceramide mediates radiation-induced death of endothelium. *Crit. Care Med.* **28,** N87–N93.
15. Billis, W., Fuks, Z., and Kolesnick, R. (1998) Signaling in and regulation of ionizing radiation-induced apoptosis in endothelial cells. *Recent Prog. Horm. Res.* **53,** 85–92; discussion 93.
16. Bodmer, J. L., Schneider, P., and Tschopp, J. (2002) The molecular architecture of the TNF superfamily. *Trends Biochem. Sci.* **27,** 19–26.
17. Sartorius, U., Schmitz, I., and Krammer, P. H. (2001) Molecular mechanisms of death-receptor-mediated apoptosis. *Chembiochem* **2,** 20–29.
18. Kawabe, S., Roth, J. A., Wilson, D. R., and Meyn, R. E. (2000) Adenovirus-mediated p16INK4a gene expression radiosensitizes non-small cell lung cancer cells in a p53-dependent manner. *Oncogene* **19,** 5359–5366.
19. Kawashita, Y., Ohtsuru, A., Kaneda, Y., et al. (1999) Regression of hepatocellular carcinoma in vitro and in vivo by radiosensitizing suicide gene therapy under the inducible and spatial control of radiation. *Hum. Gene Ther.* **10,** 1509–1519.
20. Atkinson, G. and Hall, S. J. (1999) Prodrug activation gene therapy and external beam irradiation in the treatment of prostate cancer. *Urology* **54,** 1098–1104.
21. Kim, S. H., Kim, J. H., Kolozsvary, A., Brown, S. L., and Freytag, S. O. (1997) Preferential radiosensitization of 9L glioma cells transduced with HSV-TK gene by acyclovir. *J. Neurooncol.* **33,** 189–194.
22. Kim, J. H., Kim, S. H., Brown, S. L., and Freytag, S. O. (1994) Selective enhancement by an antiviral agent of the radiation-induced cell killing of human glioma cells transduced with HSV-TK gene. *Cancer Res.* **54,** 6053–6056.
23. Mauceri, H. J., Hanna, N. N., Wayne, J. D., Hallahan, D. E., Hellman, S., and Weichselbaum, R. R. (1996) Tumor necrosis factor alpha (TNF-alpha) gene therapy targeted by ionizing radiation selectively damages tumor vasculature. *Cancer Res.* **56,** 4311–4314.

24. Staba, M. J., Mauceri, H. J., Kufe, D. W., Hallahan, D. E., and Weichselbaum, R. R. (1998) Adenoviral TNF-alpha gene therapy and radiation damage tumor vasculature in a human malignant glioma xenograft. *Gene Ther.* **5,** 293–300.

25. Hallahan, D. E., Mauceri, H. J., Seung, L. P., et al. (1995) Spatial and temporal control of gene therapy using ionizing radiation. *Nat. Med.* **1,** 786–791.

26. Mauceri, H. J., Hanna, N. N., Wayne, J. D., Hallahan, D. E., Hellman, S., and Weichselbaum, R. R. (1996) Tumor necrosis factor alpha (TNF-alpha) gene therapy targeted by ionizing radiation selectively damages tumor vasculature. *Cancer Res.* **56,** 4311–4314.

27. Stevens, C. W., Zeng, M., and Cerniglia, G. J. (1996) Ionizing radiation greatly improves gene transfer efficiency in mammalian cells. *Hum. Gene Ther.* **7,** 1727–1734.

28. Stevens, C. W., Stamato, T. D., Mauldin, S. K., Getts, R. C., Zeng, M., and Cerniglia, G. J. (1999) Radiation-induced recombination is dependent on Ku80. *Radiat. Res.* **151,** 408–413.

29. Ram, Z., Walbridge, S., Shawker, T., Culver, K. W., Blaese, R. M., and Oldfield, E. H. (1994) The effect of thymidine kinase transduction and ganciclovir therapy on tumor vasculature and growth of 9L gliomas in rats. *J. Neurosurg.* **81,** 256–260.

30. Tanaka, T., Yamasaki, H., and Mesnil, M. (2001) Stimulation of intercellular communication of poor-communicating cells by gap-junction-competent cells enhances the HSV-TK/GCV bystander effect in vitro. *Int. J. Cancer* **91,** 538–542.

31. Belyakov, O. V., Malcolmson, A. M., Folkard, M., Prise, K. M., and Michael, B. D. (2001) Direct evidence for a bystander effect of ionizing radiation in primary human fibroblasts. *Br. J. Cancer* **84,** 674–679.

32. Andrade-Rozental, A. F., Rozental, R., Hopperstad, M. G., Wu, J. K., Vrionis, F. D., and Spray, D. C. (2000) Gap junctions: the "kiss of death" and the "kiss of life." *Brain Res. Brain Res. Rev.* **32,** 308–315.

33. Kaneda, Y. (2001) Improvements in gene therapy technologies. *Mol. Urol.* **5,** 85–89.

34. Donahue, J. M., Mullen, J. T., and Tanabe, K. K. (2002) Viral oncolysis. *Surg. Oncol. Clin. N. Am.* **11,** 661–680.

35. Xu, L., Pirollo, K. F., and Chang, E. H. (2001) Tumor-targeted p53-gene therapy enhances the efficacy of conventional chemo/radiotherapy. *J. Control. Release* **74,** 115–128.

36. Rainov, N. G. (2000) A phase III clinical evaluation of herpes simplex virus type 1 thymidine kinase and ganciclovir gene therapy as an adjuvant to surgical resection and radiation in adults with previously untreated glioblastoma multiforme. *Hum. Gene Ther.* **11,** 2389–2401.

37. Rainov, N. G., Kramm, C. M., Banning, U., et al. (2000) Immune response induced by retrovirus-mediated HSV-TK/GCV pharmacogene therapy in patients with glioblastoma multiforme. *Gene Ther.* **7,** 1853–1858.

38. Xu, L., Pirollo, K. F., and Chang, E. H. (1997) Transferrin-liposome-mediated p53 sensitization of squamous cell carcinoma of the head and neck to radiation in vitro. *Hum. Gene Ther.* **8,** 467–475.

39. Li, X. J., Wang, K. M., Xu, Y., et al. (2003) [Ionizing radiation-regulated killing of human hepatoma cells by liposome-mediated CDglyTK gene delivery]. *Sheng Wu Hua Xue Yu Sheng Wu Wu Li Xue Bao (Shanghai)* **35,** 64–70.

40. Carson, D. A. and Lois, A. (1995) Cancer progression and p53. *Lancet* **346,** 1009–1011.

41. Dasika, G. K., Lin, S. C., Zhao, S., Sung, P., Tomkinson, A., and Lee, E. Y. (1999) DNA damage-induced cell cycle checkpoints and DNA strand break repair in development and tumorigenesis. *Oncogene* **18,** 7883–7899.

42. Pruschy, M., Rocha, S., Zaugg, K., et al. (2001) Key targets for the execution of radiation-induced tumor cell apoptosis: the role of p53 and caspases. *Int. J. Radiat. Oncol. Biol. Phys.* **49,** 561–567.

43. Macleod, K. F., Sherry, N., Hannon, G., et al. (1995) p53-dependent and independent expression of p21 during cell growth, differentiation, and DNA damage. *Genes Dev.* **9,** 935–944.

44. Szumiel, I. (1994) Ionizing radiation-induced cell death. *Int. J. Radiat. Biol.* **66,** 329–341.

45. Kearsey, J. M., Shivji, M. K., Hall, P. A., and Wood, R. D. (1995) Does the p53 up-regulated Gadd45 protein have a role in excision repair? *Science* **270,** 1004–1005; discussion 1005–1006.

46. Smith, M. L., Chen, I. T., Zhan, Q., et al. (1994) Interaction of the p53-regulated protein Gadd45 with proliferating cell nuclear antigen. *Science* **266,** 1376–1380.

47. Spitz, F. R., Nguyen, D., Skibber, J. M., Meyn, R. E., Cristiano, R. J., and Roth, J. A. (1996) Adenoviral-mediated wild-type p53 gene expression sensitizes colorectal cancer cells to ionizing radiation. *Clin. Cancer Res.* **2,** 1665–1671.

48. Roth, J. A. (1998) Restoration of tumour suppressor gene expression for cancer. *Forum (Genova)* **8,** 368–376.

49. Horowitz, J. (1999) Adenovirus-mediated p53 gene therapy: overview of preclinical studies and potential clinical applications. *Curr. Opin. Mol. Ther.* **1,** 500–509.

50. Roth, J. A., Swisher, S. G., and Meyn, R. E. (1999) p53 tumor suppressor gene therapy for cancer. *Oncology (Huntingt.)* **13,** 148–154.

51. Kawabe, S., Munshi, A., Zumstein, L. A., Wilson, D. R., Roth, J. A., and Meyn, R. E. (2001) Adenovirus-mediated wild-type p53 gene expression radiosensitizes non-small cell lung cancer cells but not normal lung fibroblasts. *Int. J. Radiat. Biol.* **77,** 185–194.

52. Cowen, D., Salem, N., Ashoori, F., et al. (2000) Prostate cancer radiosensitization in vivo with adenovirus-mediated p53 gene therapy. *Clin. Cancer Res.* **6,** 4402–4408.

53. Nishizaki, M., Meyn, R. E., Levy, L. B., et al. (2001) Synergistic inhibition of human lung cancer cell growth by adenovirus-mediated wild-type p53 gene transfer in combination with docetaxel and radiation therapeutics in vitro and in vivo. *Clin. Cancer Res.* **7,** 2887–2897.

54. Fujiwara, T., Inoue, F., and Tanaka, N. (1997) [Human gene therapy for lung cancer]. *Nippon Rinsho* **55,** 1296–1306.

55. Fujiwara, T., Kataoka, M., Kawamata, O., and Tanaka, N. (1999) [A phase I trial of adenoviral p53 gene therapy for non-small cell lung cancer]. *Nippon Geka Gakkai Zasshi* **100,** 749–755.

56. Swisher, S. G. and Roth, J. A. (2002) Clinical update of Ad-p53 gene therapy for lung cancer. *Surg. Oncol. Clin. N. Am.* **11,** 521–535.

57. Yazawa, K., Fisher, W. E., and Brunicardi, F. C. (2002) Current progress in suicide gene therapy for cancer. *World J. Surg.* **26,** 783–789.

58. Kaminski, J. M., Kaminski, R. J., Dicker, A. P., and Urbain, J. L. (2001) Defining a future role for radiogenic therapy. *Cancer Treat. Rev.* **27,** 289–294.

59. Chhikara, M., Huang, H., Vlachaki, M. T., et al. (2001) Enhanced therapeutic effect of HSV-TK + GCV gene therapy and ionizing radiation for prostate cancer. *Mol. Ther.* **3,** 536–542.

60. Lebovics, R. S. and DeLaney, T. F. (1993) Sensitizers of photoradiation and ionizing radiation in the management of head and neck cancer. *Med. Clin. North Am.* **77,** 583–596.

61. Pu, A. T., Robertson, J. M., and Lawrence, T. S. (1995) Current status of radiation sensitization by fluoropyrimidines. *Oncology (Huntingt.)* **9,** 707–714; discussion **714,** 717–718, 721.

62. Urtasun, R. C., Kinsella, T. J., Farnan, N., DelRowe, J. D., Lester, S. G., and Fulton, D. S. (1996) Survival improvement in anaplastic astrocytoma, combining external radiation with halogenated pyrimidines: final report of RTOG 86-12, phase I–II study. *Int. J. Radiat. Oncol. Biol. Phys.* **36,** 1163–1167.

63. Ben-Hattar, J., Beard, P., and Jiricny, J. (1989) Cytosine methylation in CTF and Sp1 recognition sites of an HSV TK promoter: effects on transcription in vivo and on factor binding in vitro. *Nucleic Acids Res.* **17,** 10,179–10,190.

64. Gabel, M., Kim, J. H., Kolozsvary, A., Khil, M., and Freytag, S. (1998) Selective in vivo radiosensitization by 5-fluorocytosine of human colorectal carcinoma cells transduced with the E. coli cytosine deaminase (CD) gene. *Int. J. Radiat. Oncol. Biol. Phys.* **41,** 883–887.

65. Pederson, L. C., Buchsbaum, D. J., Vickers, S. M., et al. (1997) Molecular chemotherapy combined with radiation therapy enhances killing of cholangiocarcinoma cells in vitro and in vivo. *Cancer Res.* **57,** 4325–4332.

66. Pederson, L. C., Vickers, S. M., Buchsbaum, D. J., et al. (1998) Combined cytosine deaminase expression, 5-fluorocytosine exposure, and radiotherapy increases cytotoxicity to cholangiocarcinoma cells. *J. Gastrointest. Surg.* **2,** 283–291.

67. Vokes, E. E., Beckett, M., Karrison, T., and Weichselbaum, R. R. (1992) The interaction of 5-fluorouracil, hydroxyurea, and radiation in two human head and neck cancer cell lines. *Oncology* **49,** 454–460.

68. Kim, J. H., Kim, S. H., Kolozsvary, A., Brown, S. L., Kim, O. B., and Freytag, S. O. (1995) Selective enhancement of radiation response of herpes simplex virus thymidine kinase transduced 9L gliosarcoma cells in vitro and in vivo by antiviral agents. *Int. J. Radiat. Oncol. Biol. Phys.* **33,** 861–868.

69. Kim, J. H., Kim, S. H., Brown, S. L., and Freytag, S. O. (1994) Selective enhancement by an antiviral agent of the radiation-induced cell killing of human glioma cells transduced with HSV-TK gene. *Cancer Res.* **54,** 6053–6056.

70. Freeman, S. M., Abboud, C. N., Whartenby, K. A., et al. (1993) The "bystander effect": tumor regression when a fraction of the tumor mass is genetically modified. *Cancer Res.* **53,** 5274–5283.

71. Freeman, S. M., Whartenby, K. A., Freeman, J. L., Abboud, C. N., and Marrogi, A. J. (1996) In situ use of suicide genes for cancer therapy. *Semin. Oncol.* **23,** 31–45.

72. Imaizumi, K., Hasegawa, Y., Kawabe, T., et al. (1998) Bystander tumoricidal effect and gap junctional communication in lung cancer cell lines. *Am. J. Respir. Cell Mol. Biol.* **18,** 205–212.

73. Beltinger, C., Fulda, S., Kammertoens, T., Meyer, E., Uckert, W., and Debatin, K. M. (1999) Herpes simplex virus thymidine kinase/ganciclovir-induced apoptosis involves ligand-independent death receptor aggregation and activation of caspases. *Proc. Natl. Acad. Sci. USA* **96,** 8699–8704.

74. Beltinger, C., Fulda, S., Walczak, H., and Debatin, K. M. (2002) TRAIL enhances thymidine kinase/ganciclovir gene therapy of neuroblastoma cells. *Cancer Gene Ther.* **9,** 372–381.

75. Vrionis, F. D., Wu, J. K., Qi, P., Cano, W. G., and Cherington, V. (1996) Preservation of the bystander cytocidal effect of irradiated herpes simplex virus thymidine kinase (HSV-TK) modified tumor cells. *J. Neurooncol.* **30,** 225–236.

76. Nishihara, E., Nagayama, Y., Mawatari, F., et al. (1997) Retrovirus-mediated herpes simplex virus thymidine kinase gene transduction renders human thyroid carcinoma cell lines sensitive to ganciclovir and radiation in vitro and in vivo. *Endocrinology* **138,** 4577–4583.

77. Teh, B. S., Aguilar-Cordova, E., Vlachaki, M. T., et al. (2002) Combining radiotherapy with gene therapy (from the bench to the bedside): a novel treatment strategy for prostate cancer. *Oncologist* **7,** 458–466.

78. Herman, J. R., Adler, H. L., Aguilar-Cordova, E., et al. (1999) In situ gene therapy for adenocarcinoma of the prostate: a phase I clinical trial. *Hum. Gene Ther.* **10,** 1239–1249.

79. Rainov, N. G. (2000) A phase III clinical evaluation of herpes simplex virus type 1 thymidine kinase and ganciclovir gene therapy as an adjuvant to surgical resection and radiation in adults with previously untreated glioblastoma multiforme. *Hum. Gene Ther.* **11,** 2389–2401.

80. Hanna, N. N., Mauceri, H. J., Wayne, J. D., Hallahan, D. E., Kufe, D. W., and Weichselbaum, R. R. (1997) Virally directed cytosine deaminase/5-fluorocytosine gene therapy enhances radiation response in human cancer xenografts. *Cancer Res.* **57,** 4205–4209.

81. Rogulski, K. R., Zhang, K., Kolozsvary, A., Kim, J. H., and Freytag, S. O. (1997) Pronounced antitumor effects and tumor radiosensitization of double suicide gene therapy. *Clin. Cancer Res.* **3,** 2081–2088.

82. Hirschowitz, E. A., Ohwada, A., Pascal, W. R., Russi, T. J., and Crystal, R. G. (1995) In vivo adenovirus-mediated gene transfer of the Escherichia coli cytosine deaminase gene to human colon carcinoma-derived tumors induces chemosensitivity to 5-fluorocytosine. *Hum. Gene Ther.* **6,** 1055–1063.

83. Szary, J., Missol, E., and Szala, S. (1998) Characteristics of cytosine deaminase-5-fluorocytosine system. Enhancement of radiation cytotoxicity and bystander effect. *Adv. Exp. Med. Biol.* **451,** 121–123.

84. Robe, P. A., Princen, F., Martin, D., et al. (2000) Pharmacological modulation of the bystander effect in the herpes simplex virus thymidine kinase/ganciclovir gene therapy system: effects of dibutyryl adenosine 3',5'-cyclic monophosphate, alpha-glycyrrhetinic acid, and cytosine arabinoside. *Biochem. Pharmacol.* **60,** 241–249.

85. Freytag, S. O., Paielli, D., Wing, M., et al. (2002) Efficacy and toxicity of replication-competent adenovirus-mediated double suicide gene therapy in combination with radiation therapy in an orthotopic mouse prostate cancer model. *Int. J. Radiat. Oncol. Biol. Phys.* **54,** 873–885.

86. Weichselbaum, R. R., Hallahan, D., Fuks, Z., and Kufe, D. (1994) Radiation induction of immediate early genes: effectors of the radiation-stress response. *Int. J. Radiat. Oncol. Biol. Phys.* **30,** 229–234.

87. Sherman, M. L., Datta, R., Hallahan, D. E., Weichselbaum, R. R., and Kufe, D. W. (1990) Ionizing radiation regulates expression of the c-jun protooncogene. *Proc. Natl. Acad. Sci. USA* **87,** 5663–5666.

88. Hallahan, D. E., Virudachalam, S., Beckett, M., Sherman, M. L., Kufe, D., and Weichselbaum, R. R. (1991) Mechanisms of X-ray-mediated protooncogene c-jun expression in radiation-induced human sarcoma cell lines. *Int. J. Radiat. Oncol. Biol. Phys.* **21,** 1677–1681.

89. Hallahan, D. E., Sukhatme, V. P., Sherman, M. L., Virudachalam, S., Kufe, D., and Weichselbaum, R. R. (1991) Protein kinase C mediates X-ray inducibility of nuclear signal transducers EGR1 and JUN. *Proc. Natl. Acad. Sci. USA* **88,** 2156–2160.

90. Datta, R., Rubin, E., Sukhatme, V., et al. (1992) Ionizing radiation activates transcription of the EGR1 gene via CArG elements. *Proc. Natl. Acad. Sci. USA* **89,** 10,149–10,153.

91. Hallahan, D. E., Sukhatme, V. P., Sherman, M. L., Virudachalam, S., Kufe, D., and Weichselbaum, R. R. (1991) Protein kinase C mediates X-ray inducibility of nuclear signal transducers EGR1 and JUN. *Proc. Natl. Acad. Sci. USA* **88,** 2156–2160.

92. Sherman, M. L., Datta, R., Hallahan, D. E., Weichselbaum, R. R., and Kufe, D. W. (1990) Ionizing radiation regulates expression of the c-jun protooncogene. *Proc. Natl. Acad. Sci. USA* **87,** 5663–5666.

93. Datta, R., Taneja, N., Sukhatme, V. P., Qureshi, S. A., Weichselbaum, R., and Kufe, D. W. (1993) Reactive oxygen intermediates target CC(A/T)6GG sequences to mediate activation of the early growth response 1 transcription factor gene by ionizing radiation. *Proc. Natl. Acad. Sci. USA* **90,** 2419–2422.

94. Meyer, R. G., Kupper, J. H., Kandolf, R., and Rodemann, H. P. (2002) Early growth response-1 gene (Egr-1) promoter induction by ionizing radiation in U87 malignant glioma cells in vitro. *Eur. J. Biochem.* **269,** 337–346.

95. Datta, R., Rubin, E., Sukhatme, V., et al. (1992) Ionizing radiation activates transcription of the EGR1 gene via CArG elements. *Proc. Natl. Acad. Sci. USA* **89,** 10,149–10,153.

96. Ohno, T. (1995) [Inducible regulatable promoter—ionizing radiation-inducible promoter EGR-1]. *Tanpakushitsu Kakusan Koso* **40,** 2624–2630.

97. Cao, X., Zhang, W., and Wang, J. (1996) [An in vitro study on radiation-induced TNF gene therapy of cancer]. *Zhonghua Zhong Liu Za Zhi* **18,** 161–164.

98. Park, W. Y., Hwang, C. I., Im, C. N., et al. (2002) Identification of radiation-specific responses from gene expression profile. *Oncogene* **21,** 8521–8528.

99. Fornace, A. J. Jr., Amundson, S. A., Do, K. T., Meltzer, P., Trent, J., and Bittner, M. (2002) Stress-gene induction by low-dose gamma irradiation. *Mil. Med.* **167,** 13–15.

100. Khodarev, N. N., Park, J. O., Yu, J., et al. (2001) Dose-dependent and independent temporal patterns of gene responses to ionizing radiation in normal and tumor cells and tumor xenografts. *Proc. Natl. Acad. Sci. USA* **98,** 12,665–12,670.

101. Hallahan, D. E., Spriggs, D. R., Beckett, M. A., Kufe, D. W., and Weichselbaum, R. R. (1989) Increased tumor necrosis factor alpha mRNA after cellular exposure to ionizing radiation. *Proc. Natl. Acad. Sci. USA* **86,** 10,104–10,107.

102. Hallahan, D. E., Haimovitz-Friedman, A., Kufe, D. W., Fuks, Z., and Weichselbaum, R. R. (1993) The role of cytokines in radiation oncology. *Important Adv. Oncol.* 71–80.

103. Weichselbaum, R. R., Hallahan, D. E., Beckett, M. A., et al. (1994) Gene therapy targeted by radiation preferentially radiosensitizes tumor cells. *Cancer Res.* **54,** 4266–4269.

104. Knisely, T. L. and Niederkorn, J. Y. (1990) Emergence of a dominant cytotoxic T lymphocyte antitumor effector from tumor-infiltrating cells in the anterior chamber of the eye. *Cancer Immunol. Immunother.* **30,** 323–330.

105. Abraham, E. (1991) Effects of stress on cytokine production. *Methods Achiev. Exp. Pathol.* **14,** 45–62.

106. Hallahan, D. E., Chen, A. Y., Teng, M., and Cmelak, A. J. (1999) Drug-radiation interactions in tumor blood vessels. *Oncology (Huntingt.)* **13,** 71–77.
107. Glauner, H., Siegmund, D., Motejadded, H., et al. (2002) Intracellular localization and transcriptional regulation of tumor necrosis factor (TNF) receptor-associated factor 4 (TRAF4). *Eur. J. Biochem.* **269,** 4819–4829.
108. Baker, S. J. and Reddy, E. P. (1998) Modulation of life and death by the TNF receptor superfamily. *Oncogene* **17,** 3261–3270.
109. Hallahan, D. E., Beckett, M. A., Kufe, D., and Weichselbaum, R. R. (1990) The interaction between recombinant human tumor necrosis factor and radiation in 13 human tumor cell lines. *Int. J. Radiat. Oncol. Biol. Phys.* **19,** 69–74.
110. Old, L. J. (1985) Tumor necrosis factor (TNF). *Science* **230,** 630–632.
111. McIntosh, J. K., Mule, J. J., Travis, W. D., and Rosenberg, S. A. (1990) Studies of effects of recombinant human tumor necrosis factor on autochthonous tumor and transplanted normal tissue in mice. *Cancer Res.* **50,** 2463–2469.
112. Hallahan, D., Weichselbaum, R., Kufe, D., and Vokes, E. (1995) Phase I trial of tumor necrosis factor combined with radiotherapy. *Cancer J.* **3,** 204.
113. Rasmussen, H. S., Lempicki, M., Chu, K. W., Carey, J. W., Smidt, E. B., and Weichselbaum, R. R. (2001) PASCO.
114. Mauceri, H. J., Hanna, N. N., Beckett, M. A., et al. (1998) Combined effects of angiostatin and ionizing radiation in antitumour therapy. *Nature* **394,** 287–291.
115. Mauceri, H. J., Seung, L. P., Grdina, W. L., Swedberg, K. A., and Weichselbaum, R. R. (1997) Increased injection number enhances adenoviral genetic radiotherapy. *Radiat. Oncol. Investig.* **5,** 220–226.
116. Chung, T. D., Mauceri, H. J., Hallahan, D. E., et al. (1998) Tumor necrosis factor-alpha-based gene therapy enhances radiation cytoxicity in human prostate cancer. *Cancer Gene Ther.* **5,** 344–349.
117. Park, J. O., Lopez, C. A., Gupta, V. K., et al. (2002) Transcriptional control of viral gene therapy by cisplatin. *J. Clin. Invest.* **110,** 403–410.
118. Hanna, N., Nemunaitis, J., Cunningham, C. C., et al. (2002) *PASCO.*
119. Mundt, A. J., Nemunaitis, J., Vijayakumar, S., and Weichselbaum, R. R. (2002) TNFerade, an adenovector encoding the human tumor necrosis factor alpha gene, in soft tissue sarcoma in the extremity. *Eur. J. Cancer* **38,** 141.
120. Chambers, R., Gillespie, G. Y., Soroceanu, L., et al. (1995) Comparison of genetically engineered herpes simplex viruses for the treatment of brain tumors in a SCID mouse model of human malignant glioma. *Proc. Natl. Acad. Sci. USA* **92,** 1411–1415.
121. Stanziale, S. F., Petrowsky, H., Joe, J. K., et al. (2002) Ionizing radiation potentiates the antitumor efficacy of oncolytic herpes simplex virus G207 by upregulating ribonucleotide reductase. *Surgery* **132,** 353–359.
122. Markert, J. M., Medlock, M. D., Rabkin, S. D., et al. (2000) Conditionally replicating herpes simplex virus mutant, G207 for the treatment of malignant glioma: results of a phase I trial. *Gene Ther.* **7,** 867–874.
123. Meignier, B., Martin, B., Whitley, R. J., and Roizman, B. (1990) In vivo behavior of genetically engineered herpes simplex viruses R7017 and R7020. II. Studies in immunocompetent and immunosuppressed owl monkeys (*Aotus trivirgatus*). *J. Infect. Dis.* **162,** 313–321.
124. Advani, S. J., Chung, S. M., Yan, S. Y., et al. (1999) Replication-competent, nonneuroinvasive genetically engineered herpes virus is highly effective in the treatment of therapy-resistant experimental human tumors. *Cancer Res.* **59,** 2055–2058.
125. Chung, S. M., Advani, S. J., Bradley, J. D., et al. (2002) The use of a genetically engineered herpes simplex virus (R7020) with ionizing radiation for experimental hepatoma. *Gene Ther.* **9,** 75–80.
126. Advani, S. J., Sibley, G. S., Song, P. Y., et al. (1998) Enhancement of replication of genetically engineered herpes simplex viruses by ionizing radiation: a new paradigm for destruction of therapeutically intractable tumors. *Gene Ther.* **5,** 160–165.
127. Bradley, J. D., Kataoka, Y., Advani, S., et al. (1999) Ionizing radiation improves survival in mice bearing intracranial high- grade gliomas injected with genetically modified herpes simplex virus. *Clin. Cancer Res.* **5,** 1517–1522.
128. Rampling, R., Cruickshank, G., Papanastassiou, V., et al. (2000) Toxicity evaluation of replication-competent herpes simplex virus (ICP 34.5 null mutant 1716) in patients with recurrent malignant glioma. *Gene Ther.* **7,** 859–866.
129. Rodriguez, R., Schuur, E. R., Lim, H. Y., Henderson, G. A., Simons, J. W., and Henderson, D. R. (1997) Prostate attenuated replication competent adenovirus (ARCA) CN706: a selective cytotoxic for prostate-specific antigen-positive prostate cancer cells. *Cancer Res.* **57,** 2559–2563.
130. Bischoff, J. R., Kirn, D. H., Williams, A., et al. (1996) An adenovirus mutant that replicates selectively in p53-deficient human tumor cells. *Science* **274,** 373–376.
131. Levine, A. J. (1989) The p53 tumor suppressor gene and gene product. *Princess Takamatsu Symp.* **20,** 221–230.
132. Harada, J. N., Shevchenko, A., Pallas, D. C., and Berk, A. J. (2002) Analysis of the adenovirus E1B-55K-anchored proteome reveals its link to ubiquitination machinery. *J. Virol.* **76,** 9194–9206.
133. Biederer, C., Ries, S., Brandts, C. H., and McCormick, F. (2002) Replication-selective viruses for cancer therapy. *J. Mol. Med.* **80,** 163–175.
134. Freytag, S. O., Rogulski, K. R., Paielli, D. L., Gilbert, J. D., and Kim, J. H. (1998) A novel three-pronged approach to kill cancer cells selectively: concomitant viral, double suicide gene, and radiotherapy. *Hum. Gene Ther.* **9,** 1323–1333.

135. Rogulski, K. R., Freytag, S. O., Zhang, K., et al. (2000) In vivo antitumor activity of ONYX-015 is influenced by p53 status and is augmented by radiotherapy. *Cancer Res.* **60,** 1193–1196.

136. Dix, B. R., Edwards, S. J., and Braithwaite, A. W. (2001) Does the antitumor adenovirus ONYX-015/dl1520 selectively target cells defective in the p53 pathway? *J. Virol.* **75,** 5443–5447.

137. Petit, T., Davidson, K. K., Cerna, C., et al. (2002) Efficient induction of apoptosis by ONYX-015 adenovirus in human colon cancer cell lines regardless of p53 status. *Anticancer Drugs* **13,** 47–50.

138. Geoerger, B., Grill, J., Opolon, P., et al. (2002) Oncolytic activity of the E1B-55 kDa-deleted adenovirus ONYX-015 is independent of cellular p53 status in human malignant glioma xenografts. *Cancer Res.* **62,** 764–772.

139. Edwards, S. J., Dix, B. R., Myers, C. J., et al. (2002) Evidence that replication of the antitumor adenovirus ONYX-015 is not controlled by the p53 and p14(ARF) tumor suppressor genes. *J. Virol.* **76,** 12,483–12,490.

140. Yang, C. T., You, L., Uematsu, K., Yeh, C. C., McCormick, F., and Jablons, D. M. (2001) p14(ARF) modulates the cytolytic effect of ONYX-015 in mesothelioma cells with wild-type p53. *Cancer Res.* **61,** 5959–5963.

141. Vasey, P. A., Shulman, L. N., Campos, S., et al. (2002) Phase I trial of intraperitoneal injection of the E1B-55-kd-gene-deleted adenovirus ONYX-015 (dl1520) given on days 1 through 5 every 3 weeks in patients with recurrent/refractory epithelial ovarian cancer. *J. Clin. Oncol.* **20,** 1562–1569.

142. Reid, T., Galanis, E., Abbruzzese, J., et al. (2002) Hepatic arterial infusion of a replication-selective oncolytic adenovirus (dl1520): phase II viral, immunologic, and clinical endpoints. *Cancer Res.* **62,** 6070–6079.

143. Nemunaitis, J., Khuri, F., Ganly, I., et al. (2001) Phase II trial of intratumoral administration of ONYX-015, a replication-selective adenovirus, in patients with refractory head and neck cancer. *J. Clin. Oncol.* **19,** 289–298.

144. Ganly, I., Kirn, D., Eckhardt, G., et al. (2000) A phase I study of Onyx-015, an E1B attenuated adenovirus, administered intratumorally to patients with recurrent head and neck cancer. *Clin. Cancer Res.* **6,** 798–806.

145. Khuri, F. R., Nemunaitis, J., Ganly, I., et al. (2000) a controlled trial of intratumoral ONYX-015, a selectively-replicating adenovirus, in combination with cisplatin and 5-fluorouracil in patients with recurrent head and neck cancer. *Nat. Med.* **6,** 879–885.

146. Nemunaitis, J., Ganly, I., Khuri, F., et al. (2000) Selective replication and oncolysis in p53 mutant tumors with ONYX-015, an E1B-55kD gene-deleted adenovirus, in patients with advanced head and neck cancer: a phase II trial. *Cancer Res.* **60,** 6359–6366.

24

Nonviral Vector Systems for Cancer Gene Therapy

Greg F. Walker and Ernst Wagner

1. INTRODUCTION

There is increasing interest in nonviral systems for the delivery of genes for cancer therapy. Nonviral gene delivery has been considered an alternative to the intensely researched viral systems, although nonviral systems have several advantages. First, they are nonimmunogenic and therefore can be applied to the patient more than once; there is no limitation to the size of the deoxyribonucleic acid (DNA) that can be delivered, and the DNA vector can be engineered for specific cell targeting. Furthermore, they will offer easier synthesis and production as a pharmaceutical product. Unfortunately, nonviral vectors have poor transfection efficiency compared to viral vectors both in vitro and in vivo. However, with substantial efforts in the development of new transfection systems and better understanding of the barriers, the transfection efficiency and targeting of nonviral systems have improved significantly.

The long-standing goal of cancer gene therapy is to express such therapeutic genes specifically and effectively in target cells in vivo; however, this is the biggest hurdle in treating cancer by nonviral gene therapy. There are two general means to target gene expression in vivo. In the first, physical transfection systems, the DNA vector is directly applied locally to tissue. However, for the control of disseminated cancer cells, DNA has to be applied systemically using particle-mediated systems. Particle-mediated systems must protect the DNA from serum nucleases and deliver its load to target tissues.

Depending on the mode of application, DNA will have to overcome intracellular and extracellular barriers (Table 1). DNA internalized by endocytosis will enter the endosome; because entry of DNA into the cytosol is a prerequisite for nuclear translocation, entrapment and degradation of DNA in the endolysosomes is a major barrier to efficient gene transfer. DNA in the cytoplasm has to overcome diffusional and metabolic barriers before reaching the nuclear pore complex, the gateway of the nucleosol. Nuclear translocation of DNA requires either the disassembly of the nuclear envelope or active nuclear transport via the nuclear pore complex. In addition, particle-mediated systems have to overcome the extracellular barrier; these systems must be stabilized to remain as discrete particles in blood before reaching the target cell. To achieve this, particles must avoid interactions with plasma proteins, extracellular matrices, nontargeted cell surfaces, and self-interactions (i.e., not aggregate). Such interactions result in the particles being cleared rapidly either into the first capillary bed encountered (e.g., lung) or are scavenged from the bloodstream by phagocytic cells. For a review on the barriers to nonviral gene therapy, consult ref. *1*.

This chapter focuses on the pros and cons of physical methods for the delivery of genes to control cancer (*see* Table 2). For particle-mediated gene transfer systems, strategies for improving tumor gene expression are described, including examples of application for tumor targeting (*see* Table 3), and future directions for nonviral cancer therapy are discussed.

From: *Contemporary Cancer Research*
Cancer Gene Therapy
Edited by: D. T. Curiel and J. T. Douglas © Humana Press Inc., Totowa, NJ

Table 1
Strategies to Overcome Extracellular and Intracellular Barriers

Barrier	Strategy employed
Extracellular	
Degradation of DNA by serum nucleases or lipids or encapsulation in nanoparticles	Protect DNA by condensation with cationic polymers
Nonspecific interactions with blood components	Surface shielding with hydrophilic polymers
	Crosslinking of polymer gene carrier
Toxicity	Surface shielding by PEG, biodegradable gene carriers
Targeting of DNA to tumor cells, tumor tissues, and tumor vasculature	Specific targeting ligands (e.g., epidermal growth factor, transferrin, folate, antibodies, and so on)
	Passive targeting, long-circulating particle-based systems
Intracellular	
DNA uptake by cells	Specific targeting ligands that undergo receptor-mediated endocytosis (e.g., epidermal growth factor, transferrin)
	Physical methods (e.g., EP, US)
Endosomal escape	Membrane-active peptides (e.g., Melittin)
	Polycations "proton sponges" (e.g., PEI)
Transport from the cytosol into the nucleus	Allow cytosolic migration by keeping the particles small or use cytoskeleton-mediated transport
	Nuclear localization signal peptides/sequences
Disassembly of DNA from gene carrier	Cytosolic reduction of LMW polymers crosslinked with bioreversible bonds in DNA complex assembly (e.g., disulfide bonds)
Cytotoxicity	Avoid strongly charged DNA particles
	Biodegradable cationic gene carriers
	LMW polymers crosslinked with bioreversible bonds

2. PHYSICAL TRANSFECTION SYSTEMS

2.1. Direct Injection

Direct plasmid injection offers the advantages of safety, tolerability, and minimal manipulation; however, it has yielded relatively low levels of transfection in tumors *(2)*. Nevertheless, it has been effective in the regression of tumors in vivo by delivering a suicide gene that converts a systemically administered nontoxic prodrug into a lethal drug *(3)*. For instance, intratumoral injection of cytosine deaminase-expressing plasmid in rats bearing subcutaneous metastases induced a 65% decrease in the median tumor volume after the injection of nontoxic prodrug, 5-fluorocytosine, compared to control rats *(3)*.

Direct injection of DNA has also been applied to cancer immunotherapy by intradermal injection of a DNA melanoma vaccine that resulted in most of the mice (8 of 10) rejecting the challenge by tumor cells; most control animals developed tumors *(4)*. Song et al. *(5)* showed that the coinjection of interleukin 12 (IL-12) encoded plasmid with human carcinoembryonic antigen DNA vaccine at the muscle site in mice resulted in enhanced antitumor immunity.

2.2. Gene Gun

The principle of gene transfection with a gene gun (GG) is direct mechanical transport of the DNA into the cell using metal beads as carriers. DNA is coated on the surface of the microscopic beads and shot into the cells with a gas-propelled gun. The advantage of the GG is that it can be used to transfer

Table 2
Cancer Therapy by Physical Transfection Systems

Method	Site	Therapeutic strategy	Result
Direct injection	Tumor	Gene protein expression (e.g., cytosine deaminase) activates systemically applied prodrug (5-fluorocytosine)	Subcutaneous metastases decrease tumor volume
	Muscle	Coinjection of cytokine (IL-12) and/or vaccine plasmids (e.g., human carcinoembryonic antigen)	Enhanced antitumor immunity
Gene gun	Skin	Vaccination (e.g., HPV-16 E7 gene)	Antitumor immunity in the liver and lung metastases models
Electroporation	Muscle	Vaccine (human gp100 or mouse TRP-2 antigens)	Increased survival time of mice bearing established lung metastases
US/systemically applied lipoplex	Tumor	Cytokine (IL-12)	Inhibited tumor growth
Jet injection	Tumor	Cytokine (TNF-α)	Gene expression in tumor

genes to nondividing cells. The major limitation of GG transfer is that DNA penetration is limited to dermal applications and cannot reach deeper tissue areas.

The GG can be applied to DNA vaccination and cytokine gene therapy for cancer. The GG delivered DNA vaccines intradermally in mice, resulting in the control of liver and lung metastases *(6)*. Delivery of plasmid DNA encoding cytokines by GG significantly reduced the growth of melanoma tumors in mice and resistance to renewed tumor growth following challenge *(6)*. GG delivery of IL-12-expressing plasmid to skin resulted in fewer side effects than recombinant protein therapy *(7)*. Studies by Wang et al. *(8)* suggested that immunization of oral mucosa by GG may induce systemic antitumor immunity more efficiently than immunization of the skin.

2.3. Electroporation

Electroporation (EP) is a technique involving the application of short-duration, high-intensity electric field pulses to cells or tissue. The electrical stimulus is believed to cause the membrane to destabilize and the subsequent formation of nanometer-size pores, which can allow passage of the molecule directly into the cell cytoplasm, avoiding the inefficient endocytosis pathway. Transfection efficiency has low dependence on the cell cycle *(9)*. For effective transfection using EP, DNA first has to be injected into the tumor, followed by the application of electric pulses at given field strengths with surface electrodes at the tumor tissue.

EP has been shown to deliver marker genes to various cutaneous tumors, including bladder *(10)*, breast *(11)*, brain tumors *(12)*, and melanoma *(13)*. EP has also enhanced delivery of genes after direct injection into muscle and skin cells. In muscle, EP enhanced transgene expression by two or three orders of magnitude *(14,15)* and stimulated the immune response by an even greater factor *(16)*. Mendiratta et al. *(17)* showed that the combined muscle EP of DNA plasmids encoding human gp100 (melanoma antigen epitope) or mouse tyrosine-related protein 2 (TRP-2) antigens resulted in greater tumor rejection in 100% of the immunized mice. Furthermore, this immunotherapy led to the generation of a therapeutic immune response that significantly improved the mean survival time of mice bearing established lung metastases.

EP is considered safe, inexpensive, and simple, although again it is limited to certain applications; it represents an interesting method to enhance treatment efficiency.

Table 3
Systemic Tumor-Targeted Gene Therapy

	System	Gene	Result
Polyplexes			
Ogris, 1999 *(27)*	Tf-targeted, PEG shielded, PEI	Reporter gene	High gene expression in distant tumors
Kursa, 2003 *(32)*		TNF-α	Hemorrhagic tumor necrosis and inhibition of tumor growth
Kircheis, 2002 *(30)*	Tf-targeted, Tf-shielded, PEI	TNF-α	Hemorrhagic tumor necrosis and inhibition of tumor growth
Wolschek, 2002 *(36)*	EGF-targeted, PEG shielded, PEI	Reporter gene	Expression was predominantly found in the tumor
Lipoplexes			
Xu, 1999 *(62)*	Tf-liposme	*p53*	Tumor regression in combination with radiation
Monck, 2000 *(58)*	PEG-liposome	Reporter gene	High gene expression in distant tumors
Ramesh, 2001 *(64)*	Cationic liposome	*p53*	Reduction of primary and metastatic lung tumor growth
Ueno, 2002 *(55)*	Lipopolyplex	*E1A*	Apoptotic tumor cells, reduction in tumor volume
Rait, 2002 *(63)*	Folate-PEG-liposome	HER2 antisense	Chemosensization
Hofland, 2002 *(59)*	Folate-PEG-liposome	Reporter gene	High-gene expression in distant tumors
Nanoplex			
Hood, 2002 *(72)*	Integrin $(\alpha_v\beta_3)$-NP	A mutant Raf gene	Tumor cell apoptosis and sustained regression of established primary and metastatic tumors

2.4. Ultrasound

Ultrasound (US) has been shown to facilitate the delivery of DNA into tumor tissues in vivo. The mechanism of enhancement has yet to be determined fully; however, it is believed that US waves cause microbubbles to cavitate, which in turn causes the cells to be more permeable to macromolecules *(18)*.

US enhanced marker gene expression after DNA was intratumorally injected into cutaneous tumor models, including colon carcinoma *(19)* and prostate tumors *(20)*. Huber and Pfisterer *(20)* showed that US was not effective when naked DNA was applied systemically, presumably because of the degradation of DNA by serum nucleases.

Inhibited tumor growth was also observed when IL-12 gene was administered systemically prior to US, when the DNA was protected from nuclease attack by condensation with cationic lipid *(21)*.

A promising new approach for US is to apply vehicles such as liposomes or microparticles that encapsulate microbubbles and DNA systemically *(22)*. Microbubbles lower the energy for cavitation, and it is proposed that when the vehicle enters the region of US, the microbubbles cavitate, opening up the vehicle and releasing the DNA locally. In addition, the local cavitation of the microbubbles should make the cells more permeable for DNA uptake.

The US method of enhancing direct injection appears to have distinct advantages for cancer therapy, including the ability to target deep tissues with a minimally invasive treatment regimen.

2.5. Jet Injection

The jet injection method uses mechanical compression to force fluid (DNA in solution) through a small orifice within a fraction of a second, producing a high-pressure stream that can penetrate a number of different tissues.

Walther et al. *(23)* used a new low-volume, versatile, handheld high-speed jet injector for gene transfer into tumors. A combination of plasmids encoding a marker gene and tumor necrosis factor-α (TNF-α) gene (1 µg/µL) were jet injected into subcutaneous Lewis lung carcinoma tumors. After five injections, gene expression was widespread within tumor tissues, with a penetration depth of 5–10 mm, deeper tissue penetration than GG and other jet injection studies. Gene expression was observed in the tumors up to 120 hours after injection.

2.6. Magnetofection

The technique of magnetofection has been applied to targeted gene therapy with encouraging results *(24)*. Genes are reversibly bound to superparamagnetic nanoparticles, which then can be directed within the host by high-energy magnetic fields. The application of magnetofection in vitro resulted in much faster transfection times of minutes rather than hours. This transfection power was also observed when applied to the gastrointestinal tract and in blood vessels in vivo *(24)*. The present system could be used for the treatment of local forms of cancer; however, it is hoped the penetration effect could be expanded to deeper organs.

3. PARTICLE-BASED GENE TRANSFER SYSTEMS

Particle-based systems can be divided into three main groups involving the combination of DNA with cationic polymers (polyplex), lipids (lipoplex), or submicron colloidal systems (nanoplex). These particle-based systems are necessary primarily to both reduce the size and the charge of the DNA molecules for uptake into the cell and protect DNA against hydrolysis by serum nucleases. In general, these particle-based systems have been to shown to require several characteristics and modifications to overcome the barriers to targeted gene expression (Table 1). Particles can be formulated into small nanosize dimensions of 25 nm *(25)* or micrometer large complexes.

Targeting of particle-based systems to tumor tissue can be achieved by taking advantage of the tumor vasculature hyperpermeability and inadequate lymphatic drainage, which results in enhanced permeability and retention of circulating particles. This approach is considered a passive targeting strategy. Alternatively, active targeting can be achieved when agents are coupled to the particle-based systems that bind to receptors or antigens highly expressed on the target tumor cell. This targeting strategy is particularly attractive as an active targeting process can lead to enhanced internalization of the vector by endocytosis. Targeting principles, shielding, and intracellular trafficking, including application examples such as tumor targeting, are discussed next.

3.1. Polyplexes

A variety of polycations has been used to condense DNA: naturally occurring proteins (e.g., histones or protamines, etc.), synthesized polyamino acids (e.g., polylysine, -histidine, and -arginine), and others (e.g., polyethyleneimine [PEI], chitosan, etc.) (for review, *see* ref. *1*). The major advantage of using polyplexes is that they can be easily conjugated to targeting agents; these include proteins (e.g., transferrin, epidermal growth factor, antibodies) and small molecules (e.g., folate, galactose). Various polymer-ligand gene delivery systems have been demonstrated to facilitate receptor-cell-mediated uptake into cancer cell lines. Of the cationic polymers tested, PEI has the highest in vitro transfection efficiency, which is believed to be because of its intrinsic ability to facilitate endosomal release. One proposed mechanism for the endosomolytic activity of PEI is the so-called proton sponge hypothesis, that an osmotic imbalance is caused on endosomal acidification, resulting in the breakup of the endosome *(26)*.

Various in vivo studies have shown that a near-neutral surface of the polyplexes is essential to minimize nonspecific interactions in the blood, allowing greater circulation time for the vector to reach its target *(27,28)*. To reduce the surface charge, hydrophilic agents have been attached to the polyplex surface to provide so-called steric stabilization *(28)*. Shielding agents investigated include polyethylene glycol (PEG) *(27)*, hydroxypropyl methacrylic acid *(29)*, and the serum protein transferrin *(30)*. Shielding by PEG not only improves circulation times, but also reduces toxicity, increases solubility, and provides stability for freezing-thawing *(31)*.

Of the shielding agents, most work has been done with PEG, with several different strategies of PEGylation developed. PEG can be covalently attached after polyplex formation (postPEGylation) *(27,33)*. PostPEGylation strategies require sequential steps, and the level of PEGylation will vary from batch to batch. Another concern for surface shielding is not only shielding of the surface charge, but also the activity of the targeting ligand. To overcome this, bifunctional PEG was used, allowing the targeting ligand to be attached at the distal end of the chain, providing greater accessibility to the receptor *(33)*.

Attempts have been made to avoid postPEGylation methods by synthesizing polycation-PEG copolymers that could form particles spontaneously when condensed with DNA. Presynthesis of polycation-PEG copolymers will allow more control over levels of PEGylation, providing more defined particles. However, for many of these copolymers the hydrophilic part appears to hinder proper DNA condensation and particle formation *(34,35)*. This improper DNA condensation, however, could be overcome by the addition of unmodified low molecular weight (LMW; 22 or 25 kDa) PEI with the shielding copolymer, in this case, Tf-PEI *(33)*.

PEGylated particles were formed spontaneously by mixing DNA with a mixture of PEI22 (condensing agent), PEG-PEI (surface shielding conjugate), and the targeting conjugate, for instance, Tf-PEG-PEI or EGF-PEG-PEI *(32,36)*. The mixing ratio of the PEI conjugates and PEI strongly influence the biophysical characteristics of the DNA particles formed. This method can generate PEG-shielded DNA complexes more quickly and easily than postPEGylation strategies.

Finsinger et al. *(37)* developed a new generation of shielding copolymers that disassemble at the lower pH of the endosome, mimicking the steps of viral entry. PEG is covalently attached to a polypeptide that is anionic at physiological pH; this copolymer is electrostatically attracted to the cationic polyplex core, shielding the surface charge. On entry to the endosome, the glutamic acids become protonated, breaking up the complex. This disassembly process enhanced the transfection efficiency of polylysine/DNA in vitro.

Wagner and coworkers first demonstrated tumor-targeted gene expression in distant tumors when PEG-shielded polyplexes of PEI (800 kDa) targeted with transferrin were injected into the tail vein of mice bearing subcutaneous Neuro-2A neuroblastoma tumors *(27,38)*. Luciferase reporter gene expression was enhanced from 100- to 1000-fold in the tumors compared to the other major organs. This specific gene expression could also be achieved with transferrin-shielded polyplexes with lower molecular weight (22 and 25 kDa) PEIs as gene carriers *(38)*. This work demonstrated that transferrin could be used as an alternative shielding agent, and that the lower molecular weight PEIs, which have lower toxicity, were effective as gene carriers.

With these encouraging results, the transferrin-targeted/shielded PEI polyplexes were used to apply the therapeutic gene TNF-α systemically to mice *(30)*. Gene expression of TNF-α was localized within the tumors in three different tumor models, resulting in pronounced hemorrhagic tumor necrosis and inhibition of tumor growth, with complete tumor regressions observed in the MethA model. No systemic TNF-related toxicity was observed *(30)*. Kursa et al. *(32)* showed a similar effective therapeutic response with a cryoconserved Tf-PEG-PEI/PEG-PEI/PEI22 formulation carrying the TNF-α gene.

For the use of tumor-targeted polyplexes as a "bedside medicine," biocompatible and biodegradable polymers would be advantageous. One approach is to use LMW polymers, which are more easily eliminated by the liver or kidney; however, because of their LMW, they inefficiently compact DNA. To condense DNA efficiently without an impact on toxicity, investigators have crosslinked LMW polymers with bioreversible disulfide linkages *(39,40)*. It is proposed that on reaching the reducing environment of the cytosol, these disulfide bonds will break, releasing the LMW polymers and DNA. To achieve the high efficiencies of PEI these new formulations will require endoosmolytic activity. To provide the sulfhydryl crosslinking of LMW peptides with endosomal buffering capacity to facilitate their endosomal release, histidine amino acids were included in the peptide sequence *(40)*. As an alternative approach to using polymers with high buffer capacity at low pH, membrane-active peptides have been covalently attached to polymers to facilitate endosomal release and, in some cases, facilitate their transport into the nucleus *(41,42)*.

To extend the concept of bioreversibly linked LMW polymer polyplexes to systemic delivery, their surface charge has to be shielded. Oupicky et al. *(39)* showed that postPEGylation of LMW crosslinked polylysine polyplexes increased circulation time 10-fold. In another approach, sulfhydryl crosslinking peptides and glycopeptides were conjugated with PEG. These copolymers bound DNA, and subsequent formation of disulfide bridges between the peptides and glycopeptides resulted in stable particles. The systemic stability of these PEG-shielded polyplexes has yet to be tested.

In the literature, there are several examples of high molecular weight biodegradable polycation gene carriers; however, they suffer from poor transfection efficiencies. Lim et al. *(43)* described a new biodegradable polymer of amino esters that has transfection efficiencies in mammalian cells similar to 25-kDa PEI but with minimal cytotoxicity. The polymer consists of a branched network of amino esters with synthesis based on that of the branched 25-kDa PEI. The high activity was attributed to its ability to mediate endosome acidification efficiently. This new polymer fulfills the two main requirements for a gene carrier—efficient transfection and low toxicity—and should be a useful tool in cancer gene therapy in the future.

3.2. Lipoplexes

Cationic liposomes are the most popular liposomes for gene therapy because neutral or negatively charged liposomes have low DNA encapsulation efficiency and lower levels of transfection. Cationic liposomes usually include DOPE or cholesterol as colipids. They are able to protect DNA from serum nucleases and facilitate the uptake and release of DNA into the cytosol. With respect to the mechanism of cell uptake and cytosolic release, there is evidence that their high positive surface charge electrostatically attracts them to the negatively charged cell surface, inducing their uptake up by endocytosis *(44–47)*. The cationic lipids of the carrier are believed to facilitate their release from the endosome by interacting with the anionic lipids of the inner endosomal membrane, forming non-bilayer lipid structures *(47)*. This process has been enhanced by the inclusion of so-called helper lipids such as DOPE, which have fusogenic properties at the lower pH of the endosome *(46)*. For liposomal-mediated gene delivery, a major barrier is the entry of the DNA into the nucleus *(48)*.

In the presence of serum proteins, lipoplexes can form aggregates, limiting potential transfection sites to "first-pass" organs such as the liver, spleen, and lungs. Local administration of lipoplexes, when possible, can overcome the stability problems associated with systemic circulation and allow for more specific delivery to tumor cells.

Nabel and coworkers *(49)* first reported the intratumoral injection of plasmid DNA complexed to cationic lipids to elicit antitumor responses in mice; a similar approach was evaluated and found safe in a pilot study of humans with melanoma. Intratumoral administration of lipoplexes containing genes encoding cytokines (e.g., IL-2, TNF-α) or suicide genes (e.g., *Pseudomonas* exotoxin A) resulted in therapeutic benefits *(50,51)*. Seki et al. *(52)* showed that intratumoral transfection of therapeutic genes could be enhanced by the inclusion of transferrin in the lipoplex.

Cationic liposome-based vectors that consist of polycationic/DNA core and cationic liposome (lipopolyplex) have improved gene transfer activity both in vitro and in vivo compared with standard cationic liposomes *(53)*. The improved transfection efficiency has been attributed to these particles smaller size and provision of better protection against nucleases. Intravenous administration of lipopolyplexes containing DNA with high frequencies of unmethylated CpG induced a systemic cytokine response that inhibited the growth of established pulmonary metastases *(54)*. Ueno et al. *(55)* used a lipopolyplex system to deliver plasmid encoding for adenovirus type 5 E1A protein systemically to human xenograph tumor models for head, neck, and breast cancer, resulting in suppressed tumor growth in all three models. Such lipopolyplex systems have enabled improved DNA entrapment efficiencies for neutral and anionic liposomes *(56)*.

Because these lipopolyplexes do not carrier a strong positive charge, they are expected to have fewer nonspecific interactions with both blood components and non-target cell membranes in vivo. Furthermore, anionic lipopolyplexes have been shown to have significantly less cytotoxicity than cationic liposomes *(57)*. To provide tumor targeting and enhance uptake by endocytosis, anionic liposomes have been attached with the folate-targeting ligand *(46)*. The attachment of folate increased their formulation stability and enhanced their uptake in cancer cell lines that overexpress the folate receptor.

In another approach to stabilize cationic liposomes for systemic application, PEG has been incorporated, resulting in longer circulation times and reduced accumulation in first-pass organs *(58–60)*. PEG-stabilized cationic liposomes resulted in higher reporter gene expression at the tumor site (Lewis lung tumor in the mouse flank) *(58)*. Interestingly, Hofland et al. *(59)* showed that the addition of PEG shielding dramatically reduced accumulation and gene transfer not only to the lung but also to tumors. This is in agreement with diminished in vitro binding of PEG-shielded cationic liposomes to melanoma cells *(61)*. To minimize lung accumulation and restore gene transfer to tumors, the targeting ligand folate was attached to the distal ends of PEG *(59)*.

Systemic targeted cationic liposomal gene delivery to tumors in combination with either radiotherapy or chemotherapy has also been effective in treating cancer. Transferrin-targeted liposomes enhanced the gene expression of the p53 gene in head and neck squamous cell carcinoma xenografts *(62)*. Expression of the p53 gene restored the apoptotic pathway of the tumors, making them more sensitive to radiotherapy. Folate-targeted stabilized cationic liposomes increased uptake of the anti-HER-2 antisense oligonucleotide in breast xenograft tumors in mice. In combination with the intravenously administered chemotherapeutic agent docetaxel, there was strong inhibition of tumor growth *(63)*.

Ramesh et al. *(64)* showed that the systemic application of cationic liposomes loaded with either p53 or FHIT genes resulted in transgene expression in 25% of cells in primary tumors and 10% in disseminated tumors.

3.4. Nanoplexes

Nanoplex gene delivery has only recently been applied to nonviral cancer gene therapy. Depending on the method of preparation, nanoplexes can either be nanospheres or nanocapsules. In the case of nanospheres; the DNA is either dispersed throughout the particle or adsorbed to its surface; in nanocapsules, the DNA is incorporated inside the particle.

Several investigators have demonstrated that DNA can be absorbed to the surface of nanoparticles and taken up by cells in vitro *(65)*; however, the loading efficiency is poor, and in vivo the DNA will be exposed to nucleases and could be displaced by blood components. To increase loading and protection from nucleases, oligonucleotides have been formulated into nanocapsules of poly(alkylcyanoacrylate); furthermore, these particles retained their activity after freeze-drying *(66)*.

Another system suitable for the delivery of oligonucleotides is nanoparticles made from proteins. Oligonucleotides were successfully encapsulated in bovine serum albumin and gelatin nanospheres under the soft conditions of coacervation *(67,68)*. Encapsulation stabilized the oligonucleotides against nucleases *(67)*. Gelatin particles were crosslinked after the coacervation process by the addition of 1-ethyl-3-(3-dimethylaminopropyl)carbodiimide *(67)*. This crosslinking process also allows the attachment of targeting moieties such as transferrin, which enhanced in vitro transfection efficiency, although it was dependent on the coencapsulation of the endoosmolytic agent chloroquine *(67)*.

Mao et al. *(69)* reported chitosan-DNA nanoparticles prepared by coacervation of chitosan and DNA in acidic solution. The nanoparticles protected the encapsulated plasmid DNA from nuclease degradation. Transferrin-targeted chitosan nanoplexes containing DNA and chloroquine, however, had little effect on transfection efficiency in HeLa cells, but when targeted with KNOB protein from adenovirus, there was about a 130-fold increase in transfection. PEGylation of chitosan nanoplexes resulted in increased circulation time and storage stability *(69)*.

Cui and Mumper *(70)* showed that DNA could be entrapped in nanoparticles by a quick and simple method; hydrophobized DNA was entrapped inside nanoparticles engineered from oil-in-water microemulsion precursors. Nanoparticles coated with the polysaccharide pullulan enhanced in vitro transfection in Hep G2 cells. Encapsulation of DNA in the nanoparticles increased their circulation times in mice.

Analogous to tumor-targeted PEG-shielded polyplexes *(33)* and lipoplexes *(59,63)*, the tumor-targeting ligand was covalently attached to the distal end of the PEG, which is bound to the nanoplex *(71)*. The PEGgylated nanoparticles were prepared from copolymers of poly(lactic acid) and PEG by a multiple emulsion/solvent method. The antitransferrin receptor monoclonal antibody was attached to the distal end of the PEG chains; however, the targeting activity of these nanoparticles has yet to be determined.

Hood and coworkers *(72)* first reported the successful application of targeted nanoplexes for delivering genes systemically for the treatment of tumors. In this case, nanoplexes were targeted to the blood vessels feeding the tumors rather than the tumor itself. Polymerized lipid-based nanoparticles could specifically target the angiogenic blood vessels of tumor-bearing mice by the covalently attachment of an integrin $\alpha_v\beta_3$-targeting ligand. The targeted nanoplexes were packed with a mutant form of the *Raf-1* gene, which blocks endothelial signaling and angiogenesis. Systemic application of these nanoplexes resulted in tumor cell apoptosis and sustained regression of established primary and metastatic tumors.

Most studies to date have shown the potential of nanoplexes for gene delivery at the cellular level and several promising advantages for application to cancer nonviral gene therapy: (1) the surface of the nanoplex can be conjugated with targeting ligands; (2) they efficiently protect DNA from nucleases; (3) endosomal escape and nuclear targeting excipients can be easily included; and (4) they can be stored lyophilized.

4. FUTURE DIRECTIONS

The ultimate nonviral gene vector for cancer therapy will be biocompatible, have efficient and specific gene expression in target cells, and be manufactured in an economical way. Physical methods (Table 2) will be able to target internal organs such as the liver and deep tumors and not just peripheral tissues. This will require the development of more powerful and patient-compliant instruments of delivery that can be used in combination with surgical techniques and improved particle-based methods.

Developers of particle-based systems have essentially tried to mimic the properties of viruses with the aim of achieving their higher transfection efficiencies. For this reason, many investigators like to call their nonviral vectors artificial viruses. These so-called artificial viruses do have several features common to viruses, for instance, targeting domains, protective coating, or endosomal release agents. However, unlike viruses, they do not undergo coordinated/programmed structural changes that make them more compatible at each step toward cell transfection. Nonviral vectors of the future will be multifunctional systems most likely containing many of the strategies in Table 1; however, they will be designed to undergo intracellular processing to use these strategies more effectively, for instance, deshielding on entry into the cell, release of membrane-disrupting agents on entry to the endosome, and unpackaging of DNA from the carrier on transport to the nucleus. Such programmed changes will be coordinated by the intracellular environment of each step, for instance, the presence of specific peptidases in the endo-lysosome system, changes in pH, or reductive environment. Not only will the particle-based systems of the future be more efficient in targeting and transfection, but also they will have improved formulation and storage stability, enabling them to be used as a bedside medicine for various applications (Table 3).

REFERENCES

1. Brown, M. D., Schatzlein, A. G., and Uchegbu, I. F. (2001) Gene delivery with synthetic (nonviral) carriers. *Int. J. Pharm.* **229,** 1–21.
2. Yang, J. P. and Huang, L. (1996) Direct gene transfer to mouse melanoma by intratumor injection of free DNA. *Gene Ther.* **3,** 542–548.
3. Baque, P., Pierrefite-Carle, V., Gavelli, A., et al. (2002) Naked DNA injection for liver metastases treatment in rats. *Hepatology* **35,** 1144–1152.
4. Park, J. H., Kim, C. J., Lee, J. H., Shin, S. H., Chung, G. H., and Jang, Y. S. (1999) Effective immunotherapy of cancer by DNA vaccination. *Mol. Cells* **9,** 384–391.
5. Song, K., Chang, Y., and Prud'homme, G. J. (2000) Regulation of T-helper-1 vs T-helper-2 activity and enhancement of tumor immunity by combined DNA-based vaccination and nonviral cytokine gene transfer. *Gene Ther.* **7,** 481–492.
6. Chen, C. H., Ji, H., Suh, K. W., Choti, M. A., Pardoll, D. M., and Wu, T. C. (1999) Gene gun-mediated DNA vaccination induces antitumor immunity against human papillomavirus type 16 E7-expressing murine tumor metastases in the liver and lungs. *Gene Ther.* **6,** 1972–1981.
7. Rakhmilevich, A. L., Timmins, J. G., Janssen, K., Pohlmann, E. L., Sheehy, M. J., and Yang, N. S. (1999) Gene gun-mediated IL-12 gene therapy induces antitumor effects in the absence of toxicity: a direct comparison with systemic IL-12 protein therapy. *J. Immunother.* **22,** 135–144.
8. Wang, J., Murakami, T., Hakamata, Y., et al. (2001) Gene gun-mediated oral mucosal transfer of interleukin 12 cDNA coupled with an irradiated melanoma vaccine in a hamster model: successful treatment of oral melanoma and distant skin lesion. *Cancer Gene Ther.* **8,** 705–712.
9. Brunner, S., Furtbauer, E., Sauer, T., Kursa, M., and Wagner, E. (2002) Overcoming the nuclear barrier: cell cycle independent nonviral gene transfer with linear polyethylenimine or electroporation. *Mol. Ther.* **5,** 80–86.
10. Harimoto, K., Sugimura, K., Lee, C. R., Kuratsukuri, K., and Kishimoto, T. (1998) In vivo gene transfer methods in the bladder without viral vectors. *Br. J. Urol.* **81,** 870–874.
11. Wells, J. M., Li, L. H., Sen, A., Jahreis, G. P., and Hui, S. W. (2000) Electroporation-enhanced gene delivery in mammary tumors. *Gene Ther.* **7,** 541–547.
12. Nishi, T., Yoshizato, K., Yamashiro, S., et al. (1996) High-efficiency in vivo gene transfer using intraarterial plasmid DNA injection following in vivo electroporation. *Cancer Res.* **56,** 1050–1055.
13. Rols, M. P., Delteil, C., Golzio, M., Dumond, P., Cros, S., and Teissie, J. (1998) In vivo electrically mediated protein and gene transfer in murine melanoma. *Nat. Biotechnol.* **16,** 168–171.
14. Aihara, H. and Miyazaki, J. (1998) Gene transfer into muscle by electroporation in vivo. *Nat. Biotechnol.* **16,** 867–870.
15. Mathiesen, I. (1999) Electropermeabilization of skeletal muscle enhances gene transfer in vivo. *Gene Ther.* **6,** 508–514.
16. Widera, G., Austin, M., Rabussay, D., et al. (2000) Increased DNA vaccine delivery and immunogenicity by electroporation in vivo. *J. Immunol.* **164,** 4635–4640.
17. Mendiratta, S. K., Thai, G., Eslahi, N. K., et al. (2001) Therapeutic tumor immunity induced by polyimmunization with melanoma antigens gp100 and TRP-2. *Cancer Res.* **61,** 859–863.
18. Lauer, U., Burgelt, E., Squire, Z., et al. (1997) Shock wave permeabilization as a new gene transfer method. *Gene Ther.* **4,** 710–715.
19. Manome, Y., Nakamura, M., Ohno, T., and Furuhata, H. (2000) Ultrasound facilitates transduction of naked plasmid DNA into colon carcinoma cells in vitro and in vivo. *Hum. Gene Ther.* **11,** 1521–1528.
20. Huber, P. E. and Pfisterer, P. (2000) In vitro and in vivo transfection of plasmid DNA in the Dunning prostate tumor R3327-AT1 is enhanced by focused ultrasound. *Gene Ther.* **7,** 1516–1525.
21. Anwer, K., Kao, G., Proctor, B., et al. (2000) Ultrasound enhancement of cationic lipid-mediated gene transfer to primary tumors following systemic administration. *Gene Ther.* **7,** 1833–1839.
22. Seemann, S., Hauff, P., Schultze-Mosgau, M., Lehmann, C., and Reszka, R. (2002) Pharmaceutical evaluation of gas-filled microparticles as gene delivery system. *Pharm. Res.* **19,** 250–257.
23. Walther, W., Stein, U., Fichtner, I., Malcherek, L., Lemm, M., and Schlag, P. M. (2001) Nonviral in vivo gene delivery into tumors using a novel low volume jet-injection technology. *Gene Ther.* **8,** 173–180.
24. Scherer, F., Anton, M., Schillinger, U., et al. (2002) Magnetofection: enhancing and targeting gene delivery by magnetic force in vitro and in vivo. *Gene Ther.* **9,** 102–109.
25. Blessing, T., Remy, J. S., and Behr, J. P. (1998) Monomolecular collapse of plasmid DNA into stable virus-like particles. *Proc. Natl. Acad. Sci. USA* **95,** 1427–1431.
26. Kichler, A., Leborgne, C., Coeytaux, E., and Danos, O. (2001) Polyethylenimine-mediated gene delivery: a mechanistic study. *J. Gene Med.* **3,** 135–144.
27. Ogris, M., Brunner, S., Schuller, S., Kircheis, R., and Wagner, E. (1999) PEGylated DNA/transferrin-PEI complexes: reduced interaction with blood components, extended circulation in blood and potential for systemic gene delivery. *Gene Ther.* **6,** 595–605.
28. Oupicky, D., Ogris, M., and Seymour, L. W. (2002) Development of long-circulating polyelectrolyte complexes for systemic delivery of genes. *J. Drug Target.* **10,** 93–98.

29. Dash, P. R., Read, M. L., Fisher, K. D., et al. (2000) Decreased binding to proteins and cells of polymeric gene delivery vectors surface modified with a multivalent hydrophilic polymer and retargeting through attachment of transferrin. *J. Biol. Chem.* **275**, 3793–3802.

30. Kircheis, R., Ostermann, E., Wolschek, M. F., et al. (2002) Tumor-targeted gene delivery of tumor necrosis factor-alpha induces tumor necrosis and tumor regression without systemic toxicity. *Cancer Gene Ther.* **9**, 673–680.

31. Choi, Y. H., Liu, F., Kim, J. S., Choi, Y. K., Park, J. S., and Kim, S. W. (1998) Polyethylene glycol-grafted poly-L-lysine as polymeric gene carrier. *J. Control. Release* **54**, 39–48.

32. Kursa, M., Walker, G. F., Roessler, V., et al. (2003) Novel shielded transferrin-polyethylene glycol-polyethylenimine/DNA complexes for systemic tumor-targeted gene transfer. *Bioconjug. Chem.* **14**, 222–231.

33. Blessing, T., Kursa, M., Holzhauser, R., Kircheis, R., and Wagner, E. (2001) Different strategies for formation of pegylated EGF-conjugated PEI/DNA complexes for targeted gene delivery. *Bioconjug. Chem.* **12**, 529–537.

34. Wolfert, M. A., Schacht, E. H., Toncheva, V., et al. (1996) Characterization of vectors for gene therapy formed by self-assembly of DNA with synthetic block co-polymers. *Hum. Gene Ther.* **7**, 2123–2133.

35. Erbacher, P., Bettinger, T., Belguise-Valladier, P., et al. (1999) Transfection and physical properties of various saccharide, poly(ethylene glycol), and antibody-derivatized polyethylenimines (PEI). *J. Gene Med.* **1**, 210–222.

36. Wolschek, M. F., Thallinger, C., Kursa, M., et al. (2002) Specific systemic nonviral gene delivery to human hepatocellular carcinoma xenografts in SCID mice. *Hepatology* **36**, 1106–1114.

37. Finsinger, D., Remy, J. S., Erbacher, P., Koch, C., and Plank, C. (2000) Protective copolymers for nonviral gene vectors: synthesis, vector characterization and application in gene delivery. *Gene Ther.* **7**, 1183–1192.

38. Kircheis, R., Wightman, L., Schreiber, A., et al. (2001) Polyethylenimine/DNA complexes shielded by transferrin target gene expression to tumors after systemic application. *Gene Ther.* **8**, 28–40.

39. Oupicky, D., Carlisle, R. C., and Seymour, L. W. (2001) Triggered intracellular activation of disulfide crosslinked polyelectrolyte gene delivery complexes with extended systemic circulation in vivo. *Gene Ther.* **8**, 713–724.

40. McKenzie, D. L., Smiley, E., Kwok, K. Y., and Rice, K. G. (2000) Low molecular weight disulfide cross-linking peptides as nonviral gene delivery carriers. *Bioconjug. Chem.* **11**, 901–909.

41. Ogris, M., Carlisle, R. C., Bettinger, T., and Seymour, L. W. (2001) Melittin enables efficient vesicular escape and enhanced nuclear access of nonviral gene delivery vectors. *J. Biol. Chem.* **276**, 47,550–47,555.

42. Wagner, E. (1999) Application of membrane-active peptides for nonviral gene delivery. *Adv. Drug Deliv. Rev.* **38**, 279–289.

43. Lim, Y. B., Kim, S. M., Suh, H., and Park, J. S. (2002) Biodegradable, endosome disruptive, and cationic network-type polymer as a highly efficient and nontoxic gene delivery carrier. *Bioconjug. Chem.* **13**, 952–957.

44. Friend, D. S., Papahadjopoulos, D., and Debs, R. J. (1996) Endocytosis and intracellular processing accompanying transfection mediated by cationic liposomes. *Biochim. Biophys. Acta* **1278**, 41–50.

45. Xu, Y. and Szoka, F. C. Jr. (1996) Mechanism of DNA release from cationic liposome/DNA complexes used in cell transfection. *Biochemistry* **35**, 5616–5623.

46. Reddy, J. A. and Low, P. S. (2000) Enhanced folate receptor mediated gene therapy using a novel pH-sensitive lipid formulation. *J. Control. Release* **64**, 27–37.

47. Hafez, I. M., Maurer, N., and Cullis, P. R. (2001) On the mechanism whereby cationic lipids promote intracellular delivery of polynucleic acids. *Gene Ther.* **8**, 1188–1196.

48. Zabner, J., Fasbender, A. J., Moninger, T., Poellinger, K. A., and Welsh, M. J. (1995) Cellular and molecular barriers to gene transfer by a cationic lipid. *J. Biol. Chem.* **270**, 18,997–19,007.

49. Nabel, G. J., Nabel, E. G., Yang, Z. Y., et al. (1993) Direct gene transfer with DNA-liposome complexes in melanoma: expression, biologic activity, and lack of toxicity in humans. *Proc. Natl. Acad. Sci. USA* **90**, 11,307–11,311.

50. Clark, P. R., Stopeck, A. T., Ferrari, M., Parker, S. E., and Hersh, E. M. (2000) Studies of direct intratumoral gene transfer using cationic lipid-complexed plasmid DNA. *Cancer Gene Ther.* **7**, 853–860.

51. Yerushalmi, N., Brinkmann, U., Brinkmann, E., Pai, L., and Pastan, I. (2000) Attenuating the growth of tumors by intratumoral administration of DNA encoding *Pseudomonas* exotoxin via cationic liposomes. *Cancer Gene Ther.* **7**, 91–96.

52. Seki, M., Iwakawa, J., Cheng, H., and Cheng, P. W. (2002) p53 and PTEN/MMAC1/TEP1 gene therapy of human prostate PC-3 carcinoma xenograft, using transferrin-facilitated lipofection gene delivery strategy. *Hum. Gene Ther.* **13**, 761–773.

53. Li, S. and Huang, L. (1997) In vivo gene transfer via intravenous administration of cationic lipid-protamine-DNA (LPD) complexes. *Gene Ther.* **4**, 891–900.

54. Whitmore, M. M., Li, S., Falo, L. Jr., and Huang, L. (2001) Systemic administration of LPD prepared with CpG oligonucleotides inhibits the growth of established pulmonary metastases by stimulating innate and acquired antitumor immune responses. *Cancer Immunol. Immunother.* **50**, 503–514.

55. Ueno, N. T., Bartholomeusz, C., Xia, W., et al. (2002) Systemic gene therapy in human xenograft tumor models by liposomal delivery of the E1A gene. *Cancer Res.* **62**, 6712–6716.

56. Lee, R. J. and Huang, L. (1996) Folate-targeted, anionic liposome-entrapped polylysine-condensed DNA for tumor cell-specific gene transfer. *J. Biol. Chem.* **271**, 8481–8487.

57. Guo, W. and Lee, R. J. (2000) Efficient gene delivery using anionic liposome-complexed polyplexes (LPDII). *Biosci. Rep.* **20,** 419–432.
58. Monck, M. A., Mori, A., Lee, D., et al. (2000) Stabilized plasmid-lipid particles: pharmacokinetics and plasmid delivery to distal tumors following intravenous injection. *J. Drug Target.* **7,** 439–452.
59. Hofland, H. E., Masson, C., Iginla, S., et al. (2002) Folate-targeted gene transfer in vivo. *Mol. Ther.* **5,** 739–744.
60. Tam, P., Monck, M., Lee, D., et al. (2000) Stabilized plasmid-lipid particles for systemic gene therapy. *Gene Ther.* **7,** 1867–1874.
61. Harvie, P., Wong, F. M., and Bally, M. B. (2000) Use of poly(ethylene glycol)-lipid conjugates to regulate the surface attributes and transfection activity of lipid-DNA particles. *J. Pharm. Sci.* **89,** 652–663.
62. Xu, L., Pirollo, K. F., Tang, W. H., Rait, A., and Chang, E. H. (1999) Transferrin-liposome-mediated systemic p53 gene therapy in combination with radiation results in regression of human head and neck cancer xenografts. *Hum. Gene Ther.* **10,** 2941–2952.
63. Rait, A. S., Pirollo, K. F., Xiang, L., Ulick, D., and Chang, E. H. (2002) Tumor-targeting, systemically delivered antisense HER-2 chemosensitizes human breast cancer xenografts irrespective of HER-2 levels. *Mol. Med.* **8,** 475–486.
64. Ramesh, R., Saeki, T., Templeton, N. S., et al. (2001) Successful treatment of primary and disseminated human lung cancers by systemic delivery of tumor suppressor genes using an improved liposome vector. *Mol. Ther.* **3,** 337–350.
65. Panyam, J., Zhou, W. Z., Prabha, S., Sahoo, S. K., and Labhasetwar, V. (2002) Rapid endo-lysosomal escape of poly(DL-lactide-*co*-glycolide) nanoparticles: implications for drug and gene delivery. *FASEB J.* **16,** 1217–1226.
66. Berton, M., Allemann, E., Stein, C. A., and Gurny, R. (1999) Highly loaded nanoparticulate carrier using an hydrophobic antisense oligonucleotide complex. *Eur. J. Pharm. Sci.* **9,** 163–170.
67. Truong-Le, V. L., Walsh, S. M., Schweibert, E., et al. (1999) Gene transfer by DNA-gelatin nanospheres. *Arch. Biochem. Biophys.* **361,** 47–56.
68. Arnedo, A., Espuelas, S., and Irache, J. M. (2002) Albumin nanoparticles as carriers for a phosphodiester oligonucleotide. *Int. J. Pharm.* **244,** 59–72.
69. Mao, H. Q., Roy, K., Troung, L., et al. (2001) Chitosan-DNA nanoparticles as gene carriers: synthesis, characterization and transfection efficiency. *J. Control. Release* **70,** 399–421.
70. Cui, Z. and Mumper, R. J. (2002) Plasmid DNA-entrapped nanoparticles engineered from microemulsion precursors: in vitro and in vivo evaluation. *Bioconjug. Chem.* **13,** 1319–1327.
71. Olivier, J. C., Huertas, R., Lee, H. J., Calon, F., and Pardridge, W. M. (2002) Synthesis of pegylated immunoparticles. *Pharm. Res.* **19,** 1137–1143.
72. Hood, J. D., Bednarski, M., Frausto, R., et al. (2002) Tumor regression by targeted gene delivery to the neovasculature. *Science* **296,** 2404–2407.

25

Viral Vectors for Cancer Gene Therapy

Joanne T. Douglas and David T. Curiel

1. INTRODUCTION

Cancer gene therapy is the transfer of genetic material to the cells of an individual with the goal of eradicating cancer cells. This can be accomplished directly by transferring genetic material into the cancer cells themselves to bring about their destruction, or indirectly, either by stimulating the immune system to recognize and eliminate the cancer cells or by targeting the nonmalignant stromal cells that support the growth and metastasis of cancer cells. Each of these approaches exploits the expanding knowledge of the genetic basis of cancer, thereby allowing rationally targeted interventions at the molecular level. Thus, cancer gene therapy offers the potential to achieve a much higher level of specificity of action than afforded by conventional drug therapeutics. Cancer gene therapy therefore mandates a gene delivery vehicle, or vector, capable of delivering the therapeutic gene into the target cell such that an appropriate level of the gene product is expressed for a sufficient length of time to achieve its desired effect. Moreover, this should be accomplished within an acceptable safety margin.

There are two major classes of delivery vehicles for cancer gene therapy: viral and nonviral vectors. As a class, viral vectors possess the key advantage of efficiency: Viruses have evolved over millions of years to be highly effective at infecting cells and transferring their genetic material to the nucleus, where it is expressed. In contrast, the major obstacles to the use of nonviral vectors are their relatively poor specificity and efficiency; strategies to improve nonviral vectors for cancer gene therapy are discussed elsewhere in this book. However, viral vectors also suffer from a number of limitations, including the potential for acute toxicity in response to vector administration and the possibility that previous exposure to a virus will render a host resistant to transduction by the viral vector.

A number of different viruses have been adapted as vectors for cancer gene therapy. The underlying biology of the virus dictates the most rational application for that vector in cancer gene therapy. For example, retroviruses have been employed predominantly for gene transfer ex vivo, which involves a time-consuming and complex procedure in which the target cells are removed from the patient, genetically modified, and then reimplanted into the same recipient, whereas the attributes of other viruses favor their use for in vivo gene transfer. The properties of the virus also determine whether the vector would be more rationally employed to transduce the cancer cells themselves, for which short-term gene expression would be sufficient to achieve cell death, or to mediate long-term expression of therapeutic genes, such as genes encoding antiangiogenic factors, from stromal cells.

In this chapter, we discuss the various viral vectors employed in cancer gene therapy, focusing on how the biology of the virus informs the choice of the particular therapeutic approach, and discussing strategies to improve the vectors for clinical application.

From: *Contemporary Cancer Research*
Cancer Gene Therapy
Edited by: D. T. Curiel and J. T. Douglas © Humana Press Inc., Totowa, NJ

2. VIRAL VECTORS

2.1. Retroviral Vectors

Several mammalian and avian C-type retroviruses have been exploited as vectors for cancer gene therapy, including Moloney murine leukemia virus (MuLV), gibbon ape leukemia virus, spleen necrosis virus, and avian sarcoma and leukosis viruses. A mature C-type retroviral particle is spherical, roughly 100 nm in diameter, and surrounded by an envelope consisting of a lipid membrane bilayer into which glycoproteins are inserted. The retroviral genome is a homodimer of linear, positive-sense, single-stranded ribonucleic acid (RNA), with the size of each monomer 7 to 13 kb. The distinguishing characteristic of the life cycle of retroviruses is the reverse flow of genetic information from this RNA genome to double-stranded deoxyribonucleic acid (DNA), the provirus, which is integrated into the chromosomal DNA of an infected cell, thereby allowing the retrovirus to maintain a persistent infection *(1)*.

The life cycle of retroviruses accounts for their use as gene therapy vectors. To enter a cell and initiate infection, all retroviruses require an interaction between the viral envelope glycoprotein and a specific cell surface receptor; the viral envelope glycoprotein therefore dictates the type of cells that can be infected. Once virus particles have bound to the receptor, the virion and host membranes fuse, and the virion core is delivered into the cytoplasm of the infected cell, where the RNA genome is reverse transcribed to form double-stranded linear DNA *(1)*. Nuclear entry of the viral DNA is absolutely dependent on disruption of the nuclear membrane during the process of mitosis *(2)*. Hence, retroviral vectors can only infect actively dividing cells, a feature that limits their application for cancer gene therapy.

The retroviral DNA then integrates into the host DNA to form the provirus. The integrated provirus is collinear with the product of reverse transcription and consists of a 5' long terminal repeat (LTR), about 8 kb of intervening viral sequences encoding the structural proteins (Gag, Pol, and Env), and a 3' LTR. Transcription of the provirus is initiated from a promoter within the 5' LTR and proceeds through the genome. The messenger RNA (mRNA) is polyadenylated and processed using signals in transcribed regions from the 3' LTR. A portion of the transcripts is exported directly from the nucleus and serves as the genome to be packaged into the progeny virion particle. Another portion of the mRNA is translated to form the structural proteins. Progeny virions are assembled at the plasma membrane, and the RNA genome is incorporated by virtue of interactions between specific RNA sequences near the 5' end of the genome, termed the packaging or Psi sequences, and specific residues in the Gag protein. The progeny then bud off from the cell membrane and are released *(1)*.

Retroviral vectors are constructed from the DNA form, corresponding to the integrated provirus. Because the *cis*-acting sequences are located in the terminal regions, the central sequences encoding the structural proteins can be removed from the virus and replaced by the transgene of interest, which can therefore be up to 8 kb long. The proteins needed for production of infectious viral particles are supplied in *trans* in packaging/producer cells in which the vector DNA is transcribed into RNA and packaged into viral particles. The biosafety of retroviral vectors has been improved by expressing the *trans*-acting viral proteins from separate constructs within the packaging cell lines to increase the number of separate recombination events that would be necessary to generate replication-competent retroviruses. The latest packaging cell lines can produce retroviral vector titers above 10^7 transducing units per milliliter.

The first cancer gene therapy clinical trials, dating to 1990 *(3)*, employed retroviral vectors in ex vivo immunotherapy strategies that took advantage of the ability of the vector RNA genome to be reverse transcribed in the transduced cells, followed by stable integration of the DNA into the host genome to mediate long-term expression of the therapeutic gene. This ex vivo approach was an appropriate application of retroviral vectors because the viral titers that could be achieved at that time were not sufficient to permit in vivo administration. Moreover, the fact that retroviral vectors were sensitive to inactivation by complement mandated an ex vivo approach.

In these immunotherapy trials, the target cells were removed from the cancer patient, transduced with a retroviral vector carrying a cytokine gene, expanded in culture, and then readministered to the patient to induce an antitumor immune response. A number of target cells were employed in these early protocols, including tumor-infiltrating lymphocytes *(4)*, cancer cells *(5,6)*, and fibroblasts *(7,8)*, together with a variety of therapeutic genes, such as tumor necrosis factor *(4,5)*; interleukins 2 *(9)*, 4 *(7)*, and 12 *(8)*; and granulocyte-macrophage colony-stimulating factor *(6)*. Autologous T cells or dendritic cells expressing major histocompatibility complex class II antigens or receptors directed against tumor-specific antigens, such as TAG-72, have been evaluated in phase I/II clinical trials *(10)*. Although these immunotherapy approaches have been safe, there has not been a clear demonstration of an effective cure.

The ability of retroviral vectors to selectively transduce dividing cells provided the rationale for a strategy designed to treat glioblastoma by targeting gene expression to actively dividing brain tumor cells while avoiding normal, nonmitotic, parenchymal brain tissue. In this approach, murine retroviral producer cell lines producing vectors expressing the herpes simplex virus thymidine kinase (HSV*tk*) suicide gene were stereotactically injected directly into the brain tumors of patients *(11)*. Patients were then treated with the prodrug ganciclovir (GCV), a nucleoside analog phosphorylated by HSV*tk* to form a nucleotidelike precursor that inhibits DNA replication, thereby leading to cell death. The selective toxic effect of GCV on proliferating cells therefore superimposed a second level of tumor targeting on top of the selective transduction of actively dividing glioblastoma cells by the retroviral vector. In 1997, a randomized multicenter trial designed to compare the efficacy of surgery, radiation, and injection of murine cells producing the HSV*tk* vector followed by intravenous GCV against the efficacy of surgery and radiation in the treatment of newly diagnosed, previously untreated glioblastoma became the first cancer gene therapy trial to advance to phase III *(12)*. However, it has been determined that human cancer cells cycle rather slowly, so that only a small fraction of the target tumor cells is actually dividing at any given time; consequently, the large percentage of quiescent cells undermines the utility of this strategy.

A number of modifications have been made to retroviral vectors to improve their usefulness for cancer gene therapy. Improved packaging cell lines based on human cells have been developed to allow the production of complement-resistant particles, which therefore have the potential for intravenous administration. To achieve a higher level of transgene expression than can be achieved from the 5' LTR and/or to achieve specific expression in target cell types and tissues, heterologous promoters can be placed internally in the retroviral transcription unit to drive transgene transcription. Work is also under way to understand the mechanism by which retroviral vectors integrated into the chromatin of the host cell become subject to transcriptional silencing so that rational strategies can be designed to circumvent this problem.

The integration of the DNA genome into regions of open chromatin affords the risk of insertional mutagenesis, as recently reported in a clinical trial for X-linked severe combined immunodeficiency, in which retrovirus-mediated γc chain transfer into autologous bone marrow cells in two very young patients led to uncontrolled clonal proliferation of mature T cells caused by insertion of the vector near the promoter of the proto-oncogene *LMO2 (13)*. Although disease- and protocol-specific factors may have played a role in this event, it is clear that greater understanding of the mechanisms of retroviral integration could facilitate the design of safer vectors.

Perhaps the major obstacle to the use of retroviral vectors in human cancer gene therapy is that the viral envelope glycoprotein dictates the host range of the vector. Thus, MuLV-based vectors containing the ecotropic envelope protein can infect only mouse cells; vectors containing the amphotropic envelope protein can infect both mouse and nonmouse cells. Importantly, virions containing these envelope proteins can be concentrated only with a very low efficiency and labor-intensive protocols and cannot withstand the shear forces of ultracentrifugation. Fortunately, the process of virion assembly means that it is possible to substitute one envelope glycoprotein for another, a process known as pseudotyping (*see* p. 384). In this regard, MuLV can be pseudotyped with the G protein of the vesicular stomatitis virus (VSV-G) *(14)*. Such VSV-G-pseudotyped vectors can be concentrated 100- to 300-fold by ultracentrifugation to titers above 10^9 transducing units per milliliter. However, VSV-G mediates viral entry by membrane fusion via the interaction with phospholipid components of the cell membrane; therefore, it has a broad host range. Hence, it is apparent that a major advance in the utility of retroviral vectors for cancer gene therapy would accrue from the development of strategies to allow the efficient and specific transduction of target cancer cells in vivo.

Transductional targeting of avian leukosis viruses has been accomplished by a molecular bridge consisting of the extracellular domain of the cellular receptor for the virus fused to a ligand, such as epidermal growth factor or vascular endothelial growth factor *(15,16)*. The receptors for avian leukosis virus are well suited to this strategy because they are simple type 1 transmembrane proteins with extracellular domains that can be produced as soluble forms that retain the ability to bind the virus and stimulate cellular entry. In contrast, the receptors for most other retroviruses have multiple membrane-spanning domains that render them inappropriate for use in a receptor–ligand molecular bridge.

Other targeted retroviral vectors have been engineered by insertion of ligands *(17)* or single-chain antibodies *(18)* into the envelope glycoprotein. In many cases, however, this modification prevents the conformational change required for membrane fusion and cell entry that is triggered by receptor binding. Consequently, the infectious titer of targeted retroviral vectors is often considerably less than the titer of retroviruses with wild-type envelope glycoproteins. To some extent, this problem can be overcome by incorporating wild-type envelope proteins into targeted retroviral particles in addition to the modified envelope proteins *(19)*. Alternatively, a protease-cleavable linker peptide can be inserted between the displayed ligand and the viral envelope glycoprotein, so that cleavage of the ligand at the target site restores the native configuration of the envelope protein, allowing efficient membrane fusion and productive infection *(20)*.

A retroviral vector with a targeting modification in its envelope glycoprotein has been approved for the first clinical gene therapy trial employing vascular delivery of a retroviral vector. Dr. Heinz-Josef Lenz and colleagues at the University of Southern California, Keck School of Medicine, will conduct a tumor site-specific phase I/II evaluation of the safety and efficacy of hepatic arterial infusion of a matrix-targeted retroviral vector bearing a dominant-negative cyclin G1 construct as a treatment for colorectal carcinoma metastatic to liver *(21)*. Rather than target specific cancer cells, this vector is designed to target an area of pathology, namely, the sites of exposed collagen with the lesions created by growing tumors *(19)*. The hypothesis is that, by binding the vector to the exposed collagen, the rapidly proliferating cancer cells in proximity will be more efficiently transduced. Binding of the vector to collagen is accomplished by incorporating a discrete collagen-binding domain of von Willebrand factor into the amphotropic MuLV envelope protein. Importantly, the matrix-targeted vector possesses near wild-type amphotropic infectivity. The results of the clinical trial are keenly awaited so that the potential of this targeted injectable retroviral vector for human gene therapy can be evaluated.

2.2. Adenoviral Vectors

Adenoviruses possess a nonenveloped icosahedral protein shell or capsid 70–100 nm in diameter surrounding an inner DNA-containing core. The 20 facets of the capsid are each composed of 12 copies of the trimeric hexon protein, which is the most abundant component of the virion and performs a structural role. Each vertex of the capsid is composed of a pentameric penton base protein in association with a trimeric fiber protein that projects from the viral surface and ends with a globular knob domain. The fiber and penton base both play important roles in the initial steps of the virus–cell interaction during infection. The core of the adenoviral particle contains the viral genome, a linear, double-stranded DNA molecule approximately 36 kb long. The *cis*-acting origins of replication of the viral DNA are located in the first 50 base pairs (bp) of the 100- to 140-bp inverted terminal repeat

(ITR) sequences located at each end of the genome. The ITR sequences play an important role in replication of the DNA. A terminal protein is covalently attached to each of the 5' termini of the DNA and serves as a primer for DNA replication. The left end of the genome also includes a *cis*-acting packaging signal that directs the interaction of the viral DNA with its encapsidating proteins *(22)*.

Human adenoviruses are classified into six species based on the percentage of guanine and cytosine in the DNA molecules and the ability to agglutinate red blood cells *(22)*. They are further subdivided into more than 50 serotypes, primarily on the basis of neutralization assays. The majority of recombinant adenoviral vectors are based on human adenovirus serotypes 2 (Ad2) and 5 (Ad5) of species C, which cause a mild respiratory disease in humans and are nononcogenic.

The rational design of adenoviral vectors is based on an understanding of the infectious cycle of the parental viruses. The entry of adenoviruses into susceptible cells requires two distinct, sequential steps—binding and internalization—each mediated by the interaction of a specific capsid protein with a cellular receptor. The initial high-affinity binding of Ad2 and Ad5 to the primary cellular receptor, the so-called coxsackie and adenovirus receptor (CAR), occurs via the globular knob domain of the fiber capsid protein *(23–26)*. CAR appears to function purely as a docking site for the virus on the cell surface; the cytoplasmic and transmembrane domains of the molecule are not essential for adenoviral infection *(27)*. Subsequent internalization of the virus by receptor-mediated endocytosis is potentiated by the interaction of Arg-Gly-Asp (RGD) peptide sequences in the penton base protein with secondary host cell receptors, integrins $\alpha_v\beta_3$ and $\alpha_v\beta_5$ *(28,29)*. The virion escapes from the endosome, the capsid is disrupted, and the virus is transported to the nuclear membrane. The genome then passages through the nuclear pore into the nucleus, where the primary transcription events are initiated.

Expression of the adenoviral genes is temporally regulated. E1A is the first transcription unit to be expressed after the adenoviral chromosome enters the nucleus of an infected cell; its expression requires only cellular proteins. The E1A proteins activate transcription from the other adenoviral early regions and induce the host cell to enter the S phase of the cell cycle. The E1B gene encodes two proteins (E1B 19K and E1B 55K) that inhibit apoptosis and further modulate cellular metabolism to render the cell more susceptible to viral replication. The E2 transcription unit encodes three proteins involved in viral DNA replication. The E3 region encodes multiple proteins designed to inhibit pathways of cell death induced by the host innate and cellular immune response to the infected cell. The E3 proteins are dispensable for the replication of adenoviruses in tissue culture. The E4 gene products perform a range of functions, with distinct proteins playing roles in viral DNA replication, viral mRNA transport and splicing, shut off of host protein synthesis, and regulation of apoptosis *(22)*.

The expression of the early adenoviral genes sets the stage for replication of the viral DNA. Replication of the adenoviral DNA starts at the origins of replication in the ITR sequences at either end of the chromosome, with the terminal protein serving as a primer. The expression of the late adenoviral genes commences with the onset of DNA replication. The late gene products are expressed after processing a 20-kb transcript from the major late promoter, which is attenuated during transcription of the early genes. This primary transcript undergoes multiple splicing events to generate five families of late mRNAs encoding proteins that are part of the viral capsid or are involved in the encapsidation and assembly of viral particles in the host cell nucleus. Encapsidation of the viral DNA is directed by the packaging signal at the left end of the chromosome. This process is accompanied by alterations in the nuclear infrastructure and the permeabilization of the nuclear membrane, facilitating the egress of the progeny viruses into the cytoplasm. The plasma membrane subsequently disintegrates, and the progeny are released from the cell *(22)*.

A number of characteristics of human Ad2 and Ad5 spawned their development as vectors for cancer gene therapy. Adenoviruses can infect a broad range of cell types, including both dividing and nonmitotic cells, and have evolved an extremely efficient mechanism for delivery of their genome to the nucleus. The genome remains extrachromosomal, which minimizes the risk of insertional mutagenesis. Vectors derived from serotypes 2 and 5 can be purified to high titers (up to 10^{13} virus particles per milliliter), which means that it is practical to employ them in vivo. Adenoviruses possess the important attribute of stability in the bloodstream, which means that adenoviral vectors can potentially be employed for gene delivery following intravenous administration. Adenoviral vectors are rendered replication-deficient by deletion of the E1 region of the genome, which means they are capable of propagation only in specially designed complementing cell lines. So-called first-generation E1-deleted Ad2 and Ad5 vectors can accommodate up to 7.5 kb of foreign DNA, and the capacity of the vectors can be expanded by additional deletions of the viral genes. The promise of adenovirus-based gene delivery vehicles has, in turn, led to the development of a range of techniques by which their genomes can be manipulated and recombinant vectors generated with relative ease.

Based on these key features, adenoviral vectors have been widely employed in cancer gene therapy strategies in both preclinical and clinical studies. In fact, the number of cancer gene therapy clinical trials employing adenoviral vectors now exceeds those using retroviral vectors. These trials have been designed to exploit the ability of adenoviral vectors to accomplish efficient in vivo gene delivery. Adenoviral vectors have been employed to deliver a variety of therapeutic genes in the context of mutation compensation and molecular chemotherapy approaches, including the tumor suppressor genes p53 *(30)* and p16 *(31)*, antisense DNA, ribozymes and single-chain antibodies *(32,33)*, and the suicide genes HSV*tk* and cytosine deaminase. In the absence of a vector capable of targeted, tumor cell-specific gene delivery on systemic administration, clinical trials involving adenovirus-mediated gene transfer have concentrated on those cancers that would benefit from improved local or regional control of tumor growth, including squamous cell carcinoma of the head and neck; brain, bladder, and ovarian cancers; locally advanced prostate cancer; and nonmetastatic stages of non-small cell lung cancer and breast cancer.

In general, the results of adenovirus-mediated cancer gene therapy have been disappointing, with only limited efficacy observed in preclinical and clinical studies. A number of studies have shown that primary cancer cells express only low levels of CAR *(34)*, and it has been demonstrated that the therapeutic efficacy of adenoviral vectors is restricted by the inability of the vectors to infect tumor cells expressing low levels of CAR *(35)*. This therefore suggests that the efficacy of adenoviral vectors for cancer gene therapy could be improved by modifying the viruses to allow efficient infection via a CAR-independent pathway. Modification of adenoviral tropism is accomplished by alteration of the knob domain of the adenoviral fiber capsid protein to redirect binding to an alternative cellular receptor. Because adenoviruses use two distinct capsid proteins for cell binding and entry, modifications to the fiber protein, which is responsible for binding to the primary cellular receptor, will not adversely affect internalization, which is mediated by binding of the viral penton base protein to cellular integrins.

Targeted adenoviral vectors have been constructed by two general strategies *(36)*. In one approach, the vector is complexed with molecular bridges, either chemical conjugates *(37)* or recombinant fusion proteins *(38)*, with specificity for both the vector and a cellular receptor. A truly targeted vector can be generated by designing the vector-specific component of the bispecific molecule to ablate native viral tropism, for example, a neutralizing antifiber antibody *(37)* or a soluble form of CAR *(38)*. This approach has the advantage that a single targeting moiety can be employed with different vectors, but it suffers from the problem that the two components, vector and targeting molecule, must be generated separately, limiting its attractiveness for clinical application.

An alternative approach to targeting involves the genetic modification of the vector, thus forming a single-component system *(39)*. Although the most commonly used adenovirus vectors for gene therapy are based on species C serotypes 2 and 5, which recognize CAR, other adenovirus serotypes recognize a different primary cellular receptor. This has led to the hypothesis that CAR-independent gene transfer could be accomplished by substituting fiber genes from the Ad2 or Ad5 backbone with genes encoding homologous fiber proteins from alternate adenovirus serotypes, a process known as pseudotyping. Although pseudotyping an Ad5-based vector with fiber proteins from serotypes such as Ad3 *(40)* and Ad35 *(41)* of species B has allowed efficient, CAR-independent gene transfer to cancer cells, the approach is still limited by its reliance on the expression of a native adenoviral receptor by the target cells. This limitation can be overcome by incorporating cell-specific targeting ligands into the fiber to redirect adenoviral infection.

To date, the majority of genetically modified adenoviral vectors incorporating targeting peptide ligands possess expanded tropism; they retain the ability to recognize the native primary receptor, CAR. Adenoviral vectors containing the α_v integrin-specific RGD peptide motif have been shown to increase the efficiency of gene delivery by up to three orders of magnitude to a variety of CAR-deficient primary human cancer cells in vitro without increasing gene transfer to normal, CAR-positive cells *(42)*. A major advantage of such vectors with enhanced infectivity is that a given level of gene transfer can be achieved with a lower viral dose compared with the untargeted vector. Because the viral dose is directly related to toxicity, this has important implications for safety.

The improvement in infectivity observed with these vectors translates into enhanced therapeutic benefit in preclinical animal models, supporting their evaluation in human clinical trials. The Gene Therapy Center at the University of Alabama at Birmingham is currently employing this vector backbone in phase I clinical trials for ovarian cancer *(43)* and recurrent cancer of the oral cavity and oropharynx. These trials are the first to employ tropism-modified adenoviral vectors in human patients. It is hypothesized that the tropism-modified vectors will allow augmented transfer of the HSV*tk* and cytosine deaminase genes at lower vector doses, thereby leading to increased efficacy and reduced toxicity.

Now that the amino acid residues responsible for binding CAR have been identified, site-directed mutagenesis of the fiber protein will permit the engineering of vectors lacking native tropism but possessing specificity for target receptors. A more radical approach to the construction of truly targeted adenoviral vectors involves the replacement of the knob domain of the fiber with a targeting moiety. The technical challenge is to retain trimerization of the modified fiber protein so that mature viral particles can be assembled. This has been achieved by replacing the fiber with the trimeric fibritin protein from bacteriophage T4 *(44)*, a maneuver that has allowed the trimeric CD40L protein to be incorporated as a targeting motif *(45)*.

An additional level of specificity for the target cancer cell can be achieved by placing the therapeutic gene under the transcriptional control of a tissue- or tumor-selective promoter. Because both transductional and transcriptional targeting approaches by themselves tend to be "leaky," the combination of two complementary targeting approaches leads to enhanced specificity for the target cells *(46)*.

It is anticipated that the further improvements in the area of transductionally targeted adenoviral vectors will ultimately lead to a targeted, injectable vector capable of transducing disseminated cancer cells on vascular administration. This will require additional obstacles to be overcome, including the uptake of systemically administered vectors by the liver. An increasing understanding of the role of both hepatocytes and Kupffer cells in hepatic sequestration of adenoviral vectors should lead to rational strategies by which this can be overcome. It is also recognized that there are physical barriers to adenoviral transduction of target cancer cells.

An additional obstacle to the clinical use of adenoviral vectors for cancer gene therapy is the presence of neutralizing antibodies, which may limit vector readministration (or the initial administration of vector in a host with preexisting neutralizing antibodies because of previous exposure to the virus). However, this challenge can be addressed by the process of "serotype switching," which involves substituting capsid proteins from one serotype with those from another serotype to avoid recognition by the neutralizing antibodies *(47)*. In this regard, modification of adenoviral tropism by incorporation of the RGD peptide motif into the knob has also been shown to allow efficient infection in the presence of neutralizing antifiber antibodies that block infection by vectors with wild-type fiber proteins *(48)*. Alternatively, the adenoviral vector can be coated with a polymer to prevent recognition by neutralizing antibodies *(49)*.

It is becoming increasingly apparent that mutation compensation and molecular chemotherapy strategies for cancer gene therapy are inherently limited by the technical problem of transducing all the cells in a solid tumor. Although the exploitation of bystander effects or the combination of cancer gene therapy with conventional cancer treatments, such as chemotherapy and radiation therapy, may in part overcome this problem, replication-defective vectors remain incapable of delivering therapeutic genes to more than a small proportion of cancer cells in a three-dimensional tumor mass. Considerable attention has therefore switched to the idea of employing adenoviral vectors in immunotherapy applications that exploit their ability to transduce dendritic cells, as discussed in detail elsewhere in this book.

2.3. Adeno-Associated Virus Vectors

Adeno-associated viruses (AAVs) are so called because they were first identified in association with adenoviruses in tissue culture. They are human parvoviruses that require a helper virus, such as adenovirus, to mediate a productive infection. An AAV particle has an icosahedral protein capsid 25 nm in diameter surrounding a single minus- or plus-strand DNA genome around 4.7 kb long. The genome consists of two genes, each producing multiple polypeptides: *rep*, which is required for viral genome replication, structural gene expression, and integration into the host genome; and *cap*, which encodes the structural capsid proteins. The genes are flanked by *cis*-acting ITR sequences 145 nucleotides long that are vital for the rescue, replication, packaging, and integration of the viral genome. To date, eight different human AAV serotypes with different tissue tropisms have been identified, none of which cause disease. Most AAV vectors employed in gene therapy have been based on serotype 2.

AAV infects cells via a receptor-mediated pathway. AAV-2 vectors use heparan sulfate proteoglycan as the primary receptor *(50)* and fibroblast receptor type 1 *(51)* and integrin $\alpha_v\beta_5$ *(52)* as coreceptors. On entry into cells, AAV is rapidly transported through endosomes to the nucleus, where the genome is released. Following this, the single-stranded vector genome is converted to transcriptionally active double-stranded intermediates. This step is achieved by either second-strand synthesis of the single-stranded viral genome or annealing of complementary sequences from viral particles containing positive or negative strands. The double-stranded AAV viral genome integrates into a specific region of human chromosome 19. Thus, the key features of AAV that led to its development as a gene therapy vector are genomic integration and long-term gene expression.

When used as a vector, the *rep* and *cap* genes are replaced by a transgene and its associated regulatory sequences, including promoter and polyadenylation signal. The packaging capacity of AAV is about 5.0 kb, which limits the utility of this vector system for some gene therapy applications. The production of the recombinant vector requires that rep and cap proteins are provided in *trans*, along with helper virus gene products such as adenovirus E1A, E1B, E2A, E4, and VA proteins. Initial methods for the production of AAV vectors involved the cotransfection of human 293, HeLa, or KB cells with an AAV helper plasmid and a plasmid containing the transgene cassette flanked by the AAV ITR sequences, followed by infection of these cells with wild-type adenovirus. Approximately 48–72 hours after the transfection/infection, the cells were lysed, and extracts containing AAV vectors were used after heat inactivation at 56°C to destroy contaminating adenovirus. DNaseI digestion was used to remove unencapsidated and input plasmid genome.

Advances in the production and purification of AAV vector have included the generation of packaging cell lines, the use of helper plasmids containing the necessary adenoviral genes to eliminate the possibility of wild-type adenovirus contaminating AAV preparations, and new column chromatographic methods of vector purification. These improvements have resulted in high-titer AAV vector yields of up to 10^{15} particles per milliliter, necessary for in vivo studies, including human clinical trials.

An advantage of AAV vectors is that they lack any viral coding sequences and therefore do not induce a cellular immune response (although neutralizing antibodies can be induced that may limit readministration of the vector). However, because AAV vectors do not express the *rep* gene, they do not have the ability to integrate into the host cell genome in a site-specific manner; the double-stranded vector genome remains as an episome or integrates randomly into host chromosomes, raising the risk of insertional mutagenesis. Maximal gene expression from AAV vectors occurs after a period of several weeks, presumably in part because of the requirement for the single-stranded DNA genome to be converted to the transcriptionally active double-stranded form.

Gene therapy strategies designed to transfer therapeutic genes into the cancer cells themselves to bring about their destruction do not necessitate the use of a vector capable of long-term gene expression. The properties of AAV vectors suggest that they would be well suited for use in cancer gene therapy strategies mandating long-term, stable gene expression of therapeutic proteins that target the nonmalignant stromal cells that support the growth and metastasis of cancer cells. In this regard, it has been hypothesized that AAV vector-mediated delivery would afford the potential for sustained release of antiangiogenic substances, thereby obviating the need for chronic administration of recombinant factors. A further attractive feature of this approach is that is not necessary to achieve expression of the antiangiogenic factors within the target tumor endothelial cells themselves. Instead, an organ that is readily transduced by AAV vectors, such as the liver or muscle, can be turned into a "factory" to secrete the antiangiogenic proteins into the bloodstream. Although not yet at the stage of clinical trials, AAV-mediated expression of the antiangiogenic factor angiostatin has shown promise in a preclinical study; it effectively suppressed human glioma growth in the brain of nude mice *(53)*.

The long-term gene expression mediated by AAV vectors has also been exploited in cancer immunotherapy studies; active immunization of rodents was achieved by ex vivo AAV-mediated transfer to cytokines to autologous tumor cells, which were then reimplanted into the host animals *(54)*. The ability of AAV-2 vectors to transduce immature monocyte-derived dendritic cells ex vivo has been demonstrated *(55)*. This affords the possibility of retaining the AAV-delivered transgene during the process of differentiation and then expressing it by the mature dendritic cells. It has been reported that dendritic cells that have been modified to become resistant to apoptosis exhibit enhanced immunostimulatory activity in vivo *(56)*. Based on this observation, it has been suggested that AAV vectors could be employed to transduce immature dendritic cells with antiapoptotic genes, the expression of which in the mature dendritic cells could confer an extended life-span *(55)*.

Dendritic cells from individual human subjects vary in their susceptibility to transduction by AAV-2 vectors, suggesting that there is a need for vectors capable of exploiting alternative cell surface receptors. The existence of a number of human and AAV serotypes with different tissue tropisms provides the basis for exploiting this naturally occurring diversity to develop vectors with an enhanced ability to transduce the desired target cells. The recent elucidation of the atomic structure of the AAV-2 capsid *(57)* should facilitate the rational design of targeting approaches based on the insertion of targeting ligands into the AAV-2 capsid, although the small size of the AAV particle may preclude the incorporation of anything larger than small peptides. To date, candidate sites for insertion of targeting peptides into the AAV-2 capsid have been chosen on the basis of predicted homology with the known structure of the capsid of the related B-19 parvoviruses. Although heparan sulfate proteoglycan-independent infection of target cells by AAV-2 vectors with expanded tropism has been demonstrated, this has generally been achieved at the expense of efficiency.

Although AAV is considered nonpathogenic, during the course of a study designed to determine the long-term efficacy of AAV-mediated gene therapy initiated in newborn mice with the lysosomal storage disease mucopolysaccharidosis type VII, a significant incidence of hepatocellular carcinomas and angiosarcomas was discovered *(58)*. It appears that this was most probably because of factors related to the underlying disease rather than AAV-mediated gene transfer. However, there is a need for long-term in vivo studies to evaluate rigorously the tumorigenic potential of AAV.

2.4. Other Viral Vectors

Vectors based on other viruses have been less extensively employed in cancer gene therapy.

2.4.1. Vaccinia Vectors

The poxvirus vaccinia has been widely used clinically for smallpox vaccination, a historical precedent that favored the development of vaccinia as a vector in the context of immunotherapy. Vaccinia virus is a large virus with a double envelope surrounding an 186-kb DNA genome *(59)*. Vectors have been constructed by substituting nonessential gene sequences with up to three genes of interest, although there does not seem to be a limit on the size of genes that can be incorporated into the vaccinia vector genome.

Vaccinia vectors have been employed in human clinical trials to deliver genes encoding tumor-associated antigens and cytokines, either individually or in combination *(60)*. The vectors have been administered by various routes, including intratumoral, subcutaneous, and intradermal. A disadvantage of vaccinia vectors is that they are replication-competent viruses, which is a safety concern in immunosuppressed cancer patients. The problem of toxicity in immunocompromised patients has been addressed by developing vectors based on other poxviruses, such as fowl pox and canary pox, that do not replicate in human cells *(61)*. However, vaccinia and other poxvirus vectors express a large number (150 to 200) of viral proteins in addition to the cytokine or tumor-associated antigen of interest. Consequently, the antiviral immune responses tend to dominate the antitumor immune response, an observation that has dampened enthusiasm for these vectors.

2.4.2. Herpes Simplex Virus Type 1 Vectors

Herpes simplex virus type 1 (HSV-1) is another large virus (180–200 nm diameter) employed in cancer gene therapy. The virion is surrounded by a trilaminar lipid envelope in which are embedded viral glycoproteins with various functions, including receptor-mediated cellular entry. A matrix of proteins, called the tegument, forms a layer between the envelope and the underlying icosadeltahedral capsid. The genome is a linear, double-stranded DNA molecule 152 kb long *(62)*. Approximately half of the 84 known HSV-1 genes are nonessential for virus replication in cell culture, which affords multiple sites for the insertion of foreign genes that can be independently regulated *(63)*. Replication-defective HSV-1 vectors, which cannot produce infectious progeny and therefore have reduced toxicity to infected cells, can be generated by deleting one or more of the immediate early genes essential for virus replication. Growth of these vectors therefore requires complementing cell lines that express the deleted genes.

Interest in developing replication-defective HSV-1 vectors for gene therapy was initially based on the natural life cycle, in which the parental virus is able to persist after primary infection in a latent state within neuronal cells for the lifetime of the host. However, this biological property lacks relevance to cancer gene therapy. Instead, the chief advantage of replication-defective HSV-1 vectors for cancer gene therapy has derived from their large cloning capacity, which has been exploited to allow the simultaneous delivery of multiple therapeutic genes. This may be particularly useful to deliver distinct therapeutic genes to the heterogeneous population of cells within a solid tumor. Strategies to develop HSV-1 vectors capable of cell-specific gene delivery are complicated by the complex pathway of infection, which involves the interaction of a number of different viral glycoproteins with cell surface molecules.

2.4.3. Lentiviral Vectors

Lentiviruses are a class of retroviruses that, in contrast to the C-type retroviruses, have the ability to infect nondividing cells. The field of lentiviral vector-mediated cancer gene therapy is in its infancy, but a consideration of the biology of lentiviruses suggests that these vectors could most rationally be applied in the context of strategies mandating long-term gene expression. Hence, lentiviral vectors could be exploited for antiangiogenic gene therapy or used to transduce dendritic cells for cancer immunotherapy.

3. FUTURE DIRECTIONS

Key to the realization of the full potential of cancer gene therapy is the development of viral vectors capable of efficient gene transfer specifically to disseminated cancer cells on systemic administration. Considerable efforts are currently being expended on studies to generate such targeted, injectable vectors that will be capable of selectively transducing metastatic cells. Moreover, it is now becoming increasingly apparent that anatomical barriers will also need to be overcome to enhance the utility of viral vectors in the context of systemic delivery. Future work should lead to the derivation of truly targeted viral vectors suitable for a variety of clinical applications requiring highly efficient, cell-specific delivery of therapeutic genes in vivo.

REFERENCES

1. Goff, S. P. (2001) Retroviridae: the retroviruses and their replication. In *Fields Virology*, 4th ed. (Knipe, D. M., Howley, P. M., Griffin, D. E., et al., eds.), Lippincott, Williams, and Wilkins, Philadelphia, PA, pp. 1871–1940.
2. Miller, D. G., Adam, M. A., and Miller, A. D. (1990) Gene transfer by retrovirus vectors occurs only in cells that are actively replicating at the time of infection. *Mol. Cell. Biol.* **10,** 4239–4242.
3. Rosenberg, S. A., Aebersold, P., Cornetta, K., et al. (1990) Gene transfer into humans—immunotherapy of patients with advanced melanoma, using tumor-infiltrating lymphocytes modified by retroviral gene transduction. *N. Engl. J. Med.* **323,** 570–578.
4. Rosenberg, S. A. (1990) Protocol 9007-003. Gene therapy of patients with advanced cancer using tumor infiltrating lymphocytes transduced with the gene coding for tumor necrosis factor. Available on-line at: http://www4.od.nih.gov/oba/rac/PROTOCOL.pdf.
5. Rosenberg, S. A. (1990) Protocol 9110-010. Immunization of cancer patients using autologous cancer cells modified by insertion of the gene for tumor necrosis factor (TNF). Available on-line at: http://www4.od.nih.gov/oba/rac/PROTOCOL.pdf.
6. Chang, A. E. (1993) Protocol 9312-065. Adoptive immunotherapy of cancer with activated lymph node cells primed in vivo with autologous tumor cells transduced with the GM-CSF gene. Available on-line at: http://www4.od.nih.gov/oba/rac/PROTOCOL.pdf.
7. Lotze, M. T. and Rubin, J. T. (1992) Protocol 9209-033. Gene therapy of cancer: A pilot study of IL-4 gene modified antitumor vaccines. Available on-line at: http://www4.od.nih.gov/oba/rac/PROTOCOL.pdf.
8. Lotze, M. T. (1994) Protocol 9406-081. IL-12 gene therapy using direct injection of tumor with genetically engineered autologous fibroblasts. Available on-line at: http://www4.od.nih.gov/oba/rac/PROTOCOL.pdf.
9. Rosenberg, S. A. (1990) Protocol 9110-011. Immunization of cancer patients using autologous cancer cells modified by insertion of the gene for interleukin-2 (IL-2). Available on-line at: http://www4.od.nih.gov/oba/rac/PROTOCOL.pdf.
10. Venook, A. and Warren, R. S. (1997) Protocol 9707-198. A phase I/II study of autologous CC49-zeta gene-modified T cells and alpha-interferon in patients with advanced colorectal carcinomas expressing the tumor-associated antigen, TAG-72. Available on-line at: http://www4.od.nih.gov/oba/rac/PROTOCOL.pdf.
11. Ram, Z., Culver, K. W., Oshiro, E. M., et al. (1997) Therapy of malignant brain tumors by intratumoral implantation of retroviral vector-producing cells. *Nat. Med.* **3,** 1354–1361.
12. Stockhammer, G., Brotchi, J., Leblanc, R., et al. (1997) Gene therapy for glioblastoma multiforme: in vivo tumor transduction with the herpes simplex thymidine kinase gene followed by ganciclovir. *J. Mol. Med.* **75,** 300–304.
13. Hacein-Bey-Abina, S., Von Kalle, C., Schmidt, M., et al. (2003) LMO2-associated clonal T cell proliferation in two patients after gene therapy for SCID-X1. *Science* **302,** 415–419.
14. Emi, N., Friedmann, T., and Yee, J. K. (1991) Pseudotype formation of murine leukemia virus with the G protein of vesicular stomatitis virus. *J. Virol.* **65,** 1202–1207.
15. Snitkovsky, S. and Young, J. A. (1998) Cell-specific viral targeting mediated by a soluble retroviral receptor-ligand fusion protein. *Proc. Natl. Acad. Sci. USA* **95,** 7063–7068.
16. Snitkovsky, S., Niederman, T. M., Mulligan, R. C., and Young, J. A. (2001) Targeting avian leukosis virus subgroup A vectors by using a TVA-VEGF bridge protein. *J. Virol.* **75,** 1571–1575.
17. Kasahara, N., Dozy, A. M., Kan, Y. W., Russell, S. J., Hawkins, R. E., and Winter, G. (1994) Tissue-specific targeting of retroviral vectors through ligand-receptor interactions. *Science* **266,** 1373–1376.
18. Russell, S. J., Hawkins, R. E., and Winter, G. (1993) Retroviral vectors displaying functional antibody fragments. *Nucleic Acids Res.* **21,** 1081–1085.
19. Gordon, E. M., Chen, Z. H., Liu, L., et al. (2001) Systemic administration of a matrix-targeted retroviral vector is efficacious for cancer gene therapy in mice. *Hum. Gene Ther.* **12,** 193–204.
20. Peng, K. W., Morling, F. J., Cosset, F. L., Murphy, G., and Russell, S. J. (1997) A gene delivery system activatable by disease-associated matrix metalloproteinases. *Hum. Gene Ther.* **8,** 729–738.
21. Lenz, H.-J. (2000) Protocol 0010-417. Tumor site specific phase I/II evaluation of safety and efficacy of hepatic arterial infusion of a matrix-targeted retroviral vector bearing a dominant negative cyclin G1 (dnG1) construct as treatment for colorectal carcinoma metastatic to liver. Available on-line at: http://www4.od.nih.gov/oba/rac/PROTOCOL.pdf.
22. Shenk, T. E. (2001) Adenoviridae: the viruses and their replication. In *Fields Virology*, 4th ed. (Knipe, D. M., Howley, P. M., Griffin, D. E., et al., eds.), Lippincott, Williams, and Wilkins, Philadelphia, PA, pp. 2265–2300.

23. Henry, L. J., Xia, D., Wilke, M. E., Deisenhofer, J., and Gerard, R. D. (1994) Characterization of the knob domain of the adenovirus type 5 fiber protein expressed in *Escherichia coli. J. Virol.* **68,** 5239–5246.

24. Louis, N., Fender, P., Barge, A., Kitts, P., and Chroboczek, J. (1994) Cell-binding domain of adenovirus serotype 2 fiber. *J. Virol.* **68,** 4104–4106.

25. Bergelson, J. M., Cunningham, J. A., Droguett, G., et al. (1997) Isolation of a common receptor for Coxsackie B viruses and adenoviruses 2 and 5. *Science* **275,** 1320–1323.

26. Tomko, R. P., Xu, R., and Philipson, L. (1997) HCAR and MCAR: the human and mouse cellular receptors for subgroup C adenoviruses and group B Coxsackieviruses. *Proc. Natl. Acad. Sci. USA* **94,** 3352–3356.

27. Wang, X. and Bergelson, J. M. (1999) Coxsackievirus and adenovirus receptor cytoplasmic and transmembrane domains are not essential for Coxsackievirus and adenovirus infection. *J. Virol.* **73,** 2559–2562.

28. Bai, M., Campisi, L., and Freimuth, P. (1994) Vitronectin receptor antibodies inhibit infection of HeLa and A549 cells by adenovirus type 12 but not by adenovirus type 2. *J. Virol.* **68,** 5925–5932.

29. Wickham, T. J., Mathias, P., Cheresh, D. A., and Nemerow, G. R. (1993) Integrins alpha v beta 3 and alpha v beta 5 promote adenovirus internalization but not virus attachment. *Cell* **73,** 309–319.

30. Swisher, S. G. and Roth, J. A. (2002) Clinical update of Ad-p53 gene therapy for lung cancer. *Surg. Oncol. Clin. N. Am.* **11,** 521–535.

31. Gingrich, J. R. (1999) Protocol 9909-338. A tolerance and efficacy study of neoadjuvant intraprostatic GTx-001 followed by radical prostatectomy in patients with locally advanced prostate cancer. Available on-line at: http://www4. od.nih.gov/oba/rac/PROTOCOL.pdf.

32. Alvarez, R. D., Barnes, M. N., Gomez-Navarro, J., et al. (2000) A cancer gene therapy approach utilizing an anti-erbB-2 single-chain antibody-encoding adenovirus (AD21): a phase I trial. *Clin. Cancer Res.* **6,** 3081–3087.

33. Deshane, J., Siegal, G. P., Alvarez, R. D., et al. (1995) Targeted tumor killing via an intracellular antibody against erbB-2. *J. Clin. Invest.* **96,** 2980–2989.

34. Miller, C. R., Buchsbaum, D. J., Reynolds, P. N., et al. (1998) Differential susceptibility of primary and established human glioma cells to adenovirus infection: targeting via the epidermal growth factor receptor achieves fiber receptor-independent gene transfer. *Cancer Res.* **58,** 5738–5748.

35. Kim, M., Zinn, K. R., Barnett, B. G., et al. (2002) The therapeutic efficacy of adenoviral vectors for cancer gene therapy is limited by a low level of primary adenovirus receptors on tumour cells. *Eur. J. Cancer* **38,** 1917–1926.

36. Barnett, B. G., Crews, C. J., and Douglas, J. T. (2002) Targeted adenoviral vectors. *Biochim. Biophys. Acta* **1575,** 1–14.

37. Douglas, J. T., Rogers, B. E., Rosenfeld, M. E., Michael, S. I., Feng, M., and Curiel, D. T. (1996) Targeted gene delivery by tropism-modified adenoviral vectors. *Nat. Biotechnol.* **14,** 1574–1578.

38. Dmitriev, I., Kashentseva, E., Rogers, B. E., Krasnykh, V., and Curiel, D. T. (2000) Ectodomain of Coxsackievirus and adenovirus receptor genetically fused to epidermal growth factor mediates adenovirus targeting to epidermal growth factor receptor-positive cells. *J. Virol.* **74,** 6875–6884.

39. Krasnykh, V. N., Douglas, J. T., and van Beusechem, V. W. (2000) Genetic targeting of adenoviral vectors. *Mol. Ther.* **1,** 391–405.

40. Kanerva, A., Mikheeva, G. V., Krasnykh, V., et al. (2002) Targeting adenovirus to the serotype 3 receptor increases gene transfer efficiency to ovarian cancer cells. *Clin. Cancer Res.* **8,** 275–280.

41. Mizuguchi, H. and Hayakawa, T. (2002) Adenovirus vectors containing chimeric type 5 and type 35 fiber proteins exhibit altered and expanded tropism and increase the size limit of foreign genes. *Gene* **285,** 69–77.

42. Dmitriev, I., Krasnykh, V., Miller, C. R., et al. (1998) An adenovirus vector with genetically modified fibers demonstrates expanded tropism via utilization of a Coxsackievirus and adenovirus receptor-independent cell entry mechanism. *J. Virol.* **72,** 9706–9713.

43. Barnes, M. N. (2000) Protocol 0005-398. A phase I study of a tropism modified adenovirus vector for intraperitoneal delivery of therapeutic genes in ovarian and extraovarian cancer patients. Available on-line at: http://www4.od.nih.gov/ oba/rac/PROTOCOL.pdf.

44. Krasnykh, V., Belousova, N., Korokhov, N., Mikheeva, G., and Curiel, D. T. (2001) Genetic targeting of an adenovirus vector via replacement of the fiber protein with the phage T4 fibritin. *J. Virol.* **75,** 4176–4183.

45. Belousova, N., Korokhov, N., Krendelshchikova, V., et al. (2003) Genetically targeted adenovirus vector directed to CD40-expressing cells. *J. Virol.* **77,** 11,367–11,377.

46. Barnett, B. G., Tillman, B. W., Curiel, D. T., and Douglas, J. T. (2002) Dual targeting of adenoviral vectors at the levels of transduction and transcription enhances the specificity of gene expression in cancer cells. *Mol. Ther.* **6,** 377–385.

47. Mastrangeli, A., Harvey, B. G., Yao, J., et al. (1996) "Sero-switch" adenovirus-mediated in vivo gene transfer: circumvention of anti-adenovirus humoral immune defenses against repeat adenovirus vector administration by changing the adenovirus serotype. *Hum. Gene Ther.* **7,** 79–87.

48. Blackwell, J. L., Li, H., Gomez-Navarro, J., et al. (2000) Using a tropism-modified adenoviral vector to circumvent inhibitory factors in ascites fluid. *Hum. Gene Ther.* **11,** 1657–1669.

49. Fisher, K. D., Stallwood, Y., Green, N. K., Ulbrich, K., Mautner, V., and Seymour, L. W. (2001) Polymer-coated adenovirus permits efficient retargeting and evades neutralising antibodies. *Gene Ther.* **8,** 341–348.

50. Summerford, C. and Samulski, R. J. (1998) Membrane-associated heparan sulfate proteoglycan is a receptor for adeno-associated virus type 2 virions. *J. Virol.* **72,** 1438–1445.
51. Qing, K., Mah, C., Hansen, J., Zhou, S., Dwarki, V., and Srivastava, A. (1999) Human fibroblast growth factor receptor 1 is a co-receptor for infection by adeno-associated virus 2. *Nat. Med.* **5,** 71–77.
52. Summerford, C., Bartlett, J. S., and Samulski, R. J. (1999) AlphaVbeta5 integrin: a co-receptor for adeno-associated virus type 2 infection. *Nat. Med.* **5,** 78–82.
53. Ma, H. I., Guo, P., Li, J., et al. (2002) Suppression of intracranial human glioma growth after intramuscular administration of an adeno-associated viral vector expressing angiostatin. *Cancer Res.* **62,** 756–763.
54. Coveney, E., Clary, B., Iacobucci, M., Philip, R., and Lyerly, K. (1996) Active immunotherapy with transiently transfected cytokine-secreting tumor cells inhibits breast cancer metastases in tumor-bearing animals. *Surgery* **120,** 265–272.
55. Ponnazhagan, S., Mahendra, G., Curiel, D. T., and Shaw, D. R. (2001) Adeno-associated virus type 2-mediated transduction of human monocyte-derived dendritic cells: implications for ex vivo immunotherapy. *J. Virol.* **75,** 9493–9501.
56. Josien, R., Li, H. L., Ingulli, E., et al. (2000) TRANCE, a tumor necrosis factor family member, enhances the longevity and adjuvant properties of dendritic cells in vivo. *J. Exp. Med.* **191,** 495–502.
57. Xie, Q., Bu, W., Bhatia, S., et al. (2002) The atomic structure of adeno-associated virus (AAV-2), a vector for human gene therapy. *Proc. Natl. Acad. Sci. USA* **99,** 10,405–10,410.
58. Donsante, A., Vogler, C., Muzyczka, N., et al. (2001) Observed incidence of tumorigenesis in long-term rodent studies of rAAV vectors. *Gene Ther.* **8,** 1343–1346.
59. Moss, B. (2001) Poxviridae: the viruses and their replication. In *Fields Virology*, 4th ed. (Knipe, D. M., Howley, P. M., Griffin, D. E., et al., eds.), Lippincott, Williams, and Wilkins, Philadelphia, PA, PP. 2849–2884.
60. Kwak, H., Horig, H., and Kaufman, H. L. (2003) Poxviruses as vectors for cancer immunotherapy. *Curr. Opin. Drug Discov. Dev.* **6,** 161–168.
61. Baxby, D. and Paoletti, E. (1992) Potential use of non-replicating vectors as recombinant vaccines. *Vaccine* **10,** 8–9.
62. Roizman, B. and Knipe, D. M. (2001) Herpes simplex viruses and their replication. In *Fields Virology,* 4th ed. (Knipe, D. M., Howley, P. M., Griffin, D. E., et al., eds.), Lippincott, Williams, and Wilkins, Philadelphia, PA, pp. 2399–2460.
63. Krisky, D. M., Marconi, P. C., Oligino, T. J., et al. (1998) Development of herpes simplex virus replication-defective multigene vectors for combination gene therapy applications. *Gene Ther.* **5,** 1517–1530.

26

Bacterial Systems for Tumor-Specific Gene Therapy

J. Martin Brown, Shie-Chau Liu, Jan Theys, and Philippe Lambin

1. BACTERIA FOR GENE THERAPY?

This chapter describes the power of genetically engineered bacteria in cancer therapy. In the applications we consider, the bacteria are genetically engineered to carry a specific gene into tumors, and on this basis, it can be considered gene therapy. However, if gene therapy is defined as the introduction of a gene, or part of a gene, into the cancer cells (or normal cells), then using recombinant bacteria as anticancer vectors is not gene therapy. Bacteria are not vectors for the introduction of genes into mammalian cells. However, they can and do concentrate in tumors by various means and can carry a gene of interest to produce a protein of choice in tumors. This can be a powerful adjunct to cancer therapy.

In this chapter, we consider two specific approaches to bacteria in gene therapy. First, we consider necrosis-targeted therapy, of which species of the obligate anaerobe *Clostridium* is the prototypical agent. Second, we consider non-necrosis-directed gene therapy, of which modified *Salmonella* is the prototype.

2. CLOSTRIDIAL VECTORS FOR GENE THERAPY

2.1. Hypoxia and Necrosis in Solid Tumors

Necrotic regions are a common, if not a universal, feature of human solid tumors. Although this is rarely quantitated, Dang and colleagues reported that all 20 liver metastases of colorectal carcinoma 1 cm^3 or larger had 25–75% of their volume occupied by necrosis *(1)*. These necrotic regions typically occur at a distance from functioning blood vessels beyond the diffusion distance of oxygen *(2)*, as demonstrated also in the in vitro spheroid model *(3)*. Because these necrotic regions typically develop because of prolonged lack of oxygen, they are usually intimately associated with hypoxic, but viable, cells. These hypoxic regions in tumors are best demonstrated by polarographic oxygen electrodes, and measurements with such electrodes have shown that the majority of primary tumors or metastases of the head and neck, cervix, and brain and melanomas, sarcomas, and anal, prostate and pancreatic cancers have regions that are severely hypoxic *(4–11)*. Moreover, the fact that hypoxic cells are resistant to killing by ionizing radiation and are more slowly proliferating than well-oxygenated cells makes them resistant to treatment by radiotherapy and chemotherapy *(12,13)*.

2.2. Certain Species of Clostridia Colonize Solid Tumors

The genus *Clostridium* comprises a large and heterogeneous group of Gram-positive, spore-forming bacteria that become vegetative and grow only in the absence (or at very low levels) of oxygen. Malmgren and Flanigan were the first to demonstrate that intravenous injection of spores of *Clostridium tetani* colonized solid tumors by observing that tumor-bearing mice died of tetanus within 48 hours of intravenous injection of *C. tetani* spores, whereas non-tumor-bearing animals were unaffected

From: *Contemporary Cancer Research*
Cancer Gene Therapy
Edited by: D. T. Curiel and J. T. Douglas © Humana Press Inc., Totowa, NJ

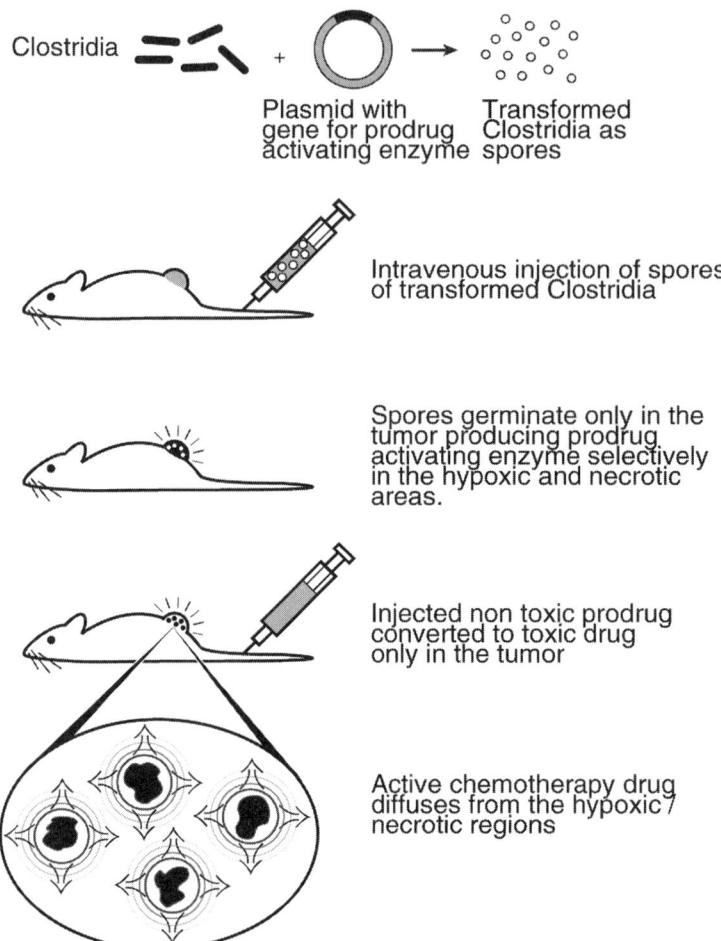

Clostridia + Plasmid with gene for prodrug activating enzyme → Transformed Clostridia as spores

Intravenous injection of spores of transformed Clostridia

Spores germinate only in the tumor producing prodrug activating enzyme selectively in the hypoxic and necrotic areas.

Injected non toxic prodrug converted to toxic drug only in the tumor

Active chemotherapy drug diffuses from the hypoxic/ necrotic regions

Fig. 1. Diagrammatic representation of tumor-specific targeting of chemotherapy using obligate anaerobes.

(14). Mose and Mose *(15,16)* later reported that a nonpathogenic clostridial strain, *Clostridium butyricum* M-55, localized and germinated in solid Ehrlich tumors, causing extensive lysis without any concomitant effect on normal tissues. Such observations were soon confirmed and extended by a number of investigators using tumors in mice, rats, hamsters, and rabbits *(17,18)* and were followed by clinical studies with cancer patients *(19–21).* Although the anaerobic bacteria did not significantly alter tumor control or eradication, these clinical reports established the safety of this approach as well as the fact that colonization of human tumors occurs following intravenous injection of clostridial spores.

2.3. Clostridia-Directed Enzyme Prodrug Therapy

The studies mentioned in Section 2.2. showing the specific colonization of tumors by nonpathogenic clostridial species prompted the suggestion first made in 1994 that they could be used as a tumor-specific gene delivery system *(22).* The tumor-targeted strategy we proposed is to inject spores of nonpathogenic clostridia genetically engineered to produce a specific protein potentially harmful to the tumor when the spores germinate. Because germination to the vegetative form will occur only in the hypoxic/necrotic regions, the protein should be produced only in the tumor. We have suggested that the best way to exploit this strategy is to use the amplifying effect of enzymes to convert a nontoxic prodrug into a toxic drug (Fig. 1). Essentially, clostridia-directed enzyme prodrug therapy (CDEPT)

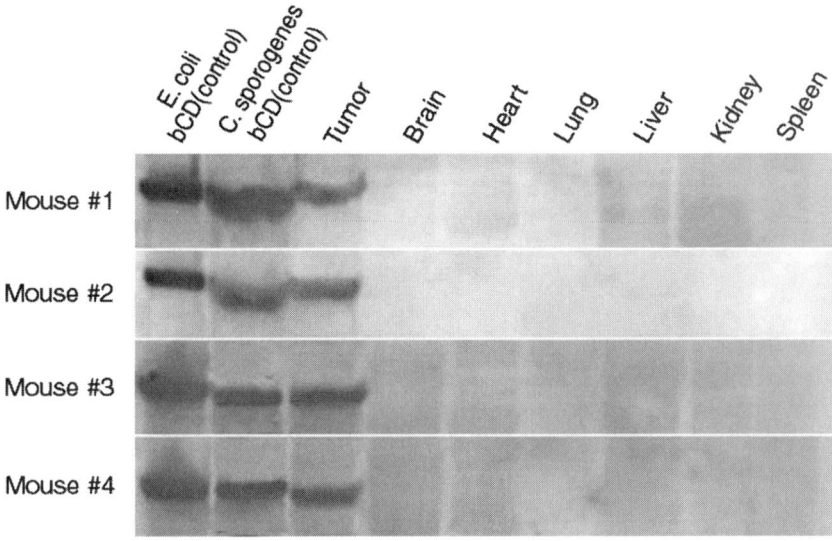

Fig. 2. Immunoblot for CD in cell extracts from SCCVII tumors and from several normal tissues from the same mice injected intravenously 7 days prior to animal sacrifice with spores of CD-transformed *C. sporogenes*. The tumors were approx 100 mg at the time of intravenous injection; 100 μg of cell extract from the tumor and normal mouse tissues were loaded on the gel. Shown also are cell extracts from CD-transformed *E. coli* and *C. sporogenes* with 1 and 20 μg cell extract loaded, respectively. bCD, bacterial cytosine deaminase (from *E. coli*). (From ref. *28* with permission.)

is a variation of the antibody-directed enzyme prodrug therapy (ADEPT) approach that is under active investigation by a number of investigators *(23,24)*.

In early studies with this approach, we showed that the *Escherichia coli* enzyme cytosine deaminase (CD) could be expressed in the clostridial species *Clostridium beijerinckii* and could convert the non-toxic prodrug 5-fluorocytosine (5-FC) to the toxic anticancer drug 5-fluorouracil (5-FU) in vitro *(25)*. In addition we, showed that injection of spores of recombinant *C. beijerinckii* expressing the *E. coli* enzyme nitroreductase (NTR) into tumor-bearing mice produced NTR protein solely in the tumors *(26)*. We have demonstrated similar tumor-specific expression of CD in rat tumors following intravenous injection of genetically engineered spores of *Clostridium acetobutylicum (27)*. These studies, therefore, established the proof of principle that a foreign protein of choice can be expressed exclusively in transplanted tumors in rodents following systemic injection of the recombinant clostridial spores.

However, early animal studies with genetically engineered *C. beijerinckii* failed to produce antitumor activity when the relevant prodrug was injected systemically (5-FC for CD-expressing tumors and CB1954 for NTR-expressing tumors). This lack of antitumor activity almost certainly resulted from insufficient levels of prodrug-activating enzymes in the tumors because of low levels of viable clostridia in the tumors. Indeed, *C. beijerinckii* produced only 10^5 to 10^6 bacteria per gram of tumor *(26)*, whereas other clostridial species, such as *Clostridium sporogenes* and *C. acetobutylicum* have a greater colonization efficiency, with levels of 10^8 or more bacteria per gram of tumor in experimental tumors *(28,29)*. However, up to very recently, attempts to transform clostridia with high tumor colonization have proved unsuccessful.

We have succeeded in transforming *C. sporogenes* with enzyme-producing constructs. This was made possible by our novel finding that these bacteria secrete high levels of DNAase, which degrades the plasmid vector before it is taken up by the cell *(28)*. We have shown that intravenous injection into tumor-bearing mice of spores of *C. sporogenes* transformed in this way with an expression plasmid for *E. coli* CD produced tumor-specific expression of the CD protein (Fig. 2). Importantly, we found

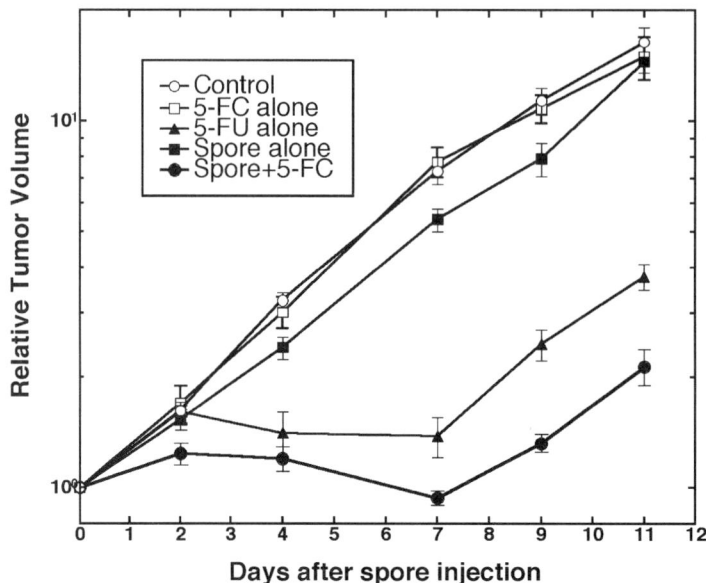

Fig. 3. Growth delay produced by daily (five times per week) injections of 5-FC (500 mg/kg body weight per day) in SCCVII tumors injected on day 0 with 10^8 spores of CD-transformed *C. sporogenes*. Shown also is the growth delay produced by a similar injection schedule of the MTD of 5-FU in the same experiment. Data from five mice per group with the error bars showing SEM for each group. (From ref. *28* with permission.)

significant antitumor efficacy of systemically injected 5-FC following intravenous injection of these recombinant spores *(28)* (Fig. 3).

These data demonstrate that systemically applied recombinant clostridial spores with a nontoxic prodrug can produce significant and specific antitumor activity.

2.4. CDEPT Has Significant Advantages Over ADEPT and Gene-Directed Enzyme Prodrug Therapy

Both ADEPT and gene-directed enzyme prodrug therapy (GDEPT) are viable approaches to achieve locally high concentrations of anticancer drugs in tumors and are appropriately receiving significant effort in both preclinical and clinical studies. However, we believe that CDEPT has a number of intrinsic advantages, discussed next.

2.4.1. Lack of an Immune Response

An immune response against the antibody/enzyme conjugates used has been a major problem with ADEPT *(30)*. However, clostridial spores elicit an undetectable immune response, and when the spores germinate into vegetative bacteria, they are present in necrotic areas in the tumor, which are immune-privileged sites. In fact, it has been found in both clinical *(19)* and preclinical studies *(31)* that multiple treatments are effective. In studies with intravenous injection of *C. sporogenes* and *C. ace-tobutylicum*, we found no loss of bacteria numbers in experimental tumors for up to 14 and 17 days, respectively, following a single intravenous injection of spores *(28,29)*.

2.4.2. Advantageous Intratumor Distribution

The necessity of delivering enzyme/antibody conjugates, or vectors for GDEPT, through the bloodstream makes it likely that the highest concentrations of enzyme will be perivascular. However, the resistant cells in the tumor are likely to be the nonproliferating hypoxic cells distant from the vasculature and often close to necrosis. In contrast, the prodrug-activating enzymes from clostridia will be at their highest concentration in areas adjacent to necrosis and far from blood vessels. Not only does this guarantee the highest active drug concentrations in the distant cells, but also it minimizes the problem of leakage of activated drug back into the blood vessels, a problem that has been reported for ADEPT *(32)*.

2.4.3. The Same Construct Will Be Universally Applicable to All Cancer Patients

As opposed to ADEPT, which requires either tumor-specific or possibly patient-specific enzyme/ antibody conjugates, the clostridial approach, because it depends only on tumor necrosis, will have universal applicability. In a publication on the potential of clostridia to target human tumors, Dang and colleagues reported that all 20 liver metastases of colorectal carcinoma 1 cm^3 or larger had 25–75% of their volume occupied by necrosis *(1)*.

2.4.4. Higher Ratios of Tumor-to-Normal Tissue Targeting

Major problems with ADEPT and GDEPT are that tumor targeting cannot be 100% effective. In most cases, the majority of the injected material will not be localized in the tumor, but in the reticular endothelial system. This necessitates efforts to clear such nonbound material. On the other hand, with clostridia, it appears that 100% of the novel protein expressed from the recombinant clostridia is within the tumor.

2.5. Combination With Vascular-Targeting Agents

Because of the need for hypoxic necrotic areas in tumors for vegetative growth of obligate anaerobes, it would seem that the CDEPT approach would not be effective in small tumors lacking necrosis. However, recent studies with vascular-targeting agents promise not only to enhance the efficacy of clostridial therapy in medium-size tumors, but also to raise the exciting possibility that the minimum tumor size for efficacy can be substantially reduced. Although the prototype vascular-targeting agent flavone acetic acid has been studied in preclinical work for over 12 years, it is only recently that this approach has shown promise in the clinic. Two classes of compounds show both preclinical and clinical activity: DMXAA (5,6-dimethylxanthenone-4-acetic acid), which acts primarily by inducing tumor necrosis factor (TNF) in tumors *(33,34)*, and tubulin-binding agents such as combretastatin 4A and an analog ZD 6126 currently under development by AstraZeneca *(35,36)*. The mechanism of action of these agents is rapid selective occlusion of tumor blood vessels, leading to necrosis within 16–24 hours.

These effects of vascular-targeting agents increase both the tumor colonization efficiency of intravenously injected clostridial spores *(37)* and the antitumor activity of nonrecombinant clostridia *(1)*. The reason for the increased tumor colonization by clostridia is the large increase in tumor necrosis caused by these vascular-targeting agents. Not only does this increase the number of active clostridia per tumor, but also it reduces the volume of viable tumor tissue that needs to be exposed to the product of the vegetative clostridia.

Thus, vascular-targeting agents could be an important adjunct to CDEPT, not only in potentiating its effectiveness in medium-to-large tumors, but also in extending its range into very small tumors.

2.6. Radioresponsive Promoters

To increase the specificity of this tumor-directed delivery system further, the gene of interest may be placed under the control of a radio-induced promoter. This will result in an activation of the promoter after irradiation of the tumor, leading to spatial and temporal control of gene expression (i.e., expression of the therapeutic genes will be limited to the irradiated tissues only).

We have investigated whether radio-induced genes exist in *Clostridium* and at what dose of irradiation these genes are activated. In bacteria, the SOS repair system, which consists of more than 20 genes, is activated by radiation-induced single-strand DNA breaks *(38)*. We found that the central gene, *recA*, was activated by ionizing irradiation in *Clostridium* at the clinically relevant dose of 2 Gy *(39)*.

To determine if the therapeutic protein by *Clostridium* could be increased by irradiation, we constructed a shuttle vector that contained the *recA* promoter upstream of the therapeutic cytokine murine tumor necrosis factor-α (mTNF-α). To obtain secretion of mTNF-α, the coding sequence was preceded by the signal sequence of the *eglA* gene. After either one or two 2-Gy doses, there was a significant increase in mTNF-α secretion 3.5 hours after irradiation compared to nonirradiated controls *(40)*.

However, with the *recA* promoter, there was some expression of mTNF-α under nonirradiated conditions because of basal activity of the promoter. Therefore, we examined whether basal transcription could be suppressed by adding an extra repressor-binding site, or Cheo box, to the promoter region. Under basal conditions, the repressor DinR binds to this repressor-binding site, limiting transcription of the SOS genes. After activation by radiotherapy, both binding sites would become free, and repression would be relieved. This would lead to an increase in transcription of the SOS genes, including *recA*, after radiotherapy. Addition of an extra Cheo box to the *recA* promoter resulted in a 412% increase of secreted mTNF-α after irradiation, although only a 44% yield increase was obtained using the wild-type promoter. Hence, the Cheo box sequence is the radioresponsive element and can be used to decrease basal transcription or to increase transcription on induction *(41)*.

The next step was to test if the Cheo box sequence could be used to bring a constitutive promoter under the control of irradiation. To this end, the Cheo box sequence was incorporated in the promoter region of the constitutive *eglA* promoter. This led to a 242% increase in mTNF-α secretion after irradiation with 2 Gy. These data show that the Cheo box is functional outside its natural sequence and can be used to bring other promoters under the control of ionizing irradiation *(41)* (Fig. 4).

In summary, specificity and safety can be even further increased using radio-inducible promoters to drive gene expression. Because radiotherapy preferentially kills well-oxygenated cells and *Clostridium*-mediated protein delivery is likely to give maximum killing of hypoxic cells, the combination of the two is a logical approach in cancer therapy.

2.7. Will CDEPT Work in the Clinic?

The initial successful studies of clostridial spores with experimental animals were followed by studies with cancer patients in which 10^9 to 10^{10} spores were injected intravenously to each individual *(19–21)*. Typically, a low-grade fever occurred from 1 to 3 days following injection, with further increase in temperature from days 5–8, which coincided with lysis in the tumor. In subsequent clinical studies with 49 patients with malignant gliomas, Heppner and colleagues injected clostridial spores into the carotid artery on the side of the tumor *(21)*. All tumors showed lysis, following which the tumors were removed surgically. These clinical studies demonstrated that spores of nonpathogenic strains of clostridia could be given safely, that the spores germinate in the necrotic regions of tumors, and that lysis of the tumors can occur.

In summary, we believe that CDEPT has established its likelihood of effectiveness in the clinic.

3. *BIFIDOBACTERIUM LONGUM*: AN ALTERNATIVE TO *CLOSTRIDIUM*?

Another anaerobic bacterium that can selectively germinate and grow in the hypoxic regions of solid tumors after intravenous injection is *Bifidobacterium longum (42)*. This is a Gram-positive anaerobe found in the lowest small intestine and large intestine of humans and other animals. Studies with mice with B16 melanoma or Lewis lung tumors have shown tumor-specific proliferation with minimal levels in normal tissues from 24 hours after injection. As with clostridia, the proliferation of the bacteria is in the necrotic areas of the tumor. *B. longum* has been successfully transformed with a shuttle vector described by Matsumura and coworkers *(43)*, and these transformed bacteria colonize tumors similarly to the wild-type bacterium. However, results published to date showed that levels of only $1–4 \times 10^6$ bacteria per gram of tumor are obtained. In addition, work of Dang and colleagues

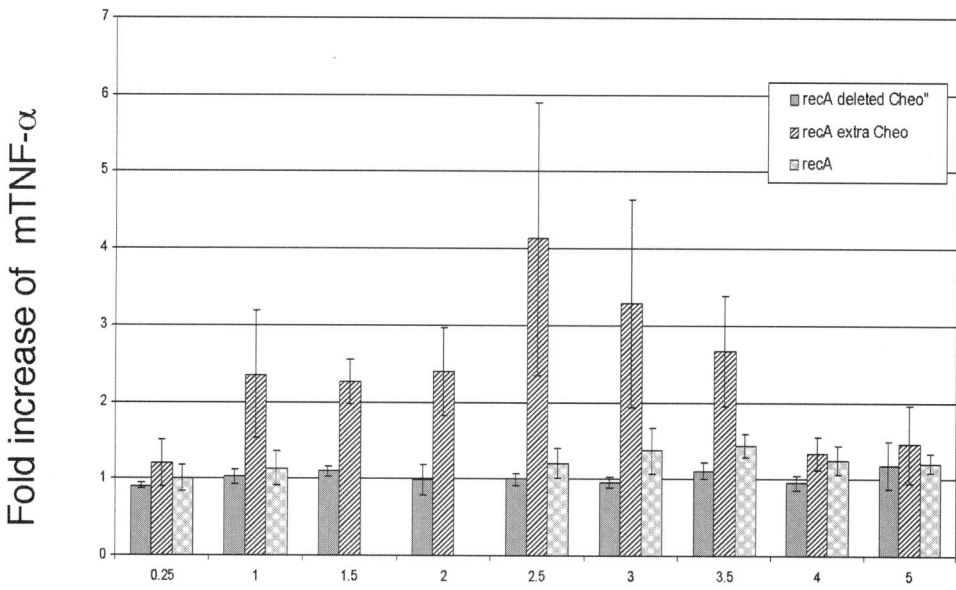

Time following irradiation(hours)

Fig. 4. Fold increase in mTNT-α in *C. acetobutylicum* DSM792 pIMP-*recA-mTNF*-α (dotted bars), pIMP-*recA* deleted *Cheo-mTNF*-α (gray bars) and pIMP-*recA*-extra *Cheobox-mTNF*-α (hatched bars) as a function of time after a single 2-Gy dose. Data from three independent experiments; the bars show standard deviations. (From ref. *29* with permission.)

showed that, following intravenous injection of *B. longum*, the growing bacteria were tightly clustered within colonies in the necrotic areas rather than distributed throughout the necrotic regions *(1)*. Thus, the rather low colonization efficiency and the tendency to clump rather than distribute within necrotic areas would appear to make *B. longum* inferior to the optimum strains of clostridia for enzyme prodrug therapy.

4. MODIFIED *SALMONELLA*-DEPENDENT TARGETING TO TUMORS

4.1. Salmonellae Accumulate in Solid Tumors

Genetically engineered stains of *Salmonella* strains have also been proposed for tumor-selective gene therapy. These are capable of both selective amplification within tumors and of expression of genes encoding therapeutic proteins *(44)*. Salmonellae are motile facultative anaerobes that grow well in both the oxygenated and the hypoxic regions of tumors.

To overcome its pathogenicity, *Salmonella typhimurium* has been attenuated by chromosomal deletion of the *purI* and *msbB* genes. The *purI* deletion created a requirement for an external source of adenine *(44)*. The deletion of the *msbB* gene reduced the toxicity associated with lipopolysaccharide by preventing the addition of a terminal myristyl group to the lipid A domain *(45)*. Unlike other lipid gene mutations, disruption of the *msbB* gene resulted in a stable strain that grows at physiological temperatures. The mutation lowered the toxicity in mice by reducing the induction of proinflammatory cytokines and nitric oxide synthase. The *purI* and *msbB* mutations are genetically stable and do not contain antibiotic resistance markers *(46)*. The resulting attenuated *msbB⁻*, *purI⁻ S. typhimurium* strain was designated VNP20009.

Biodistribution experiments with wild-type *S. typhimurium* and a purine auxotrophic clone (*purI⁻*), selected to be hyperinvasive in vitro, demonstrated differential replication in transplanted tumors, with tumor:liver ratios ranging between 250:1 and 9000:1 at 2 days postinoculation. *(44)*. The mechanisms for this accumulation are not clearly understood, but are thought to be the result of both bacterial- and tumor-related factors. Within the tumor, areas of necrosis and apoptosis may provide additional nutrients, such as purines required by the organism. In addition, the tumor may provide an environment that inhibits the clearance of *Salmonella*. Data demonstrating that several tumors express transforming growth factor-β and that transforming growth factor-β can inhibit fas-ligand-induced neutrophil activation and infiltration support the contention that bacterial clearance mechanisms may be inhibited within tumors *(47)*. Tumor types that have been shown to be targeted by *Salmonella* include melanoma, lung, colon, breast, kidney, and liver.

A further modification to theVNP20009 strain was made by constructing *msbB⁻* mutants to minimize TNF-α-mediated septic shock, which could be a significant limitation for safe use in humans. Compared with the parental *Salmonella*, this deletion avoided the high levels of TNF-α, increased the median lethal dose by 10,000-fold, and retained tumor accumulation in the absence of TNF-α induction *(48)*. Four to five days after a single intravenous injection of 1×10^6 CFU/mouse, VNP20009 proliferation and accumulation were routinely detected at levels up to 2×10^9 CFU/g tumor. The amount in the liver ranged from 3×10^4 up to 2×10^6 CFU/g. Immunohistochemical studies indicated that the attenuated salmonellae were distributed homogeneously throughout the entire tumor and could be detected from the periphery into the necrotic region of the tumors.

In parallel, using two different rat tumor models, we suggested the use of an optimal therapeutic dose for administration of VNP20009, dependent on VNP20009 concentration, administration route, and tumor volume, to establish a potential therapeutic window. Derived tumor:liver ratios using the optimal therapeutic dose increased as a function of time and reached a maximum on day 20 (more than 10^7:1), a time at which no bacteria were detectable in the liver. Importantly, we also showed that VNP20009 can circulate and accumulate to high levels at distal tumor sites, following direct intratumoral administration at a single tumor site, under conditions in which liver VNP20009 levels remain low *(49)*.

Biodistribution and genetic stability studies of VNP20009 in normal C57BL/6 mice or cynomolgus monkeys at various doses have indicated that VNP20009 has an excellent safety profile, including genetically stable attenuated virulence (stable after more than 140 generations of growth) and reduction of septic shock potential and antibiotic susceptibility *(46)*. Preclinical toxicology studies in monkeys revealed that toxicity attributed to intravenous administration of VNP20009 was confined to the liver and spleen and was mild. VNP20009 was not pathogenic in monkeys (maximum tolerated dose [MTD] = 1×10^9 CFU/monkey), pigs (MTD = 3×10^9 CFU/pig), or mice (MTD = 1×10^6 CFU/mouse).

In addition to its selective tumor accumulation, VNP20009 has been shown to have innate antitumor effects in a limited number of tumor models. The genetic basis of this anticancer phenotype has been found to be dependent on a major *Salmonella* virulence regulon, SPI-2 *(50)*. However, the mechanisms still remain unknown. In combination with irradiation, VNP20009 has been shown to produce supra-additive effects, suggesting that the combination of these genetically engineered salmonellae with radiotherapy could be a beneficial treatment for solid tumors *(51)*.

4.2. Use of Attenuated Salmonellae as a Protein Delivery Vector

As with clostridial species, the main potential of attenuated salmonellae is not with the bacteria alone, but with the "arming" with a gene that can express a protein in the tumor that will aid in treatment. The potential use of attenuated salmonellae as a protein delivery vector (so-called TAPET) was shown by intravenous administration of the bacteria expressing green fluorescent protein, CD *(52)*, or thymidine kinase *(44)* into tumor-bearing mice. Preclinical data demonstrated similar biological characteristics (pharmacokinetics, tissue distribution, shedding, intrinsic antitumor efficacy) for TAPET-CD (VNP20009 expressing an *E. coli* CD gene) compared to VNP20009. Preclinical toxicology for TAPET-CD revealed it was relatively nontoxic at doses producing antitumor effects in rodents and well tolerated in monkeys, with only occasional mild clinical signs, increased hepatic enzyme function values, and splenic enlargement *(53)*. The TAPET-CD/5-FC combination had an MTD in monkeys of 1×10^{10} CFU/monkey for TAPET-CD and 500 mg/kg for 5-FC.

We and others have demonstrated tumor-selective accumulation of TAPET-CD at levels of up to 10^9 CFU/g 4–5 days after intravenous injection into tumor-bearing mice or rats *(49,52)*. In contrast, bacterial levels in normal tissues, such as liver, were usually lower than 10^6 CFU/g. CD enzyme expressed in the attenuated salmonellae is functional, as shown by the presence of 5-FU in tumors after administering 5-FC to tumor-bearing animals. TAPET-CD, when used together with 5-FC, caused tumor growth inhibition in mice bearing colon tumor xenografts *(54)*. These results suggest that avirulent salmonellae expressing prodrug-converting enzymes could be useful for converting nontoxic prodrugs to toxic metabolites in tumors.

Various other therapeutic proteins have been cloned and expressed in VNP20009, including TNF-α, endostatin, and platelet factor 4 fragment. Yuhua and colleagues have described the use of an attenuated Salmonella strain, genetically engineered to express IL-12 or granulocyte-macrophage colony-stimulating factor (GM-CSF), as a vehicle for oral gene therapy against murine tumors *(55)*. Following administration of recombinant Salmonella, soluble cytokines that contributed to an increased number of cytotoxic T cells and prolongation of survival, were detected in murine sera. This type of oral gene therapy resulted in a high degree of protection against the development of two unrelated murine tumors.

4.3. Clinical Experience With Attenuated Salmonella

An initial phase I clinical trial in patients with advanced metastatic cancer was performed using the first-generation vector of *S. typhimurium* (VNP20009) attenuated by chromosomal deletion of the *purI* and *msbB* genes without a therapeutic gene *(56)*. In cohorts of 3 to 6 patients, 24 patients with metastatic melanoma and 1 patient with metastatic renal cell carcinoma received 30-minute intravenous bolus infusions containing 10^6 to 10^9 CFU/m^2 of VNP20009. Patients were evaluated for dose-related toxicities, selective replication within tumors, and antitumor effects. The results showed that the MTD was 3×10^8 CFU/m^2. Dose-limiting toxicity was observed in patients receiving 10^9 CFU/m^2, which included thrombocytopenia, anemia, persistent bacteremia, hyperbilirubinemia, diarrhea, vomiting, nausea, elevated alkaline phosphatase, and hypophosphatemia. VNP20009 induced a dose-related increase in the circulation of proinflammatory cytokines, such as interleukin 1 (IL-1), TNF-α, IL-6, and IL-12. However, focal tumor colonization was observed in only 2 patients receiving 10^9 CFU/m^2 and in 1 patient receiving 3×10^8 CFU/m^2. Unlike the observations with transplanted tumors in rodents, none of the patients experienced objective tumor regression, including those patients with colonized tumors. One possible reason for the relatively poor tumor colonization was the much more rapid clearance of bacteria from the peripheral blood than that found in rodents, and future clinical studies using longer infusions are planned. However, the reasons for the different colonization in transplanted rodent tumors and in human spontaneous tumors needs further investigation.

Because of the promising preclinical data, TAPET-CD is currently under evaluation in a phase I clinical trial using direct tumor injection of the armed *Salmonella* followed by oral administration of 5-FC *(57)*.

5. FUTURE DIRECTIONS

To date, antitumor efficacy has been demonstrated using one enzyme (CD) with the prodrug 5-FC, which it converts into the active anticancer 5-FU. However, 5-FU is a drug primarily active against proliferating cells, so there is a strong need for work with other enzymes that can convert prodrugs into more active anticancer agents. Thus, one avenue for future work is exploration of other enzyme/ prodrug combinations. Another avenue that should be explored is the combination of CDEPT with antivascular agents. Because these agents cause massive vascular shutdown and necrosis and have already been shown to increase the colonization of clostridia in experimental tumors, further work is needed to explore the potential of such combinations. Not only should this be performed in experimental tumors of standard size, but also it should be expanded to include small metastases, which normally do not have necrosis and so would not normally be colonized by obligate anaerobes. If systemic administration of antivascular agents such as DMXAA and combretastatin can produce necrosis in small metastases, they would then be susceptible to treatment with CDEPT.

Finally, phase I clinical trials need to be performed with the CDEPT approach. These have already been performed with attenuated salmonellae, but the lack of robust colonization by this organism has lessened enthusiasm for this approach. There is reason to believe, however, that genetically modified clostridia will not suffer the same problems because studies with nongenetically modified clostridia in the 1970s and 1980s demonstrated high levels of colonization and tumor lysis following intravenous injection of clostridial spores. Colonization and measurement of levels of novel enzymes and conversion of prodrug to active drug (for example, 5-FC to 5-FU) could readily be performed in a relatively small phase I clinical study. Positive results from such a study would augur well for larger scale applications of CDEPT.

REFERENCES

1. Dang, L. H., Bettegowda, C., Huso, D. L., Kinzler, K. W., and Vogelstein, B. (2001) Combination bacteriolytic therapy for the treatment of experimental tumors. *Proc. Natl. Acad. Sci. USA* **98,** 15,155–15,160.
2. Thomlinson, R. H. and Gray, L. H. (1955) The histological structure of some human lung cancers and the possible implications for radiotherapy. *Br. J. Cancer* **9,** 539–549.
3. Groebe, K. and Vaupel, P. (1988) Evaluation of, oxygen diffusion distances in human breast cancer xenografts using tumor-specific in vivo data: role of various mechanisms in the development of tumor hypoxia. *Int. J. Radiat. Oncol. Biol. Phys.* **15,** 691–697.
4. Becker, A., Hansgen, G., Bloching, M., Weigel, C., Lautenschlager, C., and Dunst, J. (1998) Oxygenation of squamous cell carcinoma of the head and neck: comparison of primary tumors, neck node metastases, and normal tissue. *Int. J. Radiat. Oncol. Biol. Phys.* **42,** 35–41.
5. Brizel, D. M., Rosner, G. L., Prosnitz, L. R., and Dewhirst, M. W. (1995) Patterns and variability of tumor oxygenation in human soft tissue sarcomas, cervical carcinomas, and lymph node metastases. *Int. J. Radiat. Oncol. Biol. Phys.* **32,** 1121–1125.
6. Brizel, D. M., Dodge, R. K., Clough, R. W., and Dewhirst, M. W. (1999) Oxygenation of head and neck cancer: changes during radiotherapy and impact on treatment outcome. *Radiother. Oncol.* **53,** 113–117.
7. Vaupel, P. W. and Hockel, M. (1995) Oxygenation status of human tumors: a reappraisal using computerized pO2 histography. In *Tumor Oxygenation* (Vaupel, P. W., Kelleher, D. K., and Gunderoth, M., eds.), Gustav Fischer Verlag, Stuttgart, Germany, pp. 219–232.
8. Rampling, R., Cruickshank, G., Lewis, A. D., Fitzsimmons, S. A., and Workman, P. (1994) Direct measurement of pO2 distribution and bioreductive enzymes in human malignant brain tumors. *Int. J. Radiat. Oncol. Biol. Phys.* **29,** 427–431.
9. Sundfor, K., Lyng, H., Kongsgard, U. L., Trope, C., and Rofstad, E. K. (1997) Polarographic measurement of pO2 in cervix carcinoma. *Gynecol. Oncol.* **64,** 230–236.
10. Movsas, B., Chapman, J. D., Horwitz, E. M., et al. (1999) Hypoxic regions exist in human prostate carcinoma. *Urology* **53,** 11–18.
11. Koong, A. C., Mehta, V. K., Le, Q. T., et al. (2000) Pancreatic tumors show high levels of hypoxia. *Int. J. Radiat. Oncol. Biol. Phys.* **48,** 919–922.
12. Brown, J. M. and Giaccia, A. J. (1998) The unique physiology of solid tumors: opportunities (and problems) for cancer therapy. *Cancer Res.* **58,** 1408–1416.
13. Wouters, B. G., Weppler, S. A., Koritzinsky, M., et al. (2002) Hypoxia as a target for combined modality treatments. *Eur. J. Cancer* **38,** 240–257.
14. Malmgren, R. A. and Flanigan, C. C. (1955) Localization of the vegetative form of *Clostridium tetani* in mouse tumors following intravenous spore administration. *Cancer Res.* **15,** 473–478.
15. Mose, J. R. and Mose, G. (1959) Onkolyseversuche mit apathogenen anaeroben Sporenbildnern am Ehrlich Tumor des Maus. *Z. Krebsforsch.* **63,** 63–74.

16. Mose, J. R. and Mose, G. (1964) Oncolysis by clostridia. I. Activity of *Clostridium butyricum* (M-55) and other non-pathogenic clostridia against the Ehrlich carcinoma. *Cancer Res.* **24,** 212–216.
17. Thiele, E. H., Arison, R. N., and Boxer, G. E. (1964) Oncolysis by clostridia. III. Effects of clostridia and chemotherapeutic agents on rodent tumors. *Cancer Res.* **24,** 222–233.
18. Engelbart, K. and Gericke, D. (1964) Oncolysis by clostridia V. Transplanted tumors of the hamster. *Cancer Res.* **24,** 239–243.
19. Carey, R. W., Holland, J. F., Whang, H. Y., Neter, E., and Bryant, B. (1967) Clostridial oncolysis in man. *Eur. J. Cancer* **3,** 37–46.
20. Heppner, F. and Mose, J. R. (1978) The liquefaction (oncolysis) of malignant gliomas by a nonpathogenic clostridium. *Acta Neurol.* **12,** 123–125.
21. Heppner, F., Mose, J., Ascher, P. W., and Walter, G. (1983) Oncolysis of malignant gliomas of the brain. *13th Int. Cong. Chemother.* **226,** 38–45.
22. Lemmon, M. J., Elwell, J. H., Brehm, J. K., et al. (1994) Anaerobic bacteria as a gene delivery system to tumors. *Proc. Am. Assoc. Cancer Res.* **35,** 374.
23. Bagshawe, K. D., Sharma, S. K., Springer, C. J., and Rogers, G. T. (1994) Antibody directed enzyme prodrug therapy (ADEPT). A review of some theoretical, experimental and clinical aspects. *Ann. Oncol.* **5,** 879–891.
24. Syrigos, K. N. and Epenetos, A. A. (1999) Antibody directed enzyme prodrug therapy (ADEPT): a review of the experimental and clinical considerations. *Anticancer Res.* **19,** 605–613.
25. Fox, M. E., Lemmon, M. J., Mauchline, M. L., et al. (1996) Anaerobic bacteria as a delivery system for cancer gene therapy: activation of 5-fluorocytosine by genetically engineered clostridia. *Gene Ther.* **3,** 173–178.
26. Lemmon, M. L., Van Zijl, P., Fox, M. E., et al. (1997) Anaerobic bacteria as a gene delivery system that is controlled by the tumor microenvironment. *Gene Ther.* **4,** 791–796.
27. Theys, J., Landuyt, W., Nuyts, S., et al. (2001) Specific targeting of cytosine deaminase to solid tumors by engineered *Clostridium acetobutylicum. Cancer Gene Ther.* **8,** 294–297.
28. Liu, S. C., Minton, N. P., Giaccia, A.J., and Brown, J. M. (2002) Anticancer efficacy of systemically delivered anaerobic bacteria as gene therapy vectors targeting tumor hypoxia/necrosis. *Gene Ther.* **9,** 291–296.
29. Nuyts, S., Van Mellaert, L., Theys, J., Landuyt, W., Lambin, P., and Anne, J. (2002) Clostridium spores for tumor-specific drug delivery. *Anticancer Drugs* **13,** 115–125.
30. Melton, R. G. and Sherwood, R. F. (1996) Antibody-enzyme conjugates for cancer therapy. *J. Natl. Cancer Inst.* **88,** 153–165.
31. Gericke, D., Dietzel, F., Konig, W., Ruster, I., and Schumacher, L. (1979) Further progress with oncolysis due to apathogenic clostridia. *Zentralbl. Bakteriol. (Orig. A)* **243,** 102–112.
32. Martin, J., Stribbling, S. M., Poon, G. K., et al. (1997) Antibody-directed enzyme prodrug therapy: pharmacokinetics and plasma levels of prodrug and drug in a phase I clinical trial. *Cancer Chemother. Pharmacol.* **40,** 189–201.
33. Joseph, W. R., Cao, Z., Mountjoy, K. G., Marshall, E. S., Baguley, B. C., and Ching, L. M. (1999) Stimulation of tumors to synthesize tumor necrosis factor-alpha in situ using 5,6-dimethylxanthenone-4-acetic acid: a novel approach to cancer therapy. *Cancer Res.* **59,** 633–638.
34. Zhao, L., Ching, L. M., Kestell, P., and Baguley, B. C. (2002) The antitumour activity of 5,6-dimethylxanthenone-4-acetic acid (DMXAA) in TNF receptor-1 knockout mice. *Br. J. Cancer* **87,** 465–470.
35. Tozer, G. M., Prise, V. E., Wilson, J., et al. (1999) Combretastatin A-4 phosphate as a tumor vascular-targeting agent: early effects in tumors and normal tissues. *Cancer Res.* **59,** 1626–1634.
36. Goto, H., Yano, S., Zhang, H., et al. (2002) Activity of a new vascular targeting agent, ZD6126, in pulmonary metastases by human lung adenocarcinoma in nude mice. *Cancer Res.* **62,** 3711–3715.
37. Theys, J., Landuyt, W., Nuyts, S., et al. (2001) Improvement of *Clostridium* tumour targeting vectors evaluated in rat rhabdomyosarcomas. *FEMS Immunol. Med. Microbiol.* **30,** 37–41.
38. Miller, R. V. and Kokjohn, T. A. (1990) General microbiology of recA: environmental and evolutionary significance. *Annu. Rev. Microbiol.* **44,** 365–394.
39. Nuyts, S., Theys, J., Landuyt, W., Van Mellaert, L., Lambin, P., and Anne, J. (2001) Increasing specificity of antitumor therapy: cytotoxic protein delivery by non-pathogenic clostridia under regulation of radio-induced promoters. *Anticancer Res.* **21,** 857–861.
40. Nuyts, S., Van Mellaert, L., Theys, J., et al. (2001) Radio-responsive recA promoter significantly increases TNFalpha production in recombinant clostridia after 2 Gy irradiation. *Gene Ther.* **8,** 1197–1201.
41. Nuyts, S., Van Mellaert, L., Barbe, S., et al. (2001) Insertion or deletion of the Cheo box modifies radiation inducibility of *Clostridium* promoters. *Appl. Environ. Microbiol.* **67,** 4464–4470.
42. Yazawa, K., Fujimori, M., Amano, J., Kano, Y., and Taniguchi, S. (2000) Bifidobacterium longum as a delivery system for cancer gene therapy: selective localization and growth in hypoxic tumors. *Cancer Gene Ther.* **7,** 269–274.
43. Matsumura, H., Takeuchi, A., and Kano, Y. (1997) Construction of *Escherichia coli-Bifidobacterium longum* shuttle vector transforming *B. longum* 105-A and 108-A. *Biosci. Biotechnol. Biochem.* **61,** 1211–1212.
44. Pawelek, J. M., Low, K. B., and Bermudes, D. (1997) Tumor-targeted *Salmonella* as a novel anticancer vector. *Cancer Res.* **57,** 4537–4544.

45. Khan, S. A., Everest, P., Servos, S., et al. (1998) A lethal role for lipid A in *Salmonella* infections. *Mol. Microbiol.* **29,** 571–579.
46. Clairmont, C., Lee, K. C., Pike, J., et al. (2000) Biodistribution and genetic stability of the novel antitumor agent VNP20009, a genetically modified strain of *Salmonella typhimurium. J. Infect. Dis.* **181,** 1996–2002.
47. Chen, J. J., Sun, Y., and Nabel, G. J. (1998) Regulation of the proinflammatory effects of Fas ligand (CD95L). *Science* **282,** 1714–1717.
48. Low, K. B., Ittensohn, M., Le, T., et al. (1999) Lipid A mutant *Salmonella* with suppressed virulence and TNFalpha induction retain tumor-targeting in vivo. *Nat. Biotechnol.* **17,** 37–41.
49. Mei, S., Theys, J., Landuyt, W., Anne, J., and Lambin, P. (2002) Optimization of tumor-targeted gene delivery by engineered attenuated *Salmonella typhimurium. Anticancer Res.* **22,** 3261–3266.
50. Pawelek, J. M., Sodi, S., Chakraborty, A. K., et al. (2002) *Salmonella* pathogenicity island-2 and anticancer activity in mice. *Cancer Gene Ther.* **9,** 813–818.
51. Platt, J., Sodi, S., Kelley, M., et al. (2000) Antitumour effects of genetically engineered Salmonella in combination with radiation. *Eur. J. Cancer* **36,** 2397–2402.
52. Zheng, L. M., Luo, X., Feng, M., et al. (2000) Tumor amplified protein expression therapy: *Salmonella* as a tumor-selective protein delivery vector. *Oncol. Res.* **12,** 127–135.
53. Lee, K. C., Zheng, L. M., Margitich, D., Almassian, B., and King, I. (2001) Evaluation of the acute and subchronic toxic effects in mice, rats, and monkeys of the genetically engineered and *Escherichia coli* cytosine deaminase gene-incorporated *Salmonella* strain, TAPET-CD, being developed as an antitumor agent. *Int. J. Toxicol.* **20,** 207–217.
54. King, I., Bermudes, D., Lin, S., et al. (2002) Tumor-targeted *Salmonella* expressing cytosine deaminase as an anti-cancer agent. *Human Gene Ther.* **13,** 1225–1233.
55. Yuhua, L., Kunyuan, G., Hui, C., et al. (2001) Oral cytokine gene therapy against murine tumor using attenuated *Salmonella typhimurium. Int. J. Cancer* **94,** 438–443.
56. Toso, J. F., Gill, V. J., Hwu, P., et al. (2002) Phase I study of the intravenous administration of attenuated *Salmonella typhimurium* to patients with metastatic melanoma. *J. Clin. Oncol.* **20,** 142–152.
57. Cunningham, C. and Nemunaitis, J. (2001) A phase I trial of genetically modified *Salmonella typhimurium* expressing cytosine deaminase (TAPET-CD, VNP20029) administered by intratumoral injection in combination with 5-fluoro-cytosine for patients with advanced or metastatic cancer. Protocol no: CL-017. Version: April 9, 2001. *Hum. Gene Ther.* **12,** 1594–1596.

27

Molecular Imaging of Cancer Gene Therapy

Harvey R. Herschman

1. INTRODUCTION

Applications of noninvasive imaging in cancer gene therapy research and clinical practice fall into three categories. First, "tagged" tumor cells can be used to monitor cell fates in vivo. Target tumor cells can be labeled for noninvasive imaging, either by transfer of ex vivo-labeled tumor cells to host animals or by the development of transgenic animal models in which target tumor cells express reporters that can be noninvasively imaged. The response of imagable target tumor cells to chemotherapy, immunotherapy, gene therapy, cell therapy, and multimodality therapies can then be noninvasively monitored (1). Although an important tool in preclinical cancer research studies in general and gene therapy research in particular, the use of noninvasive imaging to monitor the fate of tagged target tumor cells is not extensively reviewed here.

In the second application of noninvasive imaging to cancer gene therapy, conventional imaging technologies are used to monitor the therapeutic effects of somatically transferred genes on the processes of tumor growth and progression (e.g., by gamma camera imaging, magnetic resonance imaging [MRI]), tumor vascularization (e.g., by MRI, ultrasound), and tumor metabolism (e.g., by positron emission tomography [PET]). This application of noninvasive imaging is extensively discussed in the review by Haberkorn and Altmann (2).

The final application of noninvasive imaging technology to cancer gene therapy monitors the delivery of therapeutic vectors and the location, magnitude, and duration of expression of ectopically expressed therapeutic genes to establish correlations between (1) therapeutic gene expression and (2) measures of tumor response. Therapeutic gene delivery and expression, with a few exceptions, have not been monitored in cancer gene therapy studies. This situation is akin to trying to evaluate the effectiveness of new chemotherapies without monitoring the pharmacokinetics or pharmacodynamics of the new chemotherapeutic agent.

This chapter emphasizes noninvasive imaging of gene expression from somatic gene delivery systems. Because of the rapid developments in imaging instrumentation, alternative noninvasive imaging modalities that have been adapted to molecular imaging, increasing choices in reporter genes (Section 5.) that can be used for noninvasive imaging, and the growing interest and application of noninvasive imaging technologies to increasing areas of biology, a number of reviews on noninvasive molecular imaging have appeared in the past several years. References 2–14 provide alternative reviews (and views) of this topic and more detailed descriptions of specific areas.

2. THE NEED FOR NONINVASIVE IMAGING IN GENE THERAPY

Other chapters in this book discuss in detail the goals, tools, results, and current limitations of cancer gene therapy. It is clear that one of the greatest problems facing advancement of gene therapy for cancer

From: *Contemporary Cancer Research*
Cancer Gene Therapy
Edited by: D. T. Curiel and J. T. Douglas © Humana Press Inc., Totowa, NJ

is the need to monitor the location, duration, and magnitude of expression of therapeutic genes, whatever the mechanism and route of their delivery. Without the ability to monitor noninvasively, repetitively, and quantitatively the expression of presumptive therapeutic genes, researchers and clinicians are stymied in their attempts to improve the efficacy of gene therapy by determining the correlations between expression of therapeutic genes with tumor detection, regression, and elimination. Only by noninvasive, in vivo imaging will we be able to determine whether we have properly targeted the cells that require therapeutic modification or be certain that only the appropriate target tumor or effector cells express the therapeutic gene. If the gene therapy protocols in question require temporal regulation of therapeutic gene expression, we need to be able to monitor the correlation between regulated expression and therapeutic outcome. Similarly, if the magnitude of therapeutic gene expression must be adjusted for optimal efficacy, we must be able to monitor this process. Therapeutic modalities can be envisioned in which the level of ectopic gene expression must be modulated as the recipient responds to the therapy; monitoring of such modulation of therapeutic gene expression will require noninvasive imaging procedures.

Preclinical animal studies are fundamental in developing refinements of gene delivery for clinical applications of gene therapy. Because they mature rapidly, reproduce easily, are well characterized genetically, and can have their genomes manipulated by recombinant deoxyribonucleic acid (DNA) technology, mice are the primary experimental platform for preclinical gene therapy studies. Murine models are used to investigate vector design, routes of vector administration, adjuvant and combination therapies, and other variables that may improve somatic gene transfer and appropriate therapeutic gene expression. Imaging researchers in the gene therapy arena are therefore faced with two challenges: (1) development of assays for noninvasive, quantitative, and repetitive imaging of the location, magnitude, and duration of gene expression in small animal models and (2) development of imaging technologies that provide similar information in a clinical setting.

3. IMAGING VECTOR DELIVERY

Clearly, the first question to consider in somatic gene transfer experiments and application is the targeting of the gene delivery vector—cell, virus, liposome, or plasmid—to the tissue and/or cell population of choice. The most obvious approach to this problem is radionuclide labeling of the vector itself and in vivo detection by nuclear imaging techniques. For example, cells labeled with ^{99m}Tc have been monitored by gamma camera imaging *(15)*, and cells labeled with ^{64}Cu-pyruvaldehyde-bis (N^4-methylthiosemicarbazone) have been monitored by microPET *(16)*. Lipophilic ^{111}indium-oxine complex-labeled *(17)* and ^{99m}Tc-labeled *(18)* viruses have been used to monitor viral delivery. Weissleder and colleagues developed general methods to label plasmid DNAs with ^{99m}Tc *(10,19)*. MRI techniques have also been explored to monitor cancer gene therapy delivery vehicles; cells labeled with supermagnetic iron oxide particles coupled to the HIV-tat peptide can be tracked by MRI *(20)*. These labeling techniques for cells, viruses, liposomes, and DNA are generic and can be applied to vector delivery systems for any therapeutic gene.

Although useful, the ability to track in vivo the physical location of a vector delivery system does not provide information on the functional delivery of new genetic information to somatic targets. Tracking delivery of a vector does not reveal the level of gene expression in targeted vs nontargeted tissues or the duration of gene expression following targeting. Consequently, vector-labeling procedures are used primarily in understanding the early steps in vector targeting.

4. USING REPORTER GENES TO IMAGE GENE EXPRESSION

Reporter gene analysis utilizes surrogate coding regions that encode rapidly and sensitively assayed protein products to monitor expression from chimeric gene constructs in which expression is driven by promoter regions of either experimental interest or utility. In the context of either somatic gene delivery or cell therapy, reporter proteins expressed from appropriate promoters, by incorporating these constructs into the gene delivery system, can be used to monitor efficacy of gene delivery vehicles.

The chloramphenicol acetyl transferase (CAT) *(21,22)* and β-galactosidase (β-gal) *(23,24)* reporter genes were used extensively by cell biologists and investigators during the initial development of gene therapy vectors. The disadvantage of CAT and β-gal as reporter genes is the requirement that recipients be sacrificed or biopsied for analysis. To perform temporal gene expression studies in vivo in animal models, several animals at each time-point must be sacrificed and assayed. CAT and β-gal clearly cannot be used to monitor somatic gene delivery in patients. Secreted reporter proteins (e.g., alkaline phosphatase) facilitate serial, noninvasive monitoring of reporter gene expression in blood, but at the expense of knowing the site of reporter gene expression. Reporter genes with products that can be monitored by optical techniques, such as luciferase *(5)*, green fluorescent protein (GFP) *(13)*, and β-lactamase *(25)*, have been used by cell biologists for cell culture studies. As described in Section 5.3., in vivo analysis of optical reporter genes has emerged as an important new set of paradigms for noninvasive imaging.

5. REPORTER GENES FOR IN VIVO IMAGING

It is clear that, to monitor the efficacy of expression from somatically transferred genes in patients, noninvasive measurement of reporter gene expression is required. Moreover, the ability to monitor the location, magnitude, and duration of reporter gene expression noninvasively, quantitatively, and repetitively would greatly facilitate advances in preclinical animal models of somatic gene delivery. Advances in molecular biology, imaging instrumentation, radiochemistry, and conventional chemistry have made it possible to use a variety of modalities, including radionuclide, MRI, and optical detection systems, to monitor reporter gene expression in living animals following somatic gene transfer.

5.1. Imaging Reporter Genes With Radionuclide Probes

In principle, it should be possible to develop radionuclide-labeled small molecule binding/imaging probes for any target protein. Such probe molecules could then be used for in vivo imaging. Although target-specific probes exist for a number of protein targets, general development of protein-specific probes is not currently possible in practice. However, reporter genes that utilize radionuclide-labeled tracer probes can be used to monitor gene expression in vivo, allowing investigators to infer the expression of linked therapeutic genes. Reporter gene systems that employ radionuclide probes currently utilize receptors that sequester labeled ligands, enzymes that convert radiolabeled substrates to trapped products, or transporters that sequester radiolabeled probes inside cells. Using gamma camera imaging, single-photon emission computed tomography (SPECT), and PET, radiolabeled tracers can be used repeatedly, noninvasively, and quantitatively to image the location, magnitude, and duration of reporter gene expression.

5.1.1. The Dopamine D_2 Receptor as an In Vivo Reporter Gene

The dopamine D_2 receptor (D2R) is expressed principally in the striatum of the brain. Several radionuclide-labeled probes for the D2R, including [^{11}C]raclopride *(26–28)*, N-[^{11}C]methylspiperone *(29)*, 3-(2-[^{18}F]fluoroethyl)spiperone (FESP) *(30,31)*, and [^{123}I]iodobenzamide derivatives *(32)*, have been developed to facilitate imaging of this receptor by gamma camera imaging, SPECT, and PET.

Because the D2R is expressed at high concentrations only in the striatum and a number of radiolabeled ligands have been developed for this receptor, ectopic D2R expression has been developed as a noninvasive reporter gene system. We cloned the D2R, under the control of the cytomegalovirus (CMV) early promoter, into a replication-defective adenovirus *(33)*. Systemically administered adenovirus results primarily in infection and gene expression in the murine liver because of hepatic filtration properties and the high level of expression of the coxsackie and adenovirus receptor (CAR) in this tissue.

Mice were injected intravenously with Ad.D2R or Ad.βgal, a replication-defective adenovirus expressing the β-gal gene as a reporter. Two days later, the mice were injected via the tail vein with FESP. FESP distribution was measured by microPET imaging after an additional 3 hours. Substantial hepatic fluorine-18 retention was observed in the mouse injected with Ad.D2R. In contrast, relatively little hepatic fluorine-18 accumulation occurred in the mouse that received Ad.βgal. Varying amounts of Ad.D2R were injected into mice, and the levels of D2R expression, determined by microPET analysis of FESP retention, in living mice were compared with D2R levels determined by [^{3}H]spiperone binding to liver extracts following sacrifice of the animals. The microPET-measured FESP retention values were strongly correlated ($r^2 = 0.89$) with the in vitro binding assays. Noninvasive, in vivo analysis of the D2R reporter gene expression in living animals by microPET measurement of FESP retention accurately reflected in vitro analysis of ectopic D2R expression levels.

One potential problem in the use of receptors as reporter genes is that their ectopic expression might change the physiology of target cells. When agonist ligands bind to the D2R, a G-protein-coupled signal transduction system is activated, resulting in a reduction of cyclic adenosine 5'-mono-phosphate levels in cells. However, specific mutations in the D2R receptor have been described that uncouple ligand binding from activation of this G-protein complex signaling pathway *(34,35)*. My group created Ad.D2R80A, an adenovirus expressing one of these "uncoupled" mutants and demonstrated (1) that cells infected in culture with Ad.D2R80A do not lower cyclic adenosine 5'-mono-phosphate levels in response to dopamine exposure, but bind [^{3}H]spiperone as well as cells infected with Ad.D2R; and (2) that, for mice injected with Ad.D2R vs Ad.D2R80A, no difference in hepatic FESP accumulation was observed *(36)*. Although D2R80A does not activate G-protein-coupled signaling following agonist binding, D2R80A and D2R are equally effective as PET reporter genes. The D2R80A/FESP reporter gene/reporter probe system should be very beneficial in monitoring somatic gene transfer and cell therapy.

5.1.2. The Herpes Virus Simplex Type 1
Thymidine Kinase Gene as an In Vivo Reporter Gene

The herpes virus simplex type 1 thymidine kinase (HSV1-TK) enzyme, like its murine and human TK orthologues, phosphorylates thymidine. However, uracil derivatives such as 5-iodo-2'-fluoro-2'-deoxy-1-β-D-arabino-furanosyl-uracil (FIAU) and acycloguanosines (e.g., acyclovir, ganciclovir [GCV], penciclovir [PCV]) are much more effectively phosphorylated by HSV1-TK than by mammalian TKs. Like thymidine, FIAU and the acycloguanosines are transported into cells, where they serve as substrates for the HSV1-TK enzyme. However, once phosphorylated, these prodrugs are no longer able to exit the cell. Cellular kinases convert the monophosphates of acyclovir, GCV, PCV, and FIAU to their di- and triphosphate derivatives. The phosphorylated acycloguanosines and FIAU kill cells, either by inhibiting DNA polymerase or—if they are incorporated into DNA—by acting as chain-terminating nucleotides. Tjuvajev and colleagues suggested that radiolabeled substrates for HSV1-TK might serve as reporter probes to monitor the in vivo expression of HSV1-TK enzyme activity noninvasively following ectopic expression of the HSV1-tk gene *(37,38)*.

The Sloan-Kettering group pioneered the use of radionuclide FIAU derivatives as reporter probes to image HSV1-tk gene expression, using [^{131}I]FIAU, [^{123}I]FIAU, and [^{124}I]FIAU for gamma camera, SPECT, and PET analyses. They first used gamma camera imaging to detect [^{131}I]FIAU retention in grafted tumors, following retroviral transfer and expression of HSV1-TK *(38)*. Subsequently, [^{124}I]FIAU was employed to image HSV1-TK expression by PET in stably transfected tumor grafts *(39)*. These studies are reviewed in detail in ref. *3*.

The University of California at Los Angeles group adopted an alternative approach to imaging the HSV1-tk reporter gene. Because of the greater resolution and sensitivity of PET analyses and the relative ease of preparing fluorinated tracer molecules vs iodinated derivatives, emphasis was placed on fluorinated acycloguanosines. In the initial study, a replication-deficient adenovirus, Ad.HSV-tk, in which the reporter gene is expressed from the CMV early promoter, was injected intravenously into mice. The positron-emitting TK substrate 8-[^{18}F]fluoro-9-[(1,3-dihydroxy-2-propoxy)methyl]guanine (fluoroganciclovir, FGCV) was synthesized *(40)* and administered both to these mice and to mice injected with a control virus, Ad.βgal, expressing the β-gal gene. Using microPET, hepatic FGCV retention was demonstrated in the Ad.HSV1-tk injected animals *(41)*.

Because PCV is a more effective HSV1-TK substrate than GCV, a positron-emitting PCV analogue, 8-[^{18}F]fluoro-9-[4-hydroxy-3-(hydroxymethyl)but-1-yl]guanine (fluoropenciclovir, FPCV), was synthesized and used to image HSV1-tk expression. FPCV is several times more effective than FGCV in detecting HSV1-TK expression *(42)*. A number of other fluorine-18-labeled acycloguanosines, including 9-[3-[^{18}F]-fluoro-1-hydroxy-2-propoxy)methyl]guanine (FHPG) *(43)*, and 9-[(4-[^{18}F]-fluoro-3-hydroxymethylbutyl)guanine (FHBG) *(44,45)*, have also been developed and tested as reporter probes for HSV1-TK enzyme, using PET analysis. Comparative studies suggested that FHBG is a better substrate for *HSV1-tk* than FHPG *(45–47)*. Studies in human volunteers demonstrated that FHBG has properties suggesting that it will be compatible as a PET radiotracer to image the *HSV1-tk* reporter gene *(48)*.

5.1.2.1. MUTANT *HSV1-TK* REPORTER GENES

The acycloguanosines are not naturally occurring HSV1-TK substrates; they were developed as pharmacological agents. Black et al. *(49)*, to develop more effective therapeutic agents, identified mutant HSV1-TK enzymes that could more effectively utilize acycloguanosines as substrates. They created, by site-directed mutagenesis, mutant HSV1-TK enzymes and screened these proteins for mutants more effectively able to use acycloguanosines as substrates for phosphorylation and less effectively utilize thymidine. It seemed likely that their mutant TK enzymes might also be able to use fluorinated forms of the acycloguanosines more effectively and, consequently, be more effective reporter genes for PET imaging of gene expression. This is the case; the TK enzyme produced from the HSV1-sr39tk mutant gene is able to phosphorylate FGCV, FPCV, FHPG, and FHBG more effectively than is wild-type TK in cell culture studies. When Ad.HSV1-tk is compared with Ad.HSV1-sr39tk, a replication-deficient adenovirus expressing this mutant enzyme, the sensitivity of the Ad. HSV1-sr39tk/FHBG system is about an order of magnitude greater than the sensitivity of the Ad.HSV1-tk/FGCV system.

5.1.2.2. COMPARISONS OF POSITRON-EMITTING HSV1-TK SUBSTRATES FOR PET IMAGING

Brust et al. *(50)* compared [^{124}I]FIAU and FHPG as probes using subcutaneous xenografts of tumors expressing the wild-type enzyme in nude mice. Tjuvajev et al. *(51)* performed a similar direct comparison of [^{124}I]FIAU, FHPG, and FHBG. Their data demonstrated that [^{124}I]FIAU is a more efficient probe than FHBG or FHPG for the wild-type HSV1-TK enzyme in this context. In contrast to the acycloguanosines, FIAU is not more effectively utilized as a substrate by HSV1-sr39TK. The half-life of [^{124}I]FIAU is 4.2 days vs 110 minutes for ^{18}F. For applications for which clearance of the HSV1-TK substrate limits resolution or sensitivity of PET imaging, [^{124}I]FIAU may be a preferred alternative to image HSV1-TK. On the other hand, synthesis of ^{124}I is more difficult than preparation of ^{18}F, potentially limiting the utility of [^{124}I]FIAU as an imaging agent.

Comparison of a number of 5-substituted 2'-deoxy-2'-fluoro-1-β-D-arabinofuranosiluracil derivatives suggested that 5-fluoro-2'-deoxy-2'-fluoro-1-β-arabinofuranosyluracil may be a better substrate for HSV1-TK than FIAU or FHBG *(52)*. If the preliminary results with 5-fluoro-2'-deoxy-2'-fluoro-1-β-arabinofuranosyluracil are confirmed by more extensive in vivo analysis, using this HSV1-TK substrate may combine the sensitivity of the radioiodinated uracil analogues with the comparative ease of synthesis of the radiofluorinated acycloguanosines.

Positron-emitting radioiodinated uracil probes may be more appropriate substrates for PET imaging of HSV1-tk gene expression for some applications; positron-emitting radiofluorinated acycloguanosines or uracil derivatives may be preferable for other applications. Parallel chemical refinement of radiolabeled probes and genetic manipulation of reporter genes should continuously improve the HSV1-TK system in particular and noninvasive radionuclide reporter gene imaging systems in general.

5.1.3. The Somatostatin Receptor as an In Vivo Reporter Gene

Like the D2R, somatostatin receptors (SSTrs) are seven membrane pass proteins coupled to G-protein signaling complexes. Although there are six SSTr genes, the human subtype 2 receptor (hSSTr2) has been the subtype primarily used as a reporter gene for noninvasive imaging. The endogenous hSSTr2 gene is expressed most extensively in the pituitary, but is also active in the pancreas, kidney, lung, gastrointestinal tract, and several other tissues.

The hSSTr2 binds naturally occurring somatostatin peptides as well as a series of synthetic somatostatin analogues (e.g., octretide, P829, p2045). A number of clinically approved agents, including ^{111}In-labeled octreotide (Octreoscan) and ^{99m}Tc-labeled P829 (NeoTect/NeoSpect), are used to image, by gamma camera imaging, neuroendocrine and lung tumors that express endogenous hSSTr *(14)*. Several PET tracers ($[^{64}$Cu]TETA-octreotide *(53)*, $[^{68}$GA]DOTA-D-Phe^1-Tyr^3-octreotide *(54)*, $[^{68}$Ga] DOTATOC *(55)*) for hSSTrs have also been described.

The hSSTr2 gene has been incorporated into adenovirus vectors, expressed from the CMV promoter, and used to image, by gamma camera, virally directed reporter gene expression in xenografts of human tumors in nude mice after intravenous injection of $[^{99m}$Tc]P2045, $[^{111}$I]octreotide, and $[^{99m}$Tc] P829. In side-by-side experiments, $[^{99m}$Tc]P2045 appears to be the most effective reporter probe *(14)*.

Like the D2R, ligand binding to the SSTr2 generates a G-protein-linked signal. Under most conditions, the signal generated by ligand binding to the SSTr is antiproliferative. Indeed, it has been suggested that the antiproliferative effect of SSTr activation could potentially be used as an anticancer therapy *(56)*. Although it has been argued that ligand signaling from the hSSTr2 used as a reporter gene could have an additional therapeutic benefit, it is also possible that signaling from an ectopic, activated SSTr might result in deleterious physiological effects on the targeted cell or tissue. In contrast to the D2R80A reporter gene, no hSSTr2 mutant in which ligand binding and cell signaling have been uncoupled has been examined as a reporter gene.

Like the HSV1-TK reporter, the hSSTr2 protein has also been employed as a therapeutic gene. Several somatostatin analogues have been conjugated with radionuclides (e.g., ^{90}Y, ^{131}I, ^{153}Sm, ^{177}Lu, ^{188}Re) to deliver therapeutic doses of radiation to tumors that express the hSSTr. Although most applications have been for therapy of tumors that naturally express SSTrs, adenovirus delivery and subsequent treatment with radionuclide-labeled somatostatin ligands have been studied in human tumor xenografts in nude mice *(57)*, as described more extensively next.

5.1.4. The Sodium Iodide Symporter as an In Vivo Reporter Gene

The sodium iodide symporter (NIS) is a 13-transmembrane domain protein expressed primarily in the basolateral membrane of thyroid follicular cells. The NIS protein facilitates the transport of iodide into these cells, where the iodide is organified and used to iodinate thryoglobulin. In addition to facilitating the uptake of various radionuclide forms of iodide (e.g., ^{123}I, ^{124}I, ^{125}I, ^{131}I), the NIS protein also facilitates the accumulation of $[^{99m}$Tc]O$_4$. Although the NIS gene is expressed primarily in the thyroid, it is also active in the salivary glands, gastric mucosa, and mammary gland *(58)*. However, in these last tissues, the iodide is not organified *(7)*.

Following heterologous NIS expression in either transiently or stably transfected cells, substantial active iodide transport could be demonstrated in cultured cells despite the absence in these cells of the enzyme systems responsible for organifying the transported iodide. These data suggested that ectopic NIS gene expression might be valuable, in both therapeutic and imaging roles, in gene therapy experiments. Xenografts of cells stably transfected with the NIS gene *(59)* can be imaged with both $[^{99m}$]TcO$_4$ and ^{123}I gamma camera scintography.

Several laboratories have created replication-defective adenoviruses in which the NIS gene is expressed from the CMV promoter. Following intratumoral injection with Ad.NIS, xenografted SiHa tumors can be imaged by conventional gamma camera imaging after intraperitoneal injection of [123]I. Stomach, bladder, and thyroid gland uptake of the radionuclide probe was also observed *(60)*. Similarly, functional NIS activity could be demonstrated in xenografted human glioma cells *(61)* and in xenografts of human prostate LNCaP tumor cells *(62)* following intratumoral injection of replication-defective adenoviruses expressing the NIS gene from a CMV promoter. The NIS gene is likely to see substantial increased utility as a noninvasive imaging tool because of the variety of clinically approved reporter probes currently available. Chung *(58)* published a comprehensive review of the NIS gene as both a therapeutic agent and an imaging reagent.

5.2. Imaging Reporter Gene Expression With MRI

In principle, MRI has the advantage of providing very high spatial resolution to image reporter gene expression. However, to obtain such resolution in reasonable times, very high concentrations of substances with appropriate paramagnetic properties must be introduced into the target cells. Weissleder and colleagues used a modified transferrin ligand, to which monocrystalline iron oxide nanoparticles were linked, to image a xenografted tumor expressing an ectopically expressed transferrin receptor reporter gene. Transferrin receptor-dependent accumulation of the superparamagnetic ligand is sufficient to permit imaging of the xenografted tumor (reviewed in ref. *8*).

MRI reporter gene imaging procedures that exploit enzymatic reactions that target "caged" paramagnetic chelates have also been described. The caged chelates are exposed to water following enzyme cleavage. Access of the paramagnetic chelate to water is blocked by a substrate removed by enzyme cleavage. Enzymatic removal of the blocking substrate permits the paramagnetic chelate to interact with water protons, increasing the MR signal. The β-gal substrate, 1-(2-(b-galactopyranosyloxy)propyl)-4,7,10-tris(carboxymethyl)1,4,7,10 tetraaza-cyclododecane gadolinium(III), after injection into *Xenopus laevis* embryos, can be cleaved by ectopically expressed β-gal to generate an excellent MR image in a living embryo *(63)*. The technique, however, is limited because the substrate cannot be systemically administered to experimental animals in sufficient concentration for MR imaging. To date, enzymatically activated MR procedures for imaging reporter gene expression following somatic gene delivery have not been described. Consult refs. *8* and *10* for more detailed discussions of imaging of reporter gene expression with MR.

5.3. Imaging Reporter Gene Expression With Optical Techniques

Optical imaging of appropriate reporter genes, such as GFP *(64–66)*, β-lactamase *(25)*, and the luciferases *(67)*, has had enormous impact on molecular and cell biology. GFP fusion proteins have characterized the subcellular distribution of a wide number of cellular proteins and helped elucidate issues of subcellular protein targeting and ligand-induced redistribution of cell proteins. Firefly luciferase (ffluc) and *Renilla* luciferase (rluc) have been extensively used in cell culture studies as reporter genes to characterize both the transcriptional regulatory properties of a wide variety of genes and the signal transduction mechanisms that activate gene expression in response to extracellular signals.

Several new technologies, including video, digital, and charge-coupled device (CCD) cameras have been developed to monitor light emission from living animals and used to assay noninvasively the in vivo expression of GFP and luciferase reporter genes. Noninvasive optical imaging of reporter gene expression has substantial advantages, including ease of use, lack of any radioactive probe, relatively low background signal (at least for the luciferase reporter genes), relative simplicity of use, and low cost relative to radionuclide and MR approaches. However, optical imaging techniques are limited by fluorophore quenching effects, depth-dependent photon attenuation, scatter, and resolution issues in contrast to radionuclide and MR techniques and are likely to be employed in the clinic only in specialized applications.

In vivo optical imaging techniques are very powerful tools for imaging small animals, however, and are rapidly gaining popularity and utility in the preclinical studies of animal cancer models, somatic gene therapy research, and cell therapy studies. Optical imaging studies will provide extensive information in these preclinical models and guide the design of gene and cell therapy/imaging systems utilized in clinical research and practice. These new optical imaging systems are complementary to radionuclide and MR imaging systems and should facilitate transition from preclinical studies to clinical applications.

5.3.1. GFP as an In Vivo Reporter Gene

GFP use has seen spectacular growth in cell biology to image intracellular location and trafficking of fusion proteins in living cells. GFP has the distinct advantage that the reporter protein is intrinsically fluorescent. Consequently, no reporter probe is required, in contrast to studies with radionuclide imaging techniques (Section 5.1.) or luciferase reporter genes (Sections 5.3.2. and 5.3.3.). However, the wavelengths required to excite the GFP protein and the light emitted by GFP following excitation are both absorbed extensively by tissues. Consequently, GFP-based imaging studies work well in vivo only near the skin (e.g., with subcutaneous tumors in nude mice) or by using "skin flap" procedures to expose internal organs *(68)*. A variety of tumor xenografts in which tumor cells stably express GFP in nude mouse hosts have been used to track tumor growth, metastases, and response to therapies *(69–71)*. Adenovirus-expressing GFP can be tracked for both site and duration of expression *(72)*.

The use of surgical windows and more sophisticated imaging techniques such as confocal laser scanning microscopy and multiphoton laser scanning microscopy, which enhance signal and reduce background fluorescence *(73)*, permit a more extensive examination of GFP expression in deeper regions of the animal. Using these techniques, cellular interactions in cancer such as tumor induction of stromal vascular endothelial growth factor activation, liposomal extravasation from tumor blood vessels, and measurements of tumor blood vessel permeability can be demonstrated and quantitated in living animals *(74)*.

As the technologies for detection of GFP fluorescence grow, applications of this reporter gene technology to animal models of cancer detection, progression, and treatment will increase. However, substantial application to monitoring of cancer therapeutics in the clinic is not likely for GFP imaging given the penetration restrictions of exciting light and the tissue absorption of fluorescent emissions.

5.3.2. Firefly Photinus pyralis *Luciferase as an In Vivo Reporter Gene*

Luciferase is a generic name for a group of enzymes that share the property of emitting visible light as a product of their enzymatic activities; many of the luciferases do not share any sequence homology. The firefly *Photinus pyralis* luciferase gene (ffluc) has been by far the most extensively used luciferase for cell and molecular biology studies. Light is produced through the action of ffluc with its substrate luciferin in the presence of magnesium and adenosine triphosphate.

Firefly luciferase gene expression can also be imaged in vivo using high-sensitivity, cooled CCD cameras. The introduction of this new technology and the ease, relatively low cost, and convenience of nonradioactive ffluc imaging has led to an enormous increase in the application of this technology to noninvasive in vivo imaging. Contag et al. *(74)* reviewed the use of both ffluc and GFP to monitor tumor growth, metastasis, and response to therapy with xenografted tumor cells that stably express these optical reporter genes. The use of gene delivery vehicles carrying ffluc as an optical reporter gene to monitor reporter gene expression is in a period of dramatic growth. Readers should expect an avalanche of new applications of this technology to the study of cancer gene therapy models in mice.

5.3.3. Sea Pansy Renilla reformis *Luciferase as an In Vivo Reporter Gene*

The *Renilla* luciferase (rluc), an enzyme distinct from ffluc, and related genes are present among coelenterates, fishes, squids, and shrimp. A distinct substrate, coelenterazine, is oxidized by rluc, resulting in bioluminescence. Coelenterazine oxidation by rluc does not require adenosine triphosphate or any other energy source. Rluc has been used extensively in cell biology and molecular biology, in conjunction with ffluc, to contrast expression of "control" and "experimental" chimeric reporter genes.

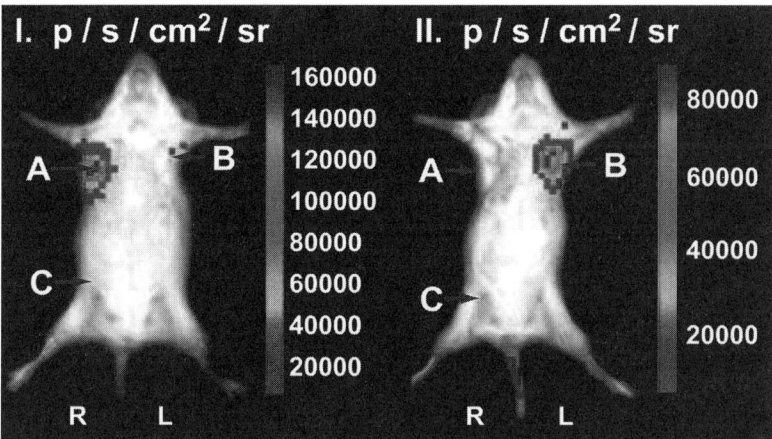

Fig. 1. Imaging firefly luciferase and sea pansy luciferase reporter genes in the same animal. Three C6 rat glioma cell lines were subcutaneously transplanted into a recipient mouse. Tumor A stably expressed the firefly luciferase gene. Tumor B stably expressed the sea pansy (*Renilla*) luciferase gene. Tumor C was a control C6 tumor, which did not express an imaging gene. In the panel on the left, the mouse was injected intraperitoneally with luciferin as substrate for the firefly luciferase, then imaged with the CCD camera. In the panel on the right, the mouse was injected intraperitoneally with coelenterazine as substrate for the sea pansy luciferase, then imaged with the CCD camera. (From ref. *75* with permission. ©2002 National Academy of Sciences, USA.)

Bhaumik and Gambhir *(75)* compared the efficacy of the ffluc/luciferin and rluc/coelentrazine reporter/substrate systems as imaging systems for in vivo monitoring of reporter gene expression. Rat C6 glioma cells transiently transfected with either rluc or ffluc were injected subcutaneously on the flanks of nude mice, and bioluminescence was monitored with a CCD camera following systemic injection of either coelenterazine and/or luciferin. Bioluminescence was observed, as expected, from the C6-ffluc xenograft following luciferin injection (Fig. 1). Similarly, bioluminescence was observed in the C6-rluc xenograft following coelenterazine injection. No crossreactivity occurred; cells expressing ffluc did not emit a detectable signal when the animal was injected with coelenterazine, and bioluminescence was not observed in cells expressing rluc following injection of luciferin.

Although quantitative studies of sensitivity need to be performed, as well as kinetic, biodistribution, and toxicology studies of coelenterazine administration, these initial experiments demonstrated the ability to carry out noninvasive optical imaging of two distinct luciferase reporter genes in the same animal. The availability of this paradigm will make comparisons of control and experimental gene expression, alternative modes of gene delivery, and similar comparative studies possible using the relatively simple and inexpensive methods of optical imaging with high-sensitivity CCD cameras.

6. CORRELATING REPORTER GENE EXPRESSION AND THERAPEUTIC GENE EXPRESSION

If reporter genes are to be useful in monitoring gene therapy procedures, there must be the ability to correlate the expression of the therapeutic and reporter genes. A number of experimental protocols to correlate expression of two genes, permitting the indirect measurement of therapeutic genes, are discussed next (*see* Fig. 2). However, several of the reporter imaging genes described here have been used as therapeutic genes, either to kill tumor cells that naturally overexpress these genes or following ectopic expression.

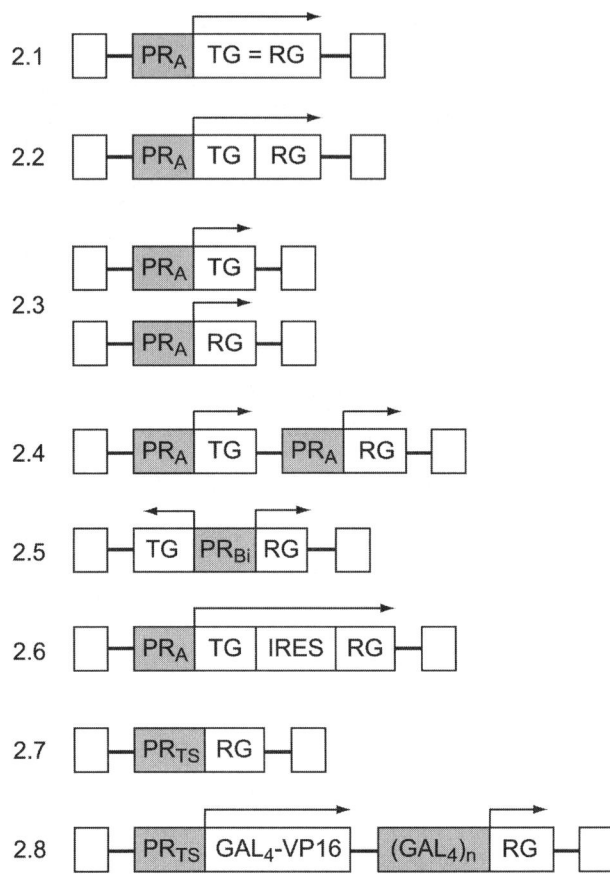

Fig. 2. Alternative methods to deliver therapeutic genes and noninvasive reporter genes for imaging. (2.1) Therapeutic genes that are also reporter genes. (2.2) Fusion genes that express a chimeric therapeutic protein/ reporter protein. (2.3) Coadministration of two otherwise identical vectors expressing a therapeutic gene and a reporter gene. (2.4) Identical promoters driving a therapeutic gene and a reporter gene. (2.5) Bidirectional promoter driving a therapeutic gene and a reporter gene. (2.6) Bicistronic message from which a therapeutic gene is expressed following the cap site, and a reporter gene is expressed from an IRES. (2.7) Expression of a reporter gene from a tissue-/tumor-specific promoter. (2.8) Expression of a reporter gene from a TSTA construct in which expression of the reporter gene is driven by an artificial promoter responsive to a chimeric transcription factor, and the chimeric transcription factor is expressed from a tissue-specific or inducible promoter. The open squares at the end of each construct represent viral long-terminal repeats. PR_A,, a promoter element such as the CMV promoter, chosen by the investigator; TG, therapeutic gene; RG, reporter gene; PR_{Bi}, bidirectional promoter; IRES, internal ribosomal entry site; PR_{TS}, tissue-specific or tumor-specific promoter; Gal_4-VP16, a chimeric gene encoding a fusion transcription factor containing the DNA-binding domain of the yeast GAL_4 transcription factor and the herpes virus VP16 transcription factor activation domain; $(GAL_4)_n$, a promoter containing multiple Gal_4-binding sites and a minimal eukaryotic promoter element, such as the TATA box of the adenovirus E4 protein *(97)*. Promoter elements are shown in gray boxes. Although these illustrations show therapeutic and reporter genes in the context of viral vectors, the constructs could be developed in the context of any gene delivery vector or therapeutic cell for somatic delivery.

6.1. Therapeutic Genes That Are Also Imaging Genes (Fig. 2.1)

The HSV1-TK enzyme converts acycloguanosine prodrugs into toxic compounds if the prodrug substrates are administered in pharmacological doses. For noninvasive imaging, when tracer levels of radionuclide-labeled HSV1-TK substrates are injected, no pharmacological effect occurs. Consequently, scenarios are possible in which investigators might first monitor *HSV1-tk* gene delivery with

FHBG or FIAU to correlate the level of HSV1-TK expression with therapeutic efficacy in response to a subsequent pharmacological regimen of acycloguanosine administration.

Similarly, somatostatin analogues coupled to radionuclide therapeutics have been used to treat tumors that naturally express SSTr genes. The expression of the hSSTr2 gene can be monitored, following delivery in a somatic gene transfer protocol, with appropriate radionuclide-labeled somatostatin imaging probes and subsequently be used for therapeutic attack by receptor-specific ligands carrying therapeutic radionuclides. Rogers et al. *(57)* imaged, by gamma camera, xenografts of human tumors injected with AdSSTr2 using [^{111}In]-DTPA-D-Phe^1-octreotide, then treated the mice with [^{90}Y]-SMT. Positive imaging and increased survival time were correlated in this study.

The ability of the thyroid gland to concentrate radioactive iodine has been exploited both to image and to treat thyroid tumors. Ectopic expression of NIS should facilitate both imaging and treatment of tumors originating from other tissues. Intracerebrally grafted gliomas expressing a retrovirally transfected NIS gene can be imaged with either ^{99m}TcO$_4$ or ^{123}I, then subsequently be successfully treated (i.e., life-span can be increased) in response to ^{131}I treatment *(76)*. Prostate xenografts expressing NIS can also be imaged, then treated with ^{131}I *(77)*.

6.2. Fusion Chimeras Between Therapeutic Genes and Reporter Genes

In a technology for noninvasive imaging of reporter genes, the therapeutic gene and the reporter gene are used to create a chimeric gene from which a protein fusion of both the therapeutic protein and the imaging protein is expressed (Fig. 2.2). Although this procedure ensures that there is a strict stochiometric correlation between the level of expressed therapeutic protein and imaging protein, it suffers from the distinct disadvantage that, for each therapeutic gene under investigation, a molecular fusion must be constructed and characterized. It is likely that the efficacy of the therapeutic protein, the imaging protein, or both will be compromised in a fusion molecule. However, expression of fusion proteins between HSV1-TK and GFP *(78,79)* and HSV1-TK, ffluc, and the neomycin resistance gene protein *(80)* has been demonstrated, and the correlation of the activity of the therapeutic and imaging components has been evaluated. In some cases, if a sufficiently active fusion of a therapeutic protein and an imaging protein can be produced, it may well be worth the effort to construct and characterize such a molecule for clinical use.

6.3. Coadministration of Vectors Expressing Reporter Genes and Therapeutic Genes

Coadministration of vectors expressing reporter genes and therapeutic genes is perhaps the simplest approach to monitoring therapeutic gene expression by inference from the expression of a reporter gene. At the same time as the therapeutic gene is delivered, one simply administers an additional vector identical to that expressing the therapeutic gene. The only difference between the two gene delivery vectors is the replacement of the coding sequence for the therapeutic gene with the coding region for the reporter imaging gene (Fig. 2.3). Although there may be substantial differences in infection and selection at an individual cell level, at the macroscopic/organismal level at which optical, MR, and radionuclide imaging is performed, such cellular phenomena are not likely to have a great effect.

Adenoviruses that express the D2R and HSV1-sr39tk PET reporter genes, but are otherwise identical, were injected intravenously, intramuscularly, or intratumorally into mice, and the expression of the two genes was monitored with FESP and FHBG, respectively. D2R and HSV1-sr39tk reporter gene expression were correlated, both for viral dose and at various times after virus injection *(81)*. Although simple in principle, coadministration may be an effective imaging procedure both in experimental contexts and in the clinic.

6.4. Dual Promoters Driving Therapeutic Genes and Reporter Genes in a Common Delivery Vehicle

In the application of dual promoters, a common somatic gene delivery vehicle is used to drive in tandem a reporter gene and an imaging gene from two copies of the same promoter (Fig. 2.4). For example, an adenovirus in which an insert containing a [CMV promoter] [hSSTr2 coding region] chimera is followed by a [CMV promoter] [HSV1-TK coding region] chimera was used by Zinn et al *(82)* to compare the expression of these two imaging genes using ^{99m}Tc-labeled P2045 to monitor hSSTr2 location and levels and [^{131}I]FIAU to monitor HSV1-TK activity in xenografted tumors. In this study, the authors were unable to demonstrate a correlation between expression of the hSSTr2 reporter gene and the *HSV1-tk* reporter gene.

6.5. Bidirectional Promoters Driving Therapeutic Genes and Reporter Genes in a Common Delivery Vehicle

Some promoter elements are "bidirectional"; they can direct expression of genes both upstream and downstream of the *cis*-acting regulatory sequence. Placement of a therapeutic gene and a reporter gene on either side of such a promoter should result in coordinate expression of the two coding units (Fig. 2.5). Baron et al. *(83)* created an artificial bidirectional promoter in which seven tetracycline regulatory subunits are placed between two CMV regulatory elements. When activated by a tetracycline-dependent transcription factor, genes in either direction were conditionally activated. This system was subsequently modified to demonstrate bidirectional, tetracycline-regulated coexpression of the GFP and β-gal reporter genes in transgenic animals *(84)*.

To demonstrate the utility of inducible, bidirectional promoters for noninvasive imaging of gene expression, Sun et al. *(85)* constructed a plasmid in which the D2R and HSV1-sr39tk coding sequences were placed on either side of this tetracycline promoter system and stably transfected HeLa cells expressing a tetracycline-regulated transcriptional activator with this plasmid. The expression of D2R and HSV1-sr39tk reporter genes was then monitored in xenografts by microPET analysis of FESP and FHBG retention. Prior to receiving doxycycline, HSV1-sr39tk and D2R expression were essentially undetectable. When doxycycline was added to the drinking water, HSV1-sr39TK and D2R reporter gene expression were coordinately induced, as measured by microPET analyses of the same tumor-bearing mice. Following doxycycline withdrawal, a third microPET scan demonstrated coordinate reduction of D2R and HSV1-sr39tk expression. These data demonstrated the potential utility of regulated, bidirectional vector delivery systems for coordinate expression of therapeutic genes and imaging genes.

6.6. Bicistronic Messages Expressing Therapeutic Genes and Reporter Genes in a Common Delivery Vehicle

Coordinate ectopic expression of two genes is most commonly accomplished using bicistronic vectors. DNA viruses (e.g., poliovirus, encephalomyocarditis virus) often express polycistronic messages, from which several proteins are translated. Proteins translated from internal positions in the polycistronic message are initiated in a cap-independent fashion at internal ribosomal entry sites (IRESs) *(86)*. In adapting this phenomenon for investigator-directed bicistronic reporter gene expression, two coding regions are engineered into a common message. One coding sequence (e.g., for a therapeutic protein) is placed proximal to an IRES (Fig. 2.6); the second coding sequence (e.g., for a reporter protein) is placed distal to the IRES. Coordinate expression of the proteins occurs, despite variations in absolute levels of transcription over time, because both proteins are translated from a common message. Measurement of one protein (e.g., the reporter protein) produced from the bicistronic message should therefore allow investigators to infer the relative levels of the second protein (e.g., the therapeutic protein) translated from this message.

Noninvasive SPECT imaging for in vivo analysis of *HSV1-tk* reporter gene activity was coupled with sacrifice and analysis of β-gal to demonstrate that noninvasive *HSV1-tk* measurement can reflect both the location and the magnitude of a second, *cis*-linked coding region in a bicistronic vector *(87)*. These experiments utilized xenografts of tumors stably expressing a retrovirally transduced bicistronic message.

Development of two PET reporter genes facilitated completely noninvasive analyses of coordinated expression of two coding units in a bicistronic vector. A plasmid was constructed that used an early CMV promoter to drive the expression of a bicistronic message in which the D2R and HSV1-sr39tk coding units were placed proximal and distal to an encephalomyocarditis virus IRES. Stably transfected C6 glioma cell xenografts were then monitored for D2R expression (by microPET analysis with FESP) and HSV1-sr39tk expression (by microPET analysis with FHBG). D2R expression (measured as FESP retention) and HSV1-sr39tk expression (measured as FHBG retention) were proportional *(88)*. This same D2R-IRES-HSV1-sr39tk construct was inserted into a replication-defective adenovirus and used to demonstrate that, following intravenous administration, hepatic expression of the two PET reporter genes was tightly coordinated ($r^2 = 0.89$) over six microPET imaging sessions spanning a 3-month period (Fig. 3) *(89)*. These data demonstrated, using only noninvasive imaging technology, that the location, magnitude, and duration of coordinate expression of two proteins can be noninvasively, quantitatively, and repetitively monitored following administration of a somatically transferred DNA delivery vehicle.

Although bicistronic vectors are currently the most widely used delivery system for coordinate expression of two proteins, they are not without problems. Attenuated expression of the coding region distal to the IRES is quite common. Moreover, the degree of attenuation may vary in differing target cells. Variable attenuation of the distal coding unit will both reduce sensitivity and alter the correlation between expression of the genes in the proximal and distal positions. These variables will have to be established for individual bicistronic systems to generate completely reliable, quantitative relationships between therapeutic and imaging cistrons.

6.7. Tissue-Specific Promoters

Somatic targeting of therapeutic genes is accomplished by one (or a combination) of two general procedures: (1) directing the tropism of the virus to a particular cell or tissue through some sort of cell-surface specific targeting and (2) use of cell-type specific promoters that will preferentially express the therapeutic gene in a specific cell type, even if the somatic gene vector delivery system is not target cell specific. Tumor cell-directed gene expression from tissue-specific promoters expressed in DNA delivery vectors (Fig. 2.7) has been reported for the α-fetoprotein promoter *(90)*, the carcino-embryonic antigen (CEA) promoter *(91)*, the tyrosinase promoter *(92)*, the prolactin promoter *(93)*, and a number of other tissue-specific regulatory elements.

The prostate-specific antigen (PSA) promoter has been one of the most widely studied cell type-specific promoters because of its cell type-specific expression in prostate cancer. Human prostate tumor LNCaP cells were stably transfected with a plasmid expressing the NIS gene from the PSA promoter. Xenografts of LNCaP(PSA-NIS) cells could be imaged by gamma camera with ^{123}I and subsequently killed by therapeutic doses of [131]I *(77)*. A replication-defective adenovirus in which the PSA promoter drives ffluc provides an easily detectable signal following injection into prostate tumor xenografts, but is expressed at only 1×10^{-5} the level of Ad.CMVffluc in murine liver when imaged in a cooled CCD camera *(94)*. The use of tissue-specific promoters to restrict somatic gene delivery expression to tumors and suppress expression in normal tissue is a burgeoning area of investigation; it is likely that molecular imaging procedures to monitor tumor-restricted gene expression noninvasively will see rapid expansion in popularity, both in preclinical models and in clinical contexts.

6.8. Two-Stage Transcriptional Activation Systems
for Somatic Cell Reporter Gene Expression

Tissue-specific promoters are, in principle, an excellent approach to targeting expression of therapeutic and imaging genes to selected targets (*see* Section 6.7.). In practice, many genes that have the advantage of tissue specificity, and even overexpression, in tumors are nevertheless transcribed at rates substantially below genes expressed from ubiquitously expressed, active promoters used in most

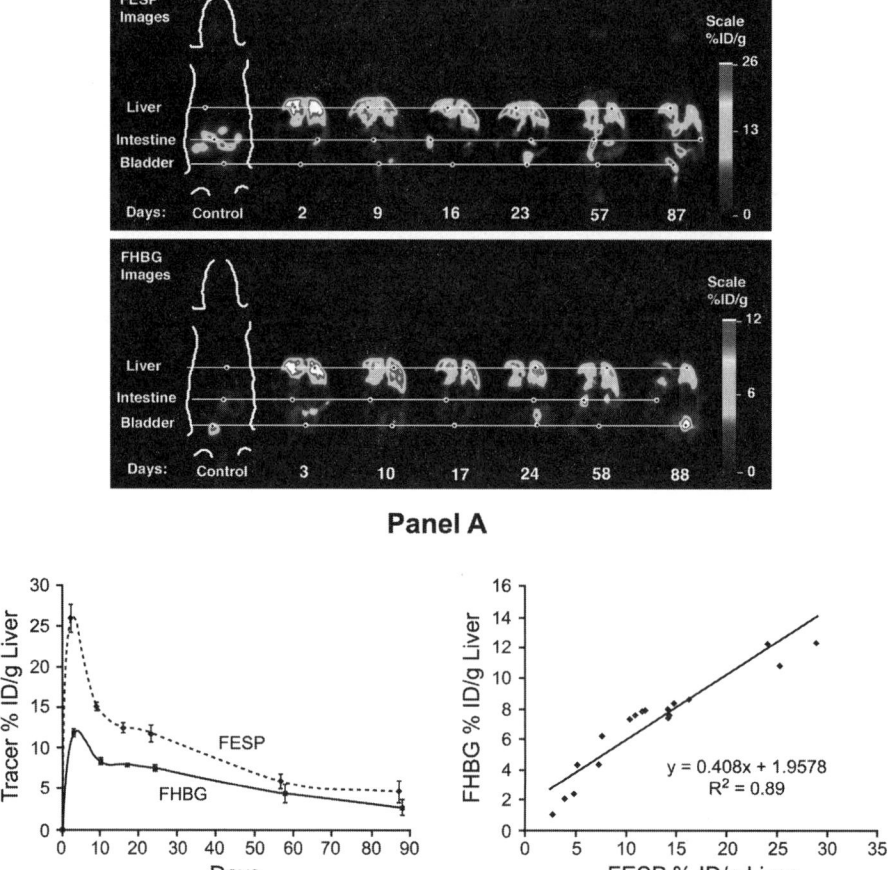

Panel A

Panel B

Panel C

Fig. 3. Repetitive imaging of the expression of the D2R and HSV1-sr39tk PET reporter genes from a bicistronic message by microPET following intravenous injection of Ad.DTm. Three Swiss Webster mice were injected by tail vein with Ad.DTm (2×10^9 pfu). Ad.DTm contains a bicistronic expression cassette driven by a CMV promoter. The bicistronic message encodes the D2R PET reporter gene proximal to an IRES and the HSV1-sr39tk reporter gene distal to the IRES. Each mouse was injected with FESP and subjected to microPET scanning on days 2, 9, 16, 23, 57, and 87 after virus injection. Each mouse was also injected with FHBG and subjected to microPET scanning on days 3, 10, 17, 24, 58, and 88 after virus injection. (A) MicroPET scans of the same mouse imaged following FESP or FHBG injection at each time-point. (B) Hepatic FESP and FHBG retention determined by microPET analysis during this 3-month experiment. Data are means + the standard errors for each FHBG or FESP measurement of the three mice. (C) The correlation between D2R PET reporter gene expression, measured as FESP retention, and HSV1-sr39TK PET reporter gene expression, measured as FHBG retention, for the six time-points measured (2/3 days, 9/10 days, 16/17 days, 23/24 days, 57/58 days, and 87/88 days after ad.DTm injection) for each of the three mice. (From ref. *89* with permission from Elsevier. Copyright 2002.)

somatic gene therapy protocols (e.g., the CMV early gene). Consequently, expression of either therapeutic or imaging genes from tissue-/tumor specific promoters may be too low either for efficient biological effectiveness or for noninvasive visualization. To amplify signals from relatively weak, but tissue-specific, promoters, a two-step transcription activation (TSTA) system has been developed *(95)*. TSTA-regulated gene expression uses two genetic components (Fig. 2.8). In one component, a cassette in which a powerful, generalized promoter for which a transcription factor is not available in most cells drives the therapeutic and/or reporter gene. In the second component, a tissue-specific and/or inducible promoter drives a unique, but otherwise unexpressed, transcription factor active on the therapeutic gene/reporter cassette.

Qiao et al. *(96)* constructed both a response cassette in which a multimerized Gal4-binding site drives the HSV1-tk gene and an induction construct in which the CEA promoter drives a chimeric transcription factor containing the GAL4 DNA-binding domain fused to the transcriptional activating domain of the herpes virus VP16 protein. In appropriate target cells that express CEA, the ectopic transcription factor expressed from the CEA promoter should stimulate HSV1-TK expression from the artificial, *cis*-acting regulatory element. These two constructs were inserted into a replication-deficient adenovirus. Using intratumoral virus injection into hepatic xenografts of a CEA-positive tumor and intravenously administered [^{131}I]FIAU as a probe for gamma camera imaging, HSV1-TK expression from this virus was compared to HSV1-TK expression from an adenovirus in which the *HSV1-tk* gene is expressed from an RSV promoter. Substantially less FIAU accumulation (e.g., HSV1-TK enzyme activity) was present in hepatic, extratumoral tissue for tumors injected with the adenovirus CEA-TSTA expression virus when compared to tumors injected with the RSV-TK-expressing virus.

A similar TSTA system was created by Zhang et al. for reporter gene expression in prostate tumor cells *(97)*. The PSA promoter is induced in response to androgen administration via the androgen receptor. The PSA promoter driving a GAL4/VP16 chimeric transcription factor and a response cassette containing multimerized Gal4-binding sites driving the ffluc reporter gene were incorporated into a common plasmid and transfected into androgen-nonresponsive HeLa cervical carcinoma cells or androgen-responsive LNCaP prostate cancer cells. Xenografts of these cells, as well as xenografts of cells transfected with CMV-ffluc and PSA-ffluc plasmids, were imaged, after luciferin injection, with a cooled CCD camera. Prior to injection, some cells were treated with androgen to activate the androgen receptor-dependent PSA promoter. The noninvasive ffluc-dependent signal intensity was 20-fold higher for the TSTA system than for CMV-driven luciferase, cell type specific and androgen sensitive. Because of its amplification and versatility, TSTA-mediated gene expression is likely to gain rapid acceptance and application in gene therapy and noninvasive gene imaging.

7. APPLICATIONS OF REPORTER GENE IMAGING IN GENE THERAPY

The use of noninvasive imaging technology is rapidly expanding in cancer gene therapy; this chapter undoubtedly will be substantially out of date regarding applications before it appears in print. However, several observations with noninvasive imaging techniques in human xenograft models are of particular translational interest and suggest important potential clinical applications for the immediate future.

7.1. Adenovirus-Expressing ffluc From a Prostate-Specific Promoter Can Identify Tumor Metastases

When Ad.CMV-ffluc is injected into human prostate tumor xenografts, robust expression is observed in the tumor. Over a 3-week period after intratumoral injection, Ad.CMV-ffluc virus "leaks" from the tumor and finds its way to the liver, where ffluc expression can be imaged with the CCD camera *(94)*. When similar prostate tumor xenografts are injected with a replication-defective adenovirus in which a derivative of the PSA promoter drives the ffluc imaging gene, similarly robust ffluc expression is observed in the tumor, but even over a 3-week period, there is relatively restricted expression in the liver. However, with time, ffluc CCD signal was observed in extratumoral sites in the back and chest. When the mice were sacrificed and individual organs were excised and examined for ffluc activity, optical signal was detected from the tumor, spine, and lungs (Fig. 4). Histological examination revealed tumor metastases in these organs.

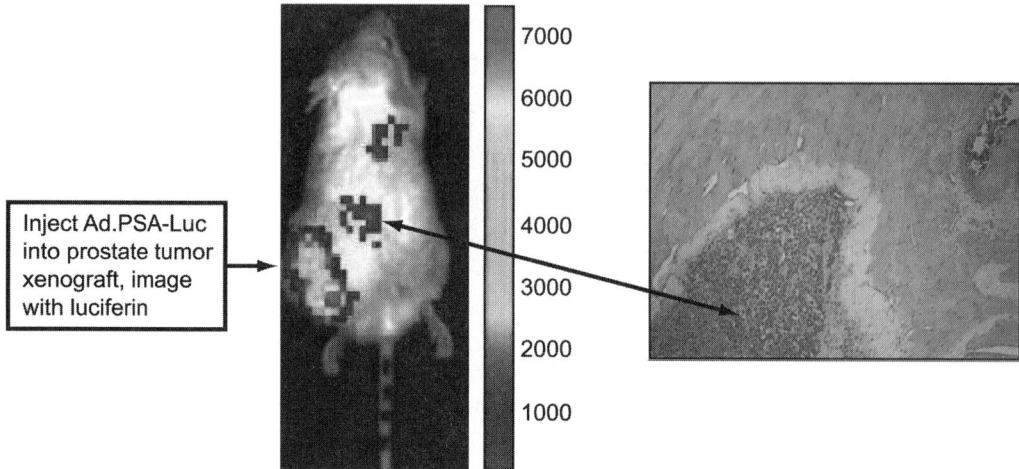

Fig. 4. An adenovirus expressing luciferase from the PSA promoter can detect prostate cancer cell metastases in a murine xenograft model. Human LAPC-4 tumor cells were xenografted into the left flank of an immune-deficient SCID mouse. After the tumors had reached a diameter of approx 7 mm, 1.8×10^9 pfu of an adenovirus expressing the ffluc gene from the PSA promoter were injected into the tumor in six doses given on 2 consecutive days. The image shown in the figure was obtained 21 days after virus injection. After virus injection, the animal was sacrificed, the spine was excised, and the tumor was stained to identify the xenografted tumor cells that had metastasized to this site. (Adapted from ref. *94* with permission.)

When animals bearing prostate tumor xenografts were injected intravenously with Ad.PSAffluc, lung metastases could be detected by optical imaging with a cooled CCD camera. These data suggest that viral vectors expressing tumor-specific, noninvasive reporter genes may be able to identify the location and size of occult metastases in human cancer patients following systemic administration and appropriate imaging.

7.2. Noninvasive Imaging of a Redirected Adenoviral Therapeutic Vector

Adenovirus preferentially targets the liver because of tissue architecture and the elevated expression of the CAR in this tissue. Many tumors, in contrast, are relatively devoid of CAR. To retarget an adenoviral HSV1-tk delivery vector for GCV therapy, Hemminki et al. *(98)* modified the adenovirus fiber to include an Arg-Gly-Asp domain, targeting the virus to $\alpha_v\beta$ integrins. An hSSTr2 receptor gene was also included in the virus, driven from a CMV promoter distinct from the CMV promoter driving the *HSV1-tk* gene (i.e., a dual-promoter gene delivery vehicle; Section 6.4.), to image the Ad.HSV1tk. hSSTr2 virus. When subcutaneous ovarian tumor xenografts were intratumorally injected with this virus and subsequently imaged with a gamma camera using [^{99m}Tc]P2045, the tumor could be imaged. These data suggest that noninvasive imaging will be clinically useful in determining the efficacy of targeted gene therapy vectors.

7.3. Monitoring Distribution and Reporter Gene Expression of Conditionally Replicating/Oncolytic Virus

The ability of adenovirus, herpes virus, and other viruses used as gene delivery vectors to replicate in and kill normal cells is a major barrier for viral therapeutic gene delivery. An alternative to ectopic gene delivery for cancer therapy is the reengineering of lytic viruses to create viral strains that preferentially replicate in and kill tumor cells and minimize the ability of these "conditionally replicating" or "oncolytic" viruses to proliferate in normal cells. Several clinical trials of oncolytic viruses are currently under way. The ability to monitor the location and intensity of viral infection repetitively and noninvasively in such therapies would be very beneficial. HSV oncolytic viral mutants marked with the *HSV1-tk* reporter gene have been used to image both human colorectal xenografts *(99)* and rat glial tumor implants into host rats *(100)*, using [^{124}I]FIAU to detect, by PET scanning, the expression of the *HSV1-tk* gene. If extended to the clinical context, noninvasive molecular imaging of reporter genes should help determine the tropism and effectiveness of oncolytic viral cancer therapy.

7.4. Noninvasive Imaging of Translational Control of Gene Expression

It is well known that methotrexate treatment increases the level of dihydrofolate reductase (DHFR) in cells as a result of gene amplification. The ability of antifolates to regulate DHFR translation from DHFR messenger ribonucleic acid has been described *(101)*. Mayer-Kuckuk et al. *(102)* created a DHFR and *HSV1-tk* chimeric gene that produces a DHFR-TK fusion protein. When tumor xenografts stably expressing the DHFR-TK fusion protein are treated with the antifolate trimetrexate, an elevated signal from the antifolate-treated animals can be noninvasively imaged by PET analysis of [^{124}I]FIAU retention after 3 days of drug administration. Translational regulation of therapeutic gene expression, although not likely to play a major role in cancer gene therapy, may find some clinical use. Fusion proteins that incorporate noninvasive imaging components could be useful in monitoring this process.

8. APPLICATIONS OF REPORTER GENE TECHNOLOGY IN CELL THERAPY

G2A is a G-protein-coupled receptor predominantly expressed in lymphocytes. Genetic ablation of G2A leads to autoimmunity. When sublethally irradiated SCID mice are transplanted with BCR-ABL-transduced G2A-deficient bone marrow cells, the animals develop tumors earlier, and the tumors progress more rapidly, resulting in shorter survival times than for mice receiving BCR-ABL-transduced bone marrow cells from wild-type animals. Histological analysis suggested that, prior to any clinical evidence of disease, the tumor cell population derived from G2A$^{-/-}$ bone marrow expands more rapidly than cells from a G2A$^{+/+}$ background; latency appears shorter, and cellular expansion appears increased. To monitor the kinetics of this process noninvasively, the tumor cells were stably transfected with a vector expressing the HSV1-sr39tk PET reporter gene, and tumor cell distribution was monitored by microPET with FHBG. Repeated imaging was used to monitor noninvasively the changing spatial and temporal distribution of BCR-ABL-driven leukemogenesis *(103)*.

Ponomarev et al. *(104)* stably transfected a human T-cell line with a vector that expresses an HSV1-TK-GFP fusion protein driven by an NFAT responsive promoter and FACS-selected cells that respond to T-cell activation stimuli by robust expression of the fusion reporter gene. Xenografts of this cell line, when stimulated by anti-CD28 and anti-CD3, can be imaged in vivo by PET analysis of [^{124}I]FIAU accumulation to monitor activation of T-cell receptor-dependent gene expression. Using cells that constitutively express both a noninvasive reporter gene (e.g., D2R80A or hSSTr2) and a noninvasive reporter gene (e.g., HSV1-tk) responsive to T-cell activation signals should permit noninvasive, repetitive monitoring of both cell targeting and antigen activation of immune lymphocyte therapy.

9. NONINVASIVE IMAGING STUDIES IN TRANSGENIC ANIMALS

Transgenic animals expressing noninvasively imaged reporter genes driven by specific gene promoters have been described for optical imaging *(105)* and for microPET analysis *(106)* and will certainly be used extensively in studies of gene expression. The use of noninvasive imaging for the analysis of transgenic mice has not yet, strictly speaking, contributed to gene therapy studies. However, it is likely that cells from transgenic mice expressing noninvasively imaged reporter genes will be used in therapy transplant studies, and that target tumor cells expressing reporter genes will be used in grafts for therapy studies. Precedent for transplant studies with cells expressing reporter genes from transgenic mice exists; myoblast transplants from mice expressing a transgenic GFP-ffluc fusion gene in a wide variety of target tissues (driven by a CMV promoter) have been monitored by optical imaging *(107)*.

Several laboratories are developing procedures to image reporter gene expression in transgenic animals noninvasively to monitor elevated signal transduction pathways activated by dominant oncogenes and to conditionally activate noninvasively imaged reporter gene expression in cells deleted for recessive oncogenes in vivo by genetic means such as CRE elimination. Noninvasive imaging in these transgenic murine models will be able to monitor tumor initiation, progression, and metastasis and the response of these tumors to chemotherapy, immunotherapy, gene therapy, cell therapy, and combined therapy modalities.

10. APPLICATIONS TO HUMAN THERAPY

At the time this chapter was prepared, only one study of the noninvasive imaging of a reporter gene in a clinical context had appeared *(108)*. As might be expected for a first trial of noninvasive imaging of reporter gene expression, this study "piggybacked" on a trial of a therapeutic gene that also doubles as an imaging gene. Five patients suffering from recurrent glioblastoma were imaged with [^{124}I]FIAU to characterize the extent of vector-mediated *HSV1-tk* gene expression in a phase I/II clinical trial. The authors concluded that "The extent of *HSV-1-tk* gene expression seemed to predict the therapeutic response." It is likely that imaging of the NIS or hSSTr reporter genes after gene transfer, followed by their exploitation for therapeutic efficacy, will soon be observed in cancer gene therapy clinical contexts. Several clinical trials employing an in vivo imaging arm that utilizes an incorporated reporter gene are in preparation, and many more are anticipated.

11. THE FUTURE OF REPORTER GENE IMAGING
AND SOMATIC GENE THERAPY

Noninvasive imaging has a long tradition in clinical practice. In contrast, until recently, these procedures have seen relatively little use in the study of cellular and molecular effects on animal models of disease—especially in studies that employ murine models. The development of new instrumentation for small animal analysis (e.g., microCT, microSPECT, microPET, animal MR instruments, and optical imaging devices), coupled with the development of noninvasively imagable reporter genes that can be repetitively and quantitatively monitored with these instruments, has provided new technologies and new paradigms for small animal research in general and cancer gene therapy research in particular. Noninvasive imaging of reporter genes in xenografted tumor cells, in cells in which oncogenes are activated in vivo, and in cells receiving gene transfer vectors provides new experimental approaches to many of the problems that need to be confronted in gene therapy preclinical studies.

There has, in the recent past, been an enormous explosion in the area of molecular imaging. Two new societies, several new journals, a host of review articles, the establishment of a number of molecular imaging centers in universities and pharmaceutical research programs, and substantial federal and private funding in this area are all testimony to the dramatic increase in the applications of noninvasive molecular imaging to all areas of biomedical research. The published literature using noninvasive molecular imaging in preclinical research is expanding exponentially, as we learned in the preparation of this chapter.

In contrast, we are only at the beginning of clinical applications, with one published report of noninvasive reporter gene imaging *(108)*. It appears that we stand on the edge of an avalanche; the lessons taught in the laboratory by noninvasive molecular imaging are on the brink of translation to the clinic, with extensive benefit for the researcher, the practicing physician, and the patient in the offering.

REFERENCES

1. Sweeney, T. J., Mailänder, V., Tucker, A. A., et al. (1999) Visualizing the kinetics of tumor-cell clearance in living animals. *Proc. Natl. Acad. Sci. USA* **96,** 12,044–12,049.
2. Haberkorn, U. and Altmann, A. (2001) Imaging methods in gene therapy of cancer. *Curr. Gene Ther.* **1,** 1–27.
3. Gambhir, S. S., Herschman, H. R., Cherry, S. R., et al. (2000) Imaging transgene expression with radionuclide imaging technologies. *Neoplasia* **2,** 118–138.

4. Herschman, H. R., MacLaren, D. C., Iyer, M., et al. (2000) Seeing is believing: non-invasive, quantitative and repetitive imaging of reporter gene expression in living animals, using positron emission tomography. *J. Neurosci. Res.* **59,** 699–705.

5. Honigman, A., Zeira, E., Ohana, P., et al. (2001) Imaging transgene expression in live animals. *Mol. Ther.* **4,** 239–249.

6. Ray, P., Bauer, E., Iyer, M., et al. (2001) Monitoring gene therapy with reporter gene imaging. *Semin. Nucl. Med.* **31,** 312–320.

7. Spitzweg C. and Morris, J. C. (2001) Approaches to gene therapy with sodium/iodide symporter. *Exp. Clin. Endocrinol. Diabetes* **109,** 56–59.

8. Allport, J. R. and Weissleder, R. (2001) In vivo imaging of gene and cell therapies. *Exp. Hematol.* **29,** 1237–1246.

9. Herschman, H. R., Barrio, J. R., Satyamurthy, N., et al. (2002) Monitoring gene therapy by positron emission tomography. In *Vector Targeting for Therapeutic Gene Delivery* (Curiel, D. T. and Douglas, J. T., eds.), Wiley-Liss, New York, pp. 661–685.

10. Bogdanov, A. Jr. and Weissleder, R. (2002) In vivo imaging of gene delivery and expression. *Trends Biotechnol.* **20,** S11–S18.

11. O'Connell-Rodwell, C. E., Burns, S. M., Bachmann, M. H., and Contag, C. H. (2002) Bioluminescent indicators for in vivo measurements of gene expression. *Trends Biotechnol.* **20,** S19–S23.

12. Greer, L. F. III and Szalay, A. A. (2002) Imaging of light emission from the expression of luciferases in living cells and organisms: a review. *Luminescence* **17,** 43–74.

13. Contag, C. H. and Bachmann, M. H. (2002) Advances in in vivo bioluminescence imaging of gene expression. *Annu. Rev. Biomed. Eng.* **4,** 235–260.

14. Zinn, K. R. and Chaudhuri, T. R. (2002) The type 2 human somatostatin receptor as a platform for reporter gene imaging. *Eur J. Nucl. Med. Mol. Imaging* **29,** 388–399.

15. Harrison, L. H. Jr., Schwarzenberger, P. O., Byrne, P. S., Marrogi, A. J., Kolls, J. K., and McCarthy, K. E. (2000) Gene-modified PA1-STK cells home to tumor sites in patients with malignant pleural mesothelioma. *Ann. Thorac. Surg.* **70,** 407–411.

16. Adonai, N., Nguyen, K. N., Walsh, J., et al. (2002) Ex vivo cell labeling with ^{64}Cu-pyruvaldehyde-bis(N^4-methyl-thiosemicarbazone) for imaging cell trafficking in mice with positron-emission tomography. *Proc. Natl. Acad. Sci. USA* **99,** 3030–3035.

17. Schellingerhout, D., Bogdanov, A. Jr., Marecos, E., Spear, M., Breakefield, X., and Weissleder, R. (1998) Mapping the in vivo distribution of herpes simplex virions. *Hum. Gene Ther.* **9,** 1543–1549.

18. Zinn, K. R., Douglas, J. T., Smyth, C. A., et al. (1998) Imaging and tissue biodistribuiton of ^{99m}Tc-labeled adenovirus knob (serotype 5). *Gene Ther.* **5,** 798–808.

19. Bogdanov, A. Jr., Tung, C. H., Bredow, S., and Weissleder, R. (2001) DNA binding chelates for nonviral gene delivery imaging. *Gene Ther.* **8,** 515–522.

20. Josephson, L., Tung, C. H., Moore, A., and Weissleder, R. (1999) High-efficiency intracellular magnetic labeling with novel superparamagnetic-Tat peptide conjugates. *Bioconjug. Chem.* **10,** 186–191.

21. Westphal, H., Overbeek, P. A., Khillan, J. S., et al. (1985) Promoter sequences of murine alpha A crystallin, murine alpha 2(I) collagen or of avian sarcoma virus genes linked to the bacterial chloramphenicol acetyl transferase gene direct tissue-specific patterns of chloramphenicol acetyl transferase expression in transgenic mice. *Cold Spring Harb. Symp. Quant. Biol.* **50,** 411–416.

22. Leite, J. P., Niel, C., and D'Halluin, J. C. (1986) Expression of the chloramphenicol acetyl transferase gene in human cells under the control of early adenovirus subgroup C promoters: effect of E1A gene products from other subgroups on gene expression. *Gene* **41,** 207–215.

23. Forss-Petter, S., Danielson, P. E., Catsicas, S., et al. (1990) Transgenic mice expressing beta-galactosidase in mature neurons under neuron-specific enolase promoter control. *Neuron* **5,** 187–200.

24. Naciff, J. M., Behbehani, M. M., Misawa, H., and Dedman, J. R. (1999) Identification and transgenic analysis of a murine promoter that targets cholinergic neuron expression. *J. Neurochem.* **72,** 17–28.

25. Zlokarnik, G., Negulescu, P. A., Knapp, T. E., et al. (1998) Quantitation of transcription and clonal selection of single living cells with beta-lactamase as reporter. *Science* **279,** 84–88.

26. Ehrin, E., Farde, L., de Paulis, T., et al. (1985) Preparation of ^{11}C-labelled Raclopride, a new potent dopamine receptor antagonist: preliminary PET studies of cerebral dopamine receptors in the monkey. *Int. J. Appl. Radiat. Isot.* **36,** 269–273.

27. Hall, H., Kohler, C., Gawell, L., Farde, L., and Sedvall, G. (1988) Raclopride, a new selective ligand for the dopamine-D$_2$ receptors. *Prog. Neuropsychopharmacol. Biol. Psychiatry* **12,** 559–568.

28. Hume, S. P., Myers, R., Bloomfield, P. M., et al. (1992) Quantitation of carbon-11-labeled raclopride in rat striatum using positron emission tomography. *Synapse* **12,** 47–54.

29. Wagner, H. N. Jr., Burns, H. D., Dannals, R. F., et al. (1983) Imaging dopamine receptors in the human brain by positron tomography. *Science* **221,** 1264–1266.

30. Barrio, J. R., Satyamurthy, N., Huang, S. C., et al. (1989) 3-(2'-[^{18}F]Fluoroethyl)spiperone: in vivo biochemical and kinetic characterization in rodents, nonhuman primates, and humans. *J. Cereb. Blood Flow Metab.* **9,** 830–839.

31. Satyamurthy, N., Barrio, J. R., Bida, G. T., Huang, S. C., Mazziotta, J. C., and Phelps, M. E. (1990) 3-(2'-[18F]Fluoro-ethyl)spiperone, a potent dopamine antagonist: synthesis, structural analysis and in-vivo utilization in humans. *Int. J. Rad. Appl. Instrum.* **41,** 113–129.

32. Kessler, R. M., Ansari, M. S., de Paulis, T., et al. (1991) High affinity dopamine D_2 receptor radioligands. 1. Regional rat brain distribution of iodinated benzamides. *J. Nucl. Med.* **32,** 1593–1600.

33. MacLaren, D. C., Gambhir, S. S., Satyamurthy, N., et al. (1999) Repetitive, non-invasive imaging of the dopamine D_2 receptor as a reporter gene in living animals. *Gene Ther.* **6,** 785–791.

34. Neve, K. A., Cox, B. A., Henningsen, R. A., Spanoyannis, A., and Neve, R. L. (1991) Pivotal role for aspartate-80 in the regulation of dopamine D_2 receptor affinity for drugs and inhibition of adenylyl cyclase. *Mol. Pharmacol.* **39,** 733–739.

35. Cox, B. A., Henningsen, R. A., Spanoyannis, A., Neve, R. L., and Neve, K. A. (1992) Contributions of conserved serine residues to the interactions of ligands with dopamine D_2 receptors. *J. Neurochem.* **59,** 627–635.

36. Liang, Q., Satyamurthy, N., Barrio, J. R., et al. (2001) Noninvasive, quantitative imaging, in living animals, of a mutant dopamine D_2 receptor reporter gene in which ligand binding is uncoupled from signal transduction. *Gene Ther.* **8,** 1490–1498.

37. Tjuvajev, J. G., Stockhammer, G., Desai, R., et al. (1995) Imaging the expression of transfected genes in vivo. *Cancer Res.* **55,** 6126–6132.

38. Tjuvajev, J. G., Finn, R., Watanabe, K., et al. (1996) Noninvasive imaging of herpes virus thymidine kinase gene transfer and expression: a potential method for monitoring clinical gene therapy. *Cancer Res.* **56,** 4087–4095.

39. Tjuvajev, J. G., Avril, N., Oku, T., et al. (1998) Imaging herpes virus thymidine kinase gene transfer and expression by positron emission tomography. *Cancer Res.* **58,** 4333–4341.

40. Namavari, M., Barrio, J. R., Toyokuni, T., et al. (2000) Synthesis of 8-[(18)F]fluoroguanine derivatives: in vivo probes for imaging gene expression with positron emission tomography. *Nucl. Med. Biol.* **27,** 157–162.

41. Gambhir, S. S., Barrio, J. R., Phelps, M. E., et al. (1999) Imaging adenoviral-directed reporter gene expression in living animals with positron emission tomography. *Proc. Natl. Acad. Sci. USA* **96,** 2333–2338.

42. Iyer, M., Barrio, J. R., Namavari, M., et al. (2001) 8-[18F]-Fluoropenciclovir: an improved reporter probe for imaging HSV1-tk reporter gene expression in vivo using positron emission tomography. *J. Nucl. Med.* **42,** 96–105.

43. Alauddin, M. M., Conti, P. S., Mazza, S. M., Hamzeh, F. M., and Lever, J. R. (1996) Synthesis of 9-[(3-[18F]fluoro-1-hydroxy-2-propoxy)methyl]guanine ([18F]FHPG): a potential imaging agent of viral infection and gene therapy using PET. *Nucl. Med. Biol.* **23,** 787–792.

44. Alauddin, M. M. and Conti, P. S. (1998) Synthesis and preliminary evaluation of 9-(4-[18F]-fluoro-3-hydroxymethyl-butyl)guanine ([18F]FHBG): a new potential imaging agent for viral infection and gene therapy using PET. *Nucl. Med. Biol.* **25,** 175–180.

45. Alauddin, M. M., Shahinian, A., Kundu, R. K., Gordon, E. M., and Conti, P. S. (1999) Evaluation of 9-[(3-18F-fluoro-1-hydroxy-2-propoxy)methyl] guanine ([18F]-FHPG) in vitro and in vivo as a probe for PET imaging of gene incorporation and expression in tumors. *Nucl. Med. Biol.* **26,** 371–376.

46. Hospers, G. A., Calogero, A., van Waarde, A., et al. (2000) Monitoring of herpes simplex virus thymidine kinase enzyme activity using positron emission tomography. *Cancer Res.* **60,** 1488–1491.

47. Hustinx, R., Shiue, C. Y., Alavi, A., et al. (2001) Imaging in vivo herpes simplex virus thymidine kinase gene transfer to tumour-bearing rodents using positron emission tomography and [18F]FHPG. *Eur. J. Nucl. Med.* **28,** 5–12.

48. Yaghoubi, S., Barrio, J., Dahlbom, M., et al. (2001) Human pharmacokinetic and dosimetry studies of [18F]-FHBG, a reporter probe for imaging herpes simplex virus type 1 thymidine kinase (HSV1-tk) reporter gene expression. *J. Nucl. Med.* **42,** 1225–1234.

49. Black, M. E., Newcomb, T. G., Wilson, H.-M. P., and Loeb, L. A. (1996) Creation of drug-specific herpes simplex virus type 1 thymidine kinase mutant for gene therapy. *Proc. Natl. Acad. Sci. USA* **93,** 3525–3529.

50. Brust, P., Haubner, R., Friedrich, A., et al. (2001) Comparison of [18F]FHPG and [124/125I]FIAU for imaging herpes simplex virus type 1 thymidine kinase gene expression. *Eur. J. Nucl. Med.* **28,** 721–729.

51. Tjuvajev, J. G., Doubrovin, M., Akhurst, T., et al. (2002) Comparison of radiolabeled nucleoside probes (FIAU, FHBG, and FHPG) for PET imaging of HSV1-*tk* gene expression. *J. Nucl. Med.* **43,** 1072–1083.

52. Alauddin, M., Shahinian, A., Fissekis, J., and Conti, P. (2002) Comparative evaluation of 2'-deoxy-2'-Fluoro-1-*b*-D-arabinofuranosiluracil and its 5-substituted derivatives as gene imaging agents. *Mol. Imaging* **1,** 222.

53. Anderson, C. J., Dehdashti, F., Cutler, P. D., et al. (2001) 64Cu-TETA-octreotide as a PET imaging agent for patients with neuroendocrine tumors. *J. Nucl. Med.* **42,** 213–221.

54. Henze, M., Schuhmacher, J., Hipp, P., et al. (2001) PET imaging of somatostatin receptors using [68GA]DOTA-D-Phe1-Tyr3-octreotide: first results in patients with meningiomas. *J. Nucl. Med.* **42,** 1053–1056.

55. Hofmann, M., Maecke, H., Borner, R., et al. (2001) Biokinetics and imaging with the somatostatin receptor PET radioligand (68)Ga-DOTATOC: preliminary data. *Eur. J. Nucl. Med.* **28,** 1751–1757.

56. Benali, N., Cordelier, P., Calise, D., et al. (2000) Inhibition of growth and metastatic progression of pancreatic carcinoma in hamster after somatostatin receptor subtype 2 (sst2) gene expression and administration of cytotoxic somatostatin analog AN-238. *Proc. Natl. Acad. Sci. USA* **97,** 9180–9185.

57. Rogers, B. E., Zinn, K. R., Lin, C. Y., Chaudhuri, T. R., and Buchsbaum, D. J. (2002) Targeted radiotherapy with [^{90}Y]-SMT 487 in mice bearing human nonsmall cell lung tumor xenografts induced to express human somatostatin receptor subtype 2 with an adenoviral vector. *Cancer* **94**, 1298–1305.

58. Chung, J.-K. (2002) Sodium iodide symporter: its role in nuclear medicine. *J. Nucl. Med.* **43**, 1188–1200.

59. La Perle, K. M. D., Shen, D., Buckwalter, T. L. F., et al. (2002) In vivo expression and function of the sodium iodide symporter following gene transfer in the MATLyLu rat model of metastatic prostate cancer. *Prostate* **50**, 170–178.

60. Boland, A., Ricard, M., Opolon, P., et al. (2000) Adenovirus-mediated transfer of the thyroid sodium/iodide symporter gene into tumors for a targeted radiotherapy. *Cancer Res.* **60**, 3484–3492.

61. Cho, J. Y., Xing, S., Liu, X., et al. (2000) Expression and activity of human Na+/I-symporter in human glioma cells by adenovirus-mediated gene delivery. *Gene Ther.* **7**, 740–749.

62. Spitzweg, C., Dietz, A. B., O'Connor, M. K., et al. (2001) In vivo sodium iodide symporter gene therapy of prostate cancer. *Gene Ther.* **8**, 1524–1531.

63. Louie, A. Y., Huber, M. M., Ahrens, E. T., et al. (2000) In vivo visualization of gene expression using magnetic resonance imaging. *Nat. Biotechnol.* **18**, 321–325.

64. Chalfie, M., Tu, Y., Euskirchen, W., Ward, W., and Prasher, D. C. (1994) Green fluorescent protein as a marker for gene expression. *Science* **263**, 802–805.

65. Naylor, L. H. (1999) Reporter gene technology: the future looks bright. *Biochem. Pharmacol.* **58**, 749–757.

66. Yang, M., Baranov, E., Jiang, P., et al. (2000) Whole-body optical imaging of green fluorescent protein-expressing tumors and metastases. *Proc. Natl. Acad. Sci. USA* **97**, 1206–1211.

67. Contag, C. H., Spilman, S. D., Contag, P. R., et al. (1997) Visualizing gene expression in living mammals using a bioluminescent reporter. *Photochem. Photobiol.* **66**, 523–531.

68. Yang, M., Baranov, E., Wang, J. W., et al. (2002) Direct external imaging of nascent cancer, tumor progression, angiogenesis, and metastasis on internal organs in the fluorescent orthotopic model. *Proc. Natl. Acad. Sci. USA* **99**, 3824–3829.

69. Ito, S., Nakanishi, H., Ikehara, Y., et al. (2001) Real-time observation of micrometastasis formation in the living mouse liver using a green fluorescent protein gene-tagged rat tongue carcinoma cell line. *Int. J. Cancer* **93**, 212–217.

70. Zhou, J. H., Rosser, C. J., Tanaka, M., et al. (2002) Visualizing superficial human bladder cancer cell growth in vivo by green fluorescent protein expression. *Cancer Gene Ther.* **9**, 681–686.

71. Bouvet, M., Wang, J., Nardin, S. R., et al. (2002) Real-time optical imaging of primary tumor growth and multiple metastatic events in a pancreatic cancer orthotopic model. *Cancer Res.* **62**, 1534–1540.

72. Yang, M., Baranov, E., Moossa, A. R., Penman, S., and Hoffman, R. M. (2000) Visualizing gene expression by whole-body fluorescence imaging. *Proc. Natl. Acad. Sci. USA* **97**, 12,278–12,282.

73. Brown, E. B., Campbell, R. B., Tsuzuki, Y., et al. (2001) In vivo measurement of gene expression, angiogenesis and physiological function in tumors using multiphoton laser scanning microscopy. *Nat. Med.* **7**, 864–868.

74. Contag, C. H., Jenkins, D., Contag, P. R., and Negrin, R. S. (2000) Use of reporter genes for optical measurements of neoplastic disease in vivo. *Neoplasia* **2**, 41–52.

75. Bhaumik, S. and Gambhir, S. S. (2002) Optical imaging of *Renilla* luciferase reporter gene expression in living mice. *Proc. Natl. Acad. Sci. USA* **99**, 377–382.

76. Cho, J.-Y., Shen, D. H. Y., Yang, W., et al. (2002) In vivo imaging and radioiodine therapy following sodium iodide symporter gene transfer in animal model of intracerebral gliomas. *Gene Ther.* **9**, 1139–1145.

77. Spitzweg, C., O'Connor, M. K., Bergert, E. R., Tindall, D. J., Young, C. Y. F., and Morris, J. C. (2000) Treatment of prostate cancer by radioiodine therapy after tissue-specific expression of the sodium iodide symporter. *Cancer Res.* **60**, 6526–6530.

78. Loimas, S., Wahlfors, J., and Janne, J. (1998) Herpes simplex virus thymidine kinase-green fluorescent protein fusion gene: new tool for gene transfer studies and gene therapy. *Biotechniques* **24**, 614–618.

79. Steffens, S., Frank, S., Fischer, U., et al. (2000) Enhanced green fluorescent protein fusion proteins of herpes simplex virus type 1 thymidine kinase and cytochrome P450 4B1: applications for prodrug-activating gene therapy. *Cancer Gene Ther.* **7**, 806–812.

80. Strathdee, C. A., McLeod, M. R., and Underhill, T. M. (2000) Dominant positive and negative selection using luciferase, green fluorescent protein and beta-galactosidase reporter gene fusions. *Biotechniques* **28**, 210–214.

81. Yaghoubi, S. S., Wu, L., Liang, Q., et al. (2001) Direct correlation between positron emission tomographic images of two reporter genes delivered by two distinct adenoviral vectors. *Gene Ther.* **8**, 1072–1080.

82. Zinn, K. R., Chaudhuri, T. R., Krasnykh, V. N., et al. (2002) Gamma camera dual imaging with a somatostatin receptor and thymidine kinase after gene transfer with a bicistronic adenovirus in mice. *Radiology* **223**, 417–425.

83. Baron, U., Freundlieb, S., Gossen, M., and Bujard, H. (1995) Co-regulation of two gene activities by tetracycline via a bidirectional promoter. *Nucleic Acids Res.* **23**, 3605–3606.

84. Krestel, H. E., Mayford, M., Seeburg, P. H., and Sprengel, R. (2001) A GFP-equipped bidirectional expression module well suited for monitoring tetracycline-regulated gene expression in mouse. *Nucleic Acids Res.* **29**, E39.

85. Sun, X., Annala, A. J., Yaghoubi, S., et al. (2001) Quantitative imaging of gene induction in living animals. *Gene Ther.* **8**, 1572–1579.

86. Martinez-Salas, E. (1999) Internal ribosome entry site biology and its use in expression vectors. *Curr. Opin. Biotechnol.* **10**, 458–464.
87. Tjuvajev, J. G., Joshi, A., Callegari, J., et al. (1999) A general approach to the non-invasive imaging of transgenes using *cis*-linked herpes simplex virus thymidine kinase. *Neoplasia* **1**, 315–320.
88. Yu, Y., Annala, A. J., Barrio, J. R., et al. (2000) Quantification of target gene expression by imaging reporter gene expression in living animals. *Nat. Med.* **6**, 933–937.
89. Liang, Q., Gotts, J., Satyamurthy, N., et al. (2002) Noninvasive, repetitive, quantitative measurement of gene expression from a bicistronic message by positron emission tomography, following gene transfer with adenovirus. *Mol. Ther.* **6**, 73–82.
90. Su, H., Lu, R., Chang, J. C., and Kan, Y. W. (1997) Tissue-specific expression of herpes simplex virus thymidine kinase gene delivered by adeno-associated virus inhibits the growth of human hepatocellular carcinoma in athymic mice. *Proc. Natl. Acad. Sci. USA* **94**, 13,891–13,896.
91. Lan, K. H., Kanai, F., Shiratori, Y., et al. (1996) Tumor-specific gene expression in carcinoembryonic antigen-producing gastric cancer cells using adenovirus vectors. *Gastroenterology* **111**, 1241–1251.
92. Siders, W. M., Halloran, P. J., and Fenton, R. G. (1996) Transcriptional targeting of recombinant adenoviruses to human and murine melanoma cells. *Cancer Res.* **56**, 5638–5646.
93. Southgate, T. D., Windeatt, S., Smith-Arica, J., et al. (2000) Transcriptional targeting to anterior pituitary lactotrophic cells using recombinant adenovirus vectors in vitro and in vivo in normal and estrogen/sulpiride-induced hyperplastic anterior pituitaries. *Endocrinology* **141**, 3493–3505.
94. Adams, J. Y., Johnson, M., Sato, M., et al. (2002) Visualization of advanced human prostate cancer lesions in living mice by a targeted gene transfer vector and optical imaging. *Nat. Med.* **8**, 891–896.
95. Nettelbeck, D. M., Jerome, V., and Muller, R. (2000) Gene therapy: designer promoters for tumour targeting. *Trends Genet.* **16**, 174–181.
96. Qiao, J., Doubrovin, M., Sauter, B. V., et al. (2002) Tumor-specific transcriptional targeting of suicide gene therapy. *Gene Ther.* **9**, 168–175.
97. Zhang, L., Adams, J. Y., Billick, E., et al. (2002) Molecular engineering of a two-step transcription amplification (TSTA) system for transgene delivery in prostate cancer. *Mol. Ther.* **5**, 223–232.
98. Hemminki, A., Zinn, K. R., Liu, B., et al. (2002) In vivo molecular chemotherapy and noninvasive imaging with an infectivity-enhanced adenovirus. *J. Natl. Cancer Inst.* **94**, 741–749.
99. Bennett, J. J., Tjuvajev, J., Johnson, P., et al. (2001) Positron emission tomography imaging for herpes virus infection: implications for oncolytic viral treatments of cancer. *Nat. Med.* **7**, 859–863.
100. Jacobs, A., Tjuvajev, J. G., Dubrovin, M., et al. (2001) Positron emission tomography-based imaging of transgene expression mediated by replication-conditional, oncolytic herpes simplex virus type 1 mutant vectors in vivo. *Cancer Res.* **61**, 2983–2995.
101. Ercikan-Abali, E. A., Banerjee, D., Waltham, M. C., et al. (1997) Dihydrofolate reductase protein inhibits its own translation by binding to dihydrofolate reductase mRNA sequences within the coding region. *Biochemistry* **36**, 12,317–12,322.
102. Mayer-Kuckuk, P., Banerjee, D., Malhotra, S., et al. (2002) Cells exposed to antifolates show increased cellular levels of proteins fused to dihydrofolate reductase: a method to modulate gene expression. *Proc. Natl. Acad. Sci. USA* **99**, 3400–3405.
103. Le, L. Q., Kabarowski, J. H. S., Wong, S., Nguyen, K., Gambhir, S. S., and Witte, O. N. (2002) Positron emission tomography imaging analysis of G2A as a negative modifier of lymphoid leukemogenesis initiated by the BCR-ABL oncogene. *Cancer Cell* **1**, 381–391.
104. Ponomarev, V., Doubrovin, M., Lyddane, C., et al. (2001) Imaging TCR-dependent NFAT-mediated T-cell activation with positron emission tomography in vivo. *Neoplasia* **3**, 480–488.
105. Zhang, W., Feng, J. Q., Harris, S. E., Contag, P. R., Stevenson, D. K., and Contag, C. H. (2001) Rapid in vivo functional analysis of transgenes in mice using whole body imaging of luciferase expression. *Transgenic Res.* **10**, 423–434.
106. Green, L. A., Yap, C. S., Nguyen, K., et al. (2002) Indirect monitoring of endogenous gene expression by positron emission tomography (PET) imaging of reporter gene expression in transgenic mice. *Mol. Imaging Biol.* **4**, 71–81.
107. Koransky, M. L., Ip, T. K., Wu, S., et al. (2001) In vivo monitoring of myoblast transplantation into rat myocardium. *J. Heart Lung Transplant.* **20**, 188–189.
108. Jacobs, A., Voges, J., Reszka, R., et al. (2001) Positron-emission tomography of vector-mediated gene expression in gene therapy for gliomas. *Lancet* **358**, 727–729.

28

Cancer-Related Gene Therapy Clinical Trials

Robert J. Korst and Ronald G. Crystal

1. INTRODUCTION

Gene therapy represents a strategy using transfer of genetic information to modify a population of target cells for therapeutic purposes. The transferred genetic material has typically included double-stranded deoxyribonucleic acid (DNA), but occasionally single-stranded DNA and even ribonucleic acid (RNA). Gene therapy represents one of the many novel "targeted" antineoplastic treatment approaches with the goal to inhibit the growth of tumor cells and spare normal cells. The use of gene therapy relevant to cancer treatment includes the in vivo genetic modification of tumors or the tumor-bearing host, as well as the ex vivo genetic manipulation of cell populations, which are then administered to the tumor-bearing host.

Many antineoplastic treatment strategies may show promise in preclinical animal models only to have a negligible antitumor effect in human cancers. The purpose of this chapter is to review the current status of clinical cancer-related gene therapy trials. We start with general concepts of cancer clinical trial design, pointing out differences and possibilities relevant to gene therapy cancer clinical trial design. We then review the published literature regarding cancer gene therapy clinical trials.

2. CANCER GENE THERAPY CLINICAL TRIAL DESIGN

The clinical evaluation of new conventional cytotoxic antineoplastic agents, usually administered systemically, has traditionally consisted of studies assessing toxicity and safety, followed by efficacy (1). Over the past several decades, phase I clinical trials conventionally were designed as dose-escalation studies for determining the maximum tolerable dose (MTD). The MTD is then evaluated in a phase II setting, during which it is established if the new agent possesses any antitumor properties utilizing well-defined end points of complete and partial response (2). Finally, if antitumor activity is demonstrated in phase II trials, the new drug is evaluated for clinical efficacy in phase III trials, in which large numbers of patients are randomized to either an experimental or a control group, with clinical parameters such as survival, quality of life, and time to progression as the established end points.

Although this paradigm is appropriate for the clinical evaluation of conventional cytotoxics, it may have only limited applicability in the realm of cancer gene therapy trials, which by the nature of the approach and its perceived risks requires the definition of novel end points during phase I and phase II evaluation. First, the majority of antineoplastic gene therapy strategies are targeted therapies, aimed at manipulating a single aspect of the malignant process, which may not result in the rapid cell death commonly seen with conventional cytotoxics. As a result, conventional definitions of complete and partial responses (e.g., radiographic regression of solid tumors) in individuals with large tumor

From: *Contemporary Cancer Research*
Cancer Gene Therapy
Edited by: D. T. Curiel and J. T. Douglas © Humana Press Inc., Totowa, NJ

burdens may not be suitable for the initial demonstration of efficacy of gene therapeutics. Second, the toxicity profile of targeted gene therapy strategies may differ from that of conventional cytotoxics, with toxicity potentially related to the gene transfer vector, transgene expression, or the method of administration of the vector. Third, because gene therapy strategies involve the transfer and expression of genetic material to the tumor-bearing host, assays testing the efficiency of gene transfer are often an important component; thus, the availability of tissue, tumor or otherwise, is required for this evaluation.

An important aspect of planning gene therapy clinical trials involves selection of the most appropriate disease in which to evaluate a particular strategy. In many cases of gene therapy aimed at a specific molecular target, the choice is made by virtue of the tumor type that expresses the given target (e.g., tumor-specific antigen-based vaccines or oncogene-inhibitory strategies). Many gene therapy strategies, however, may be potentially active in multiple tumor types, allowing the investigator to choose the most appropriate disease in which to test a given strategy. When faced with this decision, issues including ease of accrual and whether current standard therapies are effective become important. For example, a trial evaluating a relatively uncommon disease in which chemotherapy significantly prolongs survival will accrue much more slowly than one evaluating a more common, chemoresistant tumor with a poorer prognosis. Similarly, end-point analysis may be easier to interpret in the patient with chemoresistant disease because the addition of chemotherapy may confound data interpretation.

3. PHASE I CLINICAL TRIALS

Conventional cytotoxic drugs are relatively nonspecific and nonselective in their mechanisms of action, resulting in the potential for toxicity to both tumor and nontumor tissues in a dose-dependent fashion. Consequently, traditional phase I trials are designed with the primary goal of establishing the MTD to be used in subsequent efficacy studies. In contrast to conventional cytotoxics, however, most gene therapy strategies are targeted either biologically (e.g., at a target expressed mainly by tumor cells) or physically (e.g., using intratumoral vector injection) to tumors, sparing normal tissues.

In general, gene therapy strategies demonstrate therapeutic efficacy over a wider dosing range in preclinical studies compared to the steep dose–response relationship typically seen with conventional cytotoxics. As a result of these differences, establishment of the MTD, although important, is often difficult to assess in gene therapy trials and logistically may not be attainable. This phenomenon has been encountered in many of the published gene therapy trials to date.

Strategies that specifically target the tumor by either direct intratumoral injection (e.g., gene replacement, enzyme/prodrug strategies) or biologically (vaccines) have been found to be largely nontoxic (3–5). In contrast, less specifically targeted strategies that are systemically administered have been associated with dose-limiting toxicity (e.g., systemic administration of antisense oligonucleotides aimed at genes expressed by multiple tissue types (6)). A more relevant end-point for the relatively nontoxic strategies may be to assess toxicity with respect to the level of transgene expression in the tissue targeted by the vector, ensuring that significant transgene expression occurs at a nontoxic vector dose; that is, it makes little sense to increase vector doses continually if the level of transgene expression has plateaued.

Toxicity resulting from antineoplastic gene therapy strategies may potentially arise from the vector itself, the transgene product, or the method of administration of the vector. Published data generated from human studies currently suggest minimal toxicity of nonviral and viral vectors at a variety of dose ranges (7,8), with a few exceptions (9,10). The route of vector administration is also relevant, with intravascular delivery potentially more toxic than injection into other tissues (11). Other end-points relevant in phase I testing include pharmacokinetic data (e.g., serum vector levels and virus shedding) as well as the presence of replication-competent virus in trials in which replication-deficient viral vectors are used.

4. PHASE II TRIALS

For conventional cytotoxic drugs, the goal of phase II studies is to determine if any antitumor activity is induced by the new agent. Because the MTD has already been established in previous phase I trials, this is typically the dose used in phase II efficacy studies, which are classically single-arm, nonrandomized trials in patients with advanced disease. There are well-defined end-points for the measurement of tumor regression based on radiographic criteria for the shrinkage of solid tumors *(2)*.

Although radiographic evidence of tumor regression may be appropriate for the measurement of response to some gene therapy strategies (e.g., enzyme/prodrug strategy), such profound tumor regression is not characteristic of many other therapies (e.g., angiogenesis inhibitors, antimetastatics, vaccines), which may cause either more subtle decreases in tumor burden or simply stability of disease. Radiographic demonstration of disease stability is often problematic secondary to the difficulty in distinguishing inhibition of disease progression because of the experimental agent from naturally indolent disease. To circumvent this problem, studies can be conducted in diseases for which indolence is rare (e.g., small cell lung cancer), or accrual can be limited to those patients with radiographically progressive disease during prior therapy, using time to progression as the end point. Despite these approaches, surrogate end-points for the measurement of antitumor activity for targeted gene therapy trials are needed.

The use of novel, biologic end points may be appropriate to demonstrate efficacy in phase II gene therapy trials. Such end points include serum tumor marker levels, as well as evidence of transgene biologic activity measured in tumor samples following therapy. Serum tumor markers theoretically have the potential benefits of ease of acquisition and ability to carry out multiple samplings. However, their correlation with disease regression and tumor burden has not been defined clearly for many tumor types *(12,13)*. Examples of serum markers that have been used to measure efficacy in gene therapy phase II trials include prostate-specific antigen (PSA) *(14)* and carcinoembryonic antigen (CEA) *(15)*.

The biologic activity of the therapeutic transgene may also be a useful end point to measure in gene therapy trials. Examples include inhibition of target gene expression in antisense strategies, quantification of the number of tumor cells undergoing apoptosis in proapoptotic strategies, and demonstration of tumor-specific immunity in individuals in gene-based vaccine trials. Similar to serum tumor marker levels, however, correlation of changes in these end points with clinical tumor regression has been difficult to validate *(16)*. Another drawback of measuring the biologic activity of the transgene is the need for tissue acquisition, typically required both before and after the administration of the gene therapy agent. Although this may not present a problem for vaccine trials, for which peripheral blood mononuclear cells are easily obtained, the routine acquisition of tumor specimens is more problematic.

Another strategy that may be useful for obtaining efficacy data in a phase II gene therapy trial is to alter the trial design but retain the use of radiographic or clinical time to progression as the end-point. As discussed in this section, conventional phase II trials are single-arm, nonrandomized studies in patients with measurable gross disease, with the evaluation of radiographic or clinical regression as the end point. These study individuals are usually accrued in two stages, with accrual beyond the first stage dependent on the demonstration of a sufficient number of responses *(17)*.

Given the difficulties with the determination of stable disease, one of many types of randomized phase II designs may assist in the interpretation of responses. For example, study individuals can be randomly assigned to receive the standard of care or the standard of care plus a gene therapy strategy. Randomization to gene therapy or placebo is also an option. When viral vectors are to be used, randomization to the study vector or a control vector could yield important information because gene therapy vectors in the absence of a therapeutic transgene may have some antineoplastic effects *(18)*. Alternatively, a "randomized discontinuation" design can be utilized by which all study individuals are treated with the study reagent, and "responders" with stable disease are then randomly assigned to continue with the study drug or a placebo *(19)*. In both of these designs, time to progression can be the end point.

Randomized phase II trials can also be designed around surgical resection in patients with an earlier stage of disease, particularly a disease for which surgical resection alone is the standard of care. There are several advantages to this approach. First, by virtue of the resection, there is access to the tumor specimen, as well as accessory tissues such as lymph nodes, for biologic end-point analysis. Second, when surgical resection alone is the standard of care, the data are not confounded by other therapies, such as conventional chemotherapy. Finally, study individuals who are candidates for surgical resection usually have earlier stages of disease and less of a tumor burden than those individuals in "conventional" phase II trials. This may be important especially in gene-based immunologic strategies because individuals with advanced disease and significant tumor burdens have deficiencies in immune responsiveness. Trials designed around patients with earlier stage, resectable disease are ideal for biologic end-point analysis, whereas time to progression may not be an appropriate end point because it may take patients years to progress, if they progress at all.

5. PHASE III TRIALS

The goal of phase III trials in the evaluation of antineoplastic gene therapy strategies remains the same for gene therapy as that for conventional cytotoxics: evaluation for a clinical benefit of the experimental reagent. Phase III trials are large, randomized trials powered to establish a statistically significant difference between those using the experimental reagent and a control group using; the trials use end points that include overall survival, disease-free survival, time to progression, as well as symptom relief/quality of life. Reagents evaluated in these phase III trials are those shown to induce antitumor responses in previous phase II trials.

6. PUBLISHED CANCER GENE THERAPY TRIALS

Search of the English literature through the end of 2002 revealed reports describing the results from 147 separate clinical trials in cancer patients utilizing the transfer of genetic material (*see* Fig. 1 legend for details of search strategy). The majority of these trials are phase I and phase II trials and combination phase I/II trials.

The most common strategy employed in cancer gene therapy clinical trials has been immunotherapy (38% of published trials), followed by the enzyme/prodrug approach (15%), oncolytic viruses (13.5%), antisense oligonucleotides (13%), and gene replacement strategies (9.5%) (Fig. 1). Another gene therapy strategy applicable to malignant diseases is engineering bone marrow to express exogenous genes (7% of published trials), with the eventual goal of enhancing resistance to high-dose chemotherapeutic regimens.

Published results of cancer gene therapy clinical trials began appearing in the literature over a decade ago, with gene-based immunotherapy approaches comprising most of the early trials. Despite these early efforts, publications reporting the results of gene-based immunotherapy trials have steadily declined in number since their peak in 1999, when the results of 14 trials were published (Fig. 2A). Similarly, reports of trials evaluating the enzyme/prodrug strategy, as well as those aimed at the ex vivo manipulation of bone marrow, have also become less frequent since their peak in 2000 (Fig. 2B,F). In contrast, the most common type of strategy used in recently published trials was that of selectively replicating, oncolytic viruses (Fig. 2C). Similarly, the use of antisense oligonucleotides has been increasing over recent years (Fig. 2E).

Adenovirus vectors (mainly replication deficient) represent the most common gene transfer vector type used in existing published cancer gene therapy trials (Fig. 3A). These vectors have been attractive particularly for intratumoral injection, secondary to their ability to transduce a wide variety of cell types, their relatively high degree of transgene expression, and minimal toxicity arising from this route of administration. In contrast, although retrovirus systems have also been utilized for intratumoral injection (albeit to a lesser degree than adenovirus), retrovirus has been the most common vector used for the creation of cellular tumor vaccines as well as for bone marrow transduction.

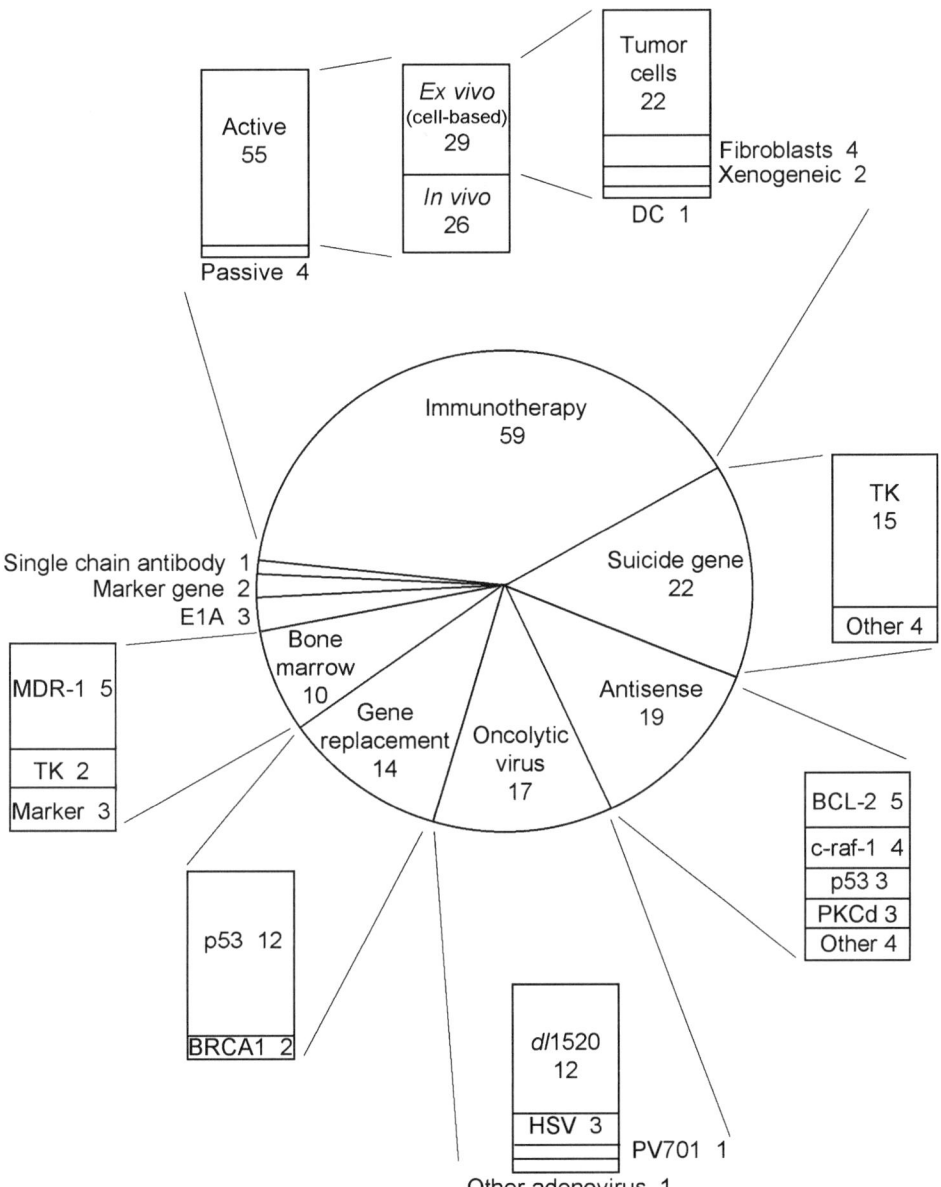

Fig. 1. A search of the English literature was performed using MEDLINE and criteria that included "gene," "cancer," "antisense," "oncolytic virus," "immunotherpy," "vaccine," "prodrug," "oligonucleotide," "oncogene," and "adoptive transfer." Reference lists from each article were also searched to ensure completeness. Abstracts, case reports, "preliminary" reports, redundant reports, and published protocols without data were omitted. The pie chart reveals the breakdown of the number of clinical trials by strategy. In addition, each "wedge" is further subcharacterized in the rectangular boxes.

In general, plasmid-based systems have been used primarily for in vivo gene therapy when the transgene is delivered intravenously, intradermally, subcutaneously, or intramuscularly. Plasmid delivery has mainly been liposome mediated or facilitated by particle bombardment ("gene gun").

Patients with a wide range of malignancies, both solid and hematologic, have been enrolled in gene therapy clinical trials (Fig. 3B). However, the most commonly investigated disease has been malignant

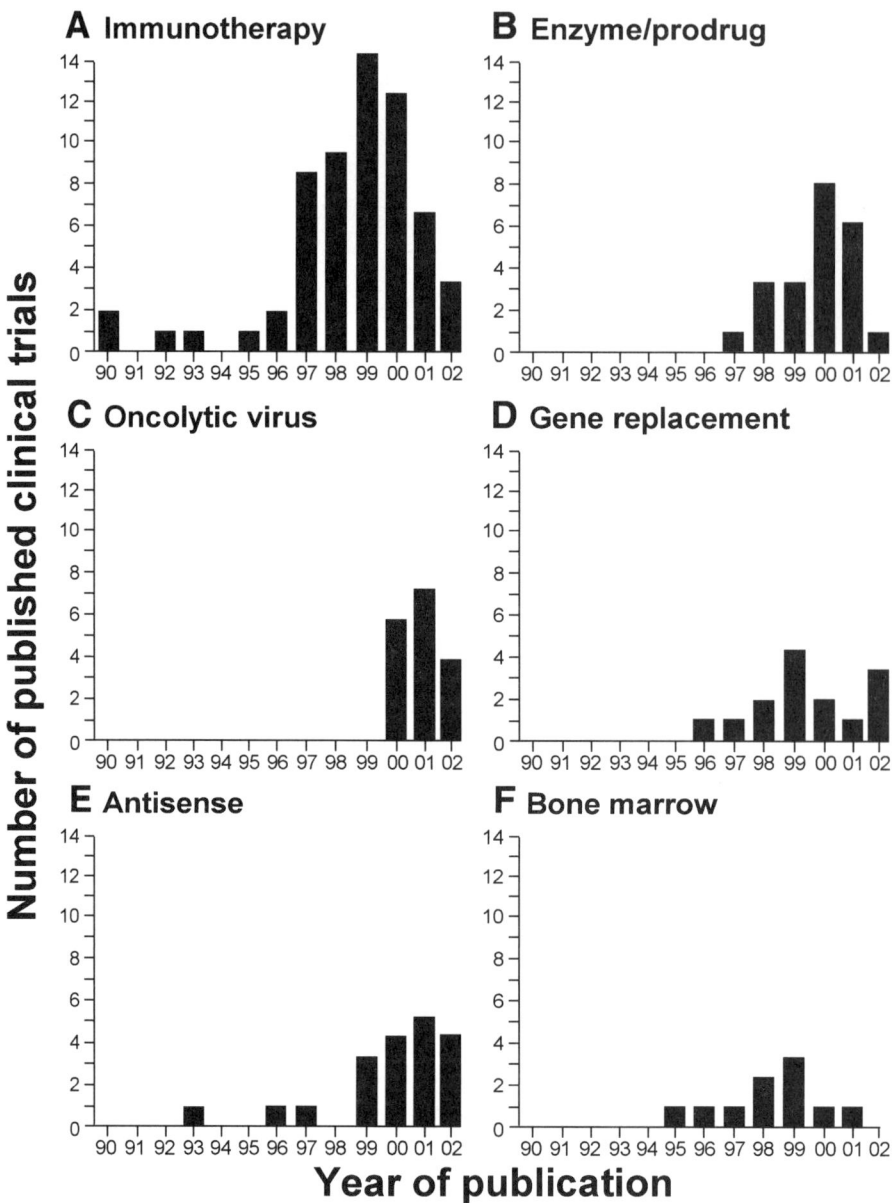

Fig. 2. Chronology of cancer gene therapy clinical trial reports according to strategy.

melanoma by virtue of its immunologic features and relatively well-characterized tumor antigen expression. These properties, combined with its relative resistance to conventional systemic therapies, have made melanoma the overwhelming choice for gene-based immunotherapy trials.

7. IMMUNOTHERAPY TRIALS

Active immunotherapy strategies, also referred to as tumor vaccines, involve the stimulation of the host's intact immune system to generate tumor-specific effector cells and/or molecules. In contrast, passive immunotherapy (adoptive transfer) refers to strategies by which effector cells or mole-

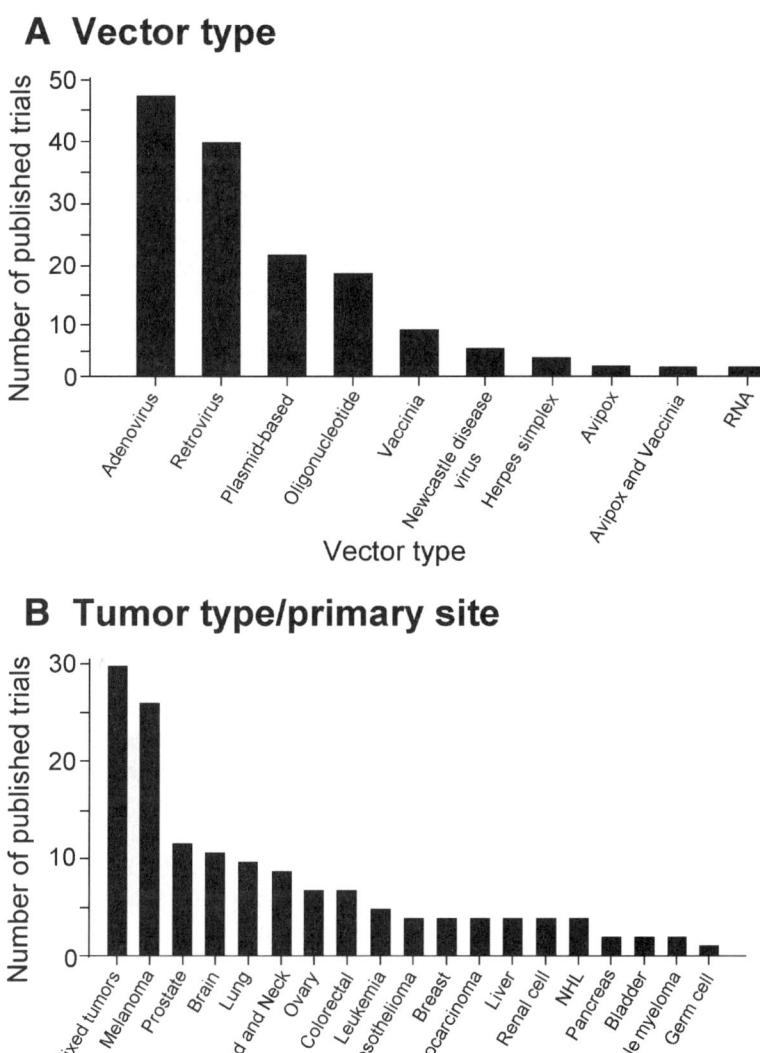

Fig. 3. The number of published cancer gene therapy clinical trial reports according to (**A**) type of vector system and (**B**) tumor type/primary site. NHL, non-Hodgkin's lymphoma.

cules are removed from tumor-bearing host(s), manipulated and/or propagated ex vivo, and administered back to the host. The majority of gene-based immunotherapy trials published to date have been active vaccine strategies, with only 4 of 59 reports involving the passive infusion of effector cells (Fig. 1). Of these 4 trials, 2 involved the use of retroviral vectors to engineer patients' lymphocytes to secrete interleukin 2 (IL-2) *(20,21)*; the other 2 were marker gene trials aimed at studying the fate of these transduced cells once they were infused back into the patients *(22,23)*. Although dramatic clinical responses were seen in a total of 2 of 20 patients in the IL-2 studies, the majority of patients in these trials exhibited disease progression despite immunotherapy, which may be related to the lack of consistent homing of the adoptively transferred cells to tumor sites *(20,21)*.

The goal of vaccination (active) strategies in the realm of immunotherapy is to enable the tumor-bearing host to produce an effective, tumor-specific, effector cell response, usually by augmenting the antigen presentation process. Antigen presentation is a complex process involving tumor-associated antigens (TAAs), multiple cell types, as well as secreted and surface-bound molecules, all of which have been targeted in gene-based immunotherapy trials. In addition to clinical response, efficacy endpoints have included the demonstration of tumor-specific cytotoxic T lymphocytes (CTLs) by a variety of techniques. It is important to note, however, that the relationship between demonstrable CTL responses and clinical responses in cancer patients has not been clearly delineated *(16)*.

Although not gene transfer *per se*, the first gene-based active immunotherapy trials involved the administration of autologous tumor cells previously exposed ex vivo to a Newcastle disease virus oncolysate as an adjuvant to surgical resection for a variety of solid tumors *(24)*. Because the vaccines were given in the minimal disease state (following resection), objective responses were not assessed. Tumor recurrence rates were thought to be lower than those seen in historical controls.

Initial trials involving formal exogenous gene transfer evaluated the toxicity of plasmid-mediated transfer of genes encoding allogeneic major histocompatibility complex proteins via intratumoral injection in patients with melanoma *(25)*. Negligible toxicity was seen, and CTLs were demonstrable in several patients, as were a few clinical responses. Other early trials were based on the outcome of studies from the 1980s, which demonstrated that the toxicity of systemically administered cytokines (e.g., IL-2, interferon-γ) precluded their use at doses high enough to provide consistent tumor regression *(26,27)*.

As a strategy to limit toxicity and take advantage of local production of these cytokines, gene transfer has been used to transduce a variety of tumor cell types to secrete cytokines and growth factors, including IL-2, IL-4, IL-7, IL-12, granulocyte-macrophage colony-stimulating factor, and interferon-γ *(28–33)*. Other immunomodulatory transgenes have also been investigated, including costimulatory molecules (such as B7.1 and CD40 ligand) *(34,35)*. Strategies have included both the in vivo manipulation of tumors (via intratumoral injection of vectors) *(28,31)* and the administration of genetically modified tumor cells *(29,30,33,35)* and even fibroblasts *(32)*. Similar to the allogeneic major histocompatibility trials, these trials resulted in nonspecific immune responses to the vaccines, such as cellular infiltrates, necrosis, and immunohistochemical changes, with tumor-specific CTLs demonstrated in some patients. Clinical responses were seen uncommonly.

The other major vaccine strategy evaluated in gene therapy clinical trials has been the transfer of genes encoding TAAs. One advantage of this approach is that the vectors can usually be administered systemically, avoiding intratumoral injections, which can be problematic for many tumor types. Transgenes investigated in clinical trials using this approach are CEA, PSA, MUC-1, and the melanoma-specific antigens MART-1 and gp100 *(36–39)*. The majority of these trials were phase I, with toxicity and various immune responses (both specific and nonspecific) as the end points, without assessment of clinical responses. One patient with melanoma who received an adenovirus-based MART-1 vaccine experienced a complete clinical response *(39)*. A novel approach to TAA gene transfer has been reported; it involved loading autologous dendritic cells with autologous total tumor RNA, resulting in tumor-specific immune responses *(40)*.

Despite the limited numbers of clinical responses, however, these trials demonstrated that immunomodulatory gene therapy for malignant disease is safe, and further investigation is warranted to establish techniques of enhancing vaccine-generated tumor immunity. Future investigation will need not only to continue to evaluate novel strategies of immune modulation, but also to focus on techniques of enhancing the immune responses to existing approaches. Novel end points need to be investigated that more clearly correlate with clinical efficacy in immunotherapeutic trials.

8. SUICIDE GENE/PRODRUG TRIALS

The paradigm consisting of genetically modifying tumors to express an enzyme that converts a relatively nontoxic prodrug to an active cytotoxic agent is referred to as the *suicide gene/prodrug strategy*

(41). Although multiple enzyme/prodrug systems have been investigated in the laboratory, the majority of clinical cancer gene therapy trials have been conducted by transducing tumors to express herpes simplex virus thymidine kinase (HSV-TK) in vivo and systemically administering the prodrug (ganciclovir), which is then phosphorylated to a cytotoxic metabolite by HSV-TK in the tumor bed (Fig. 1). Although some preclinical data suggested that suicide gene/prodrug strategies may induce a systemic, antitumor immune response *(41)*, the cytotoxic metabolites are produced locally in the tumor. The local effect of this approach is reflected in the clinical trials for HSV-TK, the majority of which have been conducted in tumors for which local control is desirable, including brain tumors, malignant pleural mesothelioma, and locally recurrent prostate cancer *(3,42,43)*. Most of these studies have been phase I designs utilizing adenovirus or retrovirus vectors and revealed the low toxicity seen with this gene therapy strategy, even at fairly high in vivo vector doses.

Although, in general, demonstration of efficacy has been lacking, some trials performed in prostate cancer have detected falling PSA levels following vector treatment *(42)*; others have shown varying degrees of delayed time to progression when compared to historical controls *(3,44)*. A controlled trial of intraoperative HSV-TK gene transfer to malignant gliomas using either adenovirus or retrovirus has been performed, revealing significantly prolonged survival in patients who received adenovirus compared to retrovirus or control vector *(45)*.

Despite these results, a phase III trial involving 248 patients with newly diagnosed glioblastoma multiforme detected no difference between either standard therapy (surgical resection plus radiotherapy) and standard therapy plus adjuvant intraoperative gene therapy using the HSV-TK system *(46)*.

Other suicide gene/prodrug strategies that have been evaluated in clinical trials have been the *Escherichia coli* cytosine deaminase/5-fluorocytosine combination for the treatment of metastatic breast cancer *(47)*, the *E. coli* nitroimidazole reductase/CB1954 system *(48)*, and cytochrome P450 2B1/ifosphamide in inoperable pancreatic cancer *(49)*. In the last study, patients received encapsulated human 293 cells genetically modified to express CP450 2B1 into the tumor vasculature. Survival was significantly prolonged compared to historical controls, and temporary tumor shrinkage was noted in most patients.

9. GENE REPLACEMENT TRIALS

Replacement of mutated tumor suppressor genes with wild-type genes has induced tumor regression in multiple animal models and has been investigated as an antineoplastic strategy in clinical trials. In the clinical arena, the majority of attention has been focused on the p53 tumor suppressor gene given its high frequency of mutation in multiple types of human cancers *(50)*. After an initial trial using a retroviral vector encoding the wild-type p53 in lung cancer patients demonstrated limited antitumor effect because of poor efficiency of transduction *(51)*, subsequent trials have focused on intratumoral injection of an adenovirus p53 vector *(4,52)*. Despite more efficient transgene expression with the adenovirus vectors (compared to retrovirus), clinical evidence of tumor regression occurred only in a small minority of patients.

Wild-type gene replacement has also been investigated using a retrovirus encoding BRCA 1 as the therapeutic transgene in patients with ovarian cancer *(53,54)*. Although a phase I trial suggested antitumor activity *(53)*, this could not be confirmed in a formal phase II trial *(54)*. Similar to p53 gene transfer, toxicity with BRCA 1 was minimal irrespective of vector type.

10. ONCOLYTIC VIRUS TRIALS

Selectively replicating viruses, without therapeutic transgenes, have received particular attention in clinical trials in the most recent 3 years of our literature review. These viruses are designed theoretically to replicate selectively in malignant cells, causing cell lysis, sparing normal tissue *(55)*. The majority of clinical trials published to date have been conducted with *dl*1520, a conditionally replicating adenovirus that replicates in cells lacking p53 function. Although phase I experience with this reagent has demonstrated minimal toxicity even when administered intravascularly at high titers, phase II assessments have revealed either minimal or no measurable antitumor effect, even though intratumoral viral replication has been demonstrated in several studies *(56–58).*

Other conditionally replicating viruses investigated in clinical trials are HSV, as well as Newcastle disease virus. HSV has been administered intratumorally, resulting in minimal vector-related toxicity in two studies of patients with malignant brain tumors *(59,60).* Both of these trials were phase I designs without efficacy data. Newcastle disease virus has been administered intravenously to a large number of patients with mixed end-stage tumors *(61).* Clinical and/or radiographic response to the virus was detected in fewer than 10% of the patients. Toxicity using this strategy was not insignificant, however, with flulike symptoms and hematologic toxicity predominating.

11. ANTISENSE TRIALS

Antisense oligonucleotides are single-stranded, short (approx 20 base pairs) molecules that are complementary to important regions of messenger RNA (mRNA) derived from a particular target gene. When bound to the mRNA, target gene expression is inhibited. The most promising targets in preclinical studies have been those genes involved in apoptosis, metastasis, cell proliferation, and angiogenesis *(6).* Published clinical trials have focused on oncogene inhibition (Hras, c-Myb), inhibitors of apoptosis (Bcl-2, insulin-like growth factor-1, tumor suppressor genes (p53), as well as cell proliferation genes (c-raf kinase, protein kinase cα, type 1 protein kinase A *(62–69).*

Early trials of this class of strategy included phase I evaluations involving a 20-mer oligonucleotide complementary to the p53 mRNA as both infusional therapy and a bone marrow purging agent in patients with leukemia, revealing minimal toxicity *(62,70).* The most extensive clinical experience, however, is with antisense inhibition of the antiapoptotic gene *Bcl-2* in patients with lymphoma, melanoma, prostate cancer, and non-small cell lung cancer. Although several objective major responses have been seen, the majority of patients had no evidence of clinical response, with thrombocytopenia the main dose-limiting toxicity *(68,71).* Similarly, although successful target inhibition of growth-potentiating kinases (type 1 protein kinase A, protein kinase cα, c-raf-1) using antisense oligonucleotides in the clinical arena has been detected, objective clinical responses have been uncommon *(63,67,69).*

12. BONE MARROW-TARGETING TRIALS

Gene therapy clinical trials targeting bone marrow have been investigated because of the interest in stem cell transplantation in patients with hematologic malignancies, but also some solid tumors. Two main strategies have been invoked: transduction of bone marrow cells with the multidrug resistance gene 1 to induce protection from myeloablative chemotherapy and transduction with "suicide" genes (HSV-TK) for potential treatment of graft-vs-host disease should it arise after transplantation. Transduction for this class of trials is performed ex vivo using retrovirus vectors. Regarding the chemoprotective strategy, although successful transduction of bone marrow cells was accomplished, evidence of multidrug resistance gene 1 gene expression was much more difficult to detect in vivo after autotransplantation *(72,73).* In contrast, Tiberghien and colleagues *(74)* were able to demonstrate the in vivo presence of circulating bone marrow cells that had been transduced with the HSV-TK gene prior to infusion. More important, the remission of graft-vs-host disease in two patients after treatment with the prodrug ganciclovir has established the potential benefit of this approach *(74).*

13. OTHER TRIALS

The adenovirus *E1A* gene has been shown to possess antineoplastic qualities thought to be mediated through a variety of mechanisms, including downregulation of HER-2/*neu* expression, induction of apoptosis, and inhibition of metastasis *(75).* Phase I clinical trials have evaluated toxicity associated with the local administration of plasmids containing the *E1A* gene complexed with liposomes into patients with breast, head and neck, and ovarian cancer *(76,77).* Toxicity was mild and mainly consisted of nausea in patients who underwent intraperitoneal administration of the vector. In a phase II trial, minimal toxicity was reported following intratumoral injection of the vector, with a small number of patients experiencing responses to varying degrees *(78)*.

In another novel approach, adenovirus-mediated delivery of a transgene encoding a single-chain antibody to erbB-2 in patients with recurrent ovarian cancer was evaluated in a phase I setting *(79)*. Toxicity was minimal, but regression of disease was not observed in any patients, although transgene expression was documented in 10 of 14 patients.

14. SUMMARY

Cancer gene therapy represents a wide range of targeted antineoplastic strategies that began testing in clinical trials over the past decade. As for other targeted therapies, the clinical trial format needs to be adjusted to account for differences between these novel approaches and conventional cytotoxic agents. These include differences in toxicity profiles as well as the dynamics of the antitumor response. Novel biologic end points and trial designs may help overcome some of these problems in designing clinical trials for gene therapy strategies. The results of cancer gene therapy clinical trials to date have demonstrated little toxicity; however, objective clinical responses are infrequent, and efficient transgene expression continues to be a challenge. Future research needs to focus not only on novel strategies and transgenes, but also on the development of novel gene transfer vectors to help overcome this inefficiency.

REFERENCES

1. Nottage, M. and Siu, L. L. (2002) Principles of clinical trial design. *J. Clin. Oncol.* **20(18, Suppl.),** 42s–46s.
2. Therasse, P., Arbuck, S. G., Eisenhauer, E. A., et al. (2000) New guidelines to evaluate the response to treatment in solid tumors. European Organization for Research and Treatment of Cancer, National Cancer Institute of the United States, National Cancer Institute of Canada. *J. Natl. Cancer Inst.* **92,** 205–216.
3. Shand, N., Weber, F., Mariani, L., et al. (1999) A phase 1–2 clinical trial of gene therapy for recurrent glioblastoma multiforme by tumor transduction with the herpes simplex thymidine kinase gene followed by ganciclovir. GLI328 European-Canadian Study Group. *Hum. Gene Ther.* **10,** 2325–2335.
4. Swisher, S. G., Roth, J. A., Nemunaitis, J., et al. (1999) Adenovirus-mediated p53 gene transfer in advanced non-small-cell lung cancer. *J. Natl. Cancer Inst.* **91,** 763–771.
5. Osanto, S., Schiphorst, P. P., Weijl, N. I., et al. (2000) Vaccination of melanoma patients with an allogeneic, genetically modified interleukin 2-producing melanoma cell line. *Hum. Gene Ther.* **11,** 739–750.
6. Jansen, B. and Zangemeister-Wittke, U. (2002) Antisense therapy for cancer—the time of truth. *Lancet Oncol.* **3,** 672–683.
7. Harvey, B. G., Maroni, J., O'Donoghue, K. A., et al. (2002) Safety of local delivery of low- and intermediate-dose adenovirus gene transfer vectors to individuals with a spectrum of morbid conditions. *Hum. Gene Ther.* **13,** 15–63.
8. Vile, R. G. and Russell, S. J. (1995) Retroviruses as vectors. *Br. Med. Bull.* **51,** 12–30.
9. Marshall, E. (1999) Clinical trials: gene therapy death prompts review of adenovirus vector. *Science* **286,** 2244–2245.
10. Verma, I. M. (2002) Success and setback: another adverse event. *Mol. Ther.* **6,** 565–566.
11. Reid, T., Warren, R., and Kirn, D. (2002) Intravascular adenoviral agents in cancer patients: lessons from clinical trials. *Cancer Gene Ther.* **9,** 979–986.
12. Saygili, U., Guclu, S., Uslu, T., Erten, O., and Dogan, E. (2002) The effect of ascites, mass volume, and peritoneal carcinomatosis on serum CA125 levels in patients with ovarian carcinoma. *Int. J. Gynecol. Cancer* **12,** 438–442.
13. Small, E. J. and Roach, M. 3rd. (2002) Prostate-specific antigen in prostate cancer: a case study in the development of a tumor marker to monitor recurrence and assess response. *Semin. Oncol.* **29,** 264–273.
14. Freytag, S. O., Khil, M., Stricker, H., et al. (2002) Phase I study of replication-competent adenovirus-mediated double suicide gene therapy for the treatment of locally recurrent prostate cancer. *Cancer Res.* **62,** 4968–4976.
15. Habib, N. A., Sarraf, C. E., Mitry, R. R., et al. (2001) E1B-deleted adenovirus (*dl*1520) gene therapy for patients with primary and secondary liver tumors. *Hum. Gene Ther.* **12,** 219–226.
16. Cormier, J. N., Salgaller, M. L., Prevette, T., et al. (1997) Enhancement of cellular immunity in melanoma patients immunized with a peptide from MART-1/melan A. *Cancer J.* **3,** 37–44.
17. Simon, R. (1989) Optimal two-stage designs for phase II clinical trials. *Control. Clin. Trials* **10,** 1–10.
18. Korst, R. J., Ailawadi, M., Lee, J. M., et al. (2001) Adenovirus gene transfer vectors inhibit lymphatic tumor metastasis independent of a therapeutic transgene. *Hum. Gene Ther.* **12,** 1639–1649.

19. Kopec, J. A., Abrahamowicz, M., and Esdaile, J. M. (1993) Randomized discontinuation trials: utility and efficiency. *J. Clin. Epidemiol.* **46,** 959–971.

20. Schmidt-Wolf, I. G., Finke, S., Trojaneck, B., et al. (1999) Phase I clinical study applying autologous immunological effector cells transfected with the interleukin-2 gene in patients with metastatic renal cancer, colorectal cancer and lymphoma. *Br. J. Cancer* **81,** 1009–1016.

21. Tan, Y., Xu, M., Wang, W., et al. (1996) IL-2 gene therapy of advanced lung cancer patients. *Anticancer Res.* **16,** 1993–1998.

22. Rosenberg, S. A., Aebersold, P., Cornetta, K., et al. (1990) Gene transfer into humans—immunotherapy of patients with advanced melanoma, using tumor-infiltrating lymphocytes modified by retroviral gene transduction. *N. Engl. J. Med.* **323,** 570–578.

23. Merrouche, Y., Negrier, S., Bain, C., et al. (1995) Clinical application of retroviral gene transfer in oncology: results of a French study with tumor-infiltrating lymphocytes transduced with the gene of resistance to neomycin. *J. Clin. Oncol.* **13,** 410–418.

24. Batliwalla, F. M., Bateman, B. A., Serrano, D., et al. (1998) A 15-year follow-up of AJCC stage III malignant melanoma patients treated postsurgically with Newcastle disease virus (NDV) oncolysate and determination of alterations in the CD8 T cell repertoire. *Mol. Med.* **4,** 783–794.

25. Nabel, G. J., Nabel, E. G., Yang, Z. Y., et al. (1993) Direct gene transfer with DNA-liposome complexes in melanoma: expression, biologic activity, and lack of toxicity in humans. *Proc. Natl. Acad. Sci. USA* **90,** 11,307–11,311.

26. Atkins, M. B., Lotze, M. T., Dutcher, J. P., et al. (1999) High-dose recombinant interleukin 2 therapy for patients with metastatic melanoma: analysis of 270 patients treated between 1985 and 1993. *J. Clin. Oncol.* **17,** 2105–2116.

27. Vial, T. and Descotes, J. (1994) Clinical toxicity of the interferons. *Drug Saf.* **10,** 115–150.

28. Galanis, E., Hersh, E. M., Stopeck, A. T., et al. (1999) Immunotherapy of advanced malignancy by direct gene transfer of an interleukin-2 DNA/DMRIE/DOPE lipid complex: phase I/II experience. *J. Clin. Oncol.* **17,** 3313–3323.

29. Nemunaitis, J., Bohart, C., Fong, T., et al. (1998) Phase I trial of retroviral vector-mediated interferon (IFN)-gamma gene transfer into autologous tumor cells in patients with metastatic melanoma. *Cancer Gene Ther.* **5,** 292–300.

30. Arienti, F., Belli, F., Napolitano, F., et al. (1999) Vaccination of melanoma patients with interleukin 4 gene-transduced allogeneic melanoma cells. *Hum. Gene Ther.* **10,** 2907–2916.

31. Mastrangelo, M. J., Maguire, H. C. Jr., Eisenlohr, L. C., et al. (1999) Intratumoral recombinant GM-CSF-encoding virus as gene therapy in patients with cutaneous melanoma. *Cancer Gene Ther.* **6,** 409–422.

32. Kang, W. K., Park, C., Yoon, H. L., et al. (2001) Interleukin 12 gene therapy of cancer by peritumoral injection of transduced autologous fibroblasts: outcome of a phase I study. *Hum. Gene Ther.* **12,** 671–684.

33. Moller, P., Sun, Y., Dorbic, T., et al. (1998) Vaccination with IL-7 gene-modified autologous melanoma cells can enhance the anti-melanoma lytic activity in peripheral blood of patients with a good clinical performance status: a clinical phase I study. *Br. J. Cancer* **77,** 1907–1916.

34. Wierda, W. G., Cantwell, M. J., Woods, S. J., Rassenti, L. Z., Prussak, C. E., and Kipps, T. J. (2000) CD40-ligand (CD154) gene therapy for chronic lymphocytic leukemia. *Blood* **96,** 2917–2924.

35. Antonia, S. J., Seigne, J., Diaz, J., et al. (2002) Phase I trial of a B7-1 (CD80) gene modified autologous tumor cell vaccine in combination with systemic interleukin-2 in patients with metastatic renal cell carcinoma. *J. Urol.* **167,** 1995–2000.

36. Eder, J. P., Kantoff, P. W., Roper, K., et al. (2000) A phase I trial of a recombinant vaccinia virus expressing prostate-specific antigen in advanced prostate cancer. *Clin. Cancer Res.* **6,** 1632–1638.

37. Conry, R. M., Khazaeli, M. B., Saleh, M. N., et al. (1999) Phase I trial of a recombinant vaccinia virus encoding carcinoembryonic antigen in metastatic adenocarcinoma: comparison of intradermal vs subcutaneous administration. *Clin. Cancer Res.* **5,** 2330–2337.

38. Scholl, S. M., Balloul, J. M., Le Goc, G., et al. (2000) Recombinant vaccinia virus encoding human MUC1 and IL2 as immunotherapy in patients with breast cancer. *J. Immunother.* **23,** 570–580.

39. Rosenberg, S. A., Zhai, Y., Yang, J. C., et al. (1998) Immunizing patients with metastatic melanoma using recombinant adenoviruses encoding MART-1 or gp100 melanoma antigens. *J. Natl. Cancer Inst.* **90,** 1894–1900.

40. Nair, S. K., Morse, M., Boczkowski, D., et al. (2002) Induction of tumor-specific cytotoxic T lymphocytes in cancer patients by autologous tumor RNA-transfected dendritic cells. *Ann. Surg.* **235,** 540–549.

41. Yazawa, K., Fisher, W. E., and Brunicardi, F. C. (2002) Current progress in suicide gene therapy for cancer. *World J. Surg.* **26,** 783–789.

42. Miles, B. J., Shalev, M., Aguilar-Cordova, E., et al. (2001) Prostate-specific antigen response and systemic T cell activation after *in situ* gene therapy in prostate cancer patients failing radiotherapy. *Hum. Gene Ther.* **12,** 1955–1967.

43. Sterman, D. H., Treat, J., Litzky, L. A., et al. (1998) Adenovirus-mediated herpes simplex virus thymidine kinase/ganciclovir gene therapy in patients with localized malignancy: results of a phase I clinical trial in malignant mesothelioma. *Hum. Gene Ther.* **9,** 1083–1092.

44. Klatzmann, D., Valery, C. A., Bensimon, G., et al. (1998) A phase I/II study of herpes simplex virus type 1 thymidine kinase "suicide" gene therapy for recurrent glioblastoma. Study Group on Gene Therapy for Glioblastoma. *Hum. Gene Ther.* **9,** 2595–2604.

45. Sandmair, A. M., Loimas, S., Puranen, P., et al. (2000) Thymidine kinase gene therapy for human malignant glioma, using replication-deficient retroviruses or adenoviruses. *Hum. Gene Ther.* **11**, 2197–2205.

46. Rainov, N. G. (2000) A phase III clinical evaluation of herpes simplex virus type 1 thymidine kinase and ganciclovir gene therapy as an adjuvant to surgical resection and radiation in adults with previously untreated glioblastoma multiforme. *Hum. Gene Ther.* **11**, 2389–2401.

47. Pandha, H. S., Martin, L. A., Rigg, A., et al. (1999) Genetic prodrug activation therapy for breast cancer: a phase I clinical trial of erbB-2-directed suicide gene expression. *J. Clin. Oncol.* **17**, 2180–2189.

48. Chung-Faye, G., Palmer, D., Anderson, D., et al. (2001) Virus-directed, enzyme prodrug therapy with nitroimidazole reductase: a phase I and pharmacokinetic study of its prodrug, CB1954. *Clin. Cancer Res.* **7**, 2662–2668.

49. Lohr, M., Hoffmeyer, A., Kroger, J., et al. (2001) Microencapsulated cell-mediated treatment of inoperable pancreatic carcinoma. *Lancet* **357**, 1591–1592.

50. Thames, H. D., Petersen, C., Petersen, S., Nieder, C., and Baumann, M. (2002) Immunohistochemically detected p53 mutations in epithelial tumors and results of treatment with chemotherapy and radiotherapy. A treatment-specific overview of the clinical data. *Strahlenther Onkol.* **178**, 411–421.

51. Roth, J. A., Nguyen, D., Lawrence, D. D., et al. (1996) Retrovirus-mediated wild-type p53 gene transfer to tumors of patients with lung cancer. *Nat. Med.* **2**, 985–991.

52. Schuler, M., Rochlitz, C., Horowitz, J. A., et al. (1998) A phase I study of adenovirus-mediated wild-type p53 gene transfer in patients with advanced non-small cell lung cancer. *Hum. Gene Ther.* **9**, 2075–2082.

53. Tait, D. L., Obermiller, P. S., Redlin-Frazier, S., et al. (1997) A phase I trial of retroviral BRCA1sv gene therapy in ovarian cancer. *Clin. Cancer Res.* **3**, 1959–1968.

54. Tait, D. L., Obermiller, P. S., Hatmaker, A. R., Redlin-Frazier, S., and Holt, J. T. (1999) Ovarian cancer BRCA1 gene therapy: phase I and II trial differences in immune response and vector stability. *Clin. Cancer Res.* **5**, 1708–1714.

55. Biederer, C., Ries, S., Brandts, C. H., and McCormick, F. (2002) Replication-selective viruses for cancer therapy. *J. Mol. Med.* **80**, 163–175.

56. Habib, N. A., Sarraf, C. E., Mitry, R. R., et al. (2001) E1B-deleted adenovirus (*dl*1520) gene therapy for patients with primary and secondary liver tumors. *Hum. Gene Ther.* **12**, 219–226.

57. Vasey, P. A., Shulman, L. N., Campos, S., et al. (2002) Phase I trial of intraperitoneal injection of the E1B-55-kd-gene-deleted adenovirus ONYX-015 (*dl*1520) given on days 1 through 5 every 3 weeks in patients with recurrent/refractory epithelial ovarian cancer. *J. Clin. Oncol.* **20**, 1562–1569.

58. Nemunaitis, J., Khuri, F., Ganly, I., et al. (2001) Phase II trial of intratumoral administration of ONYX-015, a replication-selective adenovirus, in patients with refractory head and neck cancer. *J. Clin. Oncol.* **19**, 289–298.

59. Markert, J. M., Medlock, M. D., Rabkin, S. D., et al. (2000) Conditionally replicating herpes simplex virus mutant, G207 for the treatment of malignant glioma: results of a phase I trial. *Gene Ther.* **7**, 867–874.

60. Rampling, R., Cruickshank, G., Papanastassiou, V., et al. (2000) Toxicity evaluation of replication-competent herpes simplex virus (ICP 34.5 null mutant 1716) in patients with recurrent malignant glioma. *Gene Ther.* **7**, 859–866.

61. Pecora, A. L., Rizvi, N., Cohen, G. I., et al. (2002) Phase I trial of intravenous administration of PV701, an oncolytic virus, in patients with advanced solid cancers. *J. Clin. Oncol.* **20**, 2251–2266.

62. Bishop, M. R., Iversen, P. L., Bayever, E., et al. (1996) Phase I trial of an antisense oligonucleotide OL(1)p53 in hematologic malignancies. *J. Clin. Oncol.* **14**, 1320–1326.

63. Chen, H. X., Marshall, J. L., Ness, E., et al. (2000) A safety and pharmacokinetic study of a mixed-backbone oligonucleotide (GEM231) targeting the type I protein kinase A by 2-hour infusions in patients with refractory solid tumors. *Clin. Cancer Res.* **6**, 1259–1266.

64. Luger, S. M., O'Brien, S. G., Ratajczak, J., et al. (2002) Oligodeoxynucleotide-mediated inhibition of c-myb gene expression in autografted bone marrow: a pilot study. *Blood* **99**, 1150–1158.

65. Andrews, D. W., Resnicoff, M., Flanders, A. E., et al. (2001) Results of a pilot study involving the use of an antisense oligodeoxynucleotide directed against the insulin-like growth factor type I receptor in malignant astrocytomas. *J. Clin. Oncol.* **19**, 2189–2200.

66. Cunningham, C. C., Holmlund, J. T., Geary, R. S., et al. (2001) A phase I trial of H-ras antisense oligonucleotide ISIS 2503 administered as a continuous intravenous infusion in patients with advanced carcinoma. *Cancer* **92**, 1265–1271.

67. Coudert, B., Anthoney, A., Fiedler, W., et al. (2001) Phase II trial with ISIS 5132 in patients with small-cell (SCLC) and non-small cell (NSCLC) lung cancer. A European Organization for Research and Treatment of Cancer (EORTC) Early Clinical Studies Group report. *Eur. J. Cancer* **37**, 2194–2198.

68. Jansen, B., Wacheck, V., Heere-Ress, E., et al. (2000) Chemosensitisation of malignant melanoma by BCL2 antisense therapy. *Lancet* **356**, 1728–1733.

69. Yuen, A. R., Halsey, J., Fisher, G. A., et al. (1999) Phase I study of an antisense oligonucleotide to protein kinase C-alpha (ISIS 3521/CGP 64128A) in patients with cancer. *Clin. Cancer Res.* **5**, 3357–3363.

70. Bishop, M. R., Jackson, J. D., Tarantolo, S. R., et al. (1997) Ex vivo treatment of bone marrow with phosphorothioate oligonucleotide OL(1)p53 for autologous transplantation in acute myelogenous leukemia and myelodysplastic syndrome. *J. Hematother.* **6**, 441–446.

71. Waters, J. S., Webb, A., Cunningham, D., et al. (2000) Phase I clinical and pharmacokinetic study of bcl-2 antisense oligonucleotide therapy in patients with non-Hodgkin's lymphoma. *J. Clin. Oncol.* **18,** 1812–1823.

72. Devereux, S., Corney, C., Macdonald, C., et al. (1998) Feasibility of multidrug resistance (MDR-1) gene transfer in patients undergoing high-dose therapy and peripheral blood stem cell transplantation for lymphoma. *Gene Ther.* **5,** 403–408.

73. Hesdorffer, C., Ayello, J., Ward, M., et al. (1998) Phase I trial of retroviral-mediated transfer of the human MDR1 gene as marrow chemoprotection in patients undergoing high-dose chemotherapy and autologous stem-cell transplantation. *J. Clin. Oncol.* **16,** 165–172.

74. Tiberghien, P., Ferrand, C., Lioure, B., et al. (2001) Administration of herpes simplex-thymidine kinase-expressing donor T cells with a T-cell-depleted allogeneic marrow graft. *Blood* **97,** 63–72.

75. Sang, N., Caro, J., and Giordano, A. (2002) Adenoviral E1A: everlasting tool, versatile applications, continuous contributions and new hypotheses. *Front. Biosci.* **7,** d407–d413.

76. Hortobagyi, G. N., Ueno, N. T., Xia, W., et al. (2001) Cationic liposome-mediated E1A gene transfer to human breast and ovarian cancer cells and its biologic effects: a phase I clinical trial. *J. Clin. Oncol.* **19,** 3422–3433.

77. Yoo, G. H., Hung, M. C., Lopez-Berestein, G., et al. (2001) Phase I trial of intratumoral liposome E1A gene therapy in patients with recurrent breast and head and neck cancer. *Clin. Cancer Res.* **7,** 1237–1245.

78. Villaret, D., Glisson, B., Kenady, D., et al. (2002) A multicenter phase II study of tgDCC-E1A for the intratumoral treatment of patients with recurrent head and neck squamous cell carcinoma. *Head Neck* **24,** 661–669.

79. Alvarez, R. D., Barnes, M. N., Gomez-Navarro, J., et al. (2000) A cancer gene therapy approach utilizing an anti-erbB-2 single-chain antibody-encoding adenovirus (AD21): a phase I trial. *Clin. Cancer Res.* **6,** 3081–3087.

29

Regulatory Aspects
in the Development of Gene Therapies

Rosemarie Aurigemma, Joseph E. Tomaszewski,
Sheryl Ruppel, Stephen Creekmore, and Edward A. Sausville

1. INTRODUCTION

Preclinical therapeutics development research is directed toward fulfilling two overlapping sets of goals. A set of scientific goals includes defining the best molecule or biologic construct for the task at hand, and proving the case for its development. The second set of goals addresses regulatory requirements necessary to introduce the agent into human subjects. In the case of "small molecule" drugs, in most cases the identity of the molecule and appropriate safety studies are straightforward. In contrast, the development of biologic agents, including gene therapies discussed here, presents distinct challenges. The nature of the "drug" may be an organism subject to mutation or selection of variants through recombination. Its properties may vary depending on the scale and method of its preparation, purification, and storage. How to test adequately for its safety prior to first introduction in humans may not be straightforward owing to intrinsic differences in response to the agent expected in humans as compared to animals.

The general principles, however, in allowing "first-in-human" experiences are similar for both small molecules and biologics. The ethical conduct of clinical trials in patients with a dire or life-threatening disease demands an understanding of the identity and dose of an agent that has the possibility of causing clinical benefit with adverse events expected at worst to be easily reversible and well predicted by the preclinical experience. In normal volunteers or patients who are otherwise well, evidence should be gathered that would support an initial range of doses of the test agent expected to be without substantial toxicity or long-term effects.

Thus, the successful clinical introduction of a novel therapeutic concept requires an organized approach to integrate scientific, technical, and regulatory requirements. This integration should begin in the research laboratory, as the concept becomes a candidate for the clinic, to prevent avoidable and expensive delays in clinical development. For example, if a product is created using a mammalian cell line for which viral or other contamination has not been ruled out, costly rederivation will be required before that product can be manufactured for clinical trials using current good manufacturing practices (cGMP). On the other hand, during the discovery phase, an excessive and premature concern over cGMP compliance can impede research. Therefore, a clear strategic understanding of the principles underlying regulatory issues is desirable and is the goal of this chapter.

We proceed from the experience of the Developmental Therapeutics Program (DTP) of the National Cancer Institute in the manufacture of biologicals, including gene therapy constructs for preclinical and clinical use. We outline the basis for our approach to safety testing studies to be included in an

From: *Contemporary Cancer Research*
Cancer Gene Therapy
Edited by: D. T. Curiel and J. T. Douglas © Humana Press Inc., Totowa, NJ

Table 1
Beyond a Good Idea: What the Successful Investigator
Has Already Done With a Project Leading to Commercial Development

Defined candidate biologic (or molecule)
Made comparisons with similar products
Characteristics of product are consistent with pharmaceutical requirements
Production scale is adequate
Product characterization is adequate
Laboratory reference standard exists
In vitro potency assay has been developed
Stability studies develop confidence product is a "drug"
Reproducible model systems have confirmed in vivo activity with clinical product
Early animal work includes some toxicology
Scale-up requirements practical for initial clinical trials
In general, reflects experience and scientific maturity of investigator

Investigational New Drug (IND) application to the Food and Drug Administration (FDA). We focus on studies that would allow phase I and perhaps early phase II clinical trials. In 2002, DTP contributed to over 40 different cGMP biological projects. Most of these activities were selected competitively from applications received from academic researchers or from the intramural laboratories of the National Institutes of Health (NIH).

DTP products include viruses for vaccines or gene therapy, plasmids, monoclonal antibodies, recombinant proteins, synthetic peptides, natural product fermentations, and oligonucleotides. During the 2002 fiscal year, over 30 different lots were manufactured and released under cGMP for clinical use or further cGMP manufacturing. Most products are destined for phase I or phase II clinical trials in cancer. Beyond early (phase I/II) clinical trials, technology transfer for some products has occurred, with further development through phase III now addressed by pharmaceutical companies.

Based on experience accumulated over several years, we abstracted the initial profiles of the more successful concepts (Table 1), as well as some early project characteristics that can impede clinical development (Table 2). We note correlations between the thoroughness of the early research, attention to "the rules," outlined in the references cited here, and the development of commercial interest in the product.

2. FDA/RECOMBINANT DNA ADVISORY COMMITTEE REGULATIONS REGARDING GENE THERAPY

2.1. Brief History

Gene therapy and other biologic therapeutics are regulated within the FDA by the Center for Biologics Evaluation and Research (CBER), which was created in 1972 to address products emerging from the new biotechnology. Reorganization at the FDA is currently under way that will result in regulation of many biotherapeutics by the Center for Drug Evaluation and Research, which has oversight of small molecule drugs. It is anticipated, however, that blood products, vaccines, and gene therapy products will remain with CBER. The Biological Response Modifiers Advisory Committee is a chartered advisory group with the role of advising the FDA to ensure the safety and effectiveness of biological products, including gene therapy. The Recombinant DNA Advisory Committee (RAC) also oversees gene therapy research through the NIH Office of Biotechnology Activities. The RAC was established in 1974 in response to public concerns regarding the safety of recombinant deoxyribonucleic acid (DNA) technology. Human gene transfer trials in which NIH funding is involved (either directly or indirectly) are to be submitted to the RAC for review.

Table 2
Issues Requiring Attention at the Outset of a Project

Inappropriate antibiotic selection markers (e.g., ampicillin for recombinant proteins)
Lab-scale affinity purification
Solubility problems
Low yield
Errors in genetic sequence
Extraneous genetic material
Poorly defined production systems
Inadequate purification schemes
Unvalidated or nonexistent in vitro potency assay(s)
Lack of key reagents (e.g., antibodies to desired product)
Poor biochemical characterization
Inappropriate raw materials
Raw material qualification problems
Inappropriate cell banks
Difficult or unidentified toxicology systems
Failed vendor qualification
Intellectual property concerns

In addition to the US agencies that develop the regulations that govern drug development and licensing, the International Conference on Harmonization (ICH) was formed in April 1990 involving the United States, the European Union, and Japan to address the issue of globalizing such regulations. The ICH Steering Committee meets at least twice a year to continue their agenda of updating and harmonizing regulations for medicinal products; they emphasize safety, quality, and efficacy. Expert Working Groups were formed within ICH to address specific topics related to these basic areas. Although the FDA has not formally adopted all of the ICH guidelines, these guidelines should be followed when they exist in preliminary form. For investigators planning to conduct investigational drug trials in foreign countries, it is imperative that they be familiar with, and adhere to, the regulations set forth by ICH.

2.2. Current FDA and ICH Safety Guidance Statements

In 1996–2001, a series of FDA and ICH guidance documents on characterization and preclinical safety evaluation of biotechnology-derived pharmaceuticals was developed (1–8). These guidances represent the FDA's current thinking on preclinical safety evaluation of biotechnology-derived pharmaceuticals. These are defined as products derived from characterized cells using a variety of expression systems, including bacteria, yeast, insect, plant, and mammalian cells. The active substances may include proteins and peptides, their derivatives, and products of which they are components. These materials could be derived from cell cultures or produced using recombinant DNA technology, including production by transgenic plants and animals. Examples include cytokines, enzymes, fusion proteins, growth factors, hormones, monoclonal antibodies, plasminogen activators, recombinant plasma factors, and receptors. The intended indications for use in humans may include in vivo diagnostic, therapeutic, or prophylactic uses. The principles outlined in these guidance documents may also be applicable to recombinant DNA protein vaccines, chemically synthesized peptides, plasma-derived products, endogenous proteins extracted from human tissue, and oligonucleotide drugs.

The FDA defines gene therapy as "a medical intervention based on modification of the genetic material of living cells" (9). Cells may be modified ex vivo for subsequent administration to humans or may be altered in vivo by gene therapy given directly to the patient. When the genetic manipulation is performed ex vivo on cells that are then administered to the patient, this is also considered a form of somatic cell therapy (9). "The genetic manipulation may be intended to have a therapeutic or prophylactic effect or may provide a way of marking cells for later identification. Recombinant DNA materials used to transfer genetic material for such therapy are considered components of gene therapy and as such are subject to regulatory oversight".

Specific information related to gene therapy issues is contained in the 1998 "FDA Guidance for Industry: Guidance for Human Somatic Cell Therapy and Gene Therapy" *(9)*. This guidance document updates and replaces the 1991 FDA "Points to Consider" on this subject *(9a)*. New information was intended to provide manufacturers with current information regarding regulatory concerns for production, quality control testing, and administration of recombinant vectors for gene therapy and of preclinical testing of both cellular therapies and vectors. The FDA defines somatic cell therapy as "the administration to humans of autologous, allogeneic, or xenogeneic living non-germline cells, other than transfusable blood products, for therapeutic, diagnostic, or preventive purposes."

3. PRECLINICAL SAFETY TESTING OF BIOLOGICALS

The evaluation of the safety of gene therapy products is perhaps one of the more difficult tasks that faces toxicologists in the drug development arena today. Because many of the agents, like other biologicals, are species specific and because these agents integrate into the host genome, the choice of animal models and study designs is fraught with uncertainty, and each product frequently breaks new regulatory ground. Until recently, many investigators working in this field were probably lulled into a false sense of security because of the close scrutiny that preclinical studies and clinical protocols received from the NIH RAC and the FDA. With the death of Jesse Gelsinger, a patient enrolled in a gene therapy clinical trial to correct a metabolic disease, in 1999 and the recent reports of a leukemialike disease produced in children who received gene therapy treatments to correct severe combined immunodeficiency disease (SCID) *(10–13)*, the safety of these agents is called into question more than ever.

As a result, the toxicologist is under even more pressure to design more rigorous safety evaluation programs. There have been a number of reviews in this area in recent years by toxicologists from the FDA *(14)*, industry *(15,16)*, and international workshops *(17)* that cover many of the fundamentals regarding safety evaluation of gene therapy products. These resources, in conjunction with this chapter and the various guidance documents from the FDA and the ICH *(7,9,18)*, can be used by toxicologists to develop sound safety programs. These issues are discussed in greater detail in the latter half of this chapter.

4. WHERE TO FIND REGULATORY INFORMATION

The basic foundation of regulations for drug development can be found in the Code of Federal Regulations, Title 21 Food and Drugs (21 CFR; *19-26*). In addition to Title 21, FDA maintains an extensive number of Web sites containing regulatory information that should be consulted during the development of a novel biotherapeutic. The collection of available regulatory information includes Points to Consider, Guidance Documents, Drafts, and reports from public forums and symposia as well as information on the meetings of the Biological Response Modifiers Advisory Committee. ICH also sponsors a Web site for obtaining the most recent guidelines. A free subscription to an e-mail advisory update service is also available (Table 3).

In addition to the regulatory guidelines provided by the FDA, the NIH has published, and frequently updates, the NIH Guidelines for Research Involving Recombinant DNA Molecules, which can also be found electronically (Table 3). Although published documents disseminated by the FDA and NIH are essential starting points for planning a cGMP development strategy, it is important to realize that, in this rapidly evolving field, some requirements may be reflected in public comments or a growing consensus among industry long before they are formally adopted. Furthermore, it is not unusual during the development of a new biologic to have also developed alternatives to conventional practices that are based on sound scientific data and are then implemented after discussions with the FDA.

Table 3
Web Sites for Regulatory Guidance

General FDA: www.fda.gov
    CBER: www.fda.gov/cber/index.html
    CBER guidelines: www.fda.gov/cber/guidelines.htm
General ICH: www.ich.org
    ICH guidances: www.fda.gov/cber/ich/ichguid.htm
NIH/RAC Web sites:
    Office of Biotechnology Activities: www4.od.nih.gov/oba/
    RAC: www4.od.nih.gov/oba/rac/aboutrdagt.htm
    NIH guidelines: www4.od.nih.gov/oba/rac/guidelines/guidelines.html
CBER and FDA e-mail update service:
    CBER: www.fda.gov/cber/pubinfo/elists.htm
    FDA: www.fda.gov/emaillist.html

5. BASIC REGULATORY PROCESS

Product-specific factors can influence the regulatory requirements for an investigational agent. These issues should be explored in detail with the FDA in a pre-IND meeting at which the IND sponsor presents relevant preclinical data and manufacturing and animal safety testing to support the proposed approach to clinical development. The types of further studies pertinent to the particular agent can then be proposed, and input from the agency help shape the final development plan.

Interactions should take place with regulatory authorities at intervals that will facilitate the development of a product (Table 4). A key issue frequently not understood is that regulatory demands become more stringent as a product moves from phase I (safety), through phase II (activity), to phase III (comparative efficacy) trials and licensure *(6,27–31)*. This philosophy reflects the conscious effort not to stifle innovation in early phase clinical testing, but to ensure that, by the time registration-oriented late-stage trials are contemplated, issues related to production variability, assay, and assurance of safety are mature and well-substantiated because the results of such trials could be the basis for sale of the agent to the public.

Another factor that affects the level of regulatory compliance is the nature of the study population. Products manufactured for Phase I trials in healthy normal volunteers typically must meet much stricter requirements than those studied in patients with dire, life-threatening conditions (e.g., cancer or end-stage acquired immunodeficiency syndrome). As improved technology becomes available, requirements also tend to increase *(27–31)*.

5.1. Development of a Product

The level of regulatory compliance to be followed during different stages of development is dependent on the type of biologic product and the technology available for supporting its development. Assays, methods, and technologies for monoclonal antibody development *(32)*, for instance, are better defined than the techniques available for some of the new virus vectors that are emerging. Furthermore, new technologies to support product development are also constantly evolving. The number of specific viral contaminant tests required of cGMP human cell lines, for example, has increased steadily as new pathogens are identified and assays become available.

As new scientific knowledge accumulates, novel regulatory challenges can appear. The issue of transmissible spongiform encephalopathy, for example, has resulted in stringent requirements in raw material qualifications and traceability *(33)*. To minimize the impact of regulatory changes, careful record keeping of all processes and materials involved in deriving the product is highly recommended.

Table 4
Organization of Activities and Interactions With Regulatory Authorities During Development

Phase of development	Investigator activity	FDA activity	NIH activity
Early	Demonstrated proof of concept in vitro Beginning scale-up of production and purification studies Basic assays available for identity, purity, and potency		
Preclinical	Animal model for efficacy established Assays well developed for identity, purity, and potency Animal safety studies completed Production, purification methods ready for clinical manufacturing	Pre-IND meeting	RAC review
Clinical phase I	Initial dose finding and safety studies carried out in humans Continued refinement of production and purification methods Refinement of assays Validation of stability studies in progress	30 Day review of IND	
Clinical phase II	Dose finding, initial efficacy, and further safety studies in humans Production, purification methods well defined Assay validation in progress Validation of stability assays completed	End of phase II meeting	Monitoring of safety data and clinical protocols
Clinical phase III	Comparative efficacy studies, continued collection of safety data Production scale-up and validation nearly complete Assay validation complete BLA preparation in progress	Pre-BLA submission meeting	Meetings with investigators as needed
Licensing	BLA filing Continued collection of safety data	Pre-approval inspection Comprehensive, multidisciplinary review	

Finally, because of the availability of improved techniques for characterizing certain biologicals, the FDA is reorganizing its regulatory approach in ways that are analogous to the regulation of small molecule drugs. Technical demands will rise as regulatory requirements become more standardized.

5.2. General Principles of Regulatory Requirements for a Well-Characterized Product

Beyond identification and confirmation of an interesting novel concept, a major challenge in the preclinical development of biologicals is the optimal allocation of research and development resources. Key to this is proper assessment of a candidate concept's readiness for clinical development. All applicants for the National Cancer Institute's biologicals production resources now receive a list of "generic questions" corresponding to the appropriate product type. At the beginning of a project, it is not always reasonable to expect all issues to be resolved, but the assumption is that, for a successful candidate, these issues should be in hand by the time the project is completing phase I clinical testing. Table 5 lists the generic questions for cGMP production of recombinant virus vectors.

Because it is not possible to provide a complete guide to cGMP development in a few pages, we highlight some concerns common to many projects arising from academic laboratories. These are based on DTP's experience (both successes and failures) with projects making the transition from the preclinical research phase to pilot clinical studies. Our discussion is organized primarily around the concepts of identity, purity, potency, and safety that underlie development, manufacture, and release.

5.2.1. Identity

From the viewpoint of regulatory compliance, it is essential to establish the identity of the product and the components used to generate it during manufacturing (9,22). We have noted that, frequently in proposed gene therapy or recombinant DNA-derived products submitted to us, DNA sequencing shows some deviation from the sequence published and/or submitted by the investigator, sometimes with major consequences for the project. When the DNA product, such as plasmid vaccines, will be administered to the patient, full plasmid sequencing has occasionally revealed unacceptable genetic sequences outside the open reading frame, as passengers from previous experiments, spurious promoters, frame shifts resulting in translation of nonsense sequences beyond the intended termination, and so on. DNA sequencing and repair are available at relatively low cost compared to the cost of repeating critical preclinical experiments. The FDA now requires complete sequencing of vectors of sizes up to 40 kilobases (kb) (34).

For viral vectors, genetic stability is a major concern, particularly with respect to the possible issues of recombination with generation of replication-competent viruses. Specific guidelines are provided for adenovirus, retrovirus, and lentivirus vectors (9,35,36). For other virus vectors, specific assays (e.g., neurovirulence testing of recombinant poliovirus and herpes virus vectors) are required to ensure that an attenuated phenotype is preserved after scale-up. If possible, the investigator should attempt to assess the genetic stability of the vector during preclinical studies, after administration in vivo or propagation in vitro.

In addition to the gene therapy product itself, the cells used to produce the product must be similarly identified and qualified for cGMP manufacturing. Excellent guidance documents are available for the production of master cell banks, working cell banks, and master virus banks (9,32,37). At minimum, the complete cell history should be known and documented, and the cells should be tested to verify their origin.

Peptide sequencing or mapping employing liquid chromatography-mass spectrometry is typically used to provide critical information for synthetic peptides and recombinant proteins. For recombinant vectors containing transgenes, the expression of the desired gene product should be verified, for example, by immunoassay using a specific antibody against the product.

Table 5
Generic Questions for Candidate Projects Involving Recombinant Virus Vectors

1. What amount of delivered product is desired? How are these quantities justified?
   A. Non-GMP for additional preclinical development
   B. cGMP (clinical grade)
2. Provide details of molecular construct(s), including starting materials (e.g., plasmid, relevant vector maps, detailed vector construction scheme, and so on)
3. Does the construct contain an antibiotic resistance gene or other selectable marker? Are alternative methods of selection available? Why was the proposed selection chosen?
4. Is the vector replication competent or replication defective? (For replication-selective vectors, what is the molecular basis of the selectivity and the conditions under which the vector would replicate?)
5. Does the vector have an altered cell tropism? Define. What is the effect of altered tropism on anticipated host toxicity?
6. Has this construct been sequenced? Provide a sequence in an electronic format.
7. Are data available evaluating the genetic stability of the recombinant vector? Have mutation rates been established and/or rates of reversion to either wild-type or alternate viral genomes?
8. Are data available evaluating the potential for genetic recombination with other organisms in the patient or in the environment?
9. Is the organism currently grown in a qualified cGMP cell line? If not, is there a qualified cell line available for propagation of this vector? Was the cell line genetically modified to support this vector? Provide details of its construction and any information regarding the stability of the genetic alteration in the cell line.
10. Is there a cGMP-qualified virus seed bank?
11. Provide details of the proposed production method.
12. Has this material ever been produced for laboratory or clinical studies using this production system?
13. Has this material been produced in a related or other production system? If so, please provide the details.
14. Please provide details of existing purification methods.
15. What is the average yield of the production system before and after purification? What is the largest amount of material that you have produced in your laboratory in a single production batch? Please provide average ratios obtained by this production method for virus particle/infectious unit and infectious units/cell. How does this scale to anticipated quantities for clinical trial?
16. How much material is available as a reference standard?
17. Is material available as bulk biological substance for preliminary pharmacology and toxicology studies?
18. Are there reproducible assays for the product? Please provide the following assays, if available:
    A. Identity
    B. Purity
    C. Potency
19. What are to be the release criteria for the product? How does one know that a lot of product is qualified for use?
20. In what form (lyophilized, formulated product, and so on) and fill size is the desired final product? What is the desired final product formulation?
21. Are there issues of formulation that must be resolved?
22. What is known about the product stability with respect to physical integrity and activity?
23. Do you have any information regarding the estimated costs of this production project?
24. Have you identified any possible sources of production with any commercial firms? Please provide details.
25. Are there any safety issues connected with the production, purification, and/or handling of the product?
26. What is the status of the product(s) regarding intellectual property issues?
27. Sometimes, proposed projects are an improvement or modification of an existing approach. In these cases, this information may significantly affect the analysis of feasibility, cost, and other production issues. Please provide a brief summary of the nature of any such antecedents or other approaches that appear closely related to the proposed project.
28. Have there been any meetings scheduled with regulatory agencies, such as a pre-IND meeting with the FDA or a presentation to the NIH RAC? If so, please indicate the type of meeting, the regulatory agency, and the date or proposed date.
29. If you have had a pre-IND or RAC meeting, were any issues concerning manufacturing, safety, or stability raised that will have an impact on producing your product?
30. Who will sponsor the IND for the proposed study?
31. Has a source of funding been identified for performing the clinical trial with this product?

5.2.2. Purity

Purification strategies depend on the nature of the biologic agent and expected impurities. These approaches are guided by the early development of reliable analytical techniques appropriate to the product and to the manufacturing approach. For example, purification of recombinant proteins and monoclonal antibodies for cGMP manufacture typically involve large-scale chromatography based on multiple isolation principles (e.g., charge, hydrophobicity, size, and so on). Specific contaminants, such as DNA, endotoxin, viruses from mammalian cell production systems, contaminants introduced in the manufacturing process, and the like must be quantified and may require additional specific purification measures to remove or inactivate them.

Problems in refolding or solubility, tendencies to aggregate, and product stability at intermediate holding points can be significant issues in process development for scale-up. These represent key challenges in scale-up from investigator laboratory-generated lots to a potentially suitable scale to allow clinical testing. Additional concerns include subtle degradations of proteins that can lead to undesirable immunogenicity. A major concern is the impact of each additional step on the downstream product, which should be reassessed using in vitro potency assays as well as physicochemical characterization. At major development milestones, selected in vivo models should be reexamined using purified product.

Production cells must be cGMP qualified and tested for adventitious agents and other contaminants, before initiation of production as well as at end of production. A number of cGMP-qualified cell lines and starting vectors are available commercially at relatively low cost and should be considered for use as raw materials to initiate cGMP seed banks in preference to shared materials of uncertain provenance despite the good intentions of the original provider. In the handling of cell lines, care should also be taken to avoid contamination (e.g., from media components, trypsin, or activities taking place in nearby laboratory space). Postproduction cells can be tested for specific contaminants in the presence of a viral product (e.g., using polymerase chain reaction [PCR]). In the presence of virus product, however, it is unlikely that the full set of cGMP tests (e.g., cocultivation) for adventitious agents can be performed on postproduction cells. Before initiating cGMP production, therefore, investigators should consider the parallel propagation of a mock-infected control to provide a surrogate postproduction test article.

In addition to the usual tests for sterility and purity of purified investigational product *(9,20,21)*, it is important to have an assay for residual host cell DNA. Assays for host cell proteins are not always required for all phase I products, but are required for phase II and beyond. This consideration is another reason to start with cGMP-qualified cell lines from a commercial source because host cell DNA and protein assays may already be available.

The general requirement for adventitious agent testing is given in guidance documents (e.g., ref. 9). It is important to note that some specific assays are not yet described in published FDA documents, but can enter widespread cGMP practice by sponsor-based industry consensus, liability considerations, or other factors. Endotoxin assays are available as kits, which are useful to guide laboratory process development. A qualified good laboratory practice (GLP) laboratory, however, should perform endotoxin assays for clinical product release. Specific assays may also be required to quantify process residuals from production and purification components (CsCl, antibiotics, and so on). In production facilities, particularly those where different types of gene therapy products may be produced, assays are necessary to support decontamination and cleaning, product changeover, environmental monitoring, and raw material qualification *(25,38)*. In general, all equipment that has contact with the investigational product should be verified free of contaminants before use.

Special consideration must also be given to assays to qualify virus seeds and end product for the presence of defective particles, replication-competent viruses, or defective genomes. In addition to monitoring for replication-competent and/or pathogenic vectors during manufacture, suitable assays may also be required to monitor patients receiving the therapeutic agent. In this case, levels of sensitivity for detection must be suitable for different types of patient specimens (serum, urine, sputum, and so on). Evolving requirements for long-term follow-up of gene therapy patients *(39)* should be consulted to ensure that proper assay support is maintained beyond the duration of the planned clinical trial. The FDA regulations governing the performance of assays that support the production of biologics for human use can be found in 21 CFR 211, subpart I, "Laboratory Controls" *(25)*. GLP regulations only per-tain to the performance of preclinical animal and in vitro studies *(23)*.

5.2.3. Potency

The measured activity of a biological candidate depends on the hypothesized molecular mechanism of therapeutic action (21 CFR 600.3; *9, 19*). Although it is most reassuring to see in vivo demonstration of efficacy in appropriate animal models, the efficient development of a cGMP process will strongly benefit from the availability of rapid, reliable, and reproducible in vitro assays relating to the mechanism of action in addition to assays for purity and identity. Assays based on the basic therapeutic mechanism, therefore, are critical goals of early research and development.

5.2.4. Formulation and Stability

Formulation development should begin as early as possible as suitable assays become available and experience with real-time stability accumulates. It is preferable to choose formulations from candidates likely to be acceptable to the FDA, such as those whose components are already used for licensed products. As production reaches larger scales, handling and storage considerations become increasingly important. Stability studies incorporate assays for identity, purity (including aggregation), and potency. Although they can provide some useful information, accelerated stability studies are typically not reliable for predicting real-time stability of biologics. Therefore, there is a need for real-time stability studies to be initiated as soon as possible.

Suitability of formulated product should also be assessed in the identical administration and handling conditions expected in the clinic. This may include transient exposure to conditions expected during transit to the study site and storage in an environment that closely mimics study site conditions. These may result in markedly different product behavior at the study site from that expected from the behavior of vouchered specimens at a central repository site. The results of ongoing stability studies are useful to support process development; to evaluate product at intermediate hold points in scale-up production and at product release; and to support formulation development, product storage, shipment, and handling during toxicology studies and clinical applications. As development proceeds, master specifications for release of intermediate and final product should be established and refined. The IND must indicate a schedule for real-time stability studies to be performed throughout the duration of the clinical trial.

6. ORGANIZATION OF RESEARCH ACTIVITIES TO OPTIMIZE DEVELOPMENT OPPORTUNITIES

Some key early milestones common to all product areas include the attainment of an adequate scale of high-quality, single-batch production, the availability of adequate amounts of high-quality laboratory reference standard, and the development of reliable assays for identity, purity, and potency of the product. These milestones are necessary in addition to the exploration of animal models showing safety and promising evidence of efficacy. At early stages in a project, investigators should expect substantial variability in product quality, assays, and animal models.

Ideally, therefore, a single high-quality batch should be used to establish laboratory standards, support multiple assay qualification runs, and perform replicate animal model experiments. Multiple production runs could then be performed to explore process development issues, including scale-up. In this way, fundamental issues could be explored at the research stage to prepare for development required for cGMP manufacture. Following this reasoning, our facility often manufactures high-quality GLP lots to provide a uniform supply of material for additional preclinical research and development for selected biologics of interest before making the decision to undertake cGMP production.

6.1. Good Laboratory Practices

The early establishment of certain aspects of GLP (21 CFR 58) is crucial to the advancement of a drug development project. By following simple rules of laboratory cleanliness, documentation, and segregation of materials and activities at the start of development, time can be saved by avoiding the necessity to duplicate results that were not properly performed or documented from the outset.

At the discovery phase, development of reliable assays to explore basic therapeutic mechanisms of action are just as important as the performance of animal models in laying the groundwork for future cGMP product development. Laboratory facilities and staff should be adequate to perform necessary studies. Assay protocols should be specific and reproducible. Research documentation should be kept at a GLP level with complete and secure laboratory notebooks. Records of all reagents (i.e., manufacturer, catalog number, lot number, Certificates of Analysis [COAs], and expiration dates) should be routinely archived. Even if cGMP production or testing is not contemplated in the development laboratory, fluctuations in product activity are not unusual during later scale-up, and these materials and information may be useful in resolving such issues. Key assays for product or reagent identity should be repeated at appropriate intervals.

6.2. Segregation of Laboratory Activities

Access to critical raw materials and reagents, reference standards, and cell banks should be limited. Staff should avoid comingling of research-grade, GLP, and GMP activities or reagents by labeling reagent containers and sequestering them as much as possible. Similarly, signs should be posted on dedicated equipment, and access should be limited as appropriate. If common equipment must be used, standard operating procedures should be developed to define the use and control of such equipment, to clean equipment before and after use to avoid cross-contamination, and to document the use, cleaning, and calibration of the equipment.

6.3. Raw Materials

Critical raw materials (e.g., those used in seed development or pilot product manufacture) must be traceable to their source and obtained from reliable vendors. It is beneficial when possible to use vendors subjected to commercial audits. Animal-derived reagents should be avoided; reagents such as glycerol, detergents, proteins, amino acids, and the like should preferably come from vegetable sources. If this is not possible, animal-derived reagents should come from acceptable herds in countries without endemic or questionable transmissible spongiform encephalopathy *(33)*. It is important to ensure that raw materials are stored under appropriate conditions and not used beyond their expiration date. Inventories and logbooks should be used to track use of important reagents.

Critical materials requiring special storage conditions should be stored at more than one location to prevent loss in the event of equipment failure. cGMP-qualified cell lines should be purchased from vendors if possible, but if cGMP-qualified cell lines do not exist, cell lines should be obtained directly from a reliable repository source such as the American Type Culture Collection (ATCC) and documentation should be archived. Incoming cell lines must be tested for sterility and mycoplasma contamination. Thorough records should be kept on cell passages, observations, frozen storage, and the COAs from media and other components used to grow, freeze, and otherwise manipulate the cells. Critical cell lines should be segregated to prevent cross-contamination. Stock cells should not be cultured in incubators containing virus-infected cell lines.

Vectors should be purchased from a reliable vendor, and documentation should be kept on the propagation, storage, and use, including COAs, lot numbers, and so on of the reagents used to propagate the vector. If the vector is acquired from another laboratory (i.e., is unavailable for purchase from a vendor), a detailed history should be obtained of the generation of the vector, and detailed records should be kept from that time. All genetic manipulations of the vectors should be well documented and verified by sequencing.

6.4. Reference Standards

A lab-generated reference standard is a critical raw material for a biologic. It is ideal to have a large enough stock of this reference standard to use for the duration of the development work. It is often not possible, however, to produce sufficient quantities or material of sufficient stability at the early development stages. For this reason, it may be necessary to produce fresh batches and to test them thoroughly against independent standards or the current standard before that standard is depleted or loses potency.

The same consideration should be given to other critical reagents, such as cell lines and compounds obtained from outside sources. Reference standards and key reagents should be made or obtained in adequate amounts, characterized as well as possible, and stored under conditions that will maintain stability for at least the duration of the development process. As improved manufacturing and assay processes are developed, improved reference standards will be required, but quantities of the original standards should also be preserved to provide material for later comparisons as required *(40)*. In some cases, such as for retrovirus and adenovirus vector development, the FDA has made available reference material against which all sponsors can standardize their own reference reagents.

6.5. Assays and Resources

To avoid future questions about data reliability, investigators should consider outsourcing of difficult but common technologies, such as transmission electron microscopy, tandem liquid chromatography mass spectroscopy, peptide mapping, or DNA sequencing, if these are not adequate in their facility. Product-specific assays, such as potency studies and pilot animal efficacy and toxicity studies, are likely to be performed best at the researcher's own facility, early in development. Preclinical assay protocol development and record keeping must ensure that data are useful for later IND submission. At some point in cGMP process development, consideration should be given to technology transfer of critical assays to a GLP-compliant laboratory prepared to support the repetitive studies required during cGMP process development, manufacture, release, and postrelease stability studies for the duration of the clinical trial.

6.6. Preparation of Toxicology Material

Toxicology material should ideally be manufactured using the same process used to manufacture the cGMP clinical material. Therefore, a toxicology lot is produced late in process development. If there are concerns over batch-to-batch variability, production of a single lot for both toxicology and the initial phase I trial is recommended. Typically, a toxicology lot can be available several months before the clinical lot is ready for release.

7. SPECIAL REGULATORY CONSIDERATIONS

7.1. Cellular Therapies

For studies involving autologous cells, the handling of cells must be under GMP conditions to preserve sterility and prevent cross-contamination with other cells. For allogeneic cells, it is important to use a cGMP-tested cell line with adequate traceability, including its origin, passage history, and exposure to media products that may have been derived from animal sources.

7.2. DNA Plasmids

Starting material must be routinely checked for sequence accuracy; therefore, the complete plasmid should be sequenced. It is also preferable to examine genetic stability that can lead to the introduction of coding errors and changes in protein expression. The use of penicillin-like antibiotics (β-lactams) for selection is unacceptable because of the possibility of allergic reactions in patients administered products produced using this selection system. Other antibiotics, such as kanamycin, are substituted, or alternative methods of selection are employed. Measures of DNA quality include supercoiled content, as well as assays for endotoxin, genomic DNA, and other contaminants from the production system. More in-depth guidance is available through guidance documents *(9)*.

7.3. Viral Agents

It is generally recommended by the FDA that a vector smaller than 40 kb must be completely sequenced *(34)*. As technology improves, this criterion may well be expanded to include larger vector genomes. Those vectors with genomes larger than 40 kb (e.g., herpes viruses, poxviruses) must have the transgene sequenced along with 5' and 3' flanking regions and any significant modifications to the vector backbone or sites vulnerable to alteration during molecular manipulation.

When qualified vaccine strains exist for the vector of interest (e.g., vaccinia, poliovirus) it is preferable for cGMP manufacture to derive investigational constructs using the vaccine strain if available from the NIH, ATCC, or commercial sources. For adenovirus vectors, the recent availability of an adenovirus reference standard allows for the normalization of dosing based on virus particle concentration and infectious unit (IU) titer. Current recommendations by the FDA are for a ratio of viral particle to infectious unit of less than or equal to 30:1 *(35)*.

For replication-defective adenoviruses, generation of replication-competent adenoviruses (RCA) must be measured in lots produced for clinical use. The current target requirement is fewer than 1 RCA per 3×10^{10} virus particles as measured by a cell culture/cytopathic effect method *(35)*. For viruses that are replication selective, different testing strategies (e.g., quantitative PCR) may be called for and should be discussed with the FDA. Similarly, the agency may have special considerations for viruses with altered tropism to ensure appropriate containment and prevent the generation of a replication-competent adenovirus with an expanded cell tropism. It should be noted that RCA assays must be optimized regarding the presence of defective particles and other factors that may affect the sensitivity of the assay.

Retroviruses are of special concern because of the possibility of insertional carcinogenesis. This potential safety problem is amplified if replication-competent retroviruses (RCRs) are generated *(9,36)*. The general guideline is to test at least 5% of the total virus vector supernatant produced by amplifying any RCR on a permissive cell line. In addition, 1% of the producer cells or 10^8 (whichever is less) must also be tested at the end of production by the method of coculturing on permissive cells *(36)*. As with adenovirus vectors, retrovirus vectors with tropism modifications are of special concern and may require more stringent containment and patient follow-up *(39)*. Promoter modifications may also affect the safety profile of these virus vectors.

Lentiviruses generally have the same safety concerns as retroviruses, particularly because they can replicate in a broader variety of cells (dormant as well as actively dividing cells). Although there is a retrovirus standard available through ATCC to investigators who are developing retrovirus vectors, there is no lentivirus standard currently offered. A lentivirus standard is not planned for the future primarily because of the great variability in lentivirus backbones currently under development for clinical investigations (e.g., equine, murine, human). Herpes viruses under development for clinical use either must be replication defective or, if replication competent, must be shown to be nonneurovirulent. Neurovirulence is an issue for poliovirus as well. Adeno-associated virus (AAV) vectors are of concern because, although these vectors are designed to be maintained episomally, there can be reversion to wild type, resulting in integration into the host chromosome, or the vector could be rescued in a patient with a concurrent adenovirus infection *(41)*.

Several interesting concepts seek to employ modified bacteria as the therapeutic agent. As with recombinant viruses, general issues of safety as well as specific issues of genetic stability and exchange should be considered. Stabilization of the new genetic material may be required by incorporation into the bacterial genome rather than through a plasmid that can be lost or exchanged. Strategies to incorporate new genetic material into bacterial DNA will depend on confirming the sequence accuracy of the target bacterial sequences as well as the novel genetic material. Introduction of an antibiotic resistance gene through a manufacturing step raises special concerns and can be avoided using alternative selection approaches.

8. SAFETY, TOXICOLOGY, AND BIODISTRIBUTION STUDIES
8.1. Safety Study Design Issues
8.1.1. General Toxicity Issues

Whether evaluating small molecules or biologically derived materials such as gene therapy products, the basic intent of nonclinical toxicity studies is to define the pharmacological and toxicological effects predictive of the human response, not only prior to initiation of phase I clinical trials in humans, but also throughout the entire drug development process leading ultimately to Biologics License Application (BLA). The goals of these studies include, first, to define an initial safe starting dose and dose escalation schemes for first-in-human clinical trials; second, to identify potential target organs for toxicity, biomarkers or other parameters that can be monitored in patients receiving these therapies, and to determine if this toxicity is reversible; and finally, to determine which patient populations may be at greater risk for developing toxicity to a given cellular or gene therapeutic product *(42)*.

These nonclinical studies should be designed with the following points in mind: whether the product is transduced cells, the population of cells to be administered, or the class of vector used; the most appropriate animal species and physiological state of that model most relevant for the clinical indication and product class; and the intended doses, route of administration, and treatment regimens that will be used in the clinic. Many of the questions that need to be taken into consideration and addressed during the design phase for safety studies include what is already known about the most likely toxicities related to the agent's biodistribution, local as well as systemic toxicity, immune responses (immunogenicity and immunotoxicity), the potential for insertional mutagenesis, and biological activities of the transgene product. Then specific questions that arise with the new product or use are addressed. For example, are the safety issues primarily related to the vector, the transgene product, the method of administration, the formulation/excipient, or some combination of the above? How might existing published or unpublished nonclinical or clinical data address the questions mentioned above? Safety issues that should be addressed in these studies include evaluation of the toxicity of the vector alone (irrespective of the transgene), including its potential toxicity and/or tumorigenicity (in some cases, this is apparent from previous evaluations with the same vector); toxicity of transgene expression in vivo that may not be evident from in vitro studies; occurrence and consequences of ectopic transgene expression in nontargeted tissues; occurrence and consequences of immune responses to transgene or vector proteins such as autoimmunity; and finally the possibility of germline transduction *(34)*.

Because conventional pharmacology and toxicity testing as typically used for the evaluation of small molecules may not always be appropriate to determine the safety and biologic activity of cellular and gene therapy products, issues such as species specificity of the transduced gene, permissiveness for infection by viral vectors, and comparative animal to human physiology should be considered in the design of these studies. Available animal models mimicking the disease indication may be useful in obtaining both sufficient safety and efficacy data prior to entry of these agents into clinical trials. Early pre-IND discussions with the FDA during development of a toxicology plan may prevent delays and added expenses because of inadequate data or the use of inappropriate species. Some of the questions that should be answered by preclinical pharmacology/toxicology studies are the following *(43)*: What is the relationship of the dose to the biologic activity? What is the relationship of the dose to the toxicity? Does the route and/or schedule affect activity and/or toxicity? What risks can be identified for the clinical trial?

For ex vivo gene transfer, the product is considered to be the transduced cells. The general safety test (21 CFR 610.11) must be performed on the final product. When appropriate, modified procedures may be developed according to 21 CFR 610.9. The FDA is considering proposed rule making to amend the general safety test rules and scope of applicability, especially for cell therapy products *(9)*.

Finally, it is expected that these nonclinical toxicity studies will be conducted in compliance with GLP regulations. However, there will be situations in which highly specialized assays will be required because of the nature of biotechnology-derived products, and it will not be possible to conduct these assays in full compliance with GLPs (e.g., in university or other discovery laboratories). It will be important that these areas be identified for any impact that they may have on the interpretation of toxicity data. In most cases, carefully performed studies such as this can be used to support INDs and BLAs *(7)*.

8.1.2. Animal Model/Species Selection

When selecting the animal model that will be used in the various preclinical biodistribution, pharmacology, and toxicology studies, consideration should be given to the scientific rationale for the animal species used. For example, would there be an advantage to performing the studies in rodents when larger numbers of animals might be more practical, or is there a necessity for a large animal model, such as a canine or nonhuman primate? If nonhuman primate studies are proposed, is it clear that another large animal or rodent model would not provide the same information? Would there be any utility in a genetically deficient model, and would this deficient model be more relevant to the proposed study either because of the potential for adverse immunologic consequences or because of the biological effects in the deficient condition?

Animal models of disease may not be available for every cellular or gene therapy system proposed for development. This makes species selection an even more difficult process. Preclinical pharmacological and safety testing of these agents should employ the most appropriate, pharmacologically relevant animal model available. A relevant animal species might be one in which the biological response to the therapy mimics the human response. This entails some knowledge of the pathophysiology of the disease in humans and of how faithfully it is reproduced in the animal model.

The species of animal chosen for preclinical toxicity evaluations of viral preparations should be selected for its sensitivity to infection and production of pathologic sequelae induced by the wild-type virus related to the chosen vector, as well as its utility as a model of biologic activity of the vector construct. There should be a reasonable expectation of a similar distribution of receptors or permissivity in the animal model as there is in humans. Thus, the species utilized may vary with the vector administered, the transgene expressed, the route of administration, the patient population treated, and the disease studied. Rodent models rather than nonhuman primates may be useful if they are susceptible to pathology induced by the virus class (e.g., cotton rats are semipermissive hosts for adenovirus infections) *(44)*; the use of the SCID mouse *(45)* or the cotton rat *(46)* may be suitable for the evaluation of herpes simplex virus (HSV) rather than the *Aotus* monkey. Some investigators have also suggested the use of miniature swine for evaluation of adenoviral vectors *(47,48)*. When evaluating the activity of a vector in an animal model for the clinical indication, safety data can be gathered from the same model to assess the contribution of disease-related changes in physiology or underlying pathology to the response to the vector. Some specialized circumstances illustrating these points follow.

8.1.2.1. COTTON RAT MODEL AND ADENOVIRUS

The inbred cotton rat (*Sigmodon hispidus*) has been used extensively as an animal model for research since the 1940s, when it was first used in poliomyelitis research. Since that time, it has been shown to be a semipermissive host for adenoviral infection *(44,49)*. In those studies, it was shown that the pulmonary lesions and replication pattern of the virus seen in the cotton rat paralleled those seen in humans. Virus persisted in the nasal mucosa and lung for up to 21 and 28 days, respectively, after inoculation. This was even in the presence of high-titer neutralizing antibody that was detected by day 7.

Although cotton rats have readily adapted to the laboratory environment, they have retained a number of the characteristics of their wild counterparts. These animals have a tendency to bite, panic when handled, jump out of their cages, and have a large fight-or-flight zone. Care and handling of these animals have been described by other investigators *(50,51)*.

The cotton rat has been used for the evaluation of numerous adenovirus vectors by many routes of administration, and some of these studies are described here. When early E3-deleted adenoviral vectors were evaluated in the cotton rat, it was discovered that the E3 region was not required for replication, but that this region plays a critical role in the pathogenesis of the disease in that these mutants induced a markedly greater lymphocyte and macrophage/monocyte inflammatory response in the lungs *(52)*. E3 replacement recombinants were significantly less pathogenic than E3-deleted viruses after intranasal administration *(53)*. This study also demonstrated that adenovirus replicated in BALB/c and CBA mice and produced results that were similar to those seen in cotton rats.

The intracranial administration of a replication-defective adenovirus expressing the herpes simplex virus thymidine kinase (HSV*tk*) gene at a dose of 1.0×10^9 pfu into both adenoviral immune and adenoviral naïve cotton rats resulted in only mild gliosis and trace meningitis along the injection tract and approximated a "no toxic effect" dose *(54)*. When this same vector was administered to either Wistar rats or rhesus monkeys, direct neuronal injury or a dose-related inflammatory response was seen at the injection site and in the surrounding parenchyma. There was no apparent injury to tissues not of the central nervous system in any of the three models, and all cerebral spinal fluid, blood, urine, and stool samples failed to culture for adenovirus.

In a study with a similar HSV*tk* adenovirus inoculated into cotton rats via intracardiac injection at doses up to 3×10^{10} viral particles per animal with and without ganciclovir (GCV), the only significant microscopic lesions observed were epicardial inflammation and splenic hemosiderosis *(55)*. Vector sequences persisted throughout the 14-day assay period in the heart, lung, and lymphoid organs. Infectious virions were detected for 24 hours, but these virions were only detected at the site of injection of two animals in the highest dose group.

When a similar vector was administered as either one or two subcutaneous injection cycles with 2.3×10^{12} viral particles/kg each or as a single course with 6.9×10^{13} viral particles/kg, the only significant treatment-related histopathological finding was dermatitis with mild acanthosis at the site of vector injection *(56)*. In addition to these local effects, mild hyperamylasemia, lymphocytosis, and granulocytosis were seen clinically, but no other clinical signs of toxicity or death were observed. Vector sequences were detected in the skin at the injection site and to a lesser extent in the liver, spleen, and lungs, and small amounts of vector DNA were detected in the ovaries. These were cleared rapidly, and the absence of viral sequences in the excreta and swabs of the majority of animals suggested that there was no significant replication of this adenovirus vector in this host and little shedding.

8.1.2.2. *Aotus* Monkey Model and HSV

The owl monkey (*Aotus trivirgatus* or *nancymae*) has been an excellent model for oncogenic and nononcogenic viruses such as HSV type 1 (HSV-1) and others *(57)*, and the herpes virus that infects these animals is a strain of HSV-1 *(58)*. These animals have been routinely used to test vaccines against HSV-1 and found to mimic the course of the disease in humans *(59,60)*. As a result, it was only natural that these animals be used to evaluate the safety of gene therapy vectors produced from HSV-1. However, these animals tend to be more fragile to use than other species and as a result must be handled with greater care.

G207, an attenuated, replication-competent HSV-1 recombinant, was tested for safety after intracerebral inoculation in the *Aotus (61)*. These animals received doses of either 10^7 or 10^9 pfu of G207 or 10^3 pfu of the wild-type HSV-1 strain F. Wild-type HSV-1 caused rapid mortality and symptoms consistent with HSV encephalitis, including fever, hemiparesis, meningitis, and hemorrhage in the basal ganglia. For up to 1 year after G207 inoculation, seven of the treated animals were alive and exhibited no evidence of clinical complications, indicating that this form of HSV was considerably attenuated in comparison to wild-type virus. Two animals were reinoculated with 10^7 pfu of G207 at the same stereotactic coordinates 1 year after the initial dose. These animals were alive and healthy 2 years after the second inoculation.

As a further, more comprehensive clinical evaluation, animals were subjected to cerebral magnetic resonance imaging (MRI) studies both before and after G207 inoculation. These studies failed to reveal radiographic evidence of the typical HSV-related sequelae in the brain seen in the animals treated with the wild-type virus. Microscopic examination of multiple tissues found no evidence of HSV-induced histopathology or dissemination in spite of the fact that measurable increases in serum anti-HSV titers were detected. Viral shedding and biodistribution in the *Aotus* were also evaluated using PCR analyses and viral cultures of tear, saliva, or vaginal secretion samples *(62)*. Neither infectious virus nor viral DNA was detected at any time-point up to 1 month postinoculation. Analyses of tissues obtained at necropsy at 1 month or 2 years after inoculation showed the distribution of G207 DNA was restricted to the brain, although infectious virus was not isolated in these samples.

The safety of this construct was also evaluated in the *Aotus* after intraprostatic injections *(63)*. Safety was assessed on the basis of clinical observations, viral biodistribution, virus shedding, and histopathology. None of the injected monkeys displayed evidence of clinical disease, shedding of infectious virus, or spread of the virus into other organs. No significant microscopic abnormalities were observed in the organs evaluated. The results of these studies demonstrated that G207 can be safely inoculated into either the brain or the prostate, and that the *Aotus* monkey could be successfully used in preclinical toxicological evaluations.

In addition to the studies performed with this vector in *Aotus* monkeys, BALB/c mice were also used to evaluate the safety of G207. Mice were inoculated in the same manner as the *Aotus* either intracerebrally or intraventricularly with 10^7 PFU of G207 and survived for over 20 weeks with no apparent symptoms of disease. In contrast, over 80% of animals inoculated intracerebrally with 1.5×10^3 pfu of HSV-1 wild-type strain KOS and 50% of animals inoculated intraventricularly with 10^4 pfu of wild-type strain F died within 10 days. When mice were inoculated intrahepatically with G207 $(3 \times 10^7$ pfu), all animals survived for over 10 weeks, whereas no animals survived for even 1 week after inoculation with 10^6 pfu of wild-type KOS *(64)*.

Mice were also injected in the prostate with either G207 or wild-type HSV-1 strain F and observed for 5 months *(63)*. None of the G207-injected animals exhibited any clinical signs of disease or died. However, 50% of mice injected with strain F displayed sluggishness and hunched behavior and were dead by day 13. On microscopic examination, the prostates injected with G207 were normal, whereas those injected with strain F showed epithelial flattening, sloughing, and stromal edema. These studies and those described by Whitley with the SCID mouse *(45)* point to the fact that rodents can be used in place of the owl monkey and produce adequate safety data for the evaluation of HSV-1 vectors for gene therapy.

Finally, safety data can also be obtained in well-designed efficacy studies. In many cases, mouse studies can provide similar information as studies conducted in nonhuman primates, so smaller species should not be automatically rejected. The nonhuman primate should not be relied on for use as a model simply because of the comfort of going into studies in humans only after evaluation of the toxicity of the agent in nonhuman primates. Experience has repeatedly shown for numerous classes of agents, both small molecules as well as biologicals, that no one species may be predictive of all human toxicities, and that not all human toxicities may be seen in other animal species *(65)*. Finally, certain human populations may not be predictive of all other human populations. This last fact makes predicting each and every toxicity almost impossible.

8.2. Dose, Route, and Schedule

The doses of vectors used in nonclinical studies should be selected based on preliminary efficacy/activity data from both in vitro and in vivo studies. A no-effect dose level, an overtly toxic dose, and several intermediate doses should be evaluated, along with appropriate controls, such as naïve or vehicle-treated animals. For new formulations, it is very important to include this last group to distinguish formulation-related effects from those of the agent of interest. When products are difficult to produce in large quantities and as a result are in limited supply or for products with an inherently low toxicity, a maximum tolerated dose may not be achievable; as a result, a maximum feasible dose may be administered as the highest level tested in the preclinical studies and should be so designated in appropriate reports. Although this may not be intellectually or scientifically satisfying, the data derived from such a study should at least establish the safety of the clinical starting dose. Preclinical safety/toxicity studies should include at least one dose that is equivalent to and at least one dose escalation level exceeding those proposed for the clinical trial. The multiples of the human dose required to determine adequate safety margins may vary with each class of vector employed, and the relevance of the animal model to humans and the rationale for dose selection should be provided.

Scaling of doses based on either body weight or total body surface area as appropriate facilitates comparisons across the animal species used and humans. Although most small molecule cancer therapeutics are scaled based on body surface area *(66)*, body surface area may not be appropriate for gene therapeutics. Information generated in the preclinical studies can be used to determine the margin of safety of the vector for use in the clinical trial, as well as gage an acceptable dose escalation scheme depending on the steepness of the toxicity curve.

In a cross comparison of doses for an adenoviral vector for cystic fibrosis *(14)*, very similar toxicities were seen in cotton rats, mice, hamsters, rhesus monkeys, and baboons when the agent was directly instilled into the lungs of the animals. When the doses were scaled for body surface area, the no observable adverse effect levels for the various species were remarkably similar to one another and to the first human dose at which toxicity was observed, $0.4–2.4 \times 10^9$ IU/m^2 vs 1.2×10^9 IU/m^2 for humans. The only notable exception was the rhesus monkey at 4.6×10^7 IU/m^2. Studies like this enable other investigators to make wiser choices in the selection of doses and species to evaluate.

The route of administration of vectors can have an obvious influence on toxicity in vivo because of the distribution and concentrations of the agent that are produced. For example, intravenous bolus doses can produce very high concentrations for short durations; other routes of administration, such as subcutaneous, may produce much lower concentrations and more prolonged exposure. Current practice recommends that safety evaluations in preclinical studies should be conducted by the identical route and method of administration as that proposed for the phase I clinical trial whenever possible. When this is difficult to achieve in a small animal species, a method of administration similar to that planned for use in the clinic is advised. For example, intrapulmonary instillation of adenoviral vectors by intranasal administration in cotton rats or mice is an acceptable alternative to direct intrapulmonary administration through a bronchoscope because the latter procedure is simply not feasible in rodents. If the proposed clinical route is a nonintravenous (e.g., intratumoral), it may be wise also to conduct an intravenous study to provide perhaps "worse-case" data for what may happen in the event of an accidental injection directly into a patient's blood vessel.

When possible, the schedule of administration in the animal studies should also be identical to that intended in the phase I clinical trial. This may not be feasible in certain instances because of the production of neutralizing antibodies in the animal model that might preclude repeated administration; that may not be a factor in humans. In studies in which additional agents will be administered in combination with the gene therapy agent (e.g., in suicide therapy using HSV*tk* and GCV or HSV cytosine deaminase and 5-fluorocytosine), the route and schedule should also be identical to that planned for the clinic. Evaluating the vector alone in animal models would not provide sufficient data for predicting additional toxicity that may be produced by the combination, but should be at least one arm of the planned preclinical animal studies.

8.3. Pharmacological and Toxicological End Points

At a minimum, treated animals should be monitored for general health status (clinical observations, body weight and temperature changes, changes in food and water consumption), serum biochemistry, and hematological profiles. Target organs and other critical tissues should be examined for gross and microscopic changes. The addition of other parameters to be evaluated will depend on the nature of the product studied, the species used, and the route of administration. There is no set of all-inclusive parameters that is sufficient for each and every new agent. Studies should be designed specifically for each agent, utilizing the most appropriate tests to capture as much relevant data as possible.

8.4. Immunogenicity

Because many biotechnology-derived pharmaceuticals intended for human use will be immunogenic in animals, the use of animal-derived proteins/products, if available, should be considered to define the intrinsic toxicity of the new agent. This may entail parallel development processes in which a construct relevant to the species in the safety test is developed to a point to allow a most relevant safety test to proceed. The analogous human construct then may actually be brought into the clinic supported by these results. If human material is used, measurement of antibodies associated with administration of products should always be performed when conducting repeated dose toxicity studies. These data will assist the investigator in the interpretation of the results of these studies.

Antibody responses produced in animals should be fully characterized (e.g., titer, number of responding animals, neutralizing or nonneutralizing), and their appearance should be correlated with any pharmacological and/or toxicological changes observed. More specifically, the effects of antibody formation on pharmacokinetics and/or pharmacodynamics, incidence and/or severity of adverse effects, complement activation, or the emergence of new toxic effects should be considered when interpreting the data. Attention should also be paid to the evaluation of possible pathological changes related to immune complex formation and deposition, especially in the kidney of treated animals.

The detection of antibodies in animals should not be the sole criterion for the early termination of a preclinical safety study or modification of the duration of the study unless the immune response neutralizes the pharmacological and/or toxicological effects of the biopharmaceutical in a large proportion of the animals. In most cases, the immune response to biopharmaceuticals in animals will be variable, similar to such responses in humans. If these issues do not compromise the interpretation of the data from the safety study, then no special significance should be ascribed to the antibody response.

The induction of antibody formation in animals is not necessarily predictive of a potential for antibody formation in humans. By the same token, humans may also develop serum antibodies against humanized proteins, and frequently the therapeutic response persists in their presence. The same may happen in animals if a purified protein is administered via a gene therapy viral vector. In the case of human factor IX, when the purified protein was administered to rhesus macaques, the monkeys did not make antibodies *(67)*. However, when factor IX was administered in a first-generation adenoviral vector, the animals mounted an acute phase response that produced neutralizing antibody that eliminated factor IX from the circulation *(68)*. Finally, the occurrence of severe anaphylactic responses to recombinant proteins is rare in humans. The results of guinea pig anaphylaxis tests, which are generally positive for protein products, are not considered predictive for reactions in humans; therefore, studies such as this are considered of little value for the routine evaluation of these types of products even though they are frequently performed.

Inflammatory, immune, or autoimmune responses induced by the gene product may be of concern. Animal studies should be conducted over a sufficient duration of time to allow development of such responses. Host immune responses against viral or transgene proteins may limit their usefulness for repeated administration in the clinic. The immune status of the intended recipients of a gene therapy should be considered in the risk–benefit analysis of a product, particularly for viral vectors. If exclusion of immunocompromised patients would unduly restrict a clinical protocol, immune-suppressed, genetically immunodeficient, or newborn animals may be used in preclinical studies to evaluate any potential safety risks.

8.5. Safety Pharmacology Studies

It is extremely important to investigate the potential for undesirable pharmacological activity in appropriate animal models and, when necessary, to incorporate particular monitoring for these activities in nonclinical toxicity studies and/or clinical studies. Safety pharmacology studies are designed to measure functional indices of potential toxicity. These indices may be investigated in separate studies or may be carefully incorporated into the design of nonclinical toxicity studies. The aim of these studies should be to reveal any functional effects on the major physiological systems of the body (e.g., cardiovascular, respiratory, renal, and central nervous systems) that will have a major impact on whether or how the agent is administered in the clinic. Some of these investigations may include the use of isolated organs or other test systems that do not involve the use of intact animals, such as the use of a perfused rabbit heart model for the evaluation of torsade de pointes and QT prolongation *(69,70)*. The results from all of these safety pharmacology studies may allow a mechanistically based explanation of specific organ toxicities, which should be considered carefully with respect to human use and intended indications. The use of additional biomarkers, exemplified by cardiac troponin T or I *(71,72)* for agents with potential cardiac toxicity, may be warranted in additional nonclinical animal studies and/or in clinical studies in humans.

Pharmacology studies can be divided into three main categories, depending on the nature of the effect: primary and secondary pharmacodynamic studies and safety pharmacology studies. Safety pharmacology studies are defined in the ICH guidance document (S7A) on this subject *(18)* "as those studies that investigate the potential undesirable pharmacodynamic effects of a substance on physiological functions in relation to exposure in the therapeutic range and above." This last point is particularly important in that these studies should be conducted at dose levels or serum concentrations that are therapeutic targets based on prior efficacy/activity studies. Simply conducting these studies at low doses does not provide much useful information or adequately assess the safety of the agent.

The objectives of these studies are to identify undesirable pharmacodynamic properties of a drug substance that may have relevance to its human safety and toxicity; to evaluate more fully adverse pharmacodynamic and/or pathophysiological effects of a drug substance that were previously observed in nonclinical toxicology and/or clinical studies; and to investigate the mechanism of action of the adverse pharmacodynamic effects that were either previously observed or suspected. The investigational plan developed to meet these objectives should be clearly identified and delineated by the drug development team.

For biotechnology-derived products that achieve highly specific receptor targeting, it is often sufficient to evaluate safety pharmacology end-points as a part of well-designed toxicology and/or pharmacodynamic studies; therefore, the need for separate safety pharmacology studies can be reduced or eliminated. For those bioproducts that represent a new therapeutic class and/or those products that do not achieve highly specific receptor targeting, a more extensive evaluation in separate safety pharmacology studies should be considered.

8.6. Biodistribution/Pharmacokinetic Studies

Biodistribution studies are generally performed for gene therapy products, and typical pharmacokinetic studies used for most types of drugs that measure serum or plasma levels, half-life, clearance, and the like are generally not performed. These preclinical animal biodistribution studies are designed to determine the distribution of the vector to sites other than the intended therapeutic site as an indicator of potential toxicity. The goals of these studies are generally twofold: determination of dissemination of the vector to the germline and distribution of vector to nontarget tissues. The first has been routinely accomplished by assaying total gonadal tissue. The second provides information on potential target organs of toxicity. Both may be addressed in the same preclinical study. Studies may use normal, intact animals or animal models of disease. The latter study may be more representative of the clinical setting.

Whenever possible, the intended route of administration should be employed, again with the consideration that groups of animals might also be treated intravenously as a worst-case scenario. Transfer of the gene to normal, surrounding, and distal tissues as well as the target site should be evaluated using the most sensitive detection methods possible, such as reverse transcriptase PCR, and should include evaluation of gene persistence. When aberrant or unexpected localization is observed, additional studies should be conducted to determine whether the gene is expressed and whether its presence is associated with any pathologic effects.

Biodistribution studies may not be necessary for all new agents *(73)*. With "previously defined" vectors, if there is previous experience with a similar vector, route of administration, formulation, and schedule (e.g., adenovirus type 5 vectors), if the transgene product is considered "innocuous" if expressed ectopically, and when the size of the new vector is not essentially different, biodistribution aspects of the prior agent may be referenced. On the other hand, studies may not be postponed if a new class of vector is used (i.e., there is little or no previous experience; e.g., AAV, lentivirus, others); if there is a change in the formulation (i.e., lipid carrier instead of an aqueous formulation); if the route of administration is changed to an intentional systemic route from local administration of the "established" vector; and finally, if the transgene has the potential to induce toxicity if it is aberrantly expressed in nontarget organs.

As with toxicity studies, there are a number of factors that should be taken into consideration when designing vector biodistribution studies. Regarding species selection, nonhuman primates are not always needed. Rodents may be perfectly acceptable. The animal gender should reflect the intended patient population. At least 3–5 animals per sex and group should be used as a minimum. The use of smaller animals (i.e., mice or rats) allows the inclusion of larger numbers of animals and the easy evaluation of more time points. As in other studies, the following dose groups should be included when practical: controls, the maximally feasible/clinically relevant dose, and a lower dose for establishment of the no observable adverse effect level. The route of administration should mimic intended clinical route to the greatest extent possible. Regarding animal sacrifice and/or sampling time points, an early point that reflects peak vector transduction/expression should be included, as should a later time-point determined by intended clinical use and a time-point that should reflect clearance from the gonads and nontarget organs to determine persistence. The following tissues are generally recommended: peripheral blood; gonads; injection site; highly perfused organs (to assist in determination of toxicity) such as brain, liver, lung, kidneys, heart, spleen; other tissues based on toxicity/pathology as determined by transgene (e.g., bone marrow); and those based on the route of administration, such as draining, contralateral lymph nodes. The methodology used to detect the agent should detect a sequence of the vector DNA (or ribonucleic acid) that is unique to that product and should be appropriate to detect the vector sequence adequately in tissue samples from both preclinical animal studies and samples obtained during the initial clinical trials. Many of the points presented and discussed in this section are elaborated in publicly accessible FDA documents *(43,73)*.

8.7. Dissemination, Persistence, and Shedding

Shedding of viral vectors through the skin or in excreta is of obvious concern with highly infectious viruses. To measure the dissemination, persistence, and shedding of these vectors, multiple tissues (e.g., brain, heart, lungs, spleen, liver, kidneys, ovaries, and skin) as well as bodily fluids such as urine, feces, tears, saliva, vaginal secretions, and skin swabs are taken at multiple time-points throughout the study and analyzed by real-time quantitative PCR for the presence of vector sequences. If the vector sequences are rapidly cleared and viral sequences are absent in the excreta and swabs of the majority of animals, this suggests that there was no significant replication of the vector in the host *(56,62,74)*.

8.8. Single-Dose Toxicity Studies

Even if the intended clinical schedule involves repeated doses, single-dose studies may generate useful data to describe the relationship of dose to systemic and/or local toxicity and the steepness of the dose/toxicity curve. Data from these studies can be used to select doses for repeated-dose toxicity studies. Information on dose–response relationships may be gathered through the conduct of a single-dose toxicity study or as a component of pharmacology or animal model efficacy studies. The incorporation of safety pharmacology parameters in the design of these studies should be considered, which will reduce the number of animals used, the amount of product required, and the number of studies that must be performed.

8.9. Repeated-Dose Toxicity Studies

The route and dosing regimen for these studies (e.g., daily vs intermittent dosing) should reflect the intended clinical use or exposure (e.g., once a week for 3 weeks, every other day, etc.). A recovery period should be included to determine the reversal or potential worsening of pharmacological/ toxicological effects and/or the potential for delayed toxic effects. For biopharmaceuticals that induce prolonged pharmacological/toxicological effects, recovery group animals should be monitored until reversibility is demonstrated. This may not be fundamentally obvious at the outset of the study. The duration of repeated dose studies should be based on the intended duration of clinical exposure and disease indication. This duration of animal dosing has generally been 1–3 months for most biotechnology-derived pharmaceuticals, but this probably will not be the case for most gene therapy studies. However, in the case of life-threatening diseases such as cancer, longer term studies are generally not required to support phase I trials.

8.10. Immunotoxicity Studies

One aspect of immunotoxicological evaluation includes the assessment of potential immunogenicity as described in Section 8.4. Many biotechnology-derived pharmaceuticals are intended to stimulate or suppress the immune system and therefore may affect not only humoral, but also cell-mediated immunity. Inflammatory reactions at the injection site may be indicative of a stimulatory response. It is important, however, to recognize that simple injection trauma or specific toxic effects caused by the formulation vehicle may also result in toxic changes at the injection site. In addition, the expression of surface antigens on target cells may be altered, which has implications for autoimmune potential.

8.11. Reproductive/Teratology Studies

For conventional small molecule drugs, reproductive toxicity is usually assessed in rats and rabbits. The species specificity and potential immunogenicity of biologicals has led to the increased use of nonhuman primates for this purpose. The need for reproductive and developmental toxicity studies will depend on the product, clinical indication, and intended patient population. The specific study design and dosing schedule may be modified based on issues related to species specificity, immunogenicity, biological activity, and/or a long elimination half-life.

8.12. Germline Integration

The issue of germline integration has prompted considerable public discussion *(75)*. For gene therapy products directly administered to patients, the risk of vector transfer to germ cells should be seriously considered. Animal testicular or ovarian samples should be analyzed for vector sequences by the most sensitive method available. If a signal is detected in the gonads, further studies should be conducted to determine if the sequences are present in germ cells as opposed to stromal tissues; techniques used may include, but are not limited to, cell separations, *in situ* PCR, or other techniques. Semen samples for analysis can be collected from mature animals, including mice, by well-established methods *(76,77)* for determination of vector incorporation into germ cells. Evaluation of biodistribution to the gonads may not be needed prior to all phase I clinical trials, and this issue should be considered carefully in pre-IND meetings with the FDA. The Informed Consent Form should address the lack of data and the unknown risks.

8.13. Genotoxicity Studies

Genotoxicity studies, such as the Ames salmonella assay, the micronucleus test, and the mouse lymphoma assay, which are routinely conducted for small molecule pharmaceuticals, are not applicable to biotechnology-derived pharmaceuticals, especially gene therapy products, and therefore are not needed. The administration of large quantities of peptides, proteins, or viruses may yield uninterpretable results. When there is cause for concern about the product, genotoxicity studies should be performed in available and relevant systems, including newly developed systems. The use of standard genotoxicity studies as indicated for assessing the genotoxic potential of process contaminants is not considered appropriate. If standard assays are performed for this purpose, the rationale should be provided.

8.14. Carcinogenicity Studies

Standard 2-year carcinogenicity bioassays in normal mice and rats are generally inappropriate for biotechnology-derived pharmaceuticals and probably more so for gene therapy products. This issue has received additional attention owing to the emergence of a lymphoproliferative syndrome in a potentially significant fraction of recipients of a vector designed to treat SCID syndrome *(10,11)*. This clinical result actually recapitulates to a certain degree toxicities anticipated from experience in animal models *(78)*. Thus, product-specific assessment of carcinogenic potential will still be needed for biopharmaceuticals, and studies utilized must be refined after consideration of the duration of anticipated clinical dosing, the patient population, or the biological activity of the product (e.g., retrovirus vectors, growth factors, immunosuppressive agents, etc.).

When there is a concern about carcinogenic potential, a variety of new approaches may be considered to evaluate this risk. When the potential to support or induce proliferation of transformed cells and clonal expansion leading to neoplasia is considered possible, the product should be evaluated with respect to receptor expression for the biopharmaceutical or for the transgene's expressed form in various malignant and normal human cells, especially those potentially relevant to the patient population under study. The ability of the biopharmaceutical to stimulate growth of normal and/or malignant cells expressing the relevant receptors should be determined. When in vitro studies such as this give cause for concern about carcinogenic potential, further studies in relevant animal models may be needed if these are available and relevant.

As stated in this section, when gene transfer agents must be evaluated, the standard rodent models (mice and rats) and the 2-year carcinogenicity bioassay are probably not appropriate. Daily administration of vector as is usually performed in these studies is not feasible; however, several of these vectors, including AAV, continue to express over the lifetime of the animal. The other factor that may be limiting is that the host immune response to the vector or to the transgene may either limit the toxicity, perhaps because of the development of neutralizing antibodies, or may have effects on tumor development. It will be necessary to consult with the FDA to develop product-specific studies on an individualized basis or to determine whether and which carcinogenicity studies are needed.

8.15. Local Tolerance Studies

Local tolerance to administration of the new agent should be evaluated. The formulation intended for the clinical trial should be tested unless there is a cogent reason why this would not be feasible or biologically meaningful. In most cases, the potential adverse effects of the product at the site of administration can be evaluated in the single- or repeated-dose toxicity studies that are usually conducted in the normal course of development, thus eliminating the need for separate studies.

9. SPECIAL SAFETY CONSIDERATIONS PERTAINING TO VIRAL AGENTS

9.1. Adenovirus

Adenoviral vectors can efficiently deliver genes to a wide variety of dividing and nondividing cell types both in vitro and in vivo, resulting in a high level of transient gene expression. Considerable modifications have been made in the wild-type virus to reduce infectivity and toxicity in normal tissues or to improve transduction or tropism for tumor cells. The death of Jesse Gelsinger because of several complications, including liver failure, coupled with the fact that adenovirus infections in immunocompromised oncology patients can lead to fatal hepatotoxicity *(79,80)*, and reports of serious hepatotoxicity and death in nonhuman primates treated with different adenoviral vectors make the safety evaluation of these vectors for cancer treatment paramount.

When a first-generation adenovirus vector expressing human factor IX was intravenously injected into rhesus macaques at doses from 1×10^{10} to 1×10^{11} pfu/kg, no toxicity was seen at the lower dose level, but substantial, dose-limiting liver toxicity was observed at the higher dose *(68)*. This hepatotoxicity was manifested as elevated serum transaminase levels, hyperbilirubinemia, hypoalbuminemia, and prolongation of clotting times. All evidence of liver toxicity resolved except for persistent hypofibrinogenemia in the high-dose recipient, indicating possible permanent liver damage. These data suggested a very narrow therapeutic window for this first-generation adenovirus-mediated gene transfer vector. In follow-up studies *(81)*, it was concluded that these abnormalities may be caused by direct toxic effects of the adenovirus vector itself, or may result indirectly from the accompanying acute inflammatory response marked by elevations in interleukin 6.

When another first-generation adenoviral vector expressing β-galactosidase was intravenously injected into two baboons at doses of 1.2×10^{12} or 1.2×10^{13} particles/kg, the baboon receiving the high dose developed acute symptoms, decreased platelet counts, and increased liver enzymes and became moribund at 48 hours after injection; the baboon receiving the lower dose developed no symptoms *(82)*. Again, a very narrow therapeutic index was demonstrated.

Recombinant adenoviruses infused into the portal vein of adult rhesus monkeys at a dose of 10^{13} particles/kg resulted in the formation of neutralizing antibody, severe liver toxicity, and death. Readministration of a second vector was associated with the same degree of toxicity as the first vector, but prompted a much more vigorous neutralizing antibody response *(83)*. The administration of several gene transfer vehicles and routes was studied in rhesus monkeys to develop a model for adenovirus-mediated gene transfer for liver. Vectors administered via the portal vein or saphenous vein were efficient, but this resulted in transient gene expression and was accompanied by an immune response to both vector and transgene products and acute hepatitis *(84)*.

Turning to models of intracerebral administration, baboons received intracerebral injections of either a high dose of a replication-defective adenoviral vector expressing HSV*tk* (1.5×10^9 pfu) with or without GCV or a low dose of ADV/RSV*tk* (7.5×10^7 pfu) with GCV to evaluate the safety of this regimen. Animals receiving the high-dose vector and GCV either died or became moribund and were sacrificed during the first 8 days of treatment. Necropsy of these animals revealed cavities of coagulative necrosis at the injection sites. Animals that received only the high-dose vector were clinically normal; however, lesions were detected with MRI at the injection sites corresponding to cystic cavities at necropsy. Animals that received the low-dose vector and GCV were clinically normal and exhibited small MRI abnormalities, and although no gross lesions were present at necropsy, microscopic foci of necrosis were present. Neutralizing antibodies were produced in the animals, but no shedding of the vector was found in urine, feces, or serum 7 days after intracerebral injection *(74)*.

Intrapulmonary administration uses are exemplified through the use of recombinant adenovirus vectors containing expression cassettes for human cystic fibrosis transmembrane conductance regulator, which were instilled through a bronchoscope into limited regions of lung in baboons. The only adverse effect noted was a mononuclear cell inflammatory response within the alveolar compartment of animals receiving doses of virus that were required to induce detectable gene expression. Minimal inflammation was seen at 10^7 and 10^8 pfu/mL, but at 10^9 and, more prominently, at 10^{10} pfu/mL, a perivascular lymphocytic and histiocytic infiltrate was seen *(85)*.

9.1.1. First-Generation Modified Adenoviral Vectors (E1- and E3-Deleted Vectors)

Host immune elimination of infected cells often limits gene expression in vivo to 1–2 weeks after infection *(86,87)*. In addition to a cell-mediated immune response to the adenovirus infection, a humoral response to the injected virus is often generated *(88)*. Although this humoral response may prevent the use of adenoviral vectors for repeated dosing, it may be blocked or reduced by coadministration of immunosuppressive agents or cytokines. Alternatively, the use of adenoviruses of different serotypes may allow for repeated administration, even in the presence of neutralizing antibodies *(88)*.

Harvey et al. *(89)* reported on 6 years of experience with the local administration of low (<10^9 particle units) and intermediate (10^9 to 10^{11} particle units) doses of E1$^-$/E3$^-$ adenovirus vectors to six different sites. With a group incidence of only 0.7% for major adverse events and no deaths related to administration of the adenovirus vectors, local administration of low and intermediate doses of adenovirus vectors was well tolerated.

9.1.2. Second-Generation Modified Adenoviral Vectors (E1/E2- and E1/E4-Deleted Vectors)

Second-generation adenoviral vectors, mutated in E2a, have been proposed to decrease host immune responses against transduced cells, reduce toxicity, and increase duration of expression as compared with first-generation vectors deleted only in E1. The safety of and E1-, E2a-, E3-deleted adenoviral vector (Av3H82) encoding an epitope-tagged B-domain-deleted human factor VIII complementary DNA was evaluated in cynomolgus monkeys. Animals received intravenous administration of either 6×10^{11} or 3×10^{12} particles/kg. Vector distribution was widespread, with the highest levels observed in liver and spleen. Histopathology, hematology, and serum chemistry analysis identified the liver and blood as major sites of toxicity. Transient mild serum elevations of liver enzymes were observed, along with a dose-dependent inflammatory response in the liver. In addition, mild lymphoid hyperplasia was observed in the spleen. Mild anemia and a transient decrease in platelet count were observed, as was marrow hyperplasia and extramedullary hematopoiesis *(90)*.

When vectors deleted in E1 and containing either a temperature-sensitive mutation in the E2a gene or a deletion of the E4 region were infused into the hepatic artery of nonhuman primates, minimal toxicity was seen. Histopathology showed that portal inflammation was present throughout both livers in the animals receiving the high dose. No differences were seen in the level of portal inflammation in targeted and untargeted lobes. PCR analysis detected viral DNA sequence in gonads and brain as well as many other tissues in baboons treated with high-dose vector. In baboons treated with lower doses of an E1-E4-deleted vector expressing the human ornithine transcarbamylase gene, DNA was detectable by nested PCR in liver, but not gonads, at days 29 and 61. The data suggested that intraarterial administration of recombinant adenoviral E1-E4-deleted vector is feasible and safe. *(91)*.

Toxicity of first-generation and E2a-deleted vectors expressing human α1-antitrypsin was evaluated in C3H mice after administration of increasing doses starting at 1×10^{12} particles/kg. Both vectors induced dose-dependent toxicity, including transient thrombocytopenia, elevated alanine aminotransferase, and increased hepatocyte proliferation, followed by inflammation and then hypertrophy. There were no differences in toxicity between the two vectors when measured at matching levels of human α1-antitrypsin expression. However, the E2a-deleted vector had slightly reduced hepatocyte toxicity at an intermediate particle dose *(92)*. Although these vectors are purported to be less toxic, the fact remains that the human fatality that occurred in the ornithine transcarbamylase deficiency trial at the University of Pennsylvania was an E1, E4-deleted construct *(93)*.

9.1.3. Modified Tropism Adenoviruses

The current E1-deleted adenoviruses can infect a wide variety of cells through a specific interaction between the viral fiber protein and at least one cell surface receptor. Entry of the virus into the cell is further enhanced through a specific interaction of the fiber with an integrin "coreceptor." The host's range of tissue susceptibilities to the virus can therefore be altered by various strategies so that it can bind more efficiently to the target cell surface *(94–96)*. Antibodies against tissue-specific cell surface proteins can also be coupled to the fiber protein to facilitate partial targeting of the virus *(97)*. Another approach to achieve "targeting" of the virus is the use of cell-specific promoters to drive expression of a therapeutic gene in the context of the recombinant virus *(98)*. Enhanced uptake strategies through fiber modification may present special concerns for toxicity, especially regarding hepatotoxicity when administered by an intravenous or direct hepatic artery injection. Careful comparison of a tropism-modified adenoviral vector to the nontropism-modified vector in mouse toxicity and biodistribution studies as well as nonhuman primate and toxicity studies might be desirable.

9.2. Adeno-Associated Viruses

Members of the family *Parvoviridae* AAVs are among the smallest of the DNA viruses *(99)*. Unlike autonomous parvoviruses, AAVs or dependo-viruses require coinfection with unrelated helper viruses for a productive infection to occur *(100,101)*. As recombinant vectors for gene therapy, they seem to have several advantages compared to other vectors, such as the transduction of terminally differentiated and nondividing cells *(102,103)*, relatively high stability of transgene expression *(104)*, and the potential for targeted integration *(105,106)*. From a safety point of view, AAV vectors show a lack of pathogenicity *(107–109)*, low immunogenicity *(104,110)*, and low risk of insertional mutagenesis *(111)*. Also, there did not appear to be any evidence of transduction in the gonads of rhesus monkeys *(112)*. However, AAV has a limited DNA capacity.

9.3. Herpes Simplex Virus

HSV vectors can deliver large amounts of exogenous DNA; however, cytotoxicity and maintenance of transgene expression are obvious obstacles to their use. They also have the advantages of the abilities to infect nondividing cells and to establish latency in some cell types. The ability to establish latency in neuronal cells makes HSV an attractive vector for treating neurological disorders such as Parkinson's and Alzheimer's diseases. In addition, the ability of HSV to infect efficiently a number of different cell types, such as muscle and liver, may make it an excellent vector for treating non-neurological diseases.

One problem associated with HSV-based vectors has been the toxicity of the vector in many different cell types. The generation of HSV vectors with deletions in many of the immediate early gene products, which is similar to the strategy used for adenovirus, has resulted in vectors with reduced toxicity and antigenicity as well as prolonged expression in vivo *(60–65)*.

No clinical study has been reported in detail with these vectors. Section 8.1.2. details a summary of preclinical safety considerations pertaining to use of the *Aotus* monkey in comparison to rodent species.

9.4. Retroviruses

Retrovirus vectors are replication-defective and are primarily based on the Moloney murine leukemia virus (MMLV), which is a well-studied and well-characterized retrovirus *(113,114)* with numerous advantages. They have been extensively studied, produce stable integration into the host genome, and are very efficient at gene transfer. Disadvantages include an infection that is limited to dividing cells, which makes gene transfer into nondividing cells such as hematopoietic stem cells, hepatocytes, myoblasts, and neurons an impossibility, and low titer of products.

There are four theoretical concerns that exist for retroviral-mediated gene transfer that relate to two potential delayed toxicities. These are insertional mutagenesis, recombination with endogenous retroviral sequences, transfer of exogenous genetic material, and accidental exposure to replication-competent murine retroviruses *(115)*. Because retroviral vectors can permanently integrate into the genome of the infected cell, there is a serious concern regarding insertional mutagenesis causing the development of a secondary malignancy. The presence of RCRs is of major concern because of the fact that RCRs have produced lethal malignant T-cell lymphomas in 3/10 rhesus monkeys *(78)*. These concerns resulted in a publication concerning the FDA considerations on these issues *(116)* and the issuance of a new FDA guidance on this subject in October 2000 *(36)*. Some of these concerns are no longer theoretical. The elation that this type of retroviral-mediated therapy was successful in curing a number of children with SCID *(117)* has been severely dampened by the reports of a leukemialike disease produced in two of these children *(10–13)*.

9.5. *Lentiviruses*

Unlike oncoretrovirusus such as Moloney murine leukemia virus, one subclass of retroviruses, the lentiviruses, can infect nondividing cells. This makes these viruses attractive for gene transfer. One of these viruses, human immunodeficiency virus (HIV), has been the subject of investigation by a number of groups. The most obvious concerns with using HIV for gene therapy is safety and the possible generation of replication-competent virus during vector production. This involves engineering the vector so that it is replication defective. This has been done in a number of cases by eliminating all accessory genes, such as *tat, vif, vpr, vpu,* and *nef,* from a packaging construct that still has the ability to transduce cells *(118)*. Concern about the possibility of insertional activation of cellular oncogenes by a random integration of the vector provirus into the host genome has led to the development of self-inactivating vectors *(119–122)*. The use of self-inactivating viruses significantly improves the biosafety of HIV-derived vectors because it reduces the likelihood that RCRs will originate during vector production and target cells and hampers recombination with wild-type HIV in an infected host. In an attempt to make even safer constructs, other groups are working on the development of lentiviral vectors from HIV-2 *(123)*, simian immunodeficiency virus *(124)*, bovine immunodeficiency virus *(125,126)*, and feline immunodeficiency virus *(127)*. These last vectors may be inherently more acceptable because they are not based on HIV-1. None of these newer constructs has moved toward the clinic, so there is little animal safety data and no human data on these vectors yet.

10. SUMMARY AND CONCLUSIONS

This chapter presents a range of issues that might be considered in contemplating the development of a gene therapy agent to the point of an early phase clinical trial. As no gene therapy product has yet been recognized as "safe and effective," the standard approach to these issues should be regarded very much as a "work in progress." Indeed, the nature of these agents would suggest that each new opportunity would call for its own unique set of requirements, so that a single approach will probably never "standardly" exist. Rather, the principles that underlie regulatory policy should be woven into the approach to each new agent.

In broad strokes, these involve approaches to answering the following questions: Is the identity of the agent clearly defined? Can successive batches of the material be made reproducibly in the quantity to support clinical development, and how is this known? Are the biological features of the vector, and its transgene when applicable, clearly similar in the animal species used for safety studies and in the human, at least as far as this can be ascertained? What dose is likely to be required for therapeutic effect? What level of gene expression or replication is necessary to attain a therapeutic effect? When toxicity occurs because of the agent, what is the evidence the toxicity will be reversible? Is toxicity after repeated doses of agent likely to be attenuated or magnified by immunological response to the agent? What are the consequences of long-term presence of the therapeutic agent in the recipient? Is there a danger of producing directly (as the therapeutic agent itself) or indirectly (through recombination and/or replication) an infectious agent that acts horizontally in the population or vertically across generations? How will the presence and distribution of the gene therapy agent be followed in the patient?

Sponsors are above all encouraged to see the regulatory process as a collaborative interaction with the regulatory agencies with the end not only of protecting the patient, but also of advancing the most scientifically defensible and rigorous questions to clinical trial. Far more costly than the conduct of experiments designed to be compliant with regulatory requirements is a failed or overtly injurious clinical trial. A clear understanding and a proactive approach in addressing regulatory issues outlined here will maximally ensure the likelihood of an interpretable clinical outcome. The regulatory issues outlined here must be approached with continuing appreciation of the evolving science associated with the gene therapy field. As such, requirements may evolve with the state of the science, and careful sustained contact with the regulatory agencies is important in incorporating the best and most current science into the design, conduct, and interpretation of regulatory studies.

REFERENCES*

1. ICH guidance on quality of biotechnology/biological products: derivation and characterization of cell substrates used for production of biotechnical/biological products, September 21, 1998. Available on-line at: http://www.fda.gov/cber/guidelines.htm.
2. ICH: final guideline on quality of biotechnological products: analysis of the expression construct in cells used for production of r-DNA derived protein products, February 1996. Available on-line at: http://www.fda.gov/cber/guidelines.htm.
3. ICH guidance on specifications: test procedures and acceptance criteria for biotechnological/biological products, August 18, 1999. Available on-line at: http://www.fda.gov/cber/guidelines.htm.
4. ICH Guidance for Industry Q1A (R2), stability testing of new drug substances and products, November 20, 2003. Available on-line at: http://www.fda.gov.cber/guidelines.htm.
5. ICH guidance on viral safety evaluation of biotechnology products derived from cell lines of human or animal origin, September 24, 1998. Available on-line at: http://www.fda.gov/cber/guidelines.htm.
6. ICH guidance: Q7A good manufacturing practice guidance for active pharmaceutical ingredients, September 25, 2001. Available on-line at: http://www.fda.gov/cber/guidelines.htm.
7. ICH guidance for industry: S6 preclinical safety evaluation of biotechnology-derived pharmaceuticals, July16, 1997. Available on-line at: http://www.ich.org.
8. ICH: final guidance on stability testing of biotechnological/biological products, July 10, 1996. Available on-line at: http://www.fda.gov/cber/guidelines.htm.
9. FDA guidance for industry: guidance for human somatic cell therapy and gene therapy, March 30, 1998. Available on-line at: http://www.fda.gov/cber/guidelines.htm.
10. Check, E. (2002) Gene therapy: a tragic setback. *Nature* **420,** 116–118.
10a. FDA Draft Points to Consider in Human Somatic Cell Therapy and Gene Therapy, August 27, 1991.
11. Hacein-Bey-Abina, S., von Kalle, C., Schmidt, M., et al. (2003) A serious adverse event after successful gene therapy for X-linked severe combined immunodeficiency. *N. Engl. J. Med.* **347,** 255–256.
12. Check, E. (2002) Regulators split on gene therapy as patient shows signs of cancer. *Nature* **419,** 545–546.
13. Check, E. (2003) Second cancer case halts gene-therapy trials. *Nature* **421,** 305.
14. Pilaro, A. M. and Serabian, M. A. (1999) Preclinical development strategies for novel gene therapy products. *Toxicol. Pathol.* **27,** 4–7.
15. Pilling, A. M. (1999) The role of the toxicologic pathologist in the preclinical safety evaluation of biotechnology-derived pharmaceuticals. *Toxicol. Pathol.* **27,** 678–688.
16. Dempster, A. M. (2000) Nonclinical safety evaluation of biotechnologically derived pharmaceuticals. *Biotech. Annu. Rev.* **5,** 221–258.
17. Griffiths, S. A. and Lumley, C. E. (1998) Non-clinical safety studies for biotechnology-derived pharmaceuticals: conclusions from an international workshop. *Hum. Exp. Toxicol.* **17,** 63–83.
18. ICH guidance to industry: S7A safety pharmacology studies for human pharmaceuticals, July 12, 2001. Available at: http://www.fda.gov/cber/guidelines.htm.
19. Code of Federal Regulations, Title 21, Food and Drugs, Part 610.10, Subpart B, General biological products standards; general provisions; potency, p. 61, revised as of April 1, 2002.
20. Code of Federal Regulations, Title 21, Food and Drugs, Part 610.12, Subpart B, General biological products standards; general provisions; sterility, pp. 63–67, revised as of April 1, 2002.
21. Code of Federal Regulations, Title 21, Food and Drugs, Part 610.13, Subpart B, General biological products standards; general provisions; purity, pp. 67–68, revised as of April 1, 2002.
22. Code of Federal Regulations, Title 21, Food and Drugs, Part 610.14, Subpart B, General biological products standards; general provisions; identity, pp. 68–69, revised as of April 1, 2002.
23. Code of Federal Regulations, Title 21, Food and Drugs, Part 58, Good laboratory practice for nonclinical laboratory studies, pp. 302–316, revised as of April 1, 2002.
24. Code of Federal Regulations, Title 21, Food and Drugs, Part 210, Current good manufacturing practice in manufacturing, processing, packing, or holding of drugs; general, pp. 113–115, revised as of April 1, 2002.
25. Code of Federal Regulations, Title 21, Food and Drugs, Part 211, Current good manufacturing practice for finished pharmaceuticals, pp. 115–135, revised as of April 1, 2002.

*All websites accessed 05/17/2004.

26. Code of Federal Regulations, Title 21, Food and Drugs, Part 312, Investigational new drug application, pp. 57–95, revised as of April 1, 2002.

27. FDA guidance for industry: content and format of Investigational New Drug Applications (INDs) for phase I studies of drugs, including well-characterized, therapeutic, biotechnology-derived products, November 1995. Available on-line at: http://www.fda.gov/cder/guidance/phase1.pdf.

28. FDA guidance for industry: IND's for phases 2 and 3 studies of drugs, including specified therapeutic biotechnology-derived products, chemistry, manufacturing and controls content and format, April 20, 1999. Available on-line at: http://www.fda.gov/cber/guidelines.htm.

29. FDA guidance for industry: content and format of chemistry, manufacturing, and controls information and establishment description information for a vaccine or related product, January 5, 1999. Available on-line at: http://www.fda.gov/cber/guidelines.htm.

30. FDA guidance for industry for the submission of chemistry, manufacturing, and controls information for a therapeutic recombinant DNA-derived product or a monoclonal antibody product for in vivo use, August 1996. Available on-line at http://www.fda.gov/cber/guidelines.htm.

31. FDA guidance for industry: formal meetings with sponsors and applicants for PDUFA products, March 7, 2000. Available on-line at: http://www.fda.gov/cber/guidelines.htm.

32. FDA points to consider in the manufacturing and testing of monoclonal antibody products for human use, February 28, 1997. Available on-line at: http://www.fda.gov/cber/guidelines.htm.

33. FDA letter to manufacturers of biological products: recommendations regarding bovine spongiform encephalopathy (BSE), April 19, 2000. Available on-line at: http://www.fda.gov/cber/ltr/bse041900.htm.

34. FDA Biological Response Modifiers Advisory Committee: current policy on sequence characterization of gene transfer products, November 16, 2000. Available on-line at: http://www.fda.gov/cber.

35. FDA Biological Response Modifiers Advisory Committee: adenovirus titer measurements and RCA levels, July 13, 2001. Available on-line at: http://www.fda.gov/cber.

36. FDA guidance for industry: supplemental guidance on testing for replication competent retrovirus in retroviral vector based gene therapy products and during follow-up of patients in clinical trials using retroviral vectors, October 18, 2000. Available on-line at: http://www.fda.gov/cber/guidelines.htm.

37. FDA points to consider in the characterization of cell lines used to produce biologicals, May 17, 1993. Available on-line at: http://www.fda.gov/cber/guidelines.htm.

38. FDA Dear Gene Therapy IND or Master File Sponsor Letter, March 6, 2000. Available on-line at: http://www.fda.gov/cber/ltr/gt030600.htm

39. FDA gene therapy patient tracking system final document, June 27, 2002. Available on-line at: http://www.fda.gov/cber/genetherapy/gttrack.htm.

40. FDA guidance concerning demonstration of comparability of human biological products, including therapeutic biotechnology-derived products, April 1996. Available on-line at: http://www.fda.gov/cber/gdlns/comptest.txt.

41. Third national NIH gene transfer safety symposium: safety considerations in the use of AAV vectors in gene transfer clinical trials, March 7, 2001. Available on-line at: http://www4.od.nih.gov/oba/rac/transcript 3-7-011.pdf.

42. Cornetta, K. G. and Robertson, M. J. (2000) Basic principles of gene therapy: basic principles and safety considerations. In *Principles and Practice of the Biologic Therapy of Cancer*, 3rd ed. (Rosenberg, S. A., ed.), Lippincott, New York, pp. 733–747.

43. Pilaro, A. M. (2000, November 17) Preclinical animal models in gene therapy research. Biological Response Modifiers Advisory Committee Meeting. Available on-line at: http://www.fda.gov/cber/advisory/brm/brmmain.htm

44. Pacini, D. L., Dubovi, E. J., and Clyde, W. A. Jr. (1984) A new animal model for human respiratory tract disease due to adenovirus. *J. Infect. Dis.* **150**, 92–97.

45. Whitley, R. (2000, November 16) Use of *Aotus* monkey to assess neurovirulence of replication-selective herpes vectors. Biological Response Modifiers Advisory Committee Meeting. Available on-line at: http://www.fda.gov/cber/advisory/brm/brmmain.htm.

46. Lewandowski, G., Zimmerman, M. N., Denk, L. L., Porter, D. D., and Prince, G. A. (2002) Herpes simplex type 1 infects and establishes latency in the brain and trigeminal ganglia during primary infection of the lip in cotton rats and mice. *Arch. Virol.* **147**, 167–179.

47. Torres, J. M., Alonso, C., Ortega, A., Mittal, S., Graham, F., and Enjuanes, L. (1996) Tropism of human adenovirus type 5-based vectors in swine and their ability to protect against transmissible gastroenteritis coronavirus. *J. Virol.* **70**, 3770–3780.

48. Morrissey, R. E., Horvath C., Snyder, E. A., et al. (2002) Porcine toxicology studies of SCH 58500, an adenoviral vector for the p53 gene. *Toxicol. Sci.* **65**, 256–265.

49. Prince, G. A., Porter, D. D., Jenson, A. B., Horswood, R. L., Chanock, R. M., and Ginsberg, H. S. (1993) Pathogenesis of adenovirus type 5 pneumonia in cotton rats (*Sigmodon hispidus*). *J. Virol.* **67**, 101–111.

50. Prince, G. A. (1994) The cotton rat in biomedical research. *Animal Welfare Information Center Newslett.* 5. Available on-line at: http://www.nal.usda.gov/awic/newsletters/v5n2/5n2princ.htm.

51. Ward, L. E. (2001) Handling the cotton rat for research. *Lab. Anim.* **30,** 45–50.
52. Ginsberg, H. S., Lundholm-Beauchamp, U., Horswood, R. L., et al. (1989) Role of early region 3 (E3) in pathogenesis of adenovirus disease. *Proc. Natl. Acad. Sci. USA* **86,** 3823–3827.
53. Berencsi, K., Uri, A., Valyi-Nagy, T., et al. (1994) Early region 3-replacement adenovirus recombinants are less pathogenic in cotton rats and mice than early region 3-deleted viruses. *Lab. Invest.* **71,** 350–358.
54. Smith, J. G., Raper, S. E., Wheeldon, E. B., et al. (1997) Intracranial administration of adenovirus expressing HSV-TK in combination with ganciclovir produces a dose-dependent, self limiting inflammatory response. *Hum. Gene Ther.* **8,** 943–954.
55. Rojas-Martinez, A., Wyde, P. R., Montgomery, C. A., Chen, S. H., Woo, S. L., and Aguilar-Cordova, E. (1998) Distribution, persistency, toxicity, and lack of replication of an E1A-deficient adenoviral vector after intracardiac delivery in the cotton rat. *Cancer Gene Ther.* **5,** 365–370.
56. Wildner, O. and Morris, J. C. (2002) Subcutaneous administration of a replication-competent adenovirus expressing HSV-tk to cotton rats: dissemination, dersistence, shedding, and pathogenicity. *Hum. Gene Ther.* **13,** 101–112.
57. Barahona, H., Melendez, L. V., Hunt, R. D., and Daniel, M. D. (1976) The owl monkey (*Aotus trivirgatus*) as an animal model for viral diseases and oncologic studies. *Lab. Anim. Sci.* **26,** 1104–1112.
58. Leib, D. A., Hart, C. A., and McCarthy, K. (1987) Characterization of four herpesviruses isolated from owl monkeys and their comparison with *Herpesvirus saimiri* type 1 (*Herpesvirus tamarinus*) and herpes simplex virus type 1. *J. Comp. Pathol.* **97,** 159–169.
59. Meignier, B., Jourdier, T. M., Norrild, B., Pereira, L., and Roizman, B. (1987) Immunization of experimental animals with reconstituted glycoprotein mixtures of herpes simplex virus 1 and 2: protection against challenge with virulent virus. *J. Infect. Dis.* **155,** 921–930.
60. Meignier, B., Martin, B., Whitley, R. J., and Roizman, B. (1990) In vivo behavior of genetically engineered herpes simplex viruses R7017 and R7020. II. Studies in immunocompetent and immunosuppressed owl monkeys (*Aotus trivirgatus*). *J. Infect. Dis.* **162,** 313–321.
61. Hunter, W. D., Martuza, R. L., Feigenbaum, F., et al. (1999) Attenuated, replication-competent herpes simplex virus type 1 mutant G207: safety evaluation of intracerebral injection in nonhuman primates. *J. Virol.* **73,** 6319–6326.
62. Todo, T., Feigenbaum, F., Rabkin, S. D., et al. (2000) Viral shedding and biodistribution of G207, a multimutated, conditionally replicating herpes simplex virus type 1, after intracerebral inoculation in *Aotus. Mol. Ther.* **2,** 588–595.
63. Varghese, S., Newsome, J. T., Rabkin, S. D., et al. (2001) Preclinical safety evaluation of G207, a replication-competent herpes simplex virus type 1, inoculated intraprostatically in mice and nonhuman primates. *Hum. Gene Ther.* **12,** 999–1010.
64. Sundaresan, P., Hunter, W. D., Martuza, R. L., and Rabkin, S. D. (2000) Attenuated, replication-competent herpes simplex virus type 1 mutant G207: safety evaluation in mice. *J. Virol.* **74,** 3832–3841.
65. Olson, H., Betton, G., Robinson, D., et al. (2000) Concordance of the toxicity of pharmaceuticals in humans and in animals. *Regul. Toxicol. Pharmacol.* **32,** 56–67.
66. Freireich, E. J., Gehan, E. A., Rall, D. P., Schmidt, L. H., and Skipper, H. E. (1966) Quantitative comparison of toxicity of anticancer agents in mouse, rat, hamster, dog, monkey, and man. *Cancer Chemother. Rep.* **50,** 219–244.
67. Lozier, J. N., Metzger, M. E., Donahue, R. E., and Morgan, R. A. (1999) The rhesus macaque as an animal model for hemophilia B gene therapy. *Blood* **93,** 1875–1881.
68. Lozier, J. N., Metzger, M. E., Donahue, R. E., and Morgan, R. A. (1999) Adenovirus-mediated expression of human coagulation factor IX in the rhesus macaque is associated with dose-limiting toxicity. *Blood* **94,** 3968–3975.
69. Eckardt, L., Haverkamp, W., Borggrefe, M., and Breithardt, G. (1998) Experimental models of torsade de pointes. *Cardiovasc. Res.* **39,** 178–193.
70. Eckardt, L., Haverkamp, W., Mertens, H., et al. (1998) Drug-related torsade de pointes in the isolated rabbit heart: comparison of clofilium, *d,l*-sotalol and erythromycin. *J. Cardiovasc. Pharmacol.* **32,** 425–434.
71. Jaffe, A. S. (2001) Elevations in cardiac troponin measurements: false false-positives: the real truth. *Cardiovasc. Toxicol.* **1,** 87–92.
72. Sparano, J. A., Brown, D. L., and Wolff, A. C. (2002) Predicting cancer therapy-induced cardiotoxicity: the role of troponins and other markers. *Drug Saf.* **25,** 301–311.
73. Serabian, M. A. and Pilaro, A. M. (2000, November 17) Preclinical considerations for gene transfer clinical trials: vector biodistribution. Biological Response Modifiers Advisory Committee Meeting. Available on-line at: http://www.fda.gov/cber/advisory/brm/brmmain.htm.
74. Goodman, J. C., Trask, T. W., Chen, S. H., et al. (1996) Adenoviral-mediated thymidine kinase gene transfer into the primate brain followed by systemic ganciclovir: pathologic, radiologic, and molecular studies. *Hum. Gene Ther.* **7,** 1241–1250.
75. Recombinant DNA Advisory Committee (RAC), National Institutes of Health (1999, March 11–12). Meeting summary (available on-line at: www4.od.nih.gov/oba/rac/summaries/3-99sum.htm.) and meeting minutes RAC Minutes-03/11-12/99. Available on-line at: www4.od.nih.gov/oba/rac/minutes/3-99 RAC.htm.
76. Snell, G. D., Hummel, K. P., and Abelmann, W. H. (1944) A technique for the artificial insemination of mice. *Anat. Rec.* **90,** 243–253.

77. Kile, J. C. Jr. (1951) An improved method for the artificial insemination of mice. *Anat. Rec.* **109**, 109–117.
78. Donahue, R. E., Kessler, S. W., Bodine, D., et al. (1992) Helper virus induced T cell lymphoma in nonhuman primates after retroviral mediated gene transfer. *J. Exp. Med.* **176**, 1125–1135.
79. Zahradnik, J. M., Spencer, M. J., and Porter, D. D. (1980) Adenovirus infection in the immunocompromised patient. *Am. J. Med.* **68**, 725–732.
80. Haura, E. B., Winden, M. A., Proia, A. D., and Trotter, J. E. (2002) Fulminant hepatic failure due to disseminated adenovirus infection in a patient with chronic lymphocytic leukemia. *Cancer Control* **9**, 248–253.
81. Lozier, J. N., Csako, G., Mondoro, T. H., et al. (2002) Toxicity of a first-generation adenoviral vector in rhesus macaques. *Hum. Gene Ther.* **13**, 113–124.
82. Morral, N., O'Neal, W. K., Rice, K., et al. (2002) Lethal toxicity, severe endothelial injury, and a threshold effect with high doses of an adenoviral vector in baboons. *Hum. Gene Ther.* **13**, 143–154.
83. Nunes, F. A., Furth, E. E., Wilson, J. M., and Raper, S. E. (1999) Gene transfer into the liver of nonhuman primates with E1-deleted recombinant adenoviral vectors: safety of readministration. *Hum. Gene Ther.* **10**, 2515–2526.
84. Sullivan, D. E., Dash, S., Du, H., et al. (1997) Liver-directed gene transfer in non-human primates. *Hum. Gene Ther.* **8**, 1195–1206.
85. Simon, R. H., Engelhardt, J. F., Yang, Y., et al. (1993) Adenovirus-mediated transfer of the CFTR gene to lung of nonhuman primates: toxicity study. *Hum. Gene Ther.* **4**, 771–780.
86. Yang, Y., Su, Q., and Wilson, J. M. (1996) Role of viral antigens in destructive cellular immune responses to adenovirus vector-transduced cells in mouse lungs. *J. Virol.* **70**, 7209–7212.
87. Yang, Y. and Wilson, J. M. (1995) Clearance of adenovirus-infected hepatocytes by MHC class I-restricted CD4$^+$ CTLs in vivo. *J. Immunol.* **155**, 2564–2570.
88. Mack, C. A., Song, W. R., Carpenter, H., et al. (1997) Circumvention of anti-adenovirus neutralizing immunity by administration of an adenoviral vector of an alternate serotype. *Hum. Gene Ther.* **8**, 99–109.
89. Harvey, B. G., Maroni, J., O'Donoghue, K. A., et al. (2002) Safety of local delivery of low- and intermediate-dose adenovirus gene transfer vectors to individuals with a spectrum of morbid conditions. *Hum. Gene Ther.* **13**, 15–63.
90. Brann, T., Kayda, D., Lyons, R. M., et al. (1999) Adenoviral vector-mediated expression of physiologic levels of human factor VIII in nonhuman primates. *Hum. Gene Ther.* **10**, 299–301.
91. Raper, S. E., Haskal, Z. J., Ye, X., et al. (1998) Selective gene transfer into the liver of non-human primates with E1-deleted, E2A-defective, or E1–E4 deleted recombinant adenoviruses. *Hum. Gene Ther.* **9**, 671–679.
92. O'Neal, W. K., Zhou, H., Morral, N., et al. (1998) Toxicological comparison of E2a-deleted and first-generation adenoviral vectors expressing alpha1-antitrypsin after systemic delivery. *Hum. Gene Ther.* **9**, 1587–1598.
93. Batshaw, M. L., Wilson, J. M., Raper, S., Yudkoff, M., and Robinson, M. B. (1999) Recombinant adenovirus gene transfer in adults with partial ornithine transcarbamylase deficiency (OTCD). *Hum. Gene Ther.* **10**, 2419–2437.
94. Wickham, T. J., Carrion, M. E., and Kovesdi, I. (1995) Targeting of adenovirus penton base to new receptors through replacement of its RGD motif with other receptor-specific peptide motifs. *Gene Ther.* **2**, 750–756.
95. Krasnykh, V. N., Mikheeva, G. V., Douglas, J. T., and Curiel, D. T. (1996) Generation of recombinant adenovirus vectors with modified fibers for altering viral tropism. *J. Virol.* **70**, 6839–6846.
96. Miller, R. and Curiel, D. T. (1996) Towards the use of replicative adenoviral vectors for cancer gene therapy. *Gene Ther.* **3**, 557–559.
97. Wickham, T. J., Segal, D. M., Roelvink, P. W., et al. (1996) Targeted adenovirus gene transfer to endothelial and smooth muscle cells by using bispecific antibodies. *J. Virol.* **70**, 6831–6838.
98. Kochanek, S., Clemens, P. R., Mitani, K., Chen, H. H., Chan, S., and Caskey, C. T. (1996) A new adenoviral vector: replacement of all viral coding sequences with 28 kb of DNA independently expressing both full-length dystrophin and β-galactosidase. *Proc. Natl. Acad. Sci. USA* **93**, 5731–5736.
99. Siegl, G., Bates, R. C., Berns, K. I., et al. (1985) Characteristics and taxonomy of *Parvoviridae. Intervirology* **23**, 61–73.
100. Atchison, R. W., Casto, B. C., and Hammon, W. McD. (1965) Adenovirus-associated defective virus particles. *Science* **194**, 754–756.
101. Buller, R. M., Janik, J. E., Sebring, E. D., and Rose, J. A. (1981) Herpes simplex virus types 1 and 2 completely help adenovirus-associated virus replication. *J. Virol.* **40**, 241–247.
102. Kotin, R. (1994) Prospects for the use of adeno-associated virus as a vector for human gene therapy. *Hum. Gene Ther.* **5**, 793–801.
103. Flotte, T. R. and Carter, B. J. (1995) Adeno-associated virus vectors for gene therapy. *Gene Ther.* **2**, 357–362.
104. Flotte, T. R., Afione, S. A., Conrad, C., et al. (1993) Stable in vivo expression of the cystic fibrosis transmembrane conductance regulator with an adeno-associated virus vector. *Proc. Natl. Acad. Sci. USA* **90**, 10,613–10,617.
105. Kotin, R. M., Siniscalco, M., Samulski, R. J., et al. (1990) Site-specific integration by adeno-associated virus. *Proc. Natl. Acad. Sci. USA* **87**, 2211–2215.
106. Kotin, R. M., Menninger, J. C., Ward, D. C., and Berns, K. I. (1991) Mapping and direct visualisation of region-specific viral DNA integration site on chromosome 19q13-qter. *Genomics* **10**, 831–834.
107. Blacklow, N. R., Hoggan, M. D., Kapikian, A. Z., Austin, J. B., and Rowe, W. P. (1968) Epidemiology of adeno-associated virus infection in a nursery population. *Am. J. Epidemiol.* **88**, 368–378.

108. Blacklow, N. R., Hoggan, M. D., Sereno, M. S., et al. (1971) A seroepidemiologic study of adenovirus-associated virus infection in infants and children. *Am. J. Epidemiol.* **94,** 359–366.

109. Blacklow, N. R. (1988) Adeno-associated viruses of humans. In *Parvoviruses and Human Disease* (Pattison, J., ed.), CRC Press, Boca Raton, FL, pp. 165–174.

110. Chiorini, A., Wendtner, C. M., Urcelay, H., Saffer, B., Hallek, N., and Kotin, R. M. (1995) High efficiency transfer of the T cell co-stimulatory molecule B7-2 to lymphoid cells using high-titer recombinant adeno-associated virus vectors. *Hum. Gene Ther.* **6,** 1531–1541.

111. Walsh, C. E., Liu, J. M., Xiao, X., Young, N. S., Nienhuis, A. W., and Samulski, R. J. (1992) Regulated high level expression of a human γ-globin gene introduced into erythroid cells by an adeno-associated virus vector. *Proc. Natl. Acad. Sci. USA* **89,** 7257–7261.

112. Flotte, T. R., Conrad, C., Reynolds, T., et al. (1995) Preclinical evaluation of AAV vectors expressing the human CTFR cDNA [abstract]. *J. Cell Biochem.* **21A,** 364.

113. Robbins, P. D., Tahara, H., Mueller, G., et al. (1994) Retroviral vectors for use in human gene therapy for cancer, Gaucher disease, and arthritis. *Ann. NY Acad. Sci.* **716,** 72–88.

114. Riviere, I., Brose, K., and Mulligan, R. C. (1995) Effects of retroviral vector design on expression of human adenosine deaminase in murine bone marrow transplant recipients engrafted with genetically modified cells. *Proc. Natl. Acad. Sci. USA* **92,** 6733–6737.

115. Cornetta, K. (1992) Safety aspects of gene therapy. *Br. J. Haematol.* **80,** 421–426.

116. Wilson, C. A., Ng, T.-H., and Miller, A. E. (1997) Evaluation of recommendations for replication competent retrovirus testing associated with use of retroviral vectors. *Hum. Gene Ther.* **8,** 869–874.

117. Hacein-Bey-Abina, S., Le Deist, F., Carlier, F., et al. (2002) Sustained correction of X-linked severe combined immunodeficiency by ex vivo gene therapy. *N. Engl. J. Med.* **346,** 1185–1193.

118. Kim, V. N., Mitrophanous, K., Kingsman, S. M., and Kingsman, A. J. (1998) Minimal requirement for a lentivirus vector based on human immunodeficiency virus type 1. *J. Virol.* **72,** 811–816.

119. Miyoshi, H., Blomer, U., Takahashi, M., Gage, F. H., and Verma, I. M. (1998) Development of a self-inactivating lentivirus vector. *J. Virol.* **72,** 8150–8157.

120. Mitta, B., Rimann, M., Ehrengruber, M. U., et al. (2002) Advanced modular self-inactivating lentiviral expression vectors for multigene interventions in mammalian cells and in vivo transduction. *Nucleic Acids Res.* **30,** e113.

121. Koya, R. C., Kasahara, N., Pullarkat, V., Levine, A. M., and Stripecke, R. (2002) Transduction of acute myeloid leukemia cells with third generation self-inactivating lentiviral vectors expressing CD80 and GM-CSF: effects on proliferation, differentiation, and stimulation of allogeneic and autologous anti-leukemia immune responses. *Leukemia* **16,** 1645–1654.

122. Zufferey, R., Dull, T., Mandel, R. J., et al. (1998) Self-inactivating lentivirus vector for safe and efficient in vivo gene delivery. *J. Virol.* **72,** 9873–9880.

123. Cheng, L., Chaidhawangul, S., Wong-Staal, F., et al. (2002) Human immunodeficiency virus type 2 (HIV-2) vector-mediated in vivo gene transfer into adult rabbit retina. *Curr. Eye Res.* **24,** 196–201.

124. Kobayashi, M., Iida, A., Ueda, Y., and Hasegawa, M. (2003) Pseudotyped lentivirus vectors derived from simian immunodeficiency virus SIVagm with envelope glycoproteins from paramyxovirus. *J. Virol.* **77,** 2607–2614.

125. Berkowitz, R., Ilves, H., Lin, W. Y., et al. (2001) Construction and molecular analysis of gene transfer systems derived from bovine immunodeficiency virus. *J. Virol.* **75,** 3371–3382.

126. Molina, R. P., Matukonis, M., Paszkiet, B., Zhang, J., Kaleko, M., and Luo, T. (2002) Mapping of the bovine immunodeficiency virus packaging signal and RRE and incorporation into a minimal gene transfer vector. *Virology* **304,** 10–23.

127. Lotery, A. J., Derksen, T. A., Russell, S. R., et al. (2002) Gene transfer to the nonhuman primate retina with recombinant feline immunodeficiency virus vectors. *Hum. Gene Ther.* **13,** 689–696.

Index